HANDBOOK OF
SEVERE DISABILITY

For Sale by the Superintendent of Documents, U.S. Government Printing Office
Washington, D.C., 20402

HANDBOOK OF SEVERE DISABILITY

A Text for Rehabilitation Counselors,
Other Vocational Practitioners, and
Allied Health Professionals

Edited by

WALTER C. STOLOV, M.D.
Professor

MICHAEL R. CLOWERS, PH.D.
Director, Vocational Unit

Department of Rehabilitation Medicine
University of Washington
A Rehabilitation Research and Training Center
Of the National Institute of Handicapped Research

Assisted by
Sandra R. Blair, Technical Editor
Phyllis Wood, Illustrator

1981
U.S. Department of Education
Rehabilitation Services Administration

Prepared and supported, in part, by the
Rehabilitation Services Administration,
U.S. Department of Education
Contract No. 105-76-4115
and the University of Washington
Graduate School Research Fund

Library of Congress Cataloging in Publication Data

Main entry under title:

Handbook of severe disability.
  Includes index.
   1. Physically handicapped—Rehabilitation.
2. Rehabilitation. I. Stolov, Walter C., 1928–
II. Clowers, Michael R., 1942–1979 [DNLM:
1. Counseling. 2. Handicapped. 3. Rehabilitation, Vocational.
HD7255 H2346]
RD797.H36   616   80–607924

For sale by the Superintendent of Documents,
U.S. Government Printing Office
Washington, D.C. 20402
Stock No. 017-090-00054-2

To those severely disabled by disease and injury,
in the hope that their burden may be eased
and their objectives achieved,
and to
Michael R. Clowers, Ph.D.,
who, in his short professional life,
achieved a level of excellence
in the service of the handicapped
that is a model for all of us.

CONTENTS

CONTRIBUTORS

THOMAS P. ANDERSON, M.D.
Professor
Department of Physical Medicine and Rehabilitation
University of Minnesota

GARY T. ATHELSTAN, Ph.D.
Professor and Director
Counseling Psychology Service
Department of Physical Medicine and Rehabilitation
University of Minnesota

C. WARREN BLEDSOE
Principal Consultant on Blindness (retired)
Rehabilitation Services Administration
Department of Health, Education and Welfare

HENRY L. BRAMMELL, M.D.
Associate Professor of Medicine and Physical Medicine
  and Rehabilitation
Project Director
Rehabilitation Research and Training Center
Department of Rehabilitation Medicine
University of Colorado

BEN V. BRANSCOMB, M.D.
Professor of Medicine
University of Alabama in Birmingham
School of Medicine

RENE CALLIET, M.D.
Professor and Chairman
Department of Rehabilitation Medicine
University of Southern California
School of Medicine

SANDRA S. COLE, B.A.
Health Educator
Department of Psychiatry and
Department of Physical Medicine and Rehabilitation
University of Michigan Medical School

THEODORE M. COLE, M.D.
Professor and Chairman
Department of Physical Medicine and Rehabilitation
University of Michigan Medical School

JAMES P. CONWAY, M.S.
Training Coordinator, Alcoholism Service
Long Beach General Hospital
Long Beach, CA

PAUL J. CORCORAN, M.D.
Professor and Director
Rehabilitation Research & Training Center
Department of Physical Medicine and Rehabilitation
Tufts University School of Medicine

JOEL DeLISA, M.D.
Assistant Professor
Department of Rehabilitation Medicine
University of Washington

ROBERT V. DeVITO, M.D.
Clinical Professor of Surgery
Head, Division of Plastic Surgery
University of Washington

SHELBY L. DIETRICH, M.D.
Director
Hemophilia Rehabilitation Center
Los Angeles Orthopaedic Hospital

WILLIAM H. DONOVAN, M.D.
Associate Professor
Texas Institute for Rehabilitation and Research
Baylor University

JESSIE K.M. EASTON, M.D.
Assisant Professor
Department of Physical Medicine and Rehabilitation
University of Minnesota

WILBERT E. FORDYCE, Ph.D.
Professor and Director of Research
Rehabilitation Research and Training Center
Department of Rehabilitation Medicine
University of Washington

ROY S. FOWLER, JR., Ph.D.
Associate Professor
Department of Rehabilitation Medicine
University of Washington

VERNELLE FOX, M.D.
Chief, Alcoholism Service
Long Beach General Hospital
Long Beach, CA

ROBERT T. FRASER, Ph.D.
Research Associate
Department of Rehabilitation Medicine and
Department of Neurological Surgery
University of Washington

LAWRENCE W. FRIEDMANN, M.D.
Chairman
Department of Rehabilitation Medicine
Nassau County Medical Center
Professor of Rehabilitation Medicine
State University of New York at Stony Brook

JOSEPH GOODGOLD, M.D.
Professor and Director of Research and Training
Department of Rehabilitation Medicine
New York University Medical Center

ANDREW S. HALPERN, Ph.D.
Director
Rehabilitation Research and Training Center in
    Mental Retardation
University of Oregon

DANIEL HALPERN, M.D.
Professor
Department of Physical Medicine and Rehabilitation
University of Minnesota

JOHN E. HEALEY, Jr., M.D.
Professor of Oncology and Orthopaedics and
    Rehabilitation
Universtiy of Miami School of Medicine and
Deputy Director
Division of Cancer Control and Rehabilitation
Comprehensive Cancer Center
for the State of Florida

LOREN A. HELBERG, Ph.D.
Associate Clinical Professor
Department of Rehabilitation Medicine
University of Southern California
School of Medicine

RICHARD E. HOOVER, M.D.
Chief of Ophthalmology
Greater Baltimore Medical Center
Assistant Professor of Ophthalmology
The John Hopkins University School of Medicine

CAGE S. JOHNSON, M.D.
Assistant Professor of Medicine
University of Southern California
School of Medicine

R. RAYMOND KNOWLES, M.B.
Clinical Professor
Department of Mental Health and Behavioral Science
St. Louis University

GEORGE H. KRAFT, M.D.
Professor
Department of Rehabilitation Medicine
University of Washington

H. RICHARD LAMB, M.D.
Associate Professor
Department of Psychiatry
University of Southern California
School of Medicine

CECILE MACKOTA
Director
Vocational Rehabilitation Services
San Mateo County (California)
Department of Public Health and Welfare

LEONA V. MILLER, M.D.
Director
Diabetes Institute of Southern California
Los Angeles, CA

JOHN J. NICHOLAS, M.D.
Associate Professor of Clinical Medicine
    and Clinical Orthopedics
Division of Rehabilitation Medicine
Presbyterian University Hospital
Pittsburgh, PA

EDWARD J. O'SHAUGHNESSY, M.D.
Assistant Professor
Department of Rehabilitation Medicine
University of Washington

ALVIN E. PARRISH, M.D.
   Professor of Medicine and Director
   Division of Renal Diseases
   The George Washington University Medical Center

JEROME D. SCHEIN, Ph.D.
   Professor and Director
   Deafness Rehabilitation
   Deafness Research & Training Center
   New York University

JERI SCHWEIGLER, M.S.
   Training Coordinator, Alcoholism Service
   Long Beach General Hospital
   Long Beach, CA

WALTER C. STOLOV, M.D.
   Professor and Director of Training
   Rehabilitation Research & Training Center
   Department of Rehabilitation Medicine
   University of Washington

ALLAN S. TROUPIN, M.D.
   Assistant Professor
   Director, Seizure Clinic
   Department of Neurological Surgery
   University of Washington

ARTHUR A. WARD, JR., M.D.
   Professor and Chairman
   Department of Neurological Surgery
   University of Washington

JACK M. ZISLIS, M.D.
   Assistant Professor
   Assistant Director, Rehabilitation Center
   Department of Orthopaedics and Rehabilitation
   University of Miami School of Medicine

PREFACE

The Rehabilitation Act of 1973, with its emphasis on the severely disabled, found many State vocational rehabilitation agencies ill prepared. Not enough of the counseling staff had the knowledge and the skills to deal with the vocational rehabilitation of the severely disabled. As a result, a number of training courses were developed throughout the country to equip the counselors with the necessary basic information that might allow them to successfully deal with their severely disabled clients.

In the State of Washington, the Division of Vocational Rehabilitation, through its chief medical social work consultant Mr. Thayne Wright, asked the University of Washington Rehabilitation Research and Training Center to develop and offer a course to upgrade the education of the Washington counselors in the area of severe disability. The first 5-day course was held May 20-24, 1974. Subsequently, four additional courses were held, which were not only presented to every counselor within the State of Washington, but also to counselors from the States of Alaska, Idaho, and Oregon.

As chairmen of these courses, we came to understand more completely the needs of the counselor in the area of severe disability. Preparation of a training manual for the courses became the initial framework for this text.

When the Rehabilitation Services Administration indicated interest in developing a new book on severe disability oriented toward the vocational rehabilitation counselor, we expressed interest in this area and subsequently accepted the offer to edit such a text. We viewed the project as a natural extension and continuation of our work in assisting with the training of rehabilitation counselors.

Following acceptance of the contract, an advisory committee was established and met with RSA representatives in Washington, D.C. on December 6, 1976. Persons serving on the advisory committee were: Raymond Ehrle Ph.D., President, American Rehabilitation Counseling Association; Leslie McCoy, M.D., Chief Medical Consultant, Division of Vocational Rehabilitation, West Virginia; William

Graves, Ed.D., President, National Council on Rehabilitation Education; Ann Crumpton, Past President, National Rehabilitation Counseling Association; Paul Corcoran, M.D., Professor and Chairman, Department of Physical Medicine and Rehabilitation, Tufts University; Ruth Savlowsky, Rehabilitation Group, Arlington, Virginia; Ekkehard Petring, Ph.D., Director, Region X Rehabilitation Counselor Education Program; and Guy Hubbard, Director, Division of Vocational Rehabilitation, North Carolina. Representatives of the Rehabilitation Services Administration at the meeting included: Harold Shay, Director, Division of Manpower Development; Sterling Brinkley, M.D., Chief Medical Officer; Joseph Fenton, Ed.D., Chief, Special Centers; Gregory March, Vocational Rehabilitation Consultant; Frederick Sachs, Assistant Commissioner for Program Management; William Usdane, Ph.D., Director, Bureau of Demonstrations and Manpower Development; Katherine Lloyd, M.D., Medical Officer; Elizabeth Bush, Manpower Development Specialist; and Richard Melia, Vocational Rehabilitation Program Specialist.

At the advisory committee meeting, decisions were made on the topics to be covered in the text, the authors to be invited to participate, the general format of the chapters (see p. 8), and the overall character and orientation of the text. It was decided to orient the book toward the first-year graduate student in rehabilitation counseling as a text for his course on the medical aspects of severe disability, and to the vocational counselor in the field as a reference. It became clear as the text evolved that it would also have value for others within the entire field of vocational rehabilitation, as well as for many allied health professionals and medical consultants.

As we invited authors to contribute to the project, we felt ourselves quite fortunate. All authors contacted entered into the project with enthusiasm, were reasonably prompt with their submissions, and adhered to requests and efforts to ensure that the text would be a uniform volume, rather than a collection of disjointed unrelated contributions. We are most grateful to all the authors.

We are also thankful for the fine technical editing by Sandra Blair. She was instrumental in achieving uniformity of style and presentation format, made many author contacts, monitored the production of the figures, and prepared the glossary. Editorial assistant Cheryl Dineen performed exceptional service in our bibliographical search of the literature for those key texts and articles added to the annotated bibliography at the end of each chapter. In addition, we are thankful to her and to Wilma Dlouhy for typing and retyping manuscripts during the review process.

Phyllis Wood, of the University of Washington Health Sciences Illustration Studio, produced the line illustrations for the text. We are most grateful for her fine work and her unfailing care and patience in drawing and revising the illustrations to ensure clarity and accuracy.

During our review of inital drafts, second drafts, and, in some cases, third drafts, we consulted numerous individuals within the University of Washington, the Northwest Region, and the country at large. We wish to express our appreciation to the following reviewers for their assistance in enhancing the final text: Marjorie Anderson, Ph.D., University of Washington; Sandra Belcher, Ph.D., University of Washington; David Beukelman, Ph.D., University of Washington; Stirling B. Brinkley, M.D., Rehabilitation Services Administration; JoAnn Brockway, Ph.D., University of Washington; Alan Dralle, CPO, University of Washington; Joseph Fenton, Ed.D., Rehabilitation Services Administration; William Graves, Ed. D., Mississippi State University; John L. Hampson, M.D., University of Washington; Noreen R. Haupt, State of Wisconsin Department of Health and Social Services; David Hooks, M.Ed., University of Washington; Kathleen Lloyd, M.D., Rehabilitation Services Administration; Steve Lund, C.P.O., University of Washington; Leslie McCoy, M.D., State Board of Vocational Education, West Virginia; Greg March, Rehabilitation Services Administration; Willman Massie, Rehabilitation Services Administration; Ekkhard Petring, Ph.D., Seattle University; Donald E. Rawe, Rehabilitation Services Administration; Frederick Sachs, Rehabilitation Services Administration; Martin Spickler, Rehabilitation Services Administration; J. Paul Thomas, Rehabilitation Services Administration; Susan Tollefson, R.N., University of Washington; Ann B. Trotter, Ph.D., University of Wisconsin-Milwaukee: William Usdane, Ph.D., Rehabilitation Services Administration; Johan Verhulst, M.D., University of Washington; David Wenner, Rehabilitation Services Administration; Boyce R. Williams, Rehabilitation Services Administration; and Robert J. Winn, Jr., Rehabilitation Services Administration.

We hope the counselor will find within these pages the information that may allow his clients to achieve and successfully maintain a desired employment.

Walter C. Stolov, M.D.
Michael R. Clowers, Ph.D.

Addendum

Following completion of the text but before final publication, my co-editor, Michael R. Clowers, Ph.D., passed away on October 22, 1979 after an extended illness. Both the professional and the patient-client rehabilitation communities lost a trusted colleague, advocate, and friend. Marks of his insistence that excellence prevail in the production of this text can be seen throughout its pages. It is hoped that this last major project of Dr. Clowers can serve as a living monument to his memory.

Walter C. Stolov, M.D.

1 COMPREHENSIVE REHABILITATION: EVALUATION AND TREATMENT

Walter C. Stolov, M.D.

DISABILITY

Definition

Consider the following scenario:

A colony of 100 Earth men and women, selected from the most able-bodied and intelligent applicants, lands its space ship on the planet Soil of a nearby star system. The planet is very dark due to a persistent cloud cover. The friendly Soil people quickly establish a successful method of communication. Despite some similarities and differences, both groups agree to be examined by each other's physicians.

Two days later, the Earth physicians report to their group:

The Soil people, although mildly grotesque looking and somewhat smaller than us, are quite nice and friendly. They see on this dark planet because their eyes respond to infrared light, but not to visible light. The frequency range of their vocal cords includes ours, and also extends into the inaudible high-frequency ultrasound range. The foods here consist of highly complex compounds, and their digestive system includes a double stomach. The first stomach, much like our cow's, predigests the food. The rest of the digestive system is the same as ours.

Like us, they have two arms, but theirs are shaped in the form of wings, which allow them to fly, and instead of having five fingers, the ends of their arms are flat pads. All their various utensils, of course, interface successfully with these pads. They write with special pens that lay down infrared radiation sources which, though invisible to us, they can read. They have only one leg which is as broad as our two and ends in a round, flat, pad-like structure. Walking involves a rolling motion of this pad.

The Soil people live in high-rise apartments which look almost like ours, but there are no stairs or elevators. They simply fly up into their apartments and pass through doors located on the outside walls. A combination of high-frequency sound signals, which they emit, open the door locks.

All manual labor on Soil is done by computers and by robots with physical configurations like ours. Computers are programmed and triggered by combinations of the high-frequency sounds. All children gradually learn these sound combinations in school.

The Soil physicians presented the following report to the Soil President:

The Earth people are blind; *they have no infrared vision.*

They speak of being able to see light, but we are not sure what they mean. They are partially aphasic, *as their vocal cords do not have vibration capacity at our high frequencies. Of more immediate consequence is the fact that the Earth people* cannot eat. *Their digestive system is incapable of breaking down our food products. We will have to tackle this problem soon, as their own food supply will run out in a week. Of course, as you noticed, they are* dependent in flying *and, because of their size, they are also* dependent in transfers *in and out of our cars.*

It appears that the Earth people cannot live anywhere on our planet. They say our apartments look like theirs, but asked if we had something called "stairs" or "elevators." Except perhaps for the first floor in some of our buildings, these people really have no place to live.

At first glance, the Earth people will be unable to work *on our planet. Without high frequency vocal cords, they cannot learn to operate our computers and robots. Some of them look strong enough to work alongside our robots, but I suspect they will consider this to be menial employment. Also, 25 percent of them are* severely depressed.

Mr. President, the Earth people are clearly severely and totally disabled. What shall we do?

The President replied, "Hospitalize them in our Comprehensive Rehabilitation Center, and report back to me in 6 months the outcome of the treatment."

This scene graphically illustrates the definition of disability. Disability is present, or a *person* is disabled, when a set of *functions*, either desired or required, exists, which cannot be independently performed when attempted in a specific *environment*. While the desired functions may be specific preferences of the person, the required functions may be totally dictated by the environment.

The above Earth-Soil illustration of the influence of the environment on disability has exact parallels on Earth. Our environment has been a continuing end result of the activities of perhaps one-third or less of our population who, by virtue of power, a high level of intelligence, and superior health, direct the creation of our physical plants, our institutions, our jobs, and our recreation. These institutions, jobs, and physical plants are created for use by the majority, who are much like the creators—people "in their own image."

These insitutions, jobs, and physical plants were, however, not created for use by those less able-bodied, less intelligent, sick, or disabled—the people the creators hardly ever see.

As the creators have become more sophisticated, systems have been developed to accommodate this disabled group, but somewhere "off to the side," away from the mainstream. Only recently has the concept that the disabled can be brought into the mainstream been considered, and the environment has begun to be modified to accomodate them.

Characteristics of Disability

Let us return again to the planet Soil and listen to the report given to the President 6 months after the Earth people entered the Rehabilitation Center.

Mr. President, I am happy to report that 30 percent of the Earth people have been "closed rehabilitated." All of these learned to use the apparatus we developed to convert infrared to visible light. They also learned to manage the high-frequency ultrasound radiator we developed, which they wear around their waists. Our drug industry developed a pill which allowed this group to digest our food products, although the pill is unsuccessful with the others. Half of the 30 percent became independent in flying with rocket devices, while the other half chose to have their arms amputated and prosthetic wings applied. Automobiles were built to accommodate the Earth people, who actually helped in the design. The cost of the automobiles, however, is quite high. This group is now living in the community alongside our people and, in fact, some of the Earth men and women are in love with Soil people and have talked about marriage. We have therefore initiated sex education and counseling in an effort to achieve sexual compatibility.

Twenty-five percent are still in the Rehabilitation Center and we are hopeful that they, too, will succeed. The residual problem for most of them is digestion. They all continue to need the predigestion machine, which is not yet generally available throughout the planet.

Twenty percent of the Earth people have also been discharged "partially rehabilitated," but they are not living among our people. They were unable to master the eating problem or the flying skills, and were not intelligent enough to handle the ultrasound machine. We built a handicapped housing community nearby for them. The building has stairs, elevators, and their type of lights. A sheltered workshop is also in the building, where the Earth people repair computers. As you know, this has been a task that only a small number of our Soil people care for. Some of them have chosen to work alongside our robots and appear happy in this menial labor.

Another 10 percent of the Earth people have been "closed unrehabilitated" and have been transferred to a nursing home. They were able to overcome only a few of their functional disabilities and require attendant care. The attendant turnover is quite high for, as you know, few Soil people are interested in this activity.

Unfortunately, 15 percent of the Earth people have committed suicide, some indirectly and some directly. Initially, some refused to be admitted to the Rehabilitation Center, claiming that they were not disabled. They were cared for briefly in our acute hospital, where food could be prepared, but they soon died from a combination of malnutrition and disease. The others simply found the stress too great, discharged themselves from the Rehabilitation Center against medical advice, and soon thereafter took an overdose of one of the Earth medicines they brought with them.

The above scene illustrates three important characteristics of disability:

1. There is no one-to-one correlation between a disease and the spectrum of associated disability problems. The same disease can produce separate sets of disability problems in different individuals.
2. There is no one-to-one relationship between a disease and the amount of residual disability. Disability problems can be removed even though the disease is unchanged.
3. The ability of a patient and the total health care team to remove disability in the face of chronic disease is dependent upon the patient's residual capacity for physiological and psychological adaptation. Residual strength must be evaluated and enhanced to "work around" an impairment in order to remove disability.

In our Earth-Soil scenario, the disease was "able-bodied human." On Earth, the disease is any of the many different conditions discussed in this textbook. Thus, in the case of multiple sclerosis, for example, no two patients have the *same* problems. Their individual disabilities will depend upon the functions desired or required, the environments in which these functions are to be performed, and the extent of the attack on the central nervous system by the multiple sclerosis lesions. Even if the amount of destruction within the nervous system is not altered, the functional losses can be removed in several ways. The capacity of the unaffected body systems can be enhanced, the environment can be modified, and the interface between person and environment can be altered to match residual skills to environmental demands.

Patient-Environment Interaction

Figure 1-1 illustrates the interaction between an individual (the patient or client) and his environment through the interface between the two. On the patient side is the basic chronic disease interacting with basic psychological characteristics that identify the patient as a personality. The psychological factors include those

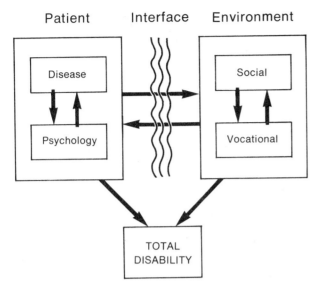

Patient   Interface   Environment

FIGURE 1-1. Schematic representation of the interaction of the patient with his environment. On the left, disease factors are reciprocally influenced by psychological factors. On the right, social factors are mutually influenced by vocational factors. The patient and his environment mutually influence each other through their interface. The Total Disability is fed by all areas.

emotional responses that may be reactive to the stress of the chronic disease. The disease and the patient's psychology are in dynamic interaction. In most of the conditions discussed in this text, changes in the basic disease can affect the patient's psychology, and changes in the patient's psychology can influence and alter the extent of disease, particularly its complications.

On the environment side of figure 1-1 there are also two components in dynamic interaction: the *social sphere* (the patient's home, family unit, social responsibilities, and interpersonal contacts) and the *vocational sphere* (the place of work, the breadth of responsibilities, and the financial and personal rewards, and also avocational and recreational pursuits). The dynamic interaction is clear. In many situations, disturbances in the equilibrium of the social sphere can interfere with vocational performance, and vice versa. Alterations in either sphere can cross the patient-environment interface and modify the patient's disease and level of psychological performance.

A patient's total disability (his disability diagnosis or complete list of disability problems) derives from factors specific to himself and to his environment. Problems may relate to the disease; to the patient's psychology, social functioning, or vocational functioning; and to the interface between the patient and the environment. Removal of disability is achieved through therapeutic attacks on the disease, through enhancement of the patient's psychology, through modification of the interface, and through direct

modification of social and vocational environmental factors.

Consider the following brief case history and list of disability problems of a patient recently admitted to a rehabilitation center for comprehensive rehabilitation:

A 19-year-old woman fractured her cervical spine in a small-plane accident, with resultant quadriplegia. Her male companion, with whom she had been living for the previous year and a half, was killed in the crash. Their relationship had been close and family oriented, since she served as "stepmother" for her companion's two small children from a prior marriage. Following the accident, responsibility for the children was legally assumed by their natural mother.

The patient was hospitalized for a short period on an acute neurosurgical service and then transferred to a comprehensive rehabilitation center for inpatient care. Her problem list following a complete comprehensive evaluation shortly after admission to the rehabilitation center included:

1. *C7 (seventh cervical vertebra) fracture dislocation*
2. *C7 complete quadriplegia*
3. *Ambulation dependent*
4. *Transfer skills dependent*
5. *Eating, dressing, personal hygiene skills dependent*
6. *Bowel incontinence*
7. *Bladder incontinence*
8. *Decreased respiratory function*
9. *Potential for pressure sore*
10. *Potential for thrombophlebitis*
11. *Immature personality*
12. *Reactive depression*
13. *Home architecture incompatible with paralysis*
14. *Financially dependent*
15. *Estranged from parents*
16. *Unemployed, no prior work history*
17. *Homemaking skills deficient*
18. *Transportation dependent*

Comparing the patient's problem list with the scheme in figure 1-1 identifies problems 1, 2, 6, 7, 8, 9, and 10 as directly involved with the patient's disease. Problems 3, 4, 5, and 18, while also a direct result of the disease, constitute her physical disabilties. Problems 11 and 12 relate to the patient's psychology, and problems 13, 14, 15, and 17 to the social sphere. Problem 16 succinctly and precisely identifies the vocational disability.

Severe Disability

The Rehabilitation Act of 1973 and subsequent amendments charged the State-Federal Vocational Rehabilitation Program to concentrate its efforts on patients and clients with severe disability. Some efforts have been made to quantify disability by defining a large number of functions and assessing a patient's degree of independence or dependence in these functions according to a numbering system. The numbers can then be totaled for each patient, and an arbitrary cutoff point can be established. Patients with total numbers above this point may be called severely disabled and those with total numbers below this point may be called minimally or mildly disabled.

Such an approach, while seemingly solving the problem of definition, is fraught with difficulties because disability is so highly individualized. Further, the relative importance of one set of functions compared to another (e.g., physical vs. social) is lost when an arbitrary numbering system is used. Applying a "weight factor" which scales the relative importance of one function to another (assuming a consensus on such a factor) would also be inadequate because the importance of one function relative to another usually varies from patient to patient.

Rather than a quantitative definition, an operational approach to defining the severity of disability may perhaps be more useful for a particular counselor and client. As already discussed, disability is removed via therapeutic techniques applied to the patient, to the environment, and to the interface. Disability problems can be characterized by the therapeutic techniques available, or perhaps unavailable.

1. A disability problem in a particular patient may be one for which a therapeutic technique is immediately available ("on the shelf") and is well-known to be capable of removing the disability problem.
2. A disability problem may be one for which a therapeutic technique is available, but it is not certain that the technique can indeed remove the disability problem.
3. A disability problem may be one for which no therapeutic technique is available that is known to be capable of removing the problem, but it is believed that one can be created.

Given these concepts of disability problems and therapeutic techniques, a definition of severe disability can be stated which may be operationally useful for any particular client or patient.

A minimally or mildly disabled individual may be viewed as one for whom therapeutic techniques, which will remove the disability and complete the rehabilitation, are well known and immediately available. The following short histories are useful examples.

A 45-year-old editor notices increasing difficulty seeing the print of the texts and manuscripts he is asked to review. He visits his ophthalmologist, who determines that the editor suffers from the commonplace farsightedness caused by the loss of elasticity in the lens of the eye with age. The physician prescribes reading glasses. The glasses are purchased, the reading difficulty is eliminated, the disability is removed, and the rehabilitation is complete.

In this example, the eyeglasses constitute the readily available therapeutic technique with a well-known capability to remove the reading disability due to this type of eye problem.

A 35-year-old outdoor carpenter suffers a fall and ruptures an intervertebral disc in his lower back. Spinal nerve irritation, back and leg pain, and leg weakness result. Back surgery is recommended to remove the pressure on the nerve. The patient has the surgery, pressure on the nerve is removed, and the back and leg pain and weakness disappear. The physician advises that the heavy carrying loads associated with outdoor carpentry work will cause early degeneration of the spine and are too strenuous for the residual capacity of the back. Lighter work activities are recommended, but are unobtainable in the outdoor carpentry field.

Vocational evaluation of the unemployed carpenter indicates that hand dexterity, which is required for indoor light cabinetmaking and refinishing, is excellent. Jobs in indoor carpentry are available, and the counselor knows that the local vocational school has a good 1-year course in cabinetmaking, refinishing, and other indoor carpentry skills. The counselor develops an educational plan with the unemployed carpenter, who completes the course, finds employment, and succeeds in his new occupation.

In this example, the readily available therapeutic technique was the local carpentry course which, when applied, removed the disability problem, "unemployment."

A 45-year old married male with fairly stable adult-onset muscular dystrophy manages quite well at home and in his office job as long as his wife assists him with dressing. The patient's upper extremity weakness interferes with shirt buttoning, belt buckling, and putting on socks, shoes, and ties. When his wife unfortunately dies, the patient is totally disabled in his dressing skills and is consequently unable to maintain employment. He is admitted to a rehabilitation center where, through clothing modifications, the use of adaptive equipment, and technique training, he achieves full independence in dressing. The disability removed, he returns home and resumes employment.

In this example, the readily available techniques were those adaptive devices and methods of performance known to enable achievement of dressing independence. Of significance in this example is the fact that it was a change within the patient's social sphere of activities that created the disability and the potential for unemployment.

In the above examples, the therapeutic techniques were readily available and known to be capable of removing the disability problems. Hence, these patients were minimally or mildly disabled.

Severe disability can also be characterized in relation to available therapeutic techniques. At least three different types of situations signify severe disability.

1. As in the above examples, the therapeutic techniques are available and known to be capable of removing a disability problem. However, the patient has several disability problems, and more than one technique must be applied. These various disability problems require simultaneous solutions and hence several professionals from different fields working together. A simple sequential application of each

technique will not be successful because a particular solution to one of the problems may interfere with the solution of another. All the professionals must therefore work together in a single setting to solve the problems effectively. In this case, the disability qualifies as severe because of the need for a center where various professionals can interact in the application of therapeutic techniques to remove the patient's disability.

2. A second situation signifying severe disability occurs when a number of possible techniques are available, but it is not known in advance that they are capable of removing the several disability problems, and therefore an extended evaluation and treatment period is necessary. In this case, there might also be several techniques potentially available for each of the individual problems, but much trial is necessary.

3. Finally, disability can be considered severe when the therapeutic techniques are not readily available, but evaluation suggests that they can be treated in therapeutic settings, working closely with the patient on their design. Some of these techniques might relate directly to the interface between the patient and the environment.

Using these three operational definitions of severe disability and the operational definition of minimal or mild disability, the counselor can decide whether or not a particular client's disability is severe. The counselor first performs and/or obtains a careful evaluation of the client's total function and a listing of all the client's disability problems. This review can be compared to the operational definitions and the examples cited above to decide whether severe or minimal disability is present. The review also serves to create the rehabilitation plan.

For example, the problem list of the 19-year-old quadriplegic on page 3 can be considered in light of the above definitions. The patient's condition can be identified as severe disability from several points of view. Available "on the shelf" therapeutic techniques, useful for dealing with problems 1–10 and possibly also 17 and 18, do exist. Their successful application, however, requires the coordinated, simultaneous efforts of physicians, rehabilitation nurses, physical therapists, occupational therapists, and possibly also orthotists.

Further, while some therapeutic techniques do exist that might be applied toward the solution of the problems 11–16, they do not have the promise of certain resolution, and several new techniques need to be created. Thus, all three operational definitions of severe disability apply in the example.

REHABILITATION

Comprehensive Evaluation

Medical evaluation. As the understanding of causes and treatment of diseases and injury increased, a number of specialties evolved within the medical profession. Some of these specialties were organized according to known causes of the disease (e.g., allergy, oncology) and others as disciplines dealing with a particular system of the body (e.g., neurology, ophthalmology). The medical evaluation of a disease may therefore involve one or more specialists, each with a specific set of skills and knowledge.

All medical evaluations include a history of the symptoms, a review of the past medical history, a historical review of each of the systems in the body capable of producing symptoms, and a review of the social, vocational, and psychological history of the patient. A physical examination of all the systems is also performed. While almost all physicians carry out the above, the different specialists bring additional insights, depending upon their expertise. Medical evaluation also includes a number of different laboratory and X-ray examinations designed to clarify a patient's problems, as well as to suggest or monitor treatment.

The current widely used medical-record system was introduced and became popular about 10 years ago. Under this new *problem-oriented format*, medical evaluation results in a list of patient problems, rather than simply a diagnosis of the suspected disease. Included in such a list might well be the known disease itself. The list, however, will also include: (a) significant consequences and complications of the disease; (b) physical function problems, which comprise the extent of the physical disability; and (c) problems in the psychological, social, and vocational spheres, as in the 19-year-old quadriplegic patient.

With this approach, therapeutics can be directed at each of the problems on the list, rather than exclusively at the disease itself. This is particularly important when the disease is chronic. In chronic disease, therapeutics do not exist for eliminating the pathology of the disease; i.e., the pathology itself may be permanent. Functional problems which might be a direct result of the disease can, however, be identified and solved through appropriate therapeutic techniques. Physicians specializing in physical medicine and rehabilitation (physiatrists, rehabilitation medicine specialists) have particular expertise in the identification of functional, psychosocial, and vocational problems which might be overlooked by other specialists whose interest is focused more on the organ system or on specific therapies.

Allied health evaluation. As already discussed, the breadth of disability problems includes not only the disease, but also issues in the patient's psychology and in his social and vocational spheres. The clear identification and need for treatment of all these has resulted in a large number of medically related health professionals who both participate in the evaluation phase and work in medical settings with attending physicians. Examples of such professionals include physical therapists, occupational therapists, rehabilitation nurses, prosthetists and orthotists, medical social workers, clinical psychologists, speech and language therapists, recreation therapists, vocational counselors, work evaluators, rehabilitation teachers and mobility instructors for the blind, bioengineers, sex therapists, and audiologists. These professionals add their own special expertise, not only to help achieve a thorough evaluation of the disability problems, but also to ensure that all available therapeutics are applied.

Comprehensive Rehabilitation Centers

A rehabilitation center is the facility that has evolved for the management of patients and clients with chronic disability problems. These institutions are usually associated with general hospitals, but they may be "free standing." Most of the centers that have the capacity to treat severe disability also have inpatient facilities for 24-hour-a-day intensive treatment. Some rehabilitation centers are only outpatient facilities and, as such, cannot handle as wide a range of problems.

Usually, each rehabilitation center develops an expertise in certain areas and certain diseases, but many are able to handle all types of problems. Highly specialized rehabilitation centers include those related to blindness, deafness, severe mental retardation, or alcoholism, to name a few. All rehabilitation centers have a certain commonality. Their staffs all include full-time physicians with special interest and training in disability and expertise in rehabilitation treatment. All also have full-time staffs of allied health professionals representing those disciplines necessary for the rehabilitation treatment of the type of patient they serve. Most offer vocational rehabilitation services by full-time vocational rehabilitation counseling staff. They are not necessarily counselors for the State Vocational Rehabilitation agency, although in many instances staff from the State agency are assigned full-time to such institutions. Vocational rehabilitation counselors in such institutions who are not actually State agency staff do relate directly to State agency personnel to ensure continuity of vocational rehabilitation after discharge from the center.

The hallmark of all rehabilitation centers with regard to any patient admitted is an initial evaluation to identify the full range of disability problems. Evaluation invariably involves participation by all the relevant professionals for the individual situation. After the evaluation, the rehabilitation team, together with the patient, develops a treatment plan for removal of the disability problems. For each problem, goals are established which characterize the anticipated end result of treatment. Formulation of goals and a treatment plan, in concert, ensures that all professionals are working with the patient toward a common end.

During the course of treatment, the rehabilitation team meets frequently to assess progress, modify goals, and alter treatment programs, as indicated by the patient's progress. Efforts are directed toward minimizing the disease, maximizing residual capacity, establishing suitable interfaces between the patient and the environment, and modifying the environment to secure an adequate match between what the patient may be able to achieve and what his environmental circumstances may demand.

Referral Information Sources

Physicians are licensed to practice, based on examination by the state in which they work. Minimum competency in a specialty, however, is not associated with any governmental license, but rather is assessed by examinations prepared by peers. These are organized by the various Specialty Boards of the American Medical Association. The Boards admit to examination applicants who have met certain minimum training standards for their specialty. Certification is then achieved through examination, usually written and oral. The *Directory of Medical Specialists,* a yearly publication available in almost all libraries, lists the training and certification of medical specialists. Appendix A lists those Specialty Boards in which certification by examination under the auspices of the American Medical Association exists.

Allied health professionals have similar standards of competency, and directories are available of licensed individuals and those who may have met local or national examinations. Appendix B presents the name and address of the major national organization of each of the allied health professional groups. Most have branches in each of the states, which publish directories of licensed practitioners. Some have national directories only. Each organization can, on request, indicate whether a particular person has met the standards established for the profession.

Appropriate rehabilitation centers for severely disabled clients within any given community can usually be identified by several sources. A voluntary organization called the Commission for Accreditation of Rehabilitation Facilities maintains a directory of rehabilitation centers for members of the group (Appendix C). Additional sources of information listed in Appendix C include the NIHR Medical Rehabilitation Research and Training Centers scattered throughout the country, and the American Congress of

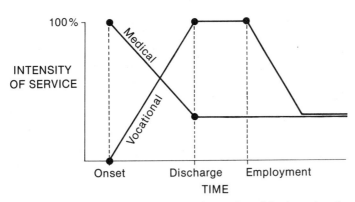

FIGURE 1-2. Schematic description of the intensity of medical and specific vocational services applicable for acute-onset severe disability requiring hospitalization. At onset, medical services dominate. At discharge, vocational services dominate until employment. Both medical and vocational services may need to be sustained for a period of time at a low level to maintain health and employment.

Rehabilitation Medicine, an organization of medical and allied health professionals actively engaged in the 'rehabilitation of the disabled. The Easter Seal Society in each city is also usually able to identify and recommend appropriate facilities.

Medical-Vocational Transition

Particularly for acute-onset, relatively "incurable" disease, or acute recurrences or complications of an ongoing chronic disease, a reciprocal relationship exists with regard to the intensity of medical services and specifically vocational services. Figure 1-2 illustrates this reciprocal relationship. At first, the medical services are intense and vocational services are minimal. With time, the intensity of the medical services decreases, while the intensity of vocational services increases. Medical services rarely decrease to zero because they usually are required to maintain achieved goals. The same, in effect, also applies to specific vocational rehabilitation services. After job placement or independent living is achieved, the intensity of vocational services tapers off. In many instances, sustaining success may require services at a lower level over an extended period of time.

In relatively few instances is a patient exposed to the rehabilitation treatment process only once. Alterations in the disease, in the environment, or in the interface may cause new or previously removed disability problems to resurface and require additional intervention. This is particularly likely for those diseases with uncertain courses or prone to develop complications. Further, as new techniques develop, patients may re-enter the treatment process to seek solutions to disability problems not previously solvable.

The Individually Written Rehabilitation Plan

The term "vocational rehabilitation services," under the State-Federal program, has come to mean "any goods or service" necessary to render a disabled individual employable. The term is not, therefore, limited to specific counseling with regard to job selection or job placement. Rather, it includes the full range of medical and allied health services which, when delivered, are expected to remove a sufficient number of disability problems to allow for employment to result. It therefore includes those services which the counselor can provide for, but might not personally be able to deliver.

Vocational rehabilitation services also include services or processes associated with extended evaluation to determine the existence of vocational potential. In such situations, the availability of therapeutic techniques may be relatively uncertain, and the extended evaluation determines whether actual therapeutic services are likely to render a disabled individual employable. Recently, there has been increasing emphasis on the value of rehabilitation services to a severely handicapped individual for whom the goal may be limited to independent living and a satisfactory avocational life.

The individually written rehabilitation plan (IWRP), a concept introduced in the Rehabilitation Act of 1973, fits in very nicely with the problem-oriented format of medical evaluation discussed above. The IWRP is, in essence, a contract or agreement between a rehabilitation counselor and a client with regard to any evaluation or treatment program that commits the counselor to restorative services, counseling services, and other appropriate services to treat disability problems. An IWRP attempts to identify a long-range rehabilitation goal, which may actually include a specific area of employment. It also identifies intermediate objectives to be accomplished on the road to the long-range goal. The intermediate objectives relate quite closely to the expectations of treatment for the various disability problems that may be uncovered in the evaluation of a client by a comprehensive rehabilitation team.

In addition to the listing of the long-range goal and intermediate objectives, an IWRP spells out the processes and the programs by which services will be delivered, by whom, and how. Such plans are not cast in stone. Periodic review between counselor and client may lead to modification of intermediate objectives, long-range goals, and techniques of treatment that prior experience may dictate. Currently, with regard to expenditure of Federal funds, long-range rehabilitation goals require an employment objective. In time, it is anticipated that the independent living objective for those very severely disabled may be a permissible long-range goal.

CHAPTER ORGANIZATION

All but five of the chapters in this text deal with those specific diseases known from experience to be instrumental in causing severe disability. The five chapters deal with issues common to most of the others and have their own special format. These five (chaps. 2, 3, 4, 21, and 32) deal with psychosocial adjustment, sexual adjustment, consequences of bed rest, reconstructive surgery, and the normal function of the six body systems which, when deranged by disease, result in severe disability. The reader is encouraged to become familiar with the normal function of these systems to enhance his understanding of the diseases themselves.

All the disease-oriented chapters are organized in a similar way. They begin with a *disease description,* which includes its natural history of evolution, its primary characteristics, and its potential complications. The description is followed by a section on the *functional disabilities,* both physical and psychosocial, associated with the disease. The physical disabilities indicate how the particular disease limits the patient's performance as a whole with regard to ambulation, transfer skills, eating skills, dressing skills, and personal hygiene skills, the group of activities usually referred to as activities of daily living (ADL). Further, if the disease produces disability in transportation and communication skills, these are also discussed. In the section of psychosocial disabilities, those potential interferences in a patient's psychological or social functioning that may be a direct result of the disease, or associated with it, are presented. *Rehabilitation potential* is then described, incorporating factors related to the disease itself and the usual expected results of treatment.

The next section in each chapter deals with *standards of evaluation.* Included in this section is what currently constitutes an optimum evaluation of the patient and his condition. It describes the physicians and allied health professionals who should be consulted to obtain a full characterization of the disease and identification of the breadth of disability problems. Significant laboratory examinations are also described, where pertinent.

The chapters then deal with the *total treatment* of the condition. Included is the current "state of the art" with regard to the medical-surgical management and treatment by allied health professionals known to be capable of modifying the disease pathology and/or affecting and removing physical and psychosocial disability problems. Maintenance management is also included if it is recommended to maintain achieved rehabilitation goals. With the information in this section and with his knowledge of his client, the counselor should be able to determine whether his client has had the benefit of all available treatment.

The final section in each chapter deals with specific *vocational implications* of the condition that a rehabilitation counselor should keep in mind when planning employment goals with his client. This section may deal with factors of education, aptitudes, interests, the environment, and physical demands as they may influence or be influenced by the disease in question.

Physical demands generally include lifting, carrying, pushing, or pulling. Lifting and carrying implies that the arms have certain capacities, and that the person has certain transport capability. Pushing or pulling implies arm or leg abilities. All four characteristics generally parallel each other, and therefore physical demands can be characterized by the lifting function alone.

With regard to physical demands, the following definitions are used throughout the text:

1. *Sedentary work* means that the lifting requirements are on the magnitude of 10 pounds (4.5 kg) maximum and usually involve smaller objects. The work is largely done sitting, although some walking or standing may be required.
2. *Light work* implies a lifting capacity of up to 20 pounds (9 kg), with significant walking or standing requirements. A heavy requirement for pushing, pulling, or leg control is also consistent with most sitting work.
3. *Medium work* implies a lifting maximum of 50 pounds (22.5 kg), with a usual lifting requirement of about 25 pounds (11.3 kg). This type of work and the two types that follow usually require walking and standing capacities.
4. *Heavy work* requires a lifting maximum of up to 100 pounds (45 kg), with the usual requirement 50 pounds (22.5 kg).
5. *Very heavy work* requires a lifting maximum of greater than 100 pounds (45 kg), with the usual

carrying capacity of 50 pounds (22.5 kg).

The chapter sections on physical demands will also discuss interferences in lower extremity functions, such as climbing, balancing, stooping, and kneeling, and in upper extremity functions, such as reaching, handling, fingering, and feeling.

Each chapter includes an annotated *bibliography,* which references only books and articles readily available in most libraries. A *glossary* is included at the end of the book. Words which have been defined in the text do not appear in the glossary, unless they occur frequently. The glossary is therefore not an exhaustive dictionary, and the counselor may wish to have a medical dictionary as well.

CONCLUSION

The challenge of providing maximal services for the severely disabled is great. The acceptance of the challenge requires knowledge, teamwork, coordination, planning, and patience. Assimilation of the material in this handbook can, at best, only equip a counselor with a few basics on which to build. Medical and rehabilitation research will soon modify these basics, eliminate some, and add others not yet imagined. The counselor must not only develop, through experience, the skill to minister successfully to the disabled, but must also maintain a continuing education program to update his knowledge and his techniques.

APPENDIX A

SPECIALTY BOARDS

The following is a list of the American Boards of the American Medical Association which certify specialists through examination. The address of their executive offices can be obtained from the American Medical Association, 535 North Dearborn Street, Chicago, Illinois 60610. Those currently certified are listed in the *Directory of Medical Specialists,* Vols. 1 & 2, Chicago, Marquis Who's Who. The *Directory* is updated annually.

American Board of Allergy and Immunology
American Board of Anesthesiology
American Board of Colon and Rectal Surgery
American Board of Dermatology
American Board of Family Practice
American Board of Internal Medicine
   Cardiovascular Disease
   Endocrinology and Metabolism (Committee)
   Gastroenterology
   Hematology (Committee)
   Infectious Disease (Committee)
   Medical Oncology (Committee)
   Nephrology (Committee)

   Pulmonary Disease
   Rheumatology (Committee)
American Board of Neurological Surgery
American Board of Nuclear Medicine
American Board of Obstetrics and Gynecology
American Board of Ophthalmology
American Board of Orthopaedic Surgery
American Board of Otolaryngology
American Board of Pathology
American Board of Pediatrics
   Pediatric Cardiology
   Pediatric Endocrinology
   Pediatric Hematology-Oncology
    (Special Competency)
   Nephrology (Special Competency)
   Neonatal-Perinatal Medicine
    (Special Competency)
American Board of Physical Medicine
  and Rehabilitation
American Board of Plastic Surgery
American Board of Preventive Medicine
American Board of Psychiatry and Neurology
   Psychiatry
   Neurology and/or Child Neurology
   Psychiatry and Neurology
   Child Psychiatry
American Board of Radiology
American Board of Surgery
American Board of Thoracic Surgery
American Board of Urology

APPENDIX B

NATIONAL OFFICES OF ALLIED HEALTH ORGANIZATIONS

American Association for Respiratory Therapy
  7411 Hines Place, Suite 101
  Dallas, TX 75235

American Association of Sex Educators,
Counselors and Therapists
  5010 Wisconsin Avenue N.W., Suite 304
  Washington, D.C. 20015

American Association of Workers for the Blind
  1511 K Street N.W.
  Washington, D.C. 20005

American Dental Associaton
  211 East Chicago Avenue
  Chicago, IL 60611

American Nurses' Association
  2420 Pershing Road
  Kansas City, MO 64138

American Occupational Therapy Association
6000 Executive Boulevard, Suite 200
Rockville, MD 20852

American Optometric Association
7000 Chippewa Street
St. Louis, MO 63119

American Orthotic and Prosthetic Association
1444 N Street N.W.
Washington, D.C. 20005

American Physical Therapy Association
1156 Fifteenth Street N.W.
Washington, D.C. 20005

American Psychological Association
1200 Seventeenth Street N.W.
Washington, D.C. 20036

American Rehabilitation Counselor Association
1607 New Hampshire Avenue N.W.
Washington, D.C. 20009

American Speech and Hearing Association
9030 Old Georgetown Road
Washington, D.C. 20014

Commission on
Rehabilitation Counselor Certification
6th Floor, 162 North State Street
Chicago, IL 60603

National Association of Social Workers
1425 H Street, Suite 600
Washington, D.C. 20005

National Rehabilitation Counseling Association
1522 K Street N.W.
Washington, D.C. 20005

APPENDIX C

VARIOUS REHABILITATION ORGANIZATIONS AND RESEARCH AND TRAINING CENTERS

Organizations

American Congress of Rehabilitation Medicine
30 North Michigan Avenue
Chicago, IL 60602
Phone: (312) 236-9512

Commission for Accreditation of Rehabilitation
Facilities
2500 North Pantano Road
Tucson, AZ 85715
Phone: (602) 886-8575

Easter Seal Society
2023 West Ogden
Chicago, IL 60612
Phone: (312) 243-8400

International Association of Rehabilitation
Facilities
5530 Wisconsin Avenue, Suite 955
Washington, D.C. 20015

National Rehabilitation Association
1522 K Street
Washington, D.C. 20005

*Department of Education-NIHR Rehabilitation
Research and Training Centers*

New York University
Medical Rehabilitation R&T Center
400 East 34th Street
New York, NY 10016

University of Minnesota
Medical Rehabilitation R&T Center
860 Mayo Building
Minneapolis, MN

University of Washington
Medical Rehabilitation R&T Center
15th Avenue N.E.
Seattle, WA 98195

Baylor College of Medicine
Medical Rehabilitation R&T Center
1333 Moursund Avenue
Houston, TX 77030

Emory University School of Medicine
Medical Rehabilitation R&T Center
1431 Clifton Road
Atlanta, GA 30322

Tufts University
Medical Rehabilitation R&T Center
171 Harrison Avenue
Boston, MA 02111

Temple University
Medical Rehabilitation R&T Center
Suite 201, 12th and Tabor Road
Philadelphia, PA 19141

The George Washington University
Medical Rehabilitation R&T Center
Room 714, Ross Hall
2300 Eye Street N.W.
Washington, D.C. 20037

University of Colorado Medical Center
Medical Rehabilitation R&T Center
  4200 Ninth Avenue, Box C242
  Denver, CO 80262

University of Wisconsin
Mental Retardation Rehabilitation R&T Center
Waisman Center on Mental Retardation
and Human Development
  2605 Marsh Lane
  Madison, WI 53706

University of Arkansas
Vocational Rehabilitation R&T Center
  346 West Avenue Annex
  Fayetteville, AR 72701

University of West Virginia
Vocational Rehabilitation R&T Center
  Suite E-1 Dunbar Plaza
  Dunbar, WV 25064

University of Oregon
Mental Retardation Rehabilitation R&T Center
  212 Clinical Services Building
  Eugene, OR 97403

New York University
Deafness Rehabilitation R&T Center
  80 Washington Square East
  New York, NY 10003

University of Alabama
Medical Rehabilitation R&T Center
  1717 Sixth Avenue South
  Birmingham, AL 35233

Northwestern University
Medical Rehabilitation R&T Center
Rehabilitation Institute of Chicago
  345 East Superior Street
  Chicago, IL 60611

Texas Tech University
Mental Retardation R&T Center
  P.O. Box 4510
  Lubbock, TX 79409

University of Wisconsin-Stout
Vocational Rehabilitation R&T Center
  Menominie, WI 54751

University of California, San Francisco
Deafness and Mental Health Rehabilitation
R&T Center
  1474 Fifth Avenue
  San Francisco, CA 94143

University of North Carolina at Chapel Hill
Blindness Rehabilitation R&T Center
  210 N. Columbia Street
  Chapel Hill, NC 25714

Boston University
Rehabilitation R&T Center in Mental Health
  1019 Commonwealth Avenue
  Boston, MA 02215

2 PSYCHOSOCIAL ADJUSTMENT TO CHRONIC DISEASE AND DISABILITY

Gary T. Athelstan, Ph.D.

ADJUSTMENT TO DISABILITY

Definition

Adjustment to disability has been defined by social scientists in various ways. Some definitions focus upon the individual and the behaviors that are learned or the roles that are assumed after onset of disability. Others adopt a sociological perspective and consider the individual in relation to society and societal units such as the family or community. This chapter will present some of the major phenomena of psychosocial adjustment to disability as they are reported in the literature and encountered in rehabilitation practice. Sexual adjustment receives special attention in chapter 21, since it is a relatively new topic in the rehabilitation literature and has been the subject of increasing interest in recent years.

Much of the research on adjustment processes in rehabilitation has been done from the perspective of a single academic discipline or to develop and test one or another theory. Nearly all such studies have contributed to our understanding of the effects of severe disabilities and how people cope with them. However, the discussion of psychosocial adjustment to disability developed in this chapter does not emphasize any particular disciplinary or theoretical viewpoint. Rather, the problems of adjustment are presented in the pragmatic terms which are familiar to disabled individuals and the counselors who work with them.

In the sections that follow, a working definition of psychosocial adjustment is presented. Special emphasis is given to developing a conceptualization of psychosocial adjustment which is consistent with the philosophy of rehabilitation. This is followed by a discussion of the process of adjustment that highlights some of the landmarks, problems, and possible phases in the process. Finally, the implications of these issues for counselors and some of the ways that counselors can intervene in the process to facilitate adjustment are discussed.

In a study of spinal cord injured patients which is currently underway at the University of Minnesota, patients were asked to tell the staff what adjustment to disability meant to them. Most of the answers expressed variations on a theme of "learning how to live with it." Others said that adjustment meant "making the most of what you have" or "trying to lead as normal a life as possible."

Rehabilitation professionals tend to define adjustment in terms of achieving the individual's maximum potential. Although this seems to be a reasonable approach, it imposes the crucial requirement of accurately measuring "potential" in order to determine how much has been realized and, consequently, how "adjusted" the individual is. Considering the drastic changes that severe disability may produce in a person's life style and functioning, correct assessment of potential can be very difficult.

Most traditional definitions of adjustment to disability in our society emphasize some form of productivity. Thus, a disabled person who is employed is generally assumed to be better adjusted to his disability than an unemployed person. However, counselors frequently encounter (a) employed disabled persons whom they consider poorly adjusted psychologically or socially; (b) poorly adjusted disabled persons who are unemployed but productive in nonvocational ways; and, occasionally, (c) seemingly unproductive and inactive disabled persons who appear to be very well adjusted. It is apparent, then, that employment, adjustment, and disability are separate, though interrelated, issues. Clearly, adjustment to disability is a very complex issue and cannot be solely defined in terms of employment; other factors must be considered as well.

A definition of psychosocial adjustment should take into account the disabled individual's satisfaction with, or acceptance of, his circumstances. This approach has the major advantage of allowing a highly individualized assessment of adjustment to disability. However, it has the disadvantage of determining the level of adjustment by what the client says rather than by what he does. Since no good methods are available to assess the validity of these self-reports, the unit of measurement becomes subjective in nature. Therefore, individuals who report being content with their circumstances, whatever they may be, must be considered well adjusted. Yet, this view can be in direct conflict with very reasonable traditional definitions. In the study mentioned above, clients were asked to rate their degree of satisfaction with their living arrangements, financial and employment status, health, social life, and sex life. In general, persons who were most active and productive, often those who were employed, tended to report being least satisfied with their situation in life.

In other words, the study found that individuals who would be considered best adjusted to their disability by traditional measures tended to be least well adjusted in terms of their self-reported acceptance of their circumstances. This could reflect, in part, a tendency of the employed and more active persons to measure themselves against a "normal" standard rather than to take satisfaction from their accomplishments in relation to other severly disabled persons. Nevertheless, the findings suggest that it would be appropriate to take into account some measure of psychological functioning or emotional status in any assessment of adjustment to disability. This means that rehabilitation counselors ought to consider the impact of their services not only on the employment status and activity level of their clients, but also on their psychosocial adjustment in the broadest sense.

When all of the theoretical formulations, research, and clinical experience with disabled persons are considered, adjustment to disability seems to be a complex, but not at all mysterious, process that normal persons undergo in trying to cope with the severe psychological stress of a major life crisis. It should be viewed as an evolutionary, changing, and highly individualized process rather than a stable state. The problems faced by the newly disabled person are those of coping with physical and psychological loss, changes in body image, social status, and earning capacity, the anxiety and grief which often accompany these changes, and the need to learn new behaviors and make concrete plans for an uncertain future. Each individual will seek personal solutions to these problems and thus define his own adjustment to disability.

PSYCHOSOCIAL EFFECTS OF DISABILITY

Since many of the psychological effects of disability are a result of the social implications, it is necessary to first consider some of the immediate consequences of disability onset. One of the most predictable effects of a visible physical disability is a *change in the social status* of the individual. Disabled persons in our society assume a special kind of minority status and occupy a socially devalued role. Numerous studies have shown that people tend to attribute negative characteristics to the disabled and that this tendency generalizes well beyond the direct effects of the disability. Visibly disabled persons are often assumed by others to be less attractive, less desirable, and less capable in ways

which are totally unrelated to their disability.

A loss of social status may also result from the indirect effects of disability, such as its *economic consequences*. The costs of acute and long-term medical care for chronic disease or disability may be so great as to deplete all of a family's assets. Furthermore, the impact of disability on an individual's earning capacity can produce a long-range change in socioeconomic status. Recent studies have shown that when the principal breadwinner of a family is disabled, an average reduction of 40 percent in total family income results.

Disability usually causes profound *changes in close social relationships*. Nagi and Clark (1964) have demonstrated the effects of disability on the family, including divorce rates, which sometimes rise, but may also decline. Also, Cogswell (1967) has shown that it is typical for predisability friendships to dissolve, an observation which is often confirmed in rehabilitation practice. In fact, in the early stages of social adjustment for paraplegics after their initial hospitalization, there is often a marked reduction of (a) social contacts; (b) frequency of entering community settings; and (c) the number of roles played. It has been suggested that much of the individual's predisability mode of social adjustment must be discarded before new roles can be assumed and a new adjustment worked out.

It should be clear from this brief discussion that the social impact of disability is great enough in itself to have psychological consequences. However, disability also has some very direct effects on behavior which may produce a variety of emotional reactions and psychological adjustment problems. A useful way to determine the impact of disability is to measure the *loss of the individual's capacity to perform certain behaviors*. The greater the loss or impairment of behaviors produced by the disability, the greater the loss of reinforcers or rewards available to the individual, and the greater the need for social relearning. Thus, adjustment to disability can be defined in operational terms relating to old behaviors which must be discarded and new behaviors which must be learned. A behavioral approach to rehabilitation is helpful in focusing on what the individual must learn to do in order to live effectively with disability.

PHASES OF ADJUSTMENT TO DISABILITY

Considering the many negative effects of disability, it is only natural that the onset of a major disability will often be accompanied by significant emotional reactions. A useful way of describing the reactions that can occur is to examine the response to crisis occurring over time. Shontz (1965) has proposed a series of five phases of adjustment: shock, realization, defensive retreat, acknowledgement, and adaptation. Each of these phases is accompanied by a characteristic emotional experience, and the predominant emotional reaction changes as a person progresses through the phases of adjustment.

The phases and their accompanying emotional reactions, which are described in the following paragraphs, are not absolute and unvarying. The stage formulation provides a reasonable basis for categorizing the behavior one often sees, but the counselor should realize that individuals' reactions are variable in time, intensity, and sequence, and some phases may occur in combination while others do not appear at all. Nevertheless, it is helpful to be alert to these reactions and sensitive to the different forms they may take, since they can affect progress in rehabilitation.

Shock

During the first few hours or days after onset of disability, the individual is usually feeling and reacting minimally and may have little awareness of what has happened. This initial phase is called shock and usually involves only muted emotional reactions. The immediate effects of serious physical illness or extensive injury may be part of the cause of shock. The counselor has little but friendship to offer during the shock phase, and that may be perceived by the client as irrelevant.

Although counseling intervention usually has little direct impact at this time, it is very helpful for the counselor to meet the client (or patient, since this initial meeting will usually be in a hospital) and begin to establish a relationship. Because of the relative lack of emotional reaction, the client may be easier to approach at this time than later, when great fear, anger, depression, or other reactions can interfere with an initial contact. This early intervention should be directed toward laying the foundation for effective counseling later, especially since most clients move relatively quickly into the next phase.

Realization

Realization is the phase in which some recognition of the reality and seriousness of the disability begins to develop. Anxiety, possibly even panic, may be the predominant emotional reaction. This fear is based on anticipation of possible death, critical losses, or unpredictable change. Its extent may or may not be consistent with the seriousness of the disability, but it is important for the counselor to recognize that the client typically feels great fear. Depression and anger may also occasionally appear during this phase.

The counselor can be helpful at this time by acknowledging and accepting the fear in an understanding way. Casual reassurance is likely to be rejected, but sincere reassurance by a counselor who has already begun to establish a relationship with the client will provide effective support for the client as he works through this crucial phase.

Defensive Retreat

The anxiety that normally follows onset of disability could easily overwhelm the individual if there were no defense mechanisms available to help him cope with the situation. Predominant among these defenses is denial. The person defends against the threat of disabilty by denying its existence or seriousness. Thus, the newly injured person may insist, "I am going to recover fully and walk out of this place," or, "Yes, I know my paralysis won't improve, but it won't make any difference." Such denial may persist or reappear occasionally long after onset of disability, usually in the form of the individual refusing to make reasonable or realistic allowances for the disability, or to accept the limitations imposed.

The counselor must recognize that denial is serving an important psychological purpose for the disabled person. Denial can be one of the most difficult barriers a counselor may meet because of the important role it plays in helping the individual control or avoid anxiety. If the counselor has not previously established a relationship with the client, even suggesting the need for counseling at this point may be very threatening. For the client to accept help would be to acknowledge that something has happened and help is needed. Insisting that the disabled person begin planning for a changed future, or in some other way directly challenging the denial of reality, may lead to a total rejection of counseling that could delay or rule out effective intervention later. It is probably also important to avoid agreeing with the client and thereby reinforcing or encouraging denial, since that could strengthen it as much as direct confrontation. If denial is not interfering with the patient's active participation in his rehabilitation program, it is usually best to leave it alone.

A very effective way for the counselor to handle denial is to work around it and try to alleviate the anxiety that produces it. The client should be informed, accurately and fully, what limitations and problems the disability creates, but this should be done in a supportive way, accompanied by realistic information about the possibilities of amelioration and rehabilitation. In other words, the bad news should not be avoided, but it need not be delivered without sensitivity.

In the later stages of adjustment, a client who recognizes and accepts the maximum level of functioning that can reasonably be achieved may still exhibit hope for total cure. This hope should not be confused with denial. Hope may in part maintain a person's motivation for rehabilitation, and should not be destroyed by the counselor. There is no cause for concern if the client is making plans and acting in a manner consistent with the limitations imposed by his disability and is making satisfactory progress toward reintegration into the community.

Acknowledgment

Acknowledgment refers to the phase in which the individual achieves an accurate understanding of the nature of the disability and the imposed limitations. Some persons may demonstrate a very thorough intellectual understanding of the disability prior to this time, but still not display full appreciation of its implications. Acknowledgment is usually marked by the onset of some degree of depression.

The depression which often accompanies recognition of the reality and seriousness of a disability is a very natural grief reaction to the losses that result. The disabled individual is generally removed for prolonged periods from his customary environment, and may abruptly lose many desired activities and behaviors and, thus, their rewarding consequences. However, rehabilitation professionals frequently assume that there is an underlying pathology or "lack of motivation" at the base of any significant depression. Consequently, they tend to attribute responsibility for depression to the disabled individual and may lack initiative or imagination in finding ways to counter it. What is worse, by providing sympathy or attention, the professional may inadvertently strengthen a maladaptive pattern of behavior.

On the other hand, professionals sometimes mistakenly insist that depression must occur. One occasionally hears the argument that if a person has not gone through a period of depression after the onset of disability, it must be due to adjustment being halted in the denial phase. The unfortunate implication of this argument is that the counselor must forcibly precipitate a depression so that adjustment can proceed to the next phase. In fact, there is no evidence that every person's adjustment must go through each of these phases, or that the phases must be experienced in any particular order. However, if the counselor has evidence that denial is present and significantly interfering with rehabilitation progress, it may be necessary to begin gently but firmly confronting the client with reality, even though this may precipitate anxiety and even some depression. Sensitive support that recognizes the stress the client feels, coupled with short-term goals successfully achieved, may well make it easier for the client to give up denial, make plans, and execute efforts that incorporate the disability.

Adaptation

Adaptation is the final phase of adjustment to disability. The term means simply that the individual has worked through any major emotional reactions to the disability, is realistic about his limitations, and is psychologically ready to make use of his potential. This is sometimes referred to as the "acceptance" phase, but it should be noted that accepting a disability does not imply a willingness to accept a diminished life or to be happy about being disabled. Rather, acceptance or adaptation means learning to live with certain limitations and to make the best use of remaining assets.

FACILITATION OF ADJUSTMENT TO DISABILITY

The emotional reactions and efforts to cope with disability shown by an individual will be determined by a combination of personal characteristics, learning history, and current circumstances. It is important for the counselor to avoid stereotyped approaches to the client. An athlete or manual laborer may reasonably be expected to experience a more adverse reaction to disability than a person whose work is mainly sedentary. However, many exceptions exist and the counselor is cautioned to set aside assumptions and perform a careful assessment of the present and potential functioning of each client in an effort to establish individual adjustment goals.

Counseling the severely disabled must be regarded as a means of helping them overcome many of the obstacles to realizing their full potential and living effectively with their disabilities. Therefore, counseling is not done primarily to produce insight, to promote self-actualization, or to restructure the personality. It may be provided partly for emotional support and to promote emotional growth, but it is mainly directed at helping the client solve some of the practical problems of adjustment. The counselor must therefore be aware of the usual course of adjustment, and intervention should be designed to facilitate the client's movement along that course.

Effective counseling is not likely to be limited to verbal interaction between the counselor and the client. It includes teaching, consultation, advising, and environmental manipulation, and may involve extensive work with many persons in addition to the disabled individual.

Resocialization

Often the first few months or even years after initial hospitalization appear to be relatively uneventful for the disabled person. Nevertheless, for many persons a subtle but critically important process of resocialization is taking place. Initially, after the onset of disability, there may be a period of apparent decline in social functioning as the client discards predisability roles and relationships. Later, the person begins a gradual process of developing new relationships and experimenting with new roles. Then gradually he begins to venture out into the community again, first visiting relatively nonthreatening, anonymous public places which are easy to leave. Subsequent outings generally involve increasing risk due to greater intimacy of the settings and the increased difficulty of leaving abruptly. Usually the last steps in the resocialization process involve settings like private parties, public places such as bars, and places of employment.

There are a number of things the counselor can do to promote resocialization. Before developing a resocialization plan, it is important for the counselor to determine the client's predisability social patterns. Since pre-existing social problems are more resistant to change than new disability-related problems, the counselor should differentiate between longstanding characteristics and problems occurring as a direct result of the disability. After determining the client's pre-existing social involvement, the counselor's efforts are best directed toward environmental manipulation rather than traditional counseling strategies.

The first thing the counselor should do to facilitate resocialization is to determine by observation and interview the specific social activities the client currently participates in. Then the counselor can judge what stage in the resocialization process the client has reached and what a reasonable next step would be. Since the stages are arranged in a hierarchy of difficulty, it is important that the counselor not encourage the client to progress too far in any one step. In addition, the client's efforts should be directed toward one area of resocialization at a time, such as development of an avocational activity or an independent living arrangement.

The counselor should define manageably small steps and assist the client directly, if necessary, in making the arrangements that will result in progress toward the stated goals. For example, the first contact with the community that some severely disabled persons might undertake could involve a visit to the counselor's office. If even that step proves to be too great at first, the counselor may want to arrange a home visit in order to establish some rapport with the client and lower the barriers to the initial effort. After a visit to the counselor's office, the next step may be to have social contacts with other disabled persons. This could be accomplished by encouraging the client to attend a club or special interest group for the handicapped. It is important for the client to know that he *can* achieve each step, and that the culmination of the steps is a goal he *wants* to attain. If there is something desirable to be gained from each step, and if the requirement for social and physical effort is minimized, the client is more likely to succeed in the plan.

Later, more demanding steps, such as enrolling in school, may be taken. Enrollment in school might be intended to provide the client with a marketable vocational skill; to provide a basis for supportive retraining, even if the vocational objective is initially in

doubt; or in some cases, to provide resocialization as an end in itself. If the counselor recognizes the progressive and hierarchical nature of resocialization and is willing to be flexible and do whatever is necessary to accomplish these steps, it should be possible to start with a client at any stage and produce movement to whatever ultimate step may be set as a goal.

Timing

In order for the counselor's intervention to be effective, he must appreciate that a considerable amount of time might be required for the rehabilitation plan to be completed, and thus realize that progress in resocialization and other aspects of adjustment can be painfully slow. Although some clients might adapt and adjust to disability relatively quickly, others might return to work after intervals exceeding 10 years after onset of disability and, naturally, others not at all.

Timing of counseling intervention is important mainly in relation to the readiness of the disabled individual to work toward rehabilitation goals. This readiness will vary over time. In an early contact, the rehabilitation counselor may find the disabled person mainly engaged in readjusting roles, struggling to "accept" the disability or "still trying to get used to it." Although these efforts may involve a very active process of adjustment, the disabled person may see this as a period in which restriction of his social life is the only obvious change taking place. Unless the counselor is sensitive to this process, neither he nor the client is likely to realize that anything significant is happening, and the client may report that he is "not ready" to undertake planning or other rehabilitation efforts. This apparent lack of readiness may persist over several contacts and, as a result, the counselor may finally mistakenly close the case due to the client's lack of motivation.

If, instead of closing the case, the counselor realizes that the seemingly uninterested client may be presently preoccupied with social and psychological adjustment processes, two avenues of effective intervention are open. The first is active intervention and provision of services explicitly aimed at facilitating psychosocial adjustment without reference to vocational goals. A second possibility is assuming a more passive stance and simply recontacting the client periodically over an extended period of time, waiting for "readiness" to develop. This approach can be more effective than is immediately apparent if the counselor takes care to make the personal contacts supportive, non-threatening, and reasonably comfortable for the client. When the client does mature to the point of being ready for professional assistance, these services are much more accessible than would be the case if a new contact had to be self-initiated at that time.

Only two demands are placed on the counselor who

takes this approach: first, he must take the little time needed, once, twice, or four times a year, to visit with the client; and second, he must persuade the counseling supervisor that this strategy can be effective and that the prospects for success warrant keeping a case open with no change in status for a longer period than usual. The result of this strategy can be a sudden and remarkable surge of "motivation" and rehabilitation progress on the part of a client who may have appeared for quite some time to have had limited rehabilitation potential.

The psychological and social phenomena described in this chapter and the techniques suggested for facilitating adjustment represent a synthesis of research and extensive professional practice. It is hoped that the guidelines and suggestions presented here will assist rehabilitation counselors in the course of working with their most severely disabled and most challenging clients.

BIBLIOGRAPHY

Albrecht GL (ed): *The Sociology of Physical Disability and Rehabilitaton.* Pittsburgh, University of Pittsburgh Press, 1976.

This book contains 11 major articles presenting psychological and sociological conceptualizations of issues and problems in rehabilitation. Although mainly academically oriented, the papers include much information of practical value to the rehabilitation counselor. WE Fordyce's chapter "A Behavioral Perspective on Rehabilitation" presents a behavioral formulation of disability, from which the reader can glean practical suggestions for the application of behavioral techniques in rehabilitation.

Athelstan, GT: A follow-up study of the psychological, social and vocational adjustment of spinal cord injured adults. *In* the Fifteenth Annual Progress Report of Rehabilitation Research and Training Center No. 2, Minneapolis, University of Minnesota, 1976.

Since this research is still in progress, its findings have not yet appeared in the formal literature. However, the annual progress reports, particularly the report of 1976, contain much useful descriptive information on a large sample of persons who have been spinal cord injured for a long period of time.

Cobb AB: *Medical and Psychological Aspects of Disability.* Springfield, IL, Thomas, 1973.

Written mainly for the vocational rehabilitation counselor, this book is a collection of papers by physicians and psychologists. Its purpose is to familiarize the professional practitioner with the principal medical and psychosocial aspects of 12 different disabilities, such as heart disease, cerebral palsy, amputations, epilepsy, deafness, and blindness.

Cogswell BE: Rehabilitation of the paraplegic: Processes of socialization. Sociological Inquiry 37:11–26, 1967.

This is a report of a rather intensive study of the postinjury social adjustment of a small group of spinal cord injured men. A conceptual formulation of the process of resocialization is presented.

Malikin D, Rusalem H (eds): *Vocational Rehabilitation of the Disabled: An Overview.* New York, New York University Press, 1969.

Just as the title states, this book provides an overview of the field of vocational rehabilitation: its history and legislative basis, philosophical viewpoints, the system, the process, and issues of practice and technique.

Nagi SZ, Clark DL: Factors in marital adjustment after disability. Journal of Marriage and the Family **26**:215–216, 1964.

A short article summarizing the factors that appear to influence marital stability after physical disability. Some of the factors are age, education, and occupation.

Neff WS (ed): *Rehabilitation Psychology.* American Psychological Association, Inc., 1200 Seventeenth Street NW, Washington, D.C. 20036, 1971.

This book consists of a set of papers presenting the state of the art in rehabilitation psychology, especially in the last 12 years. Many different points of view are presented.

The Severely Disabled. A Special Issue of the Rehabilitation Counseling Bulletin, the Journal of the American Rehabilitation Counseling Association, **18**, No. 4, 1975.

Designed to assemble current information relating to vocational rehabilitation of the severely disabled, this issue has 12 articles reporting recent research, analysis of issues, and new program developments.

Shontz FC: Reactions of crisis. Volta Review **67**:364–370, 1965.

This paper provides a conceptual view of the stages in the process of adjustment to crisis and a framework for understanding the emotional reactions that may accompany disability.

Wright BA: *Physical Disability—A Psychological Approach.* New York, Harper and Row, 1960.

This book presents a very thorough social-psychological analysis of disability and suggestions of techniques that the rehabilitation counselor can use to facilitate achievement of rehabilitation goals.

3 SIGNIFICANT BODY SYSTEMS

Joel DeLisa, M.D.
Walter C. Stolov, M.D.

NERVOUS SYSTEM

For descriptive purposes, the nervous system is divided into the central nervous system (CNS) and the peripheral nervous system (PNS). The CNS consists of the spinal cord and the brain, namely, the cerebrum, cerebellum, and brain stem, and the PNS consists of the cranial and spinal nerves. The autonomic nervous system is somewhat specialized and may be viewed as part of both the CNS and the PNS. Sometimes the term *somatic nervous system* is applied to those parts of the CNS and PNS under voluntary control and associated with the extremities and structures of the body wall (e.g., skin, bones, joints, and skeletal muscle). In contrast, the involuntary *autonomic nervous system* is associated with internal organs, blood vessels, smooth muscle, and cardiac muscle.

The main functions of the nervous system are (a) to receive sensory information from the environment and the body itself through various receptors and to transmit this information to the brain (*afferent system*); (b) to send impulses down the spinal cord and out the peripheral nerves to the various end organs to effect a motor response (*efferent system*); (c) to integrate the information obtained from all the receptors. An understanding of the nervous system is particularly relevant to chapters 5, 6, 7, 8, 9, 10, 11, 12, 15, 20, 24, and 27.

The basic functional unit of the nervous system is the *neuron*, which is responsible for transmitting this information to and from the brain. The neuron consists of a cell body and two distinct types of processes, the numerous *dendrites* and a single *axon* (fig. 3-1). The terms "axon" and "nerve fiber" are synonymous. Most axons are long and encased in a sheath of fat-like substance called *myelin* which acts as an insulator and aids in the rapid transmission of the nerve impulses away from the cell body. Dendrites are short, branched processes which receive impulses from the terminal branches of axons of other neurons and conduct them toward the cell body. The cell body contains the cell nucleus and is responsible for maintaining the health of the neuron.

The length of the path traveled by afferent or efferent information is longer than any single axon. Therefore, chains of neurons are necessary to convey

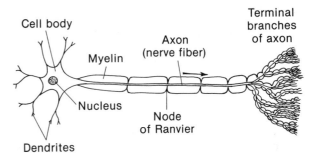

FIGURE 3-1. Basic myelinated nerve cell. Dendrites receive input from terminal branches of other axons. When sufficiently activated, the cell body transmits an electrical impulse down its axon. Myelin protects the axon and, together with nodes of Ranvier, allows for very fast conduction. Nonmyelinated, slower-conducting axons also exist. Axon diameters range from 1 to 60 $\times 10^{-4}$ cm. Arrow indicates direction of impulse travel.

messages through the entire nervous system. The message is an electrical impulse (action potential) produced by a chemical change that progresses along the axon. The system for transfer from one neuron to the next is the *synapse* (fig. 3-2). The synapse is the site at which the axon of one neuron ends near the dendrite or cell body of the next neuron. Here the electrical impulse in the axon causes the release of a chemical such as acetylcholine or dopamine, and this, in turn, causes a sequence of chemical events that results in an impulse in the next neuron.

Nerve cell bodies are usually located in groups. Within the brain and spinal cord these groups are called nuclei and constitute the *gray matter*, so-called because they have a grayish color. Outside the brain and spinal cord the groups are called ganglia. The remaining areas of the nervous system consist primarily of tracts of many axons which constitute the *white matter*, so-called because the myelin sheaths have a whitish color. Tracts that carry information of a specific type, such as pain, touch, or vision, usually have specific names.

CENTRAL NERVOUS SYSTEM

The cerebrum, cerebellum, and brain stem are contained and protected by the skull. This complex

19

mass of nervous tissue contains over seven billion nerve cells. The spinal cord is contained and protected by the vertebral column. All four structures have three membranous coverings known as *meninges* which afford further protection. From the outside in, these are the *dura mater, arachnoid mater,* and *pia mater* (fig. 3-3). The CNS literally floats in a bath of cerebrospinal fluid which occupies the space between the arachnoid mater and pia mater (*subarachnoid space*). The CNS is also cushioned internally by the cerebrospinal fluid located in cavities (ventricles) within the cerebrum and brain stem (see fig. 3-5 and 3-6). The fluid also serves as a medium through which nutrients and wastes can be exchanged between the blood and the CNS.

Cerebrum

The cerebrum, consisting of two cerebral hemispheres, is the largest part of the brain and represents about seven-eighths of the total weight of the CNS. The surface of these two cerebral hemispheres has numerous convolutions gyri. Between gyri lies an intervening furrow, the shallow *sulcus.* A very deep sulcus is a *fissure* (fig. 3-4). The outer surface of the cerebral hemispheres consists of a thin layer of gray matter, the *cortex.* The interior portion of the cerebrum consists of white matter, tracts, and nuclei (gray matter) where synapses occur. Different lobes of the hemispheres have different functions, and the cortex varies in structure from region to region depending upon the varying function. The bones of the skull have the same names as the lobes lying beneath them.

The two cerebral hemispheres are "twins," each with centers for receiving sensory (afferent) information and for initiating motor (efferent) responses. The anatomical structures of both hemispheres have the same names. Certain intellectual functions are concentrated in either the right or the left hemisphere (see chaps. 9 and 10). The left cerebral hemisphere mostly receives afferent input from, and initiates efferent activity on, the right side of the body, and the right cerebral hemisphere mostly receives afferent input from, and initiates efferent activity on, the left side of the body.

Frontal lobe.   The frontal lobe is the anterior part of each hemisphere and contains the nerve cells (Betz cells) that initiate the impulses which travel through one or more synapses to produce fine, isolated, and versatile muscle and extremity movement. These cells are referred to as the *upper motor neuron* for motor activity. The Betz cells are spatially organized in the precentral gyrus of the frontal lobe, often referred to as the *motor strip* (fig. 3-4). Their axons pass downward to the spinal cord first as the *internal capsule* and then as the *pyramidal tract.* Anterior to the motor strip are areas that are felt to deal with higher intellectual functions such as

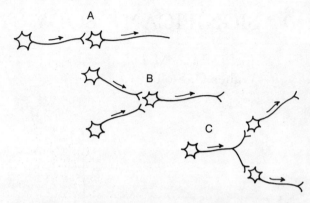

FIGURE 3-2. Schematic representation of a synapse. *(A)* Single axon synapsing with a single cell body. *(B)* Two axons synapsing with a single cell body. *(C)* One axon synapsing with two cell bodies. Arrows indicate direction of impulse travel.

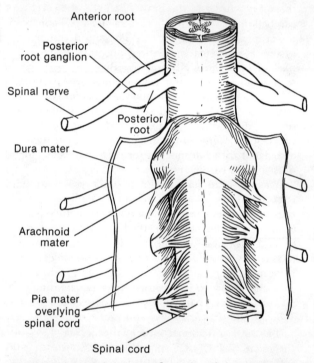

FIGURE 3-3. Posterior aspect of spinal cord showing posterior spinal roots and the coverings. Dura mater continues into sleeve of spinal root. Cerebrospinal fluid is located between the arachnoid mater and the pia mater. Note that a spinal root is really several rootlets.

abstract thinking and judgment. The cell bodies of the neurons of the first cranial nerve, the olfactory, are in the base of the frontal lobe.

Parietal lobe.   The parietal lobe is the middle portion of each hemisphere (fig. 3-4). The *postcentral gyrus* is the major sensory receptive area for the highest integration and coordination of afferent information dealing with pain, temperature, form, shape, texture, pressure, and position. Some memory functions are also subserved by the parietal lobe.

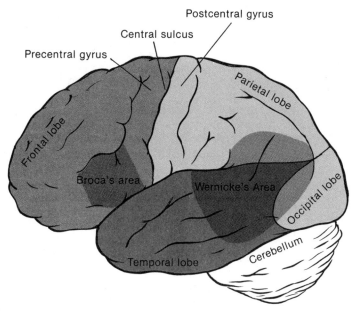

FIGURE 3-4. A left cerebral hemisphere and cerebellum showing the distribution of the cerebral cortex of the frontal, parietal, temporal, and occipital lobes. The central sulcus divides the precentral gyrus from the postcentral gyrus, and hence the frontal lobe from the parietal lobe. The location of Wernicke's area over the temporal and parietal lobes and Broca's area over the frontal and temporal lobes is shown.

Temporal lobe. The temporal lobe is under the frontal and parietal lobes (fig. 3-4). Its cortex is the primary area where auditory stimuli are received. It is also one of the centers for dreams, memory, and emotions.

Occipital lobe. The occipital lobe is in the posterior part of each hemisphere (fig. 3-4). Its cortex is the primary area where visual stimuli are received. (See p. 48 on the optic nerve and the nerve pathways for vision.)

Basal ganglia. The basal ganglia are aggregates of cell bodies (gray matter) located within the cerebral hemispheres (fig. 3-5). These ganglia constitute part of the *extrapyramidal system* which is concerned with postural adjustment and gross voluntary and automatic movements, as opposed to the fine movements controlled by the motor strip of the frontal lobe. The basal ganglia receive afferent fibers from the cerebral cortex and the thalamus. The axons from the basal ganglia synapse in the brain stem and then again at the spinal cord. The extrapyramidal system is part of an elaborate feedback system for controlling movement. Close to the basal ganglia lies the *internal capsule* which contains the important efferent motor tracts descending from the frontal lobe on their way to the spinal cord.

Thalamus. The thalamus is a large, bilateral, egg-shaped mass of gray matter also located deep and near the midline of the cerebral hemispheres (fig. 3-5). It is the main synaptic relay center for sensory messages as they travel from the peripheral sensory receptors to the sensory areas of the postcentral gyrus of the parietal cortex.

Hypothalamus. The hypothalamus is a collection of ganglia located below the thalamus and intimately associated with the pituitary gland (fig. 3-5). It has a variety of crucial functions:

1. It controls the autonomic system and hence regulates parasympathetic and sympathetic function (see below).
2. It is part of the pathway by which emotions influence body functions.
3. It secretes hormones influencing the posterior pituitary gland for maintaining body water control.
4. It secretes hormones that influence the anterior pituitary gland's release of sex, thyroid, and adrenal stimulating hormones.
5. It is part of the arousal mechanism for maintaining the waking state.
6. It is an essential part of the mechanism for regulating appetite.
7. It is crucial for the maintenance of normal body temperature.

Language areas. Language function requires an integration of visual and auditory afferent input (receptive function) with efferent motor output (expressive function). The frontal, parietal, and temporal lobes are involved. The language function is located in the left hemisphere in essentially all right-

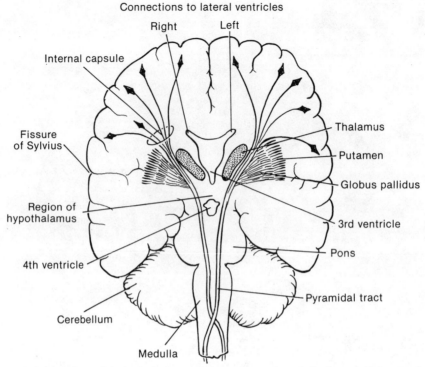

Connections to lateral ventricles

Right   Left

Internal capsule

Thalamus

Putamen

Globus pallidus

Fissure
of Sylvius

Region of
hypothalamus

3rd ventricle

Pons

4th ventricle

Pyramidal tract

Cerebellum

Medulla

FIGURE 3-5. Schematic section through the cerebrum, pons, and medulla demonstrating the deep basal ganglia and the four ventricles. Note the thalamus on either side of the third ventricle, the location of the fourth ventricle, and the pyramidal tract originating in the precentral gyrus passing its fibers through the internal capsule and crossing over to the opposite side of the medulla. The hypothalamus is located below the basal ganglia in the region of the third ventricle. The Fissure of Sylvius is a deep sulcus that separates the parietal lobe from the temporal lobe.

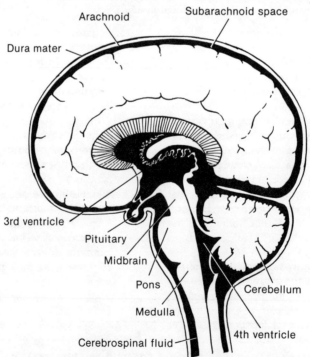

Arachnoid   Subarachnoid space

Dura mater

3rd ventricle

Pituitary

Midbrain

Pons

Cerebellum

Medulla

4th ventricle

Cerebrospinal fluid

FIGURE 3-6. Midline section through the cerebrum, cerebellum, and brain stem. This section passes through the third and fourth ventricles, both of which are midline structures. Note cerebrospinal fluid bathing the brain.

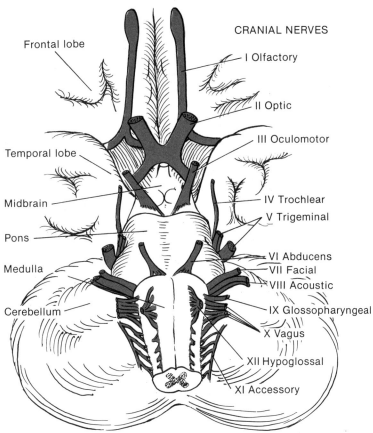

CRANIAL NERVES

Frontal lobe

I Olfactory

II Optic

III Oculomotor

Temporal lobe

Midbrain

IV Trochlear

V Trigeminal

Pons

VI Abducens

VII Facial

Medulla

VIII Acoustic

Cerebellum

IX Glossopharyngeal

X Vagus

XII Hypoglossal

XI Accessory

FIGURE 3-7. Underside view of the brain showing the brain stem and the underside of the frontal lobe. Cranial nerves I through XII are exposed in this view.

handed individuals and about 85 percent of all left-handed individuals. The receptive function is largely centered over the parietal and temporal cortex (fig. 3-4) and is called *Wernicke's Area*. Two areas of the frontal cortex contribute to the expressive function. The main one, *Broca's Area*, is located just anterior to the temporal lobe (fig. 3-4). All of these areas are intimately connected to each other by nerve fibers. Higher mental and emotional processes, such as memory and learning, require many interconnections between areas of cortex within a single hemisphere, or between the two hemispheres. The term *association areas* is given to the regions where interconnections occur.

Cerebellum

The oval-shaped cerebellum is located under the occipital lobe and posterior to the brain stem (fig. 3-4). Like the four lobes of the cerebrum, the cerebellum has an outer cortex of gray matter with numerous sulci and gyri. It also has right and left hemispheres and a central section. Almost all information to and from the cerebellum is transmitted by way of the midbrain of the brain stem. The cerebellum has three main functions:

1. Maintenance of equilibrium and balance of the trunk. Afferent input comes from the vestibular

portion of the eighth cranial nerve. Efferent messages leave the cerebellum and connect with the reticular formation of the brain stem concerned with vestibular function (equilibrium).

2. Regulation of muscle tension, spinal nerve reflexes, and posture and balance of the limbs. Afferent information arrives from muscles and tendons of the limbs. Efferent messages synapse in the brain stem to influence the extrapyramidal system to effect fine motor control.

3. Regulation of the coordination of fine limb movements originally initiated by the frontal lobe. Afferent information comes from the cerebral cortex via the pons of the brain stem. Efferent information goes back to the cerebral cortex via the thalamus for fine motor control.

Brain Stem

The brain stem is interposed between the cerebrum and the spinal cord. It contains the *midbrain* (cerebral peduncles), the *pons,* and the *medulla oblongata* (fig. 3-6). Of these three, the medulla is perhaps the most important. Vital centers for cardiac function, respiratory function, and control of the diameter of

TABLE 3-1
CRANIAL NERVES AND THEIR FUNCTIONS

Nerve Number	Name	Function
I	Olfactory[1]	Sense of smell
II	Optic[2]	Sense of vision
III	Oculomotor	Movement of eye up, down, and in toward the nose; constriction of the pupil
IV	Trochlear	Movement of eye down and out
V	Trigeminal	Muscles of mastication; sensation of skin of face, teeth, and lining of mouth and nose
VI	Abducens	Movement of eye outward
VII	Facial	Muscles of facial expression; taste to the anterior 2/3 of tongue; salivary glands secretion
VIII	Vestibulocochlear (acoustic) (a) Vestibular portion (b) Cochlear portion	Equilibrium and balance Sense of hearing
IX	Glossopharyngeal	Swallowing and speech sounds; taste to the posterior 1/3 of tongue
X	Vagus	Swallowing and speech sounds; heart rate; gastrointestinal movement
XI	Spinal accessory	Neck muscles (trapezius and sternocleidomastoid)
XII	Hypoglossal	Tongue movement; speech; swallowing movement

[1]From frontal lobe
[2]From occipital lobe

small arteries, and hence blood pressure, are located in the medulla. Reflexes controlling heart rate and breathing rate are centered here, as well as reflexes involved with vomiting, coughing, sneezing, and swallowing. The pons also participates in control of respiration and, together with the midbrain, is a reflex center for eye pupil reflexes and other eye movements.

Also scattered throughout the brain stem are cell masses termed the *recticular formation,* which is associated with initiating and maintaining wakefulness and alertness generally. Further, nerve fiber tracts to and from the cerebrum and spinal cord must pass through the brain stem.

All the functions of the brain stem are intimately associated with cranial nerves III–XII. The cell nuclei for these nerves are located in the brain stem (fig. 3-7). Unlike the cerebrum, where the left hemisphere controls right body movements and the right hemisphere controls left body movements, the cranial nerves on the left control the left side, and those on the right control the right side. Table 3-1 lists the 12 cranial nerves and their functions.

Blood Supply to the CNS

The blood supply to the brain is derived from the

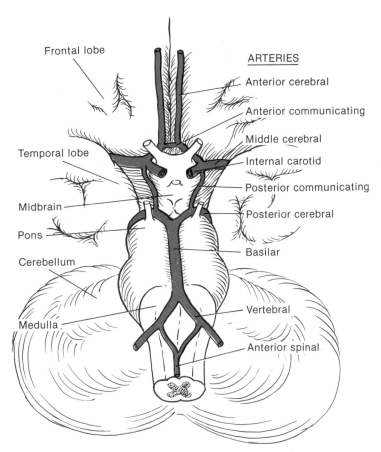

Frontal lobe

ARTERIES

Anterior cerebral

Anterior communicating

Middle cerebral

Internal carotid

Posterior communicating

Temporal lobe

Posterior cerebral

Midbrain

Pons

Basilar

Cerebellum

Vertebral

Medulla

Anterior spinal

FIGURE 3-8. Underside view of the brain demonstrating the basilar arterial system, the carotid arterial system, and the interconnections through the Circle of Willis. Note the take-off of the main branches, namely the anterior, middle, and posterior cerebral arteries. The anterior spinal artery branches off the vertebral artery to carry blood down into the spinal cord.

two *internal carotid arteries* and the two *vertebral arteries* (see fig. 3-26, p. 41). The two vertebral arteries enter the CNS between the skull and the first cervical vertebra. They join to form the *basilar artery* which continues up toward the cerebral hemispheres in front of the brain stem (fig. 3-8). The two internal carotid arteries enter the skull through two holes at its base.

On the underside of the frontal and temporal lobes, the carotid and basilar systems connect together as the *Circle of Willis*. This interconnection (anastomosis) allows the two systems to share blood, an important function. From the Circle, and mostly from the carotid system,. arise the anterior and middle *cerebral arteries*. The posterior cerebral artery is derived mostly from the basilar system.

Figure 3-9 demonstrates that the middle cerebral artery is the most important because it supplies the cortex of all four lobes. In particular, it supplies the precentral and postcentral gyri, the most important areas for movement and sensation in the frontal and parietal lobes, and also the cortex areas associated with language and vision. Figure 3-9 also shows that the

anterior cerebral artery supplies the inner surface of the frontal and parietal lobes, and the posterior cerebral artery supplies part of the temporal and occipital lobes. The blood supply to the brain stem and the cerebellum comes mostly from branches of the basilar system.

The blood supply to the spinal cord comes from the vertebral arteries which connect to form the *anterior spinal artery* (fig. 3-8), as well as from branches off the aorta at the level of the chest and abdomen.

Spinal Cord

Afferent information from the trunk and the extremities enters the CNS through the spinal peripheral nerves at various levels of the spinal cord. To reach the cerebrum, cerebellum, and brain stem, impulses travel up the spinal cord in fairly distinct tracts of nerve fibers. Similarly, to effect trunk and extremity movement, efferent impulses from the cerebrum, cerebellum, and brain stem also travel in distinct tracts within the spinal cord.

Well-defined areas of gray matter are also contained within the spinal cord where synapses occur for transmission of these afferent and efferent impulses. Anterior projections of the gray matter, termed ventral or *anterior horns,* are the location of the final synapse for efferent impulses leaving the spinal cord. The posterior projections, termed dorsal or *posterior horns,* are the location of many initial synapses for afferent information entering the spinal cord.

Figure 3-10 shows a cross-section of the spinal cord at a typical level, demonstrating the organization of anterior and posterior horns and three main tracts—the *spinothalamic tract,* which carries pain and temperature impulses to the thalamus for synaptic relay to the postcentral gyrus of the parietal lobe; the *posterior columns,* which carry position sense and pressure sense impulses to the thalamus, also for relay to the parietal lobe; and the *corticospinal* or pyramidal *tract,* which carries impulses from the precentral gyrus through the internal capsule (see fig. 3-5) of the frontal lobe to initiate muscle activity. These upper motor neurons synapse in the anterior horns with cells of the *lower motor neurons* whose axons leave the spinal cord via the spinal nerves.

PERIPHERAL NERVOUS SYSTEM

Somatic Nervous System

At the spinal level, the peripheral nervous system begins with the spinal nerves. Corresponding to each of the vertebrae there is a pair of spinal nerves, one for each side. A total of 30 pairs exist (8 cervical, 12 thoracic, 5 lumbar, and 5 sacral). Each nerve has two roots, the anterior, or ventral, motor root, and the

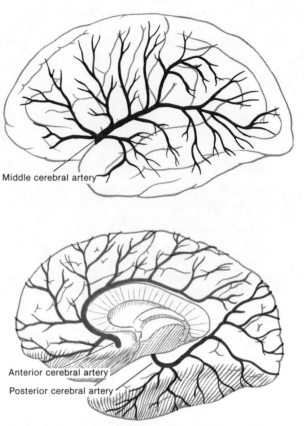

FIGURE 3-9. Distribution of anterior, middle, and posterior cerebral arteries. *(A)* Lateral (outer) aspect of left cerebral hemisphere showing middle cerebral artery serving frontal, parietal, temporal, and occipital lobes. *(B)* Medial (inner) aspect showing anterior cerebral artery serving frontal and parietal lobes, and posterior cerebral artery serving occipital and temporal lobes.

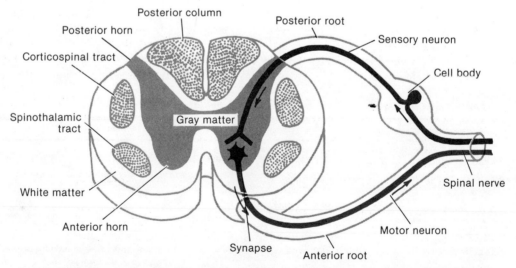

FIGURE 3-10. Cross-section of spinal cord showing the anterior and posterior horns of gray matter and three tracts: the corticospinal, spinothalamic, and posterior columns within the white matter. The afferent (sensory) and efferent (motor) neurons of a monosynaptic reflex arc and the single synapse can be seen. Arrows show direction of impulse.

posterior, or dorsal, sensory root. The anterior root contains the axons of the cell bodies in the anterior horn within the spinal cord. The posterior root has its cell bodies outside, but close to, the spinal cord in the sensory nerve ganglion. The posterior root, therefore, actually has two axons (fig. 3-10).

Each spinal nerve is numbered to correspond to the number of the vertebra near which it exits from the vertebral canal. The vertebral canal, however, is longer than the spinal cord itself. Since there are essentially the same number of spinal nerve pairs as there are vertebrae (except for the cervical segments where there are eight nerves and only seven vertebrae), some of the spinal nerves, particularly at the lower levels, have to travel down a significant distance before actually leaving the vertebral canal. In particular, beginning with the L2 vertebral level and extending downward to the S5 vertebral level, spinal nerves have to travel an increasing distance within the vertebral canal below the end of the spinal cord before they exit. From the L2 vertebral level downward, therefore, up to eight pairs of spinal nerves occupy the space within the vertebral canal. This nerve complex is referred to as the *cauda equina* (horse's tail).

All the cervical spinal nerves control movement of the shoulder and arm muscles, and receive all the sensory input from the skin, muscles, bones, and joints of the upper extremities where special receptors exist. After leaving the vertebral canal, they combine in a special way. Out of this merger, new peripheral nerves are formed, each of which may contain axons that originated from cell bodies at more than one spinal level. The merger of the cervical nerves in the neck region is called the *brachial plexus*. Table 3-2 lists the functions of the main peripheral nerves of the brachial plexus.

The thoracic spinal nerves do not recombine into plexuses. The anterior roots of the thoracic spinal nerves control the muscles of the abdomen and the back, and the posterior roots receive sensory informa-

tion from the abdominal organs, and the skin, muscles, and joints of the chest, abdomen, and upper back.

The lumbar and sacral nerves, like the cervical nerves, also combine after leaving the vertebral canal. This merger, which occurs mostly in the pelvis, is called the *lumbosacral plexus*. The lumbosacral plexus governs movement of, and receives sensory information from, the lower extremities, bladder, and anal sphincter. Table 3-3 lists the functions of the main peripheral nerves of the lumbosacral plexus.

A reflex is an automatic involuntary action of a part of the body in response to a particular stimulus. Reflexes serve a very important protective function for the body (e.g., the immediate withdrawal of a hand from a hot surface is a reflex action). A reflex has an afferent component, a nerve carrying the information of the stimulus toward the CNS, and an efferent component, a nerve carrying the impulses away from the CNS to effect the action. If only a single synapse exists between the afferent and efferent nerve, the reflex is termed a *monosynaptic reflex* (fig. 3-10). If several nerves, and hence synapses, are interposed between the afferent and efferent nerve, the reflex is termed a *polysynaptic reflex* (fig. 3-11).

Reflexes are not dependent for their existence on the cerebrum, cerebellum, or brain stem. However, nerve impulses from these centers exert a controlling influence.

The simplest spinal reflex is the tendon (stretch) reflex, a monosynaptic reflex. When the tendon is tapped, a sensory receptor in the muscle is excited and an afferent impulse travels in a sensory nerve to the spinal cord, where it enters through the posterior root. The sensory nerve axon synapses with an anterior horn cell at the same level in the spinal cord as it entered. The anterior horn cell axon carries the impulse through the anterior root of the spinal nerve and travels to the muscle whose tendon was tapped, causing the muscle to contract. A simple reflex, therefore, has an *afferent limb* (the fiber conducting the

TABLE 3-2
MAIN ACTION AND SENSATION FUNCTION OF BRACHIAL PLEXUS NERVES

Peripheral Nerve	Action	Skin Sensation
Axillary	Flex and abduct shoulder	Shoulder
Musculocutaneous	Flex elbow	Front of forearm
Radial	Extend elbow, wrist, and fingers	Back of hand and forearm
Median	Flex wrist and fingers	Palm and thumb, index and middle fingers
Ulnar	Dexterity of fingers	Palm and little finger

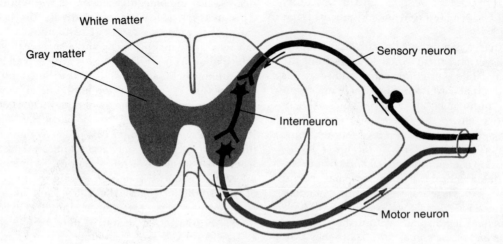

FIGURE 3-11. Cross-section of spinal cord showing example of a polysynaptic reflex. The impulse in the afferent sensory neuron synapses with a second neuron (interneuron), wholly contained within the gray matter, which then subsequently synapses with the efferent motor neuron to deliver the action response to the muscle in the periphery (compare with fig. 3-10). More than one interneuron may exist in a polysynaptic reflex. Such interneurons can also transmit an impulse up or down several levels in the spinal cord.

tendon - tap impulse), a single synapse within the spinal cord, and an *efferent limb* (the axon conducting the impulse to the muscle to produce contraction; fig. 3-10).

Reflexes also exist which govern the action of the various body organs. The dominant influence of the higher centers is to inhibit reflexes from being too active. Thus, if the spinal cord is anatomically separated from the higher centers, reflexes below the level of the separation will be hyperactive.

Autonomic Nervous System

The autonomic nervous system, while intimately connected to the brain and spinal cord, is basically a peripheral nervous system. It is fundamentally a system not under voluntary control, and it functions to regulate the activities of structures such as the stomach and intestines, the heart, the smooth muscle around arteries, the sweat glands, the salivary glands, and the bladder. The autonomic nervous system consists of two subsystems, the *sympathetic* and the *parasympathetic*. As table 3-4 indicates, the two systems are usually antagonistic.

Sympathetic nerve fibers leave the spinal cord through the anterior roots of all the thoracic spinal nerves and the first three lumbar spinal nerves. After

TABLE 3-3
MAIN ACTION AND SENSATION FUNCTION
OF LUMBOSACRAL PLEXUS NERVES

Peripheral Nerve	Action	Skin Sensation
Femoral	Extend knee	Front of thigh, and inside of leg
Sciatic	Flex knee	·············
Tibial	Flex ankle and toes	Sole of foot
Peroneal	Extend ankle and toes	Outside of leg and instep of foot
Pudendal	Anal and urethral sphincters and erection	Skin around genitals and anus

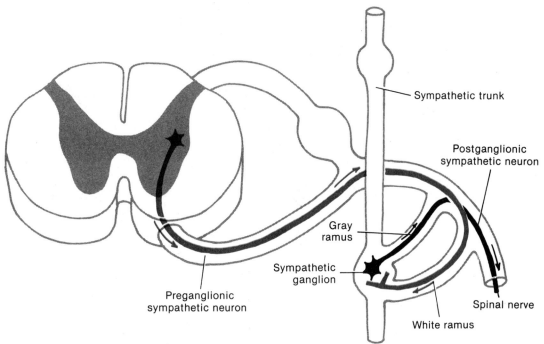

FIGURE 3-12. Cross-section of spinal cord with demonstration of the preganglionic and post-ganglionic neurons of the sympathetic nervous system. Note the synapse in the sympathetic ganglion and the postsynaptic neuron carrying the impulse back into the spinal nerve for distribution to the extremities. Postganglionic sympathetic neurons may also go directly to internal organs. A preganglionic sympathetic neuron may bypass its "own" ganglion and not synapse until reaching ganglia at other levels.

exiting from the vertebral canal, these nerve fibers branch off the spinal nerves to join a chain of ganglia that lies on either side of the vertebral column where they have their first synapse. The second sympathetic fiber (*postganglionic*) then returns to the spinal nerve to be distributed with it throughout the extremities. The

second sympathetic fiber can also proceed directly to blood vessels and to the various organs rather than returning to the spinal nerve (fig. 3-12).

The parasympathetic nervous system has basically two parts: the cranial part, which leaves the central nervous system with cranial nerves III, VII, IX, and

TABLE 3-4
FUNCTIONS OF AUTONOMIC NERVOUS SYSTEM
ON VARIOUS ORGANS

Organ	Sympathetic	Parasympathetic
Heart	Increase rate	Decrease rate
Bronchi of lungs	Dilate walls	Constrict walls
Digestive tract		
Sphincters	Increase tone	Relax tone
Peristalsis	Decrease movement	Increase movement
Sweat glands	Increase sweating	Decrease sweating
Eye	Dilate pupil	Constrict pupil
Arteries of heart	Dilate walls	Constrict walls
Peripheral arteries	Constrict walls	....
Bladder	....	Contract wall

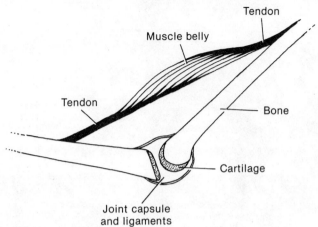

FIGURE 3-13. Schematic representation of a typical arrangement of the tissues of the musculoskeletal system.

X, and the sacral part, which leaves the spinal cord with sacral spinal nerves 2, 3, and 4. Perhaps the most important of the parasympathetic cranial nerves is the tenth, the vagus nerve, which, when activated, slows the heart rate and speeds up gastrointestinal activity. The sacral parasympathetic nerves are important for the innervation of the bladder wall muscle and for sexual function, such as erection in the male. Both the sympathetic and parasympathetic nervous systems can be influenced by hormones and the emotions.

MUSCULOSKELETAL SYSTEM

The musculoskeletal system consists of the skeletal system (bones and joints) and the skeletal muscle system (voluntary or striated muscles). These two systems are interdependent, working together to support and move the body. The functions of the musculoskeletal system are:

1. To provide a rigid support framework for the body
2. To protect vital internal body organs
3. To manufacture blood cells (the hematopoetic function)
4. To store minerals such as calcium and phosphorus
5. To provide a series of lever arms on which muscles act across joints to produce force and resulting body movement.

An understanding of the musculoskeletal system is particularly relevant to chapters 5, 8, 11, 13, 14, 15, and 26.

TISSUES

The musculoskeletal system is composed of various forms of connective tissue: cartilage, ligament, tendon, bone, and muscle. Each of these is composed of the following four basic components of connective tissue:

1. The *fibroblast* is the principal cell. It produces the building blocks that develop into the other components.
2. *Collagen* is the principal protein manufactured by the fibroblast. It forms long, thin fibrils which intertwine into fibers that have great strength and are difficult to stretch. Fibers can be organized into various configurations.
3. *Elastic fibers,* unlike collagen, are highly elastic and can be easily stretched. They are particularly abundant in the walls of the arteries.
4. *Proteoglycans* are sometimes referred to as the "ground substance." They make up the matrix, a nonliving, extracellular substance, in which fibroblasts, collagen fibers, and elastic fibers are embedded. Proteoglycans consist of complex sugars and proteins.

Depending on how these four components are combined and arranged in specific ways, cartilage, ligament, tendon, bone, muscle, or loose connective tissue is formed. Figure 3-13 shows all of these structures in their usual arrangement.

Cartilage

Cartilage has a high content of proteoglycans combined with water which gives it a gel-like consistency. It has essentially no blood supply and receives its nourishment by diffusion from nearby capillaries.

There are three types of cartilage: fibrocartilage, elastic cartilage, and hyaline cartilage. Fibrocartilage has a large concentration of collagen fibers and is dominant in intervertebral discs. Elastic cartilage has a large concentration of elastic fibers and is found in the external ear and epiglottis.

Hyaline cartilage, dominated mostly by water and proteoglycans, is the most important cartilage. It serves three main functions: (a) it forms the "original"

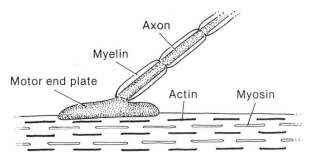

FIGURE 3-14. Very schematic representation of the terminal branch of a motor neuron attaching to a muscle fiber via the motor end plate. When the nerve's electrical impulse reaches the motor end plate, acetylcholine is released. The impulse then travels in both directions along the fiber. During contraction, the strands of actin and myosin slide past each other, thus shortening the fiber.

skeleton in the embryo, from which bone later develops; (b) it is responsible for the growth of long bones; and (c) it lines the opposing surfaces of the most important joints in the body, the synovial joints. These opposing surfaces have a protective layer of collagen fibers.

Ligaments

Ligaments are composed largely of collagen fibers and some elastic fibers arranged in a somewhat irregular pattern. They attach bone to bone, strengthen and stabilize joints, and determine the motions allowed. The ligaments are usually reinforced parts of the joint capsule, which is also a connective tissue structure.

Tendons

Tendons are also composed largely of collagen fibers, but have fewer elastic fibers than ligaments. The fibers are arranged in thick, parallel, closely packed bundles to form tough cords. They attach the contracting part of muscles to bone.

Muscles

The contracting unit of skeletal muscle, the *muscle fiber*, is a long, narrow, specialized cell with many nuclei. The many muscle fibers that make up a muscle are attached to tendons at each end. The force that develops in a muscle transmits to bone via the tendon to produce movement. Within a muscle fiber are two main proteins, *actin* and *myosin*. These proteins are long narrow strands oriented in the direction of the fiber. Where they overlap, the fiber appears dark. Where they do not overlap, the fiber appears light. These dark and light bands alternate and give the fiber, and the whole muscle, a striped or striated appearance under

the microscope.

When a muscle contracts, the actin and myosin strands slide past each other and shorten the fiber. The trigger to start this contraction comes from the motor nerve attached to each muscle fiber. The attachment occurs at the *motor end plate*. Acetylcholine is released at the motor end plate when the electrical impulse travelling in the motor nerve reaches the muscle fiber (fig.3-14). One nerve fiber branches at its end and connects with many muscle fibers. A single anterior horn cell, its axon, the terminal branches of the axon, and all the muscle fibers attached to these branches constitute a *motor unit*.

Bone

Bone is a very specialized form of connective tissue. It derives its hardness from the production and deposition of calcium crystals on the collagen fiber framework. The special cells responsible for this process, while similar to fibroblasts, are called *osteoblasts*. Bone is not a static structure. There is a dynamic balance between calcium in the bone and calcium in the blood. Constantly, new bone is produced and old bone is removed. In osteoporosis, the balance is disrupted, the removal of bone exceeds its production, and the bone becomes thin, less hard, and more easily fractured. The intestines, vitamin D, the kidney, the parathyroid gland, and sex and adrenal hormones also have important roles in this bone balance.

Bones are of two main types, flat bones (e.g., the skull), and the long bones of the extremities. Figures 3-15 and 3-16 illustrate the structure of long bone. The strength of the long bones comes from the compact cortical bone of the outer layer. The bone of the inner medullary cavity is spongy rather than compact.

The red marrow, where blood components are produced, exists within the medullary cavity of all

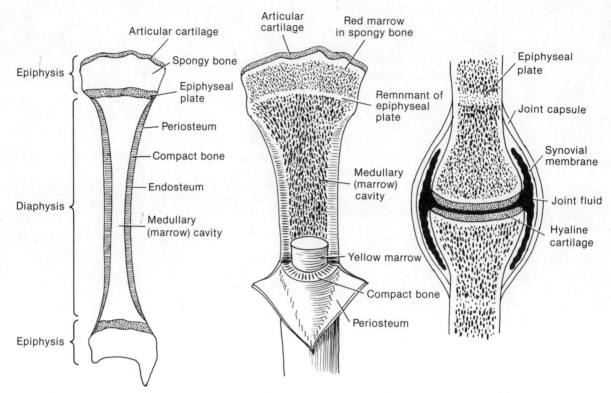

FIGURE 3-15. Longitudinal section of a long bone showing its structure. The cartilaginous epiphyseal plate is the site of long bone growth.

FIGURE 3-16. Cutaway section of an adult long bone showing the medullary cavity containing yellow marrow. In this section, only a residual line remains of the epiphyseal plate.

FIGURE 3-17. A typical synovial joint.

bones in the newborn child. During growth, the red marrow in most bone changes to yellow marrow, which is fatty and does not produce blood components. Blood-producing red marrow remains, in the adult, in the vertebrae, ribs, sternum, skull, femur, and humerus.

Each end of a long bone is called an *epiphysis*, and the *diaphysis* is the long shaft between them. At the junction of the epiphysis and the diaphysis at each end lies the *epiphyseal plate* of hyaline cartilage which is the site of long bone growth (figs. 3-15 and 3-17). The hyaline cartilage converts to bone at the diaphysial side of the plate, and reproduces itself at the epiphyseal side of the plate. Thus, the shaft gets longer. Long bone growth ceases when the hyaline cartilage stops reproducing itself and fully converts to bone.

Periosteum, a tough connective tissue with cells capable of producing compact bone, overlies the entire shaft. Flat bones are formed from periosteum alone.

Loose Connective Tissue

Loose connective tissue is a network of very loosely arranged fibroblasts, collagen, and elastic fibers in "ground substance." It lies between muscles that slide on each other, and between bone and muscle. In areas where there is much movement, such as at the shoulder and hip, identifiable spaces, or bursae, surrounded by loose connective tissue exist.

JOINTS

A joint, or articulation, is a union of usually two, but sometimes more, bones. Joints are classified into three groups according to the method of union.

Immovable (*fibrous*) joints, such as those between skull bones, unite bones by rough collagenous connective tissue. Slightly movable (*cartilagenous*) joints, such as the intervertebral disc, unite bones by cartilage. Freely movable (*synovial*) joints, such as the joints of the extremities, unite bones in a complex and specialized manner.

Figure 3-17 illustrates a typical synovial joint and its four constant features:

1. The *joint capsule* fully surrounds the joint. It is composed of connective tissue reinforced by ligaments. The capsule extends from the cortex and periosteum in the region of the epiphyseal plates of the two opposing bones.
2. The *synovial membrane*, a continuous sheet of loose connective tissue, lines the inside of the capsule, and has a thin layer of specialized synovial cells on

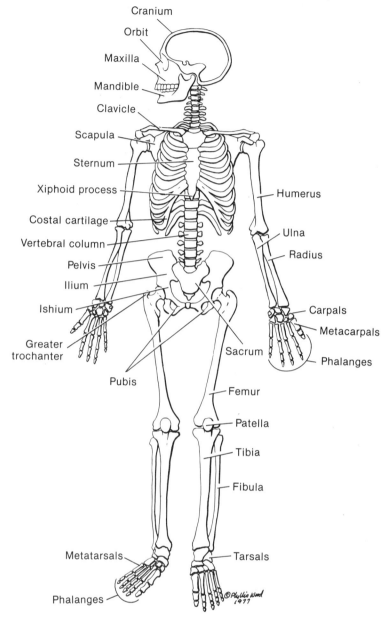

FIGURE 3-18. Anterior view of the skeleton with major bones labelled.

its surface. The synovial membrane covers all structures within the capsule except the articular cartilage.

3. The hyaline *articular cartilage* surfaces at the ends of each of the bones that make up the joint are in constant contact during movement. The cartilage receives its nourishment directly from the synovial fluid within the joint cavity. The joint cavity, therefore, has as its borders the hyaline cartilages and the synovial membrane.

4. The viscous *synovial fluid* is produced by the synovial membrane. It provides a high level of lubrication for the opposing hyaline cartilage surfaces and for the synovial membrane itself during joint movement. In the normal joint, very little fluid (less than 5 cc) exists in the cavity. The major component of synovial fluid is hyaluronic acid, a proteoglycan.

SKELETAL SYSTEM

The 206 bones of the skeleton (fig. 3-18) are divided into two subgroups, axial and appendicular. The axial skeleton, namely the head and trunk, includes the skull, the lower jaw (*mandible*), the breastbone (*sternum*), the 12 ribs, the 24 vertebrae of the vertebral

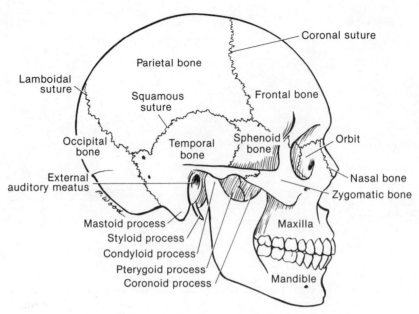

FIGURE 3-19. Major bones of the skull and facial skeleton. The sutures are immovable nonsynovial joints.

column, and the 5 fused vertebrae of the sacrum. The appendicular skeleton consists of the bones of the upper and lower extremities.

Axial Skeleton

Skull. The skulls has two parts, the bones of the cranium, which enclose and protect the brain, and the facial skeleton (fig. 3-19). The upper teeth are embedded in the maxilla and the lower teeth are embedded in the mandible. The mandible is the only freely movable bone of the skull.

Thorax. The thoracic cage consists of the sternum anteriorly, the 12 thoracic vertebrae posteriorly, and the 12 pairs of ribs, which are connected posteriorly to the thoracic vertebrae. Anteriorly, 10 ribs are connected to the sternum by cartilage and two ribs are "floating." The thoracic cage protects the lungs and the heart.

Vertebral column. The vertebral column transmits body weight from the head, thorax, and abdomen to the lower extremities and encloses and protects the delicate spinal cord. There are 7 cervical vertebrae, 12 thoracic vertebrae, 5 lumbar vertebrae, 5 sacral vertebrae, and 4 small vertebrae of the vestigial coccyx. Each vertebra has essentially the same basic components, although some special differences exist based on location and allowed movements.

Figure 3-20 shows a top view of a typical vertebra. The *vertebral body* anteriorly and the *neural arch* posteriorly encircle the *vertebral foramen*. Stacked one on top of the other, the vertebral foramina form the

vertebral canal wherein the spinal cord is contained. The neural arch is made up of the *pedicles*, the *neural arch joints*, and the *laminae*.

Figure 3-21 shows a side view of two typical vertebrae, including the intervertebral disc and the spinal cord in the vertebral canal. The anterior stacked bodies of the vertebrae form the primary weight-bearing structure of the vertebral column.

The strength of the attachments between vertebrae is achieved by several structures: (a) a long *anterior longitudinal ligament* in front of bodies and discs; (b) the disc itself; (c) a long *posterior longitudinal ligament* immediately behind bodies and discs; (d) the interlocking hyaline cartilage surfaces of the neural arch joints; and (e) the ligaments attaching spinous and transverse processes. Spinal nerves leave the vertebral canal through the intervertebral foramina between the vertebrae.

The *intervertebral discs* provide a shock-absorbing function. The disc consists of a ring of tough fibrocartilage, the *annulus fibrosis,* surrounding a central gel matrix, the *nucleus pulposus.* The nucleus pulposus gives the disc its resilience, flexibility, and shock-absorbing characteristics.

The vertebral column in the normal standing posture adopts specific curvatures (see fig. 15-3, p. 207). The orientation of the neural arch joints allows: (a) the cervical spine to rotate, flex forward, flex sideways, and extend backward; (b) the thoracic spine to rotate only; and (c) the lumbar spine to flex forward, flex sideways, and extend backward.

Sacrum. The sacrum has a dual character. It is at

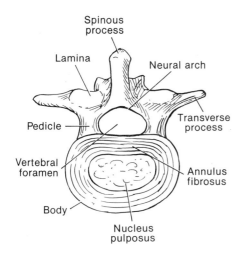

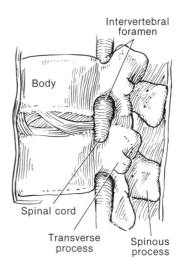

FIGURE 3-20. Top view of a typical vertebra. The vertebral foramen containing the spinal cord is bordered by the vertebral body in front, pedicles on the side, and laminae behind.

FIGURE 3-21. Side view of two typical vertebrae. They are joined in front by the intervertebral disc and in back by synovial joints (under articular capsule). Their connection is reinforced by anterior and posterior longitudinal ligaments and interspinous ligaments. A spinal nerve root exits from the vertebral canal through the intervertebral foramen.

the same time part of the vertebral column and part of the pelvis. It therefore transmits the upper body weight to the lower extremities.

Appendicular Skeleton

Upper extremity. The arms are ultimately attached to the thorax via the collarbone (*clavicle*) and shoulder bone (*scapula*). The upper arm bone (*humerus*) is united to the scapula at the shoulder joint. The scapula is attached to the thoracic cage only by muscles. The end of the clavicle close to the shoulder unites with the scapula at a synovial joint. The ultimate joint attachment of the extremity to the thorax is achieved as the other end of the clavicle connects to the sternum at the base of the neck. The elbow joint unites the humerus with the two forearm bones (*radius* and *ulna*). Three sets of joints connect the radius and ulna to the bones of the palm (*metacarpals*) via the eight small *carpal* bones of the wrist. Further, the knuckles (*metacarpophalangeal,* or MCP, joints) connect the metacarpals to the proximal *phalanx* of the fingers. Each finger has three phalanges, proximal, middle, and distal, except the thumb, which has two.

Lower extremity. The pelvis *(innominate bone)* transmits the upper body weight from the sacrum to the legs. It begins as three hipbones (*ilium, ischium,* and *pubis*) which fuse together when growth is completed. The sacrum connection is the *sacroiliac joint.* The hip joint unites the pelvic bone to the thigh bone (*femur*); the knee joint, which also includes the knee cap (*patella*), unites the femur to the two bones of the lower leg (*tibia* and *fibula*). The ankle joint unites the tibia

and fibula to the *talus.* The body weight is then transmitted to the heel (*calcaneous*), and to the balls of the feet via the other foot bones (*tarsal* and *metatarsal*). The toes have a phalangeal structure like the fingers.

SKELETAL MUSCLE SYSTEM

The two ends of a muscle are attached to different bones. All muscles, therefore, cross at least one synovial joint. Thus, when a muscle shortens, one bone is moved in relation to the other and the axis of movement is at the joint connecting the two bones. The muscle end attached to the bone closest to the body or closest to the head (proximal attachment) is usually called the *origin* of the muscle. When a muscle shortens, the origin is usually stationary. The distal attachment at the other end of the muscle is called the *insertion.* When a muscle shortens, the insertion moves.

Each muscle has its own special name. They are, however, also described by their functions. Muscles or groups of muscles which bend a limb are *flexors,* and those which straighten the limb are called *extensors* (e.g., elbow flexors, elbow extensors). Muscles which move a limb to the side away from the midline of the body are called *abductors,* and muscles which move a limb toward the midline are called *adductors* (e.g., hip abductors, hip adductors). Other functional groups are *elevators, depressors, rotators, doriflexors, plantar flexors,* and *palmar flexors* (see glossary).

Table 5-1 (p. 67) lists the major muscles and their functions, together with the spinal nerves that control the muscles. Tables 3-2 and 3-3 (p. 27, 28) list the major movements of the upper and lower extremities,

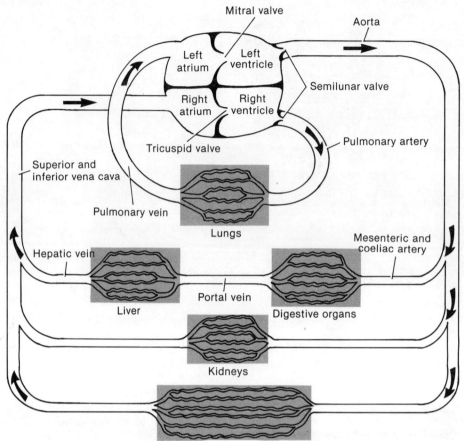

FIGURE 3-22. Schematic representation of pulmonary and systemic circulatory systems. Arrows indicate direction of blood flow. Oxygen from the lungs enters the system via the pulmonary vein. Carbon dioxide is delivered to the lungs for removal by the pulmonary artery. Food products enter the system from the digestive organs into the portal vein. Waste products are removed by the liver and kidney.

together with the peripheral nerves serving the functions.

CARDIOVASCULAR SYSTEM

The cardiovascular system distributes food, oxygen, and hormones to all the living cells and carries waste products and carbon dioxide away from the cells. The vehicle for this distribution is the blood which travels in channels, the blood vessels. The driving force for moving the blood is provided by the pumping action of the heart.

There are actually two circulations and in effect two "hearts." The *pulmonary circulation*, driven by the "right heart," delivers blood containing carbon dioxide to the lungs. The *systemic circulation*, driven by the "left heart," delivers blood containing oxygen, food, and hormones to the rest of the body.

The blood vessels leading from the heart are arteries

and the blood vessels returning blood to the heart are veins. The veins of the systemic circulation return blood carrying carbon dioxide to the right heart. This oxygen-deficient blood is then pumped to the lungs in the pulmonary circulation where the carbon dioxide is removed and oxygen is replenished. This oxygen-rich blood returns to the left heart and is pumped in the systemic circulation throughout the body. Figure 3-22 is a full schematic of the two circulations.

An understanding of the cardiovascular system is particularly relevant to chapters 9, 10, 22, 24, and 27.

BLOOD

Adults have five to six liters of blood. Forty-five percent of the blood consists of red blood cells, white blood cells, and platelets. There are five types of white blood cells: neutrophils, basophils, eosinophils, lymphocytes, and monocytes. The neutrophils and

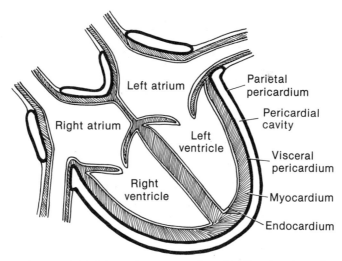

FIGURE 3-23. Schematic representation of the four chambers of the heart, the three layers of the heart wall, and the two layers of the pericardium.

lymphocytes are the most important of these five types. Some characteristics of the major cells are summarized in table 3-5.

Fifty-five percent of the blood is the *plasma*, a straw-colored solution of 90 percent water and 10 percent solutes. Protein constitutes 6–8 percent. The remaining solutes include the food substances (e.g., glucose and amino acids), waste products of metabolism (e.g., urea, creatinine), and regulatory substances, such as hormones and enzymes. Of the proteins, globulin is essential for immunity, and albumin and fibrinogen play key roles in blood clotting.

The red blood cell (erythrocyte) is filled with *hemoglobin*, a compound of protein and iron, and is the main carrier for the transport of oxygen. The erythrocyte has a life of 80–120 days.

HEART

Structure

The heart is about the size of a man's fist. Two-thirds of it lies to the left of the midline within the chest cavity between the lungs. The heart is enclosed by a double-layered loose sac, the *pericardium*. A small amount of fluid between the two layers lubricates the surfaces to allow the heart to change its shape without much friction as it pumps. The wall of the heart has three distinct layers: the outer thin membrane, the *epicardium*; the thick middle layer of cardiac muscle, the *myocardium*, which is responsible for the heart's ability to pump without stopping to rest; and the inner layer, the *endocardium* (fig. 3-23). The pumping action is achieved by contraction of the myocardium, a special form of muscle somewhat like skeletal muscle, but not under voluntary nervous control.

Chambers. The four chambers are the *right atrium, right ventricle, left atrium*, and *left ventricle* (fig. 3-23). Blood from the systemic circulation enters the right atrium through the inferior and superior *vena cava*. It passes through the *tricuspid valve* into the right ventricle. Right ventricular contraction propels the blood through the *pulmonary semilunar valve* into the *pulmonary artery* for pulmonary circulation.

TABLE 3-5
SOURCE, NUMBER, AND FUNCTION OF MAJOR BLOOD CELLS

Type	Number/mm³	Source	Function
Red blood cell	5 million	Bone marrow	Oxygen transport
Neutrophil	3,000–6,000	Bone marrow	Phagocytosis
Lymphocyte	1,500–3,000	Bone marrow spleen, lymph nodes	Production of antibodies
Platelet	250,000	Bone marrow	Blood clotting

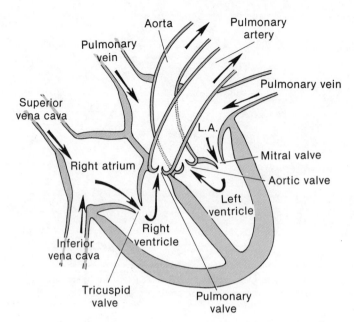

FIGURE 3-24. Schematic of the heart, showing direction of blood flow during a complete cardiac cycle. Note the location of the mitral, tricuspid, and semilunar valves.

Blood from the lungs enters the left atrium through the *pulmonary vein* and passes through the *mitral valve* into the left ventricle. Left ventricular contraction propels the blood through the *aortic semilunar valve* into the *aorta* for systemic circulation. All valves—tricuspid, mitral, and semilunar—can only pass blood in one direction in the normal situation.

The walls between the two ventricles and the two atria, the *interventricular septum* and the *interatrial septum*, block mixing of the two circulations in the normal condition.

Cardiac Cycle and Heart Sounds

Each cycle of the heart consists of two parts, *diastole* and *systole*. During diastole, all four chambers are relaxed and both atria receive and fill with blood. Systole begins first with right and left atrial contraction propelling blood through the tricuspid and mitral valves into the right and left ventricle respectively (fig. 3-24). Because a great deal of force is not needed for this, the myocardium of the atria is relatively thin. In contrast, the myocardium of the ventricles is thick. *Ventricular systole*, the main pumping action, forcefully propels blood into the pulmonary artery and aorta through the pulmonary and aortic semilunar valves. When this contraction occurs, the tricuspid and mitral valves slam shut to prevent the flow of blood back into the atria. The closure of the valves produces the first heart sound that can be heard with the stethoscope. This rush of blood out of the ventricles causes the pulse beat that can be felt at the wrist and other areas of the body where arteries are prominent. The rush of blood into the pulmonary artery and aorta distends the walls of these vessels. When ventricular contraction stops, the vessels recoil and the semilunar valves slam shut to prevent the flow of blood back into the ventricles. The closure of the semilunar valves produces the second heart sound.

Murmurs are sounds other than the two normal heart sounds which can sometimes be heard, and usually signify disease. Murmurs usually mean excessive blood turbulence caused by valve dysfunction, such as failure to open wide enough (stenosis) or failure to close completely (insufficiency).

Blood pressure recorded in the arm or leg consists of two numbers which refer to the *systolic pressure*, associated with ventricular systole, and the *diastolic pressure*, associated with diastole. Pressures are recorded in millimeters of mercury (mm Hg) and are usually recorded as a fraction—systolic pressure/diastolic pressure, e.g., 120/180. The magnitudes of the pressures are dependent not only on the force produced by the thick myocardium of the ventricles, but also by the resistance to flow produced by the progressively narrowing peripheral arterial blood vessels.

The *cardiac output* is the amount of blood pumped by the heart per minute. This is calculated by multiplying the volume ejected with each ventricular contraction (*stroke volume*) by the number of beats per minute (*heart rate*). Stroke volume varies from about 60–70cc, and heart rates can rise as high as 200. In a young individual at rest, the cardiac output is approximately five liters per minute.

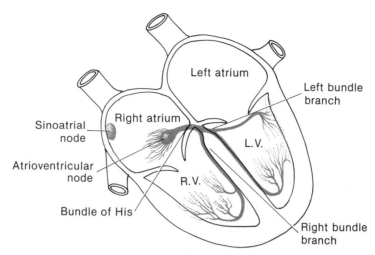

FIGURE 3-25. Schematic of the heart, showing the cardiac conducting system. The rhythm is paced by the sinoatrial node.

Cardiac Rhythm

Specialized muscle fibers within the myocardium provide the heart with an inherent capacity to contract rhythmically. Each cycle begins in a special bundle of myocardial cells (*sinoatrial node*, the "pacemaker") in the wall of the right atrium (fig. 3-25). These cells, without any stimulation, initiate electrical impulses at regular intervals. These impulses travel in the walls of the atria, causing atrial contraction, and rapidly reach the *atrioventricular node,* which also lies in the right atrial wall near the interatrial septum. Impulses delay here slightly until atrial systole is completed. From the atrioventricular node, impulses travel down two bundles of special muscle fibers (*bundle of His*) on the right and left side of the interventricular septum. The two bundles branch out as *Purkinje fibers* and spread over both ventricles, causing ventricular contraction. The electrocardiogram (ECG) records the travel time for these impulses, as well as the electrical events associated with atrial and ventricular contraction.

Pacemaker rates can be altered by the autonomic nervous system and certain hormones. Parasympathetic fibers from the vagus cranial nerve cause the sinoatrial node to slow down and sympathetic nerve fibers can cause the sinoatrial node to speed up. A number of chemicals and the hormones epinephrine and thryoid accelerate the heart rate.

VASCULAR SYSTEM

Arterial System

Major branches of the aorta distribute blood to the head, abdomen, and extremities (table 3-6). Arterial walls are composed of three layers: (a) the *intima*, a smooth thin layer of endothelial cells on which blood cannot adhere; (b) the *media*, a relatively thick middle layer comprised of smooth muscle and elastic connective tissue fibers which can distend and recoil during systole; and (c) the *adventitia*, the outer fibrous layer.

As these arteries further branch they become progressively thinner walled and smaller in diameter. The smallest divisions of the arteries are the *arterioles*, whose main component is smooth muscle. The diameter of arterioles can be altered even to the extent of closure by the sympathetic nervous system. The changes in the diameter of these vessels determine the quantity of blood delivered to capillaries. In addition, arterioles influence the blood pressure since, as their diameter changes, the resistance to blood flow changes.

The pulmonary artery and its distribution system is discussed on p. 43.

Of special importance are the right and left *coronary arteries* that supply the heart itself, in particular the myocardium (fig. 3-26). These vessels branch off the aorta as it leaves the heart. The right coronary artery serves mostly the right atrium, right ventricle, and the bottom of the left ventricle. The left coronary artery supplies the left atrium and the remainder of the left ventricle. There is, however, an interconnection (anastomosis) between the two coronary arteries, such that each vessel alone can deliver blood to the myocardium of all four chambers. Most of the blood flow in the coronary arteries occurs during diastole when the heart walls are relaxed and the aortic semilunar valves are closed.

Capillaries

The arteries lead into the microscopic capillaries which are multiply branched and lie in close approximation to the fluid bathing the living cells (*interstitial fluid*). Capillary walls are very thin, consisting only of intima, a thin lining of endothelial

TABLE 3-6
MAJOR BRANCHES OF SYSTEMIC CIRCULATION

	Name	Derived From	Serves
Head	Common carotid	Aortic arch	Brain & skull
Abdomen	Mesenteric	Descending aorta	Intestines
	Celiac	Descending aorta	Stomach, liver; spleen
	Renal	Descending aorta	Kidney
	Iliac	Descending aorta	Pelvis
Upper Extremity	Brachial (axillary)	Subclavian	Upper arm
	Radial & ulnar	Brachial	Forearm & hand
Lower Extremity	Femoral	Iliac	Thigh
	Popliteal	Femoral	Leg
	Dorsal pedis	Popliteal	Foot
	Posterior tibial	Popliteal	Foot

cells. This thin wall permits the passage of blood plasma containing dissolved nutrients and oxygen into the interstitial fluid in the vicinity of the cells, and permits the passage of waste products and carbon dioxide from the cells back into the blood stream. The outflow occurs at the arteriole end of the capillary and the inflow occurs at the venule end of the capillary. Only about 40 percent of the blood plasma that leaves the capillary at the arteriole end returns to the blood stream at the venule end. The remainder returns to the blood via the lymphatic system (see below).

Venous System

The capillaries lead into venules, which in turn unite to form veins that return blood to the heart. Veins are thin walled and the blood pressure in them is very low. Their walls have the same three layers as the arteries, but the media is much thinner. Veins from the legs, which return blood up to the heart against gravity, contain valves that function to keep the blood moving and to prevent pooling of blood and edema in the legs. The main collecting veins of any organ or part of the body are called by the same name as the main artery delivering the blood. The exceptions are the superior vena cava, which collects blood from the head and upper extremities, and the inferior vena cava, which collects blood from the rest of the body. These two vessels correspond to the aorta.

Portal System

The portal system (see fig. 3-22), while basically part of the venous system, has a unique function with regard to the liver, a most vital organ. The *portal vein* collects all the blood within the walls of the intestine. Nutrients derived from digestion diffuse into capillaries in the wall of the intestines and are therefore contained in the blood collected by the portal vein. The portal vein enters the liver and branches into venules and then into capillaries intimately associated with liver cells. In the liver, the capillaries recombine into venules and then into the *hepatic vein* which enters the inferior vena cava. This system allows the liver cells to immediately deal with the food products, performing three main functions:

1. Execution of a number of important steps in the utilization of proteins, fats, and carbohydrates
2. Storage of important substances, such as iron and various vitamins
3. Neutralization of potentially toxic products of digestion

Oxygen is delivered to the liver by the hepatic artery.

Lymphatic System

The lymphatic system is a special second pathway by which the individual cells of the body communicate with the blood. It begins as open-ended microscopic lymphatic capillaries in intimate contact with the interstitial fluid bathing all cells. The lymphatic capillaries collect interstitial fluid (*lymph*), including that part of the blood plasma that does not return to the blood capillaries and various proteins which cannot pass through the walls of blood capillaries. The lymphatic capillaries join to form lymphatic vessels of

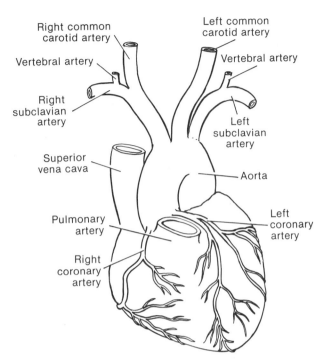

Right common
carotid artery

Left common
carotid artery

Vertebral artery

Vertebral artery

Right
subclavian
artery

Left
subclavian
artery

Superior
vena cava

Aorta

Pulmonary
artery

Left
coronary
artery

Right
coronary
artery

FIGURE 3-26. The two coronary arteries encircle the heart and supply blood to all portions of the myocardium. Each coronary artery can supply both atria and both ventricles, thus providing the heart with a safety factor in the event of disease in one of the coronary arteries. The vertebral and carotid arteries supply blood to the brain.

increasing diameter, and finally form two main vessels: (a) the *thoracic duct*, which enters the left subclavian vein after draining the interstitial fluid for most of the body; and (b) the *right lymphatic duct*, which enters into the right subclavian vein after draining the right arm and right upper trunk areas. Dispersed throughout the lymphatic system are *lymph nodes*, sometimes called glands, located in the neck (cervical nodes), in the floor of the mouth (submaxillary nodes), under the armpit (axillary nodes), and in the groin (inguinal nodes). The lymph nodes manufacture and contain lymphocytes (see table 3-5), which produce antibodies. Other cells in the lymph nodes filter out bacteria and other injurious particles, such as cancer cells.

The main forces moving lymph up toward the heart are contraction of skeletal muscles which squeeze the vessels, and the inspiration phase of respiration which provides a suction action. Further, backflow is impeded by valves in the lymphatic vessels.

PULMONARY SYSTEM

The function of the pulmonary system is to deliver oxygen to the blood and to remove carbon dioxide from the blood. Inspired air contains 21 percent oxygen and essentially no carbon dioxide, while expired air contains 16 percent oxygen and 4.5 percent carbon dioxide. Further, the temperature and water

vapor content (humidity) of inspired air is that of the immediate environment, while expired air is at body temperature and is saturated with water. Finally, inspired air may contain bacteria, dust particles, and other particulate matter, while expired air is generally free of such substances.

The actual exchange of oxygen and carbon dioxide occurs in the walls of the alveoli deep within the lungs. The nose and mouth, pharynx, larynx, trachea, right and left main bronchi and their branches, and the bronchioles distribute inspired air to the alveoli, establish appropriate air temperature and humidity, and control particulate matter. The lungs and part of the distribution system lie within the chest cavity.

Contraction of muscles in the wall of the chest cavity produces inspiration. Expiration occurs as these muscles relax. The rhythmicity of respiration is controlled by the respiratory centers in the upper part of the pons and in the medulla (see p. 23).

Dysfunction of the pulmonary system is discussed in chapter 23.

AIR DISTRIBUTION

On inspiration, air enters the nose through the nostrils (nares). Nasal hairs filter out bacteria and dust particles. As the air passes through the nose, it is warmed and humidified by the moist lining of the nose (nasal mucosa). The moist sticky mucus produced by the

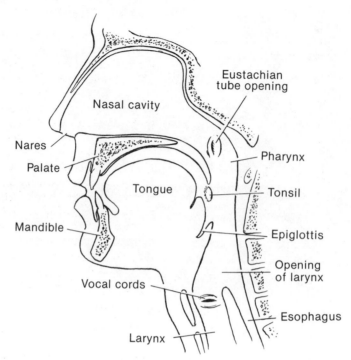

FIGURE 3-27. Section through the face and neck showing the air distribution system above the trachea: the nose, mouth, pharynx, and larynx.

mucosa also traps dust and bacteria. Less warming, humidification, and filtering occurs when air is inspired through the mouth.

Air inspired through the nose and mouth enter a common channel, the throat, or *pharynx*, a five-inch-long tube (fig. 3-27). Further warming and humidification occur as the air passes through the pharynx. The *tonsils* and *adenoids* lie within the pharynx, as does the opening of the *auditory* (*Eustachian*) *tube* which connects to the middle ear (see p. 52).

At the bottom of the pharynx, two openings exist, one into the *esophagus* for passage of food, and the other into the *larynx* for continued flow of inspired air. When food is swallowed, the opening of the larynx automatically closes. When air is inspired, it cannot enter the esophagus because its walls are collapsed. The larynx, which contains the vocal cords, is also lined with mucous membrane and has a fairly rigid wall composed of cartilage.

Inspired air continues through the larynx into the *trachea* ("windpipe"). The trachea begins in the neck and ends in the chest cavity where it branches into the right and left main *bronchi*. At this point, inspired air is considered to have entered the lungs. Multiple tree-like branches of the main bronchi subsequently distribute inspired air through the lung substance. The smallest branches are the *bronchioles*.

Rigidity of the trachea and bronchi is achieved by cartilagenous walls, which disappear at the bronchiole level. Bronchiole walls contain smooth muscle similar to that found in the walls of arterioles (see p. 39). The muscle is sufficient to collapse the bronchioles. Smooth muscle in the tracheobronchial tube may alter the diameter of the tubes, but collapse is prevented by the cartilage in the walls.

The mucosa of the trachea, bronchi, and most of the length of the bronchioles contain special cells with hairlike projections (*cilia*). The cilia "beat" rhythmically, driving mucus (which may contain bacteria and particles not previously filtered) toward the pharynx. By the time inspired air has reached the bronchioles, it is at body temperature, contains 100 percent humidity, and hopefully has been completely filtered.

The inspired air finally enters through *alveolar ducts* into *alveolar sacs*. The walls of each sac have many pockets, called *alveoli* (fig. 3-28). Some 200 million alveoli make up the bulk of the lung substance. It is in the walls of these alveoli that oxygen and carbon dioxide are exchanged with capillary blood. The total area in the walls of the alveoli in contact with the capillaries is about 753 square feet (70 m²). Nearly a liter of blood is in contact with these walls at any time.

THORAX

The thorax is enclosed by the sternum and ribs in front, ribs on the side and top, the vertebral column and ribs in back, and the diaphragm on the bottom. The diaphragm separates the chest cavity from the

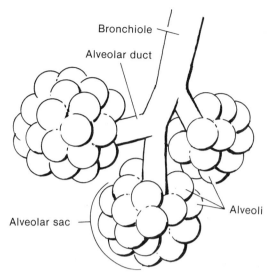

FIGURE 3-28. Schematic showing the structure of the alveolar ducts, alveolar sacs, and alveoli.

abdominal cavity and is pierced by the esophagus where it enters the abdominal cavity to connect with the stomach. The space between the ribs contains the intercostal muscles.

The thorax is firmly divided into the right and left chest cavities, which contain the right and left lungs. The left lung has two sections (the upper and lower lobes) and the right lung has three sections (the upper, middle, and lower lobes; fig. 3-29).

The septum that divides the two cavities is called the *mediastinum*. In addition to the trachea, esophagus, and various lymph nodes, the mediastinum includes the heart.

Pulmonary Circulation

As indicated on figure 3-22 (p. 36), oxygen-deficient blood carrying an excess of carbon dioxide returns to the heart through the superior and inferior vena cava. The right ventricle subsequently pumps blood through the main pulmonary artery (see fig. 3-24, p. 38), which immediately branches into the right and left pulmonary arteries to distribute this oxygen-deficient blood to the right and left lungs. Within the lung, multiple branching of the pulmonary artery occurs until the arteriole level is reached (see p. 39). The arterioles open into very small capillaries that run in the walls of the alveoli. After the gas exchange, the capillaries recombine into venules and veins. Ultimately two right pulmonary veins and two left pulmonary veins containing oxygen-rich blood enter the left atrium for distribution into the systemic circulation.

Gas Exchange

The thin walls of both the alveoli and the capillaries permit the passage of dissolved carbon dioxide and oxygen (fig. 3-30). The effective concentration of oxygen in the alveolus, and hence in the alveolar wall, is greater than the oxygen concentration in the capillary blood plasma. Oxygen therefore diffuses into the blood. The effective concentrations of carbon dioxide in the alveolar wall and the capillary blood plasma are reversed, and therefore carbon dioxide diffuses from the blood to the alveolus.

As oxygen diffuses into the plasma, the hemoglobin molecule in the red blood cell immediately takes up the

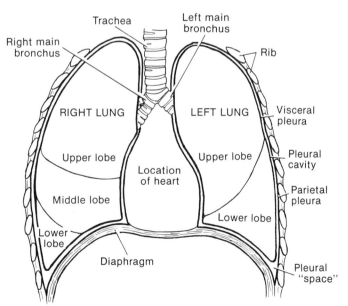

FIGURE 3-29. Main respiratory structures of the thorax: trachea, right and left main bronchi, and the lungs. Note the three lobes of the right lung and the two lobes of the left lung.

oxygen, permitting more to flow into the plasma. This unique oxygen-carrying capacity of hemoglobin within the red blood cell allows the blood to carry over 70 times more oxygen than it could carry if oxygen were simply dissolved in the plasma. Therefore, the total amount of oxygen that can be taken into the blood each minute depends mostly on: (a) the oxygen concentration difference between the alveolus and the blood; (b) the total healthy functioning surface of the alveoli; and (c) the rate of respiration.

Pleura

The right and left chest cavities are lined by a thin *pleural membrane* adherent to the ribs, intercoastal muscles, diaphragm, and mediastinum. The surface of this pleural membrane facing the lung (*parietal pleura*) is smooth and contains cells that secrete a thin layer of fluid.

A similar pleural membrane surrounds the lobes of each lung (*visceral pleura*). The outer surface of the visceral pleura facing the wall of the chest cavity also contains fluid-secreting cells. The smooth, glistening surfaces of the parietal and visceral pleurae minimize friction as the lungs expand and relax relative to the wall. Although these surfaces are usually in intimate contact, they present a potential space that can be filled under abnormal circumstances.

MECHANICS OF RESPIRATION

Inspiration

Stimuli from the respiratory center in the brain stem initiate impulses in the nerves that work the diaphragm (phrenic nerve) and the intercostal muscles (spinal nerves T2 through T12). The contraction of these muscles increases the volume of the thorax. An immediate decrease in pressure below atmospheric pressure occurs in the thorax outside the lungs. Since the pressure inside the bronchi is equal to atmospheric pressure, air rushes in as long as the nose and/or mouth are open. This same reduction in pressure within the chest cavity to below atmospheric pressure also contributes to increasing the flow of blood, particularly in the inferior vena cava into the right heart.

Expiration

At the height of inspiration, the respiratory center ceases to cause impulses in the phrenic and intercostal nerves. The stretched, elastic fibers of the lung connective tissue simply recoil. Lung volume diminishes and the air passively flows out. Expiration can be actively enhanced by contraction of abdominal muscles.

A cough is a forced expiration usually induced by an

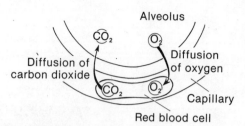

FIGURE 3-30. Schematic representation of the exchange of oxygen and carbon dioxide through the thin walls of an alveolus and a red blood cell of a capillary.

irritation in the lining of the air passages. It is usually preceded by an automatic inspiration. Immediately and automatically, the vocal cords close and seal the larynx, blocking the transfer of any air into or out of the lungs. Simultaneously, the abdominal and chest muscles contract. This contraction builds up a very high pressure within the thorax on the outside of the lungs. This pressure greatly exceeds atmospheric pressure. The vocal cords then reflexly open and air rushes out the mouth and nose. The rush of air drags the mucus lining the walls of the trachea, bronchi, and bronchioles into the pharynx.

Lung Volumes

Figure 3-31 describes the various lung volumes of importance:

1. The *tidal volume,* with the body at rest, is the amount of air (about 500 ml) taken in with each breath.
2. The *inspiratory reserve volume* is the maximum additional amount of air (about 3,000 ml) that can be taken in with a maximum inspiration effort, such as occurs at the height of maximum physical activity.
3. The *expiratory reserve volume* is the amount of air that can be further expired after passive expiration (about 1,000 ml).
4. The *vital capacity* of the lung is the sum of the above three volumes (about 4,500 to 5,000 ml) and is one of the main volumes to characterize a person's breathing capacity.
5. The *residual volume* is the amount of air that stays in the lung even after maximum expiration. The rigidity of the cartilage surrounding the trachea and bronchi does not permit their collapse, and hence the expulsion of all of the air.

Additional lung volumes which are often measured include the forced expiratory volume (FEV) and the maximum voluntary ventilation (MVV). The FEV is the volume of air that can be forcefully expired. Forced expiration is often timed to measure how fast the total FEV is exhaled. The volumes of air expired forcefully during the first, second, and third seconds are FEV_1, FEV_2, and FEV_3, respectively. The MVV is a measure of the maximum volume of air breathed in

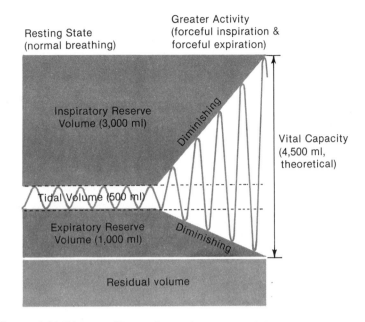

FIGURE 3-31. Diagram of lung volumes during rest and during increased activity.

and out as rapidly and forcefully as possible for 12 seconds. This value is multiplied by five to give the MVV in liters of air per minute.

Regulation of Respiration

Several factors participate in the regulation of the rate of respiration, the depth of respiration, and the rhythmicity of the inspiratory and expiratory efforts.

The controlling respiratory centers are located within the pons and medulla of the brain stem. The dominant controlling factor is the concentration of carbon dioxide (CO_2) in the blood. If the blood circulating within the respiratory centers has a high concentration of CO_2, it will stimulate the center to initiate more rapid and deeper breathing. The rapid and deeper breathing so initiated causes more CO_2 to diffuse out of the pulmonary capillaries into the alveoli and out of the system. A low concentration of CO_2 reciprocally slows down the rate and depth of respiration.

The second most important influence, particularly on the depth and rhythmicity of respiration, is nerves that are sensitive to pressures within the lung tissue. These nerve impulses reach the respiratory centers through cranial nerve X (vagus nerve). Expansion of the lungs stimulates these receptors, signaling the respiratory centers to "turn off" inspiration. When the lungs have collapsed at the end of expiration, the same receptors signal the respiratory center to begin inspiration again. This pressure reflex is called the Hering-Breuer inspiratory reflex. Other regulators of respiration are: (a) a drop in the acidity of the blood, which stimulates respiration; (b) an increase in blood pressure, which slows down respiration; and (c) a

sudden drop in blood pressure, which stimulates an increase in the rate and depth of respiration largely for the purpose of returning more blood to the heart.

Voluntary action initiated in the frontal lobe of the cerebrum can also increase or decrease the rate and depth of respiration, but a person cannot voluntarily stop breathing indefinitely. When respiration is stopped through a conscious effort, the carbon dioxide in the blood increases in concentration. This increase in carbon dioxide stimulates the respiratory center to overcome the conscious effort and forces the resumption of inspiration.

VISUAL SYSTEM

The function of the visual system is easily understood by a comparison with a camera. A camera has a shutter with a small opening in the center through which light from an object enters. If the object is bright, a smaller hole is created than if the light is dim. The camera lens is necessary to bend the light rays. For objects that are in close, a fatter, more convex ("zoom") lens is needed to bend the light more. For objects that are far away, a thinner lens is needed. The need for different shaped lenses exists because the photographic film on which the images are focused is at a fixed distance behind the lens. The camera case encloses and protects the shutter, lens, and film.

In the eye, the shutter function is performed by the *iris*, the colored part of the eye. The hole in the center of the iris is the *pupil*, through which the light enters. In bright light, the iris makes the pupil very small, and in dim light, the iris makes it large.

The lens of the eye corresponds to the lens of the

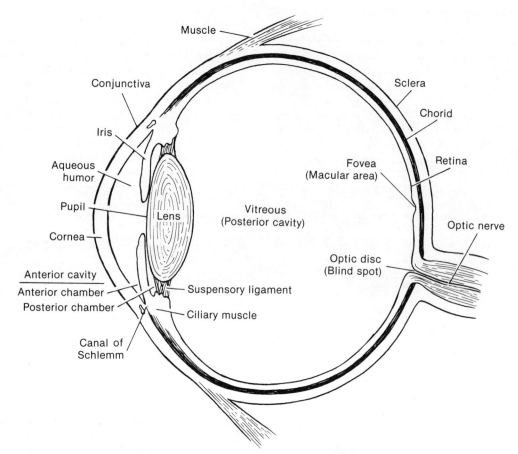

FIGURE 3-32. Schematic section of the human eye. The lens, suspensory ligament, and ciliary muscle divide the eye into anterior and posterior cavities. The iris further divides the anterior cavity into anterior and posterior chambers. Note the two extraocular muscles attached to the sclera.

camera. It has the capacity to assume a fat or thin shape through the action of the *ciliary muscle* to which it is attached.

The *retina*, at a fixed distance behind the lens, corresponds to the film of the camera, and the "developing process" is a set of complex operations that convert the image focused on the retina into nerve impulses. These impulses reach the occipital lobe of the brain where they are interpreted.

The protective camera case function in the eye is performed by the *sclera*, which is white and opaque except for the transparent *cornea* in front of the pupil and iris. The eyeball is further protected by a cushion of fat that lines the surrounding skull bones that make up the orbits (see fig. 3-19, p. 34).

In front, the sclera, cornea, and eyelids are lined by a thin, clear, skin-like layer, the *conjunctiva*. Eyelashes serve to partially keep foreign material out of the eye.

The *lacrimal glands*, above the eyeball and behind the eyelid, secrete the tears. The fluid enters through the holes in the outer aspect of the upper eyelid and drains across the eye for cleansing and lubrication. The fluid

drains into the nose through the *nasolacrimal duct* located in the inner aspect of the lower eyelid.

A defect in any of these structures can result in abnormal vision. In the following sections, individual components are discussed in sufficient detail for understanding the more common eye disorders. Chapter 29 details the treatment, rehabilitation, and vocational consequences of severe visual impairments and blindness. An understanding of the visual system is also relevant to chapters 10, 24, and 27.

CORNEA AND SCLERA

The cornea is about 10–12 mm in diameter and is curved, and hence protrudes from the rest of the eyeball (fig. 3-32). Because of this curvature, light begins to bend as it enters the cornea, even before it reaches the lens. The cornea is very clear and without blood vessels. It contains five layers and is richly supplied with nerve cells. Injuries to the cornea through disease or trauma may produce corneal opacities. If opacities are severe, corneal transplants from cadavers are possible because the cornea is nonvascular.

The white sclera, which is about 1 mm thick, completely encloses the internal structures of the eye except posteriorly, where it is pierced by the *optic nerve*. Its firm, inelastic, fibrous character maintains the form of the globe. No light passes through it.

The sclera is lined internally by the *choroid*, which consists mainly of blood vessels enmeshed in delicate connective tissue and pigmented cells, giving it a color that may range from orange to red to brownish grey. The blood vessels of the choroid nourish the lens, the posterior cavity behind the lens, and part of the retina.

IRIS AND PUPIL

The iris hangs behind the cornea immediately in front of the lens and is attached to the choroid (fig. 3-32). Its pigmented cells provide the color of the eyes. The circular muscle fibers of the iris constrict the pupil to reduce the amount of light allowed in, and radially oriented muscle fibers dilate the pupil to increase the amount of light. Reflexes initiated when light strikes the retina control these muscle contractions via cranial nerve III (oculomotor nerve). The pupil appears black because all of the light striking the retina is absorbed and none is reflected out of the eye.

LENS AND CILIARY BODY

The *ciliary body*, a muscular structure, also attaches to the choroid. In fact, the ciliary body and the iris are essentially one structure. From the ciliary body extends the *suspensory ligament* which attaches to the lens and maintains it in its proper position behind the pupil (fig. 3-32).

The lens, which is crystalline and transparent, consists of an outer cortex and an inner nucleus. The cortex is softer than the nucleus. In the young, the nucleus is small, and hence the lens is more pliable. When gazing at near objects, the ciliary muscle contracts, relaxing the suspensory ligament. The tension on the lens is thereby released, and the lens fattens. This increased curvature of the lens causes the light rays to bend more in order to focus an image on the retina. For far objects, the ciliary muscle relaxes, the suspensory ligament tightens, and the lens thins out.

With advancing age, the lens is unable to increase its curvature (presbyopia) when the suspensory ligament relaxes, and hence near objects (e.g., printed words) cannot be focused on the retina. Further, with advancing age and in some diseases, lens degeneration can occur, resulting in opacities (cataracts) which prevent light rays from reaching the retina.

The ciliary body, suspensory ligament, and the lens divide the eye into distinct anterior and posterior cavities (fig. 3-32).

ANTERIOR AND POSTERIOR CAVITIES

The anterior cavity has two chambers, anterior and posterior, separated by the iris. It contains *aqueous humor*, a fluid secreted in the posterior chamber by the ciliary body. The fluid passes through the pupil into the anterior chamber where it is absorbed at the *canal of Schlemm* (fig. 3-32). This secretion and absorption is balanced to maintain the appropriate pressure in the entire eye. A chronic interference resulting in too much production of aqueous humor and not enough absorption increases eye ball pressure (glaucoma). The increased pressure, if undetected, can lead to retinal damage and loss of vision.

The posterior cavity behind the lens contains the *vitreous humor*, a transparent, colorless gel, which consists of a mesh of clear liquid and cells but has no blood vessels. The cells are nourished from the surrounding tissues, namely, the choroid, the ciliary body, and the retina. The vitreous humor may also develop opacities which may affect vision by blocking light rays. Opacities in the vitreous humor, if present, are usually floating, and hence may not always be in the line of sight.

RETINA

The retina, a two-layered structure, is attached to almost all of the choroid. In particular, the pigmented layer is firmly fixed to the choroid. The inner layer of the retina, which contains the light-sensitive cells and the retinal blood vessels is, in essence, an expansion of the optic nerve.

The optic nerve enters the back of the eye at the *optic disc*, which itself does not contain light-sensitive cells and is therefore sometimes called the *blind spot*. Two main types of cells, *rods* and *cones* (fig. 3-33), make up the light-sensitive character of the retina.

Rods contain rhodopsin, a protein made up in part of a derivative of vitamin A. It is highly light sensitive and breaks down rapidly when exposed to light. This chemical breakdown initiates nerve impulse conduction. A short period of darkness is necessary for the rhodopsin to re-form and the rod to function again. Continuous bright light, therefore, interferes with rod function. When entering a dark environment from a bright environment, a certain amount of time for adaptation is necessary, during which rhodopsin re-forms and the rods become active again. Rods, therefore, operate most effectively in continuous dim light (night vision).

Cone cells contain iodopsin, a protein which is less sensitive than rhodopsin and requires a brighter light to break down. Daylight and color vision is therefore mostly mediated by cones.

Generally, rods are more numerous than cones, except at the *macula* (fig. 3-34). In fact, the center of the macula, the *fovea*, contains no rods and is the point

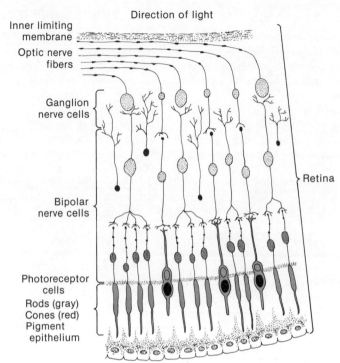

FIGURE 3-33. Layers that compose the retina. The inner limiting membrane lies nearest the inside of the eyeball and adheres to the vitreous humor. The pigment epithelium lies farthest from the inside of the eyeball and adheres to the choroid coat. Note relay of three nerve cells in the retina: photoreceptor, bipolar, and ganglion cells. Light rays pass through the vitreous humor and various layers of the retina to stimulate the rods and cones. All the individual optic nerve fibers collect at the optic disc and pierce the sclera as the optic nerve.

of clearest vision in good light. When desiring to look at a specific object in good light, the eyeball is so moved to focus the image on the fovea. To see an object better in dim light, eyeball movements occur to form the image more toward the periphery of the retina where rods are more plentiful. Diseases that produce macular degeneration therefore affect mostly direct object viewing in daylight. A vitamin A deficiency will affect mostly night vision or vision in dim light.

The main retinal artery and its branches nourish the retina and enter the eye at the optic disc. Diseases affecting retinal arteries may affect both day and night vision because of poor nutrition of rods and cones. A hemorrhage of a branch of a retinal artery may affect the function of rods or cones, depending on the location of the hemorrhage.

The distance between the lens and the retina (literally the size of the eyeball), coupled with lens factors, contribute to the common visual disturbances of near-sightedness (myopia) and far-sightedness (hyperopia). A near-sighted individual has a lengthened eyeball. Light rays from far objects focus before they reach the retina and hence appear blurred.

A far-sighted individual has a shortened eyeball. Light rays from near objects focus behind the retina and hence also appear blurred. Eyeglasses modify the bending of the light rays as necessary to ensure that focusing occurs at the retina.

Nerve impulses initiated at the rod and cone cells synapse first at the bipolar neurons within the retina (fig. 3-33). These in turn synapse with the optic nerve cells, which ultimately connect with the brain.

NERVE PATHWAYS TO THE BRAIN

When both eyes are directed toward an object, the image of the object is focused on corresponding portions of both retinas. A system then is required for the resulting impulses in each optic nerve to come together for proper interpretation by the brain.

Figure 3-35 indicates the labeling used to describe fields of vision. For each eye, that half of the retina close to the nose is called the *nasal portion* of each retina. The other half is called the *temporal portion*. Light from the tree in figure 3-35, which is on the right side of the picture (right visual field), focuses on the left side of

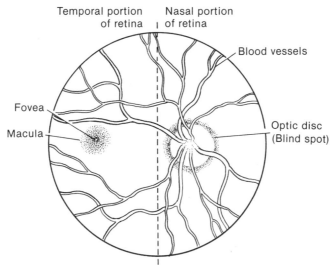

FIGURE 3-34. The retina as seen through the pupil with an ophthalmoscope in a normal human right eye. Sharpest vision occurs when the image falls on the macula, in particular on the fovea in the center. The nerve fibers are exiting at the optic disc, which is not covered by the retina. Images that focus on the optic disc are therefore not visualized ("blind spot"). Blood enters and leaves the eye at the optic disc through the central artery and the central vein.

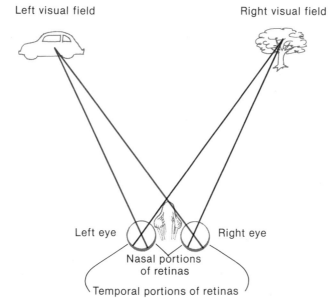

FIGURE 3-35. Note that corresponding points of focus for the tree are on the temporal portion of the retina of the left eye and the nasal portion of the retina of the right eye. Corresponding points of focus for the car are on the temporal portion of the retina of the right eye and the nasal portion of the retina of the left eye.

each retina. As the figure shows, this corresponds to the nasal portion of the right retina and the temporal portion of the left retina. Light rays from the car, which is on the left side of the picture (left visual field), focus on the temporal portion of the right retina and

the nasal portion of the left retina.

Figure 3-36 describes how images from the right visual field will all ultimately reach the left occipital lobe and how images from the left visual field will all ultimately reach the right occipital lobe. The figure

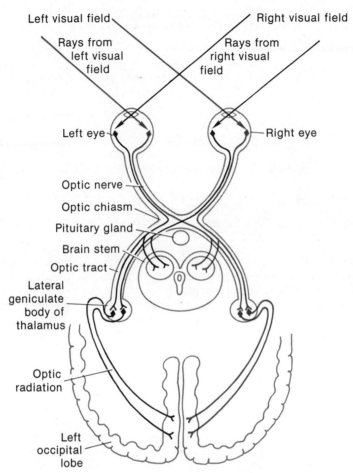

Left visual field

Right visual field

Rays from left visual field

Rays from right visual field

Left eye

Right eye

Optic nerve

Optic chiasm

Pituitary gland

Brain stem

Optic tract

Lateral geniculate body of thalamus

Optic radiation

Left occipital lobe

FIGURE 3-36. Note crossover of optic nerve fibers from both nasal retinas at the optic chiasma, with the result that the right visual field can project onto the left occipital cortex, and vice versa.

shows the fibers from the two sides of the retina traveling in each optic nerve. The two optic nerves come together under the frontal lobe and in front of the pituitary gland and join at the *optic chiasma*.

At the optic chiasma, the fibers from the nasal portion of each retina cross over and join the fibers from the temporal portion of the retina on the opposite side which carry the corresponding image. These combined fibers form the *optic tract*. Thus, the left optic tract contains nerve impulses of images from the right visual field and the right optic tract contains those from the left visual field. These fibers then synapse in the right and left lateral geniculate bodies of the thalamus. Fibers from the geniculate bodies continue as the *optic radiations* to terminate in the cortex of the right and left occipital lobes. In addition, fibers in the optic tract send branches to the brain stem to achieve coordination between the two eyes and to interact with cranial nerves III, IV, and VI (oculomotor, trochlear, and abducens) controlling the extraocular muscles.

Complete loss of the right optic radiations, such as may occur in stroke, for example, blocks vision from the left visual field for both eyes (left hemianopsia). Similarly, complete loss of the left optic radiations blocks vision from the right visual field for both eyes (right hemianopsia).

The three-dimensional perception of depth is achieved in several ways. The two eyes each see a single object from an ever-so-slightly different angle. When their two corresponding images register in the occipital lobe, these slight differences are interpreted to mean depth. Depth perception is also a learned phenomenon as we come to understand shadows, slight color changes with distance, the blocking of one object by another in front of it, and relative movement between near and far objects (parallax) as our eye surveys a scene. Thus, individuals who lose one eye still perceive depth, although not quite as accurately as with two eyes.

EYE MOVEMENTS

Each eye is moved within its orbit by six muscles that are attached to the sclera. These six muscles are

TABLE 3-7
MUSCLES OF EYE MOVEMENT

Muscle	Movement Produced	Cranial Nerve
Superior rectus	Up	Oculomotor (III)
Inferior rectus	Down	Oculomotor (III)
Medial rectus	In toward nose	Oculomotor (III)
Lateral rectus	Away from nose	Abducens (VI)
Superior oblique	Down and in	Trochclear (IV)
Inferior oblique	Up and out	Oculomotor (III)

governed by cranial nerves III, IV, and VI. The *superior rectus* and *inferior rectus* muscles mostly turn the eyeball and direct the pupil up and down, respectively. The *medial rectus* and *lateral rectus* muscles mostly turn the eyeball and direct the pupil toward the nose and away from the nose, respectively. The *superior oblique* and the *inferior oblique* muscles have more complex actions, mostly down and in and up and out, respectively. Table 3-7 summarizes these movements and the nerves operating them.

A disturbed balance in eye movements can lead to a failure of images to hit corresponding portions of the retinas and may result in double vision (diplopia). In severe losses of balance, such as might occur with paralysis, one eye might not even fix on the object at all and vision would therefore be monocular rather than binocular.

AUDITORY AND VESTIBULAR SYSTEMS

Hearing and equilibrium are usually discussed together because they derive from the same structure, the ear. The auditory system is concerned with the detection of sound waves, and the vestibular system is concerned with body balance.

Sound waves do not travel in a vacuum. They require a medium for their transmission. What actually travels is a succession of increased pressure in the medium, followed by decreased pressure, and then increased pressure again. These alternations of increased and decreased pressure (vibrations) can occur at various frequencies. Figure 3-37, using the example of a tuning fork, illustrates the traveling pressure wave. Sound waves travel 742 miles (1,187 km) per hour in air and 3,424 miles (5,478 km) per hour in water. These speeds are much slower than speeds of light. Hence, we see lightning before we hear the thunder.

The auditory system functions to conduct the sound wave to a set of special cells that sense the vibration and convert it into a nerve impulse. When the nerve impulse is transmitted to the brain, the sound is finally perceived. Not all sound vibrations can be perceived by the human ear. Only those frequencies ranging from about 20 to 20,000 cycles per second (Hz) can be perceived.

The vestibular system senses both static position and movement (acceleration and deceleration). One set of special cells senses position and a second set, movement. When stimulated, the cells produce nerve impulses which are then transmitted to the CNS.

The ear divides anatomically into three portions, termed the external ear, the middle ear, and the inner ear, which are located in special cavities within the temporal bone in the base of the skull on the underside of the cerebral hemispheres. The external and middle ears are concerned with conduction of sound waves. The inner ear contains the set of special cells for hearing and the two sets of special cells for position and movement. The nerve impulses created by these special cells reach the brain through the *vestibulocochlear nerve* (cranial nerve VIII). This is really two nerves somewhat joined together, the *cochlear nerve* for hearing and the *vestibular nerve* for equilibrium.

The following sections deal with the significant structures which, if impaired, can lead to the reduction in hearing and the sense of balance. Hearing impairments and deafness, together with their treatment, rehabilitation, and vocational implications, are discussed in chapter 30.

AUDITORY SYSTEM

External Ear

The *auricle* or *pinna,* the visible portion of the ear, is shaped to collect the sound waves, which enter the opening of the external ear canal, the *external acoustic meatus.* Sound transmits along the ear canal to the ear drum (tympanic membrane). The canal is about 1¼ inches (3.18 cm) long and contains modified sweat glands that secrete *cerumen,* a wax-like substance. Overproduction of cerumen can block transmission of sound. Figure 3-38 show the relation of the external ear to the middle ear.

Middle Ear

The middle ear continues the process of sound conduction. The air-filled cavity of the middle ear (tympanic cavity), while wholly contained within the temporal bone, connects to the throat by the auditory (Eustachian) tube. This connection makes the middle ear susceptible to infection (otitis media). The auditory tube is necessary for normal hearing. It allows the air pressure on both sides of the tympanic membrane to be equal, and this permits the membrane to vibrate maximally when sound waves impinge upon it. Normally, the walls of the auditory tube are collapsed. Swallowing and chewing actions momentarily open the tube to allow air in or out of the tympanic cavity as may be necessary for equalization of air pressure.

The tympanic membrane, which separates the external and middle ears and is considered part of the middle ear, is made up of three layers. The outer layer is like skin and the inner layer like the mucous membrane lining the nose and throat. When sound waves impinge upon the tympanic membrane, it vibrates.

A chain of three movable bones (auditory ossicles) conducts the vibration of the tympanic membrane to the inner ear. The malleus bone is directly attached to the inside layer of the tympanic membrane. A specialized joint articulates the malleus bone with the incus bone, which in turn articulates with the stapes bone. The stapes bone has a flat expanse (footplate) which fits into a hole, the oval window, in the wall of the inner ear. The three ossicles serve to transmit the vibrations of the tympanic membrane into movements of the footplate of the stapes. Figure 3-38 illustrates the relationships of the tympanic membrane, the auditory ossicles, and the auditory tube.

Inner Ear

The inner ear is an intricate fluid-filled cavity, the bony labyrinth, carved out of the temporal bone. The cavity has two connected sections, the cochlea and the semicircular canals, each with special channels within the bone. The oval window opens into the vestibule of the inner ear between the two sections.

Floating within the bony labyrinth is a complex membrane-covered sac, the membranous labyrinth. The sac fills all the channels. The fluid surrounding the sac and cushioning it is the perilymph, the fluid within the sac is the endolymph, and the sac also contains three sets of special cells. Figure 3-38 shows the cochlea, the semicircular canals, and the vestibule between them where the oval window is located.

The hearing function is subserved by the cochlea,

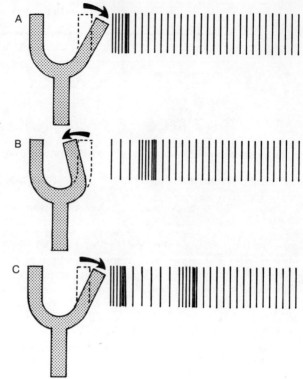

FIGURE 3-37. Schematic demonstration of traveling pressure (sound) wave using a tuning fork in an air medium. (A) Deflection of tuning fork to right compresses air molecules. (B) The pressure wave created further compresses air toward the right. The tuning fork returning to original position creates reduced pressure. (C) Deviation back to right starts second pressure wave. The distance between high pressure points is the wavelength of the sound wave. Frequency = velocity of sound/wavelength.

which is coiled to give a snail-like appearance (fig. 3-38). Figure 3-39 shows schematically how the sound wave signal is transmitted to the special hearing cells, the hair cells of the organ of Corti. Movement of the stapes creates waves in the perilymph. These transmit through the membrane of the membranous labyrinth into the endolymph. Movement of the hair cells leads to conversion of the sound vibrations into nerve impulses.

The nerve fibers carrying these impulses collect together as the cochlear nerve, entering the skull cavity through a hole in the temporal bone, the internal acoustic meatus. The nerve enters the medulla. Several synapses may occur before nerve impulses reach the auditory cortex of the temporal lobe for perception. The impulses from either ear have connections to the auditory cortices on both sides to the extent that removal of one auditory cortex does not noticeably impair the hearing of either ear.

Because of the rigid walls of the bony labyrinth of the cochlea, the waves created by the movement of the

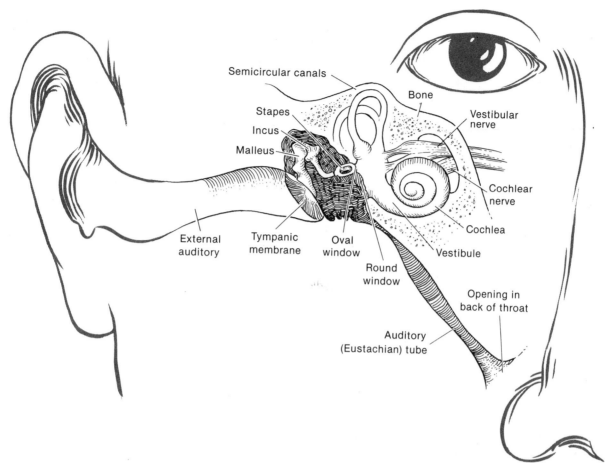

FIGURE 3-38. A section through the temporal bone to show anatomy of outer ear (pinna, external auditory canal), middle ear (tympanic membrane, malleus, incus, stapes), and inner ear (semicircular canals, cochlea, and vestibule with oval and round windows). The auditory (Eustachian) tube connects the middle ear to the back of the throat. The relative location of these structures can be appreciated from the sketched-in nose and eye.

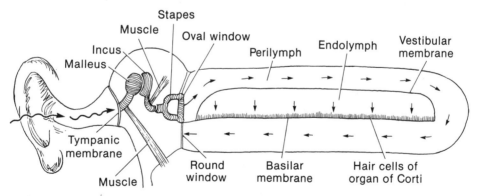

FIGURE 3-39. Schematic drawing of sound wave transmission. Sound wave vibrates the tympanic membrane, which in turn oscillates the malleus, incus, and stapes. Stapes vibrating in oval window agitates perilymph, which transmits vibration to vestibular membrane and then to endolymph to reach the hair cells of the organ of Corti. Wave dissipates at round window. Note the two muscles anchoring the malleus and incus.

stapes need to be dissipated to prevent multiple reflections. The membrane-covered *round window* in that part of the wall of the inner ear separating it from the middle ear dissipates the wave after it has excited the organ of Corti.

VESTIBULAR SYSTEM

The semicircular canals and central vestibule portion of the bony and membranous labyrinths contain the special sets of cells for sensing position and movement. The three semicircular canals are perpendicular to each other to sense movement in the three spatial dimensions. At the base of each, the membrane cavity is enlarged (*ampulla*). Within the ampulla lie hair cells called collectively the *crista ampullaris*. Depending on the plane of movement, the resultant flow of endolymph within the semicircular canals excites the appropriate hair cells. In the region of the vestibule, enlargements of the membranous labyrinth, the *utricle* and *saccule,* contain the hair cells that sense static head position. Different head positions produce different gravity effects on these hair cells. Small calcium carbonate particles (otoliths) are the ultimate stimulants of the hair cells for position.

The hair cells for both position and movement create nerve impulses. The nerve fibers carrying these impulses collect as the vestibular nerve, which enters the skull cavity through the internal acoustic meatus along with the cochlear nerve. The impulses from any one side synapse in various areas of both sides of the brain stem, cerebellum, and spinal cord. No definite connections to the cerebral cortex exist. The impulses therefore predominantly produce reflex actions. A sudden loss of balance, for example, creates endolymph movement in the semicircular canals and triggers the reflex response of leg movement or arm movement to restore balance. No interpretation by the brain (cortex) is needed to produce the corrective response.

BIBLIOGRAPHY

Basic Textbooks

Basmajian JV: *Primary Anatomy*. Ed.7, Baltimore, Williams and Wilkins, 1976.
   Basic textbook that covers all organ systems. Concise, easy to read, and well illustrated.
Gardner WD, Osburn WA: *Anatomy of the Human Body*. Ed.3, Philadelphia, Saunders, 1978.
   Excellent basic anatomy textbook that covers all organ systems. Precisely written and well illustrated. Combination motions as well as individual muscle actions are described.
Hollingshead WH: *Functional Anatomy of the Limbs and Back — A Text for Students of the Locomotor Apparatus*. Ed.4, Philadelphia, Saunders, 1976.

Jacobs SW, Ashworth C: *Structure and Function in Man*. Ed.3, Philadelphia, Saunders, 1974.
   Basic anatomy textbooks that cover all of the organ systems. Well written and illustrated. Physiology is well presented.

Atlases

Clemente C: *Anatomy — A Regional Atlas of the Human Body*. Philadelphia, Lea and Febiger, 1975.
Grant JCB: *Grant's Atlas of Anatomy*. Ed.7, Baltimore, Williams and Wilkins, 1978.
   Regional atlas of artist drawings. Most illustrations are footnoted with observations and comments that aid in understanding.
McMinn RMH, Hutchings RT: *Color Atlas of Human Anatomy*. Chicago, Year Book Medical Publishers, 1977.
   Camera pictures of dissected cadavers and skeletal bones.

4 DISABILITY CONSEQUENCES OF BED REST

Paul J. Corcoran, M.D.

INTRODUCTION

Most people are under the impression that rest is beneficial in restoring the health of an ill or injured person. Medical and nursing training has emphasized bed rest as an essential therapeutic tool. The bed is the central focus of hospitals, where policies and tradition conspire to keep patients in their beds for most of the day. Until the 1940's, strict bed rest was the routine treatment for 2 weeks after childbirth, 3 weeks after a hernia operation, and 4 weeks or more after myocardial infarction.

The shortages of personnel, resources, and hospital beds during World War II led to the startling discovery that early mobilization of the sick and injured not only was harmless but actually shortened recovery times and lessened complications. As postwar medical progress led to the survival of more and more persons with severe disabilities, rehabilitation practitioners and researchers came to realize the dangers of bed rest and the benefits of therapeutic activities. Recent research in preparation for manned space flight has produced still more evidence of the damaging effects of prolonged inactivity. Practically no body system escapes the progressive deterioration caused by bed rest.

Today it is recognized by many that rest may be necessary in the treatment of certain disorders. Prolonged continuous immobilization, on the other hand, can indeed have a disastrous net effect on the body. "Preventive rehabilitation" philosophy limits the duration of rest, and confines it only to the diseased or injured organ or part, with careful strategies to continue the functional use of the remainder of the body and mind. Practice, however, lags behind knowledge, and far too much rest is still prescribed by health practitioners or self-imposed by patients and their families. Thus the incidence of the complications described below continues to be high, especially in severe disabilities with their more lengthy periods of treatment.

As medical progress increases the survival and longevity of persons with severe physical disabilities, rehabilitation professionals will be asked to deal with increasing numbers of clients at risk from these complications. Careful preventive rehabilitation should minimize the unnecessary additional disability caused by inactivity and rest. When the complications of bed rest are present, the rehabilitation counselor should be knowledgeable about arranging for their correction. Functional abilities and work tolerance can often be improved significantly, even in clients with permanent disabilities, when these complications of inactivity are recognized and treated appropriately.

Ten organs or systems will now be considered in more detail. The common impairments which they may develop after inactivity will be described, methods of evaluation and treatment of these complications will be reviewed, and their vocational implications will be discussed.

JOINTS AND CONNECTIVE TISSUES

The "moving parts" of the body—joints, ligaments, tendons, and related muscles and skin—all have a normal range of motion which is necessary for proper performance of physical tasks. Any decrease in the normal range of motion is called a *contracture*. Contractures of muscles, tendons, joints, and skin are among the commonest complications of bed rest. Sometimes they are the anticipated but unavoidable side-effects of necessary treatment. An example would be a knee contracture after plaster immobilization to treat a fractured tibia. More often, contractures are produced unwittingly and unnecessarily: the frozen shoulder caused by use of a sling after a wrist fracture, or the hip flexion contracture after a period of bed rest (figs. 4-1 and 4-2).

The basic component of connective tissues is *collagen fibers* (see chap. 3, p. 30). Under normal circumstances, our ordinary daily activities result in frequent excursions of the moving parts through their full range of motion. This maintains the collagen fibers in a loosely coiled arrangement which permits the normal stretching of tissues during activity. Immobilization changes these loosely coiled fibers into a mass of shortened, straightened, and more densely packed fibers. The resulting limitation of the range of motion of the part is the contracture. Less than a day of

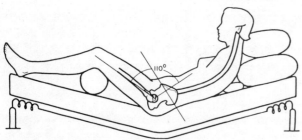

FIGURE 4-1. A person lying supine in bed sinks into the mattress, which in turn sags into the bedsprings. Pillows under the head and knees increase this flexion posture. Side-lying or sitting would reproduce the same flexed position, but prone-lying or standing would reverse it and promote straightening (full extension) of the spine and lower limbs. (Reprinted, by permission, from Krusen FH, Kottke FJ, Ellwood PM (eds): Handbook of Physical Medicine and Rehabilitation. Ed. 2, Philadelphia, Saunders, 1971.)

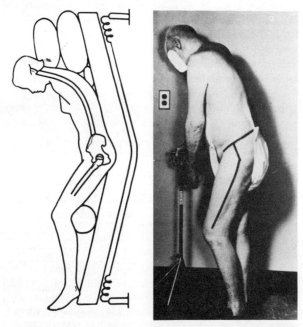

FIGURE 4-2. Flexion contractures form after prolonged bed rest without prone-lying or range-of-motion exercises. Relaxed standing is then impossible because constant muscular contraction is required to maintain the semiflexed erect posture. (Reprinted, by permission, from Krusen FH, Kottke FJ, Ellwood PM (eds): Handbook of Physical Medicine and Rehabilitation. Ed 2, Philadelphia, Saunders, 1971.)

immobilization will initiate these changes. We are all familiar with the morning stiffness after 8 hours of sleep in a curled-up position. We correct this by stretching in the opposite direction as soon as we get up. Two or three weeks of immobilization produces a much firmer contracture which may require weeks of range-of-motion exercises to correct. After 2 or 3 months of immobilization, a contracture may need

surgical correction. The rate of contracture formation is accelerated by several factors which may often coexist in the immobilized parts: edema, bleeding, infection, burns, or the healing of traumatic or surgical wounds.

Evaluation and Management

A physical therapist can measure contractures precisely with a protractor and record them on special range-of-motion charts. A physiatrist can evaluate the contracture, advise on whether surgical correction is necessary, and prescribe exercises, activities, or orthotic devices to correct them. Heating contractured tissues prior to exercise will increase their ability to stretch. One of the principal uses of deep heat produced by shortwaves, microwaves, or ultrasound (medical diathermy) is to heat deep contractures prior to range-of-motion exercises or activities. More superficial contractures (e.g., fingers, skin) can be heated with surface heat modalities such as hot water or paraffin prior to exercising. Heat also reduces pain and muscle spasm which could interfere with the exercises. Massage (manually by a physical therapist or mechanically via air-compression machines or whirlpool agitators in hot water) may help remove edema and facilitate the performance of range-of-motion exercises.

Prevention is obviously the preferred approach to contractures. The key to prevention is to carry each joint through its full range of motion at least once every 8 hours. This can be done by the nurse, a family member, or the patient himself. Proper positioning in bed is also important and can be assisted by sandbags, bedboards, and foot cushions. Intermittent lying on the abdomen (prone-lying) will help prevent hip flexion contractures. Splints can produce any desired position, but should be removed every 8 hours for range-of-motion exercises. Minimizing bed rest and encouraging self-care and diversional activities will help. An occupational therapist can position therapeutic crafts to encourage joint movements in the desired directions.

When contractures are widespread or cannot be corrected, certain vocational adjustments may be necessary. Adaptive devices, ambulation aids, or special seating may improve function. Equipment or controls at a work station may need to be relocated if the client's reach is impaired. Hip or knee contractures increase the energy cost of walking and standing, which should be considered in vocational planning.

MUSCLES

The strength of a normal muscle is determined by the amount of effort to which it is regularly subjected. Each muscle is only as strong as it needs to be for the person's life style. Increasing the force of muscular contractions will lead to an enlargement of individual muscle cells due to an increase in the amount of contractile proteins inside the cells (see chap. 3, p. 31). The resulting overall increase in muscle bulk is the familiar effect of weight lifting or heavy manual labor.

Less familiar is the *atrophy* which follows disuse of muscles. Total disuse of a muscle (as after paralysis, tendon tear, plaster casting, or severe pain on motion) will lead to the loss of about one-eighth of its strength with each passing week. A partially disused muscle which never exerts more than 20 percent of its maximum force will begin to atrophy, with a decrease in strength and size of the muscle cells, and an increase in extracellular water, fat, and collagen fibers. Regular exertion at 20–30 percent of maximum force will preserve a muscle's strength. Exercise to fatigue at greater than 30 percent of its maximum force will strengthen and hypertrophy a muscle, but work at 70 percent would be more efficient and more effective.

Persons who have had prolonged illness or inactivity will all have some degree of disuse atrophy of their muscles. The upper extremities may escape significant atrophy in a bed-bound patient if self-care activities are continued, but the weight-bearing muscles of the trunk and lower limbs usually atrophy to a greater extent. Backache and fatigue during convalescence are often due more to disuse atrophy of muscles than to the underlying disease.

Evaluation and Management

A physical therapist can evaluate muscle strength via a manual muscle test which is recorded on a special form. An evaluation by a physician skilled in rehabilitation medicine can determine the extent to which disuse atrophy is reversible. Therapeutic exercises and activities can be prescribed to strengthen muscles. Even patients in plaster casts can be taught muscle-setting, or isometric, exercises to prevent or correct disuse atrophy. When health practitioners recognize situations which could lead to disuse atrophy, preventive measures can often be instituted: therapeutic exercise, self-care and recreational activities, or mobilization with wheelchairs or ambulation aids.

Atrophy due to nerve damage with complete paralysis, unlike disuse atrophy, cannot be corrected by exercise. Partially paralyzed muscles, however, can be strengthened through exercise assisted by the physical therapist or performed with gravity eliminated by slings or hydrotherapy. For a patient with complete and permanent paralysis, much of therapy is directed toward the unaffected or normal muscles (e.g., the upper limbs in a paraplegic) to develop even greater than normal strength. Functional activities (e.g., crutch-walking or wheelchair mobility) can then be restored as the strengthened muscles of the unaffected

limbs begin to compensate for the paralysis.

The rehabilitation counselor should be alert to the possibility that prolonged bed rest, for whatever reason, may be causing unnecessary additional disability in a client. If this is suspected, the counselor should consider seeking informed medical guidance from a medical consultant to evaluate the possible need for additional treatment and to assist in the proper timing of vocational steps. True disuse atrophy should respond to therapy. Once an acceptable level of strength has been restored, a return to vocational activities will often provide the additional exercise needed for further recovery of normal strength. However, resuming vigorous activities before sufficient strength has returned may lead to sprains, pains, or accidents. Informed medical guidance should help client and counselor with the proper timing of vocational steps.

BONES

Bones are made of a framework of collagen fibers which by itself would be soft and spongy. Salts of calcium and phosphorous are deposited in this framework to produce the hard, strong characteristics of normal bone. Bones are not inert, but undergo continual deposition and reabsorption of calcium and remodeling of the fibrous framework in response to stress. The combined stresses of weight bearing and muscle pull are responsible for maintaining the normal calcium content of bones.

Bed rest and inactivity eliminate most of these stresses. The rate of calcium removal begins to exceed the rate of deposition, and within 3 days there are measurable increases in the urinary losses of calcium. The bones soften and weaken (osteoporosis), and even ordinary forces such as those encountered during wheelchair transfers, physical therapy activities, or minor falls may cause fractures. A common example of such a "pathologic fracture" is the compression fracture of a vertebra, most commonly seen in inactive elderly persons. The high calcium losses continue for several months, but usually reach a new equilibrium within a year after the onset of the paralysis or inactivity.

The excessive calcium turnover, especially during the first year of a disability, may lead to urinary tract stones. Under certain circumstances, calcium may also be deposited in soft tissues (heterotopic calcification) where it can interfere with joint or muscle function. This occurs most commonly in paralyzed limbs, such as the lower limbs of a paraplegic, and is also referred to as myositis ossificans.

Evaluation and Management

Ordinary X-rays do not demonstrate evidence of osteoporosis until more than 50 percent of the bone

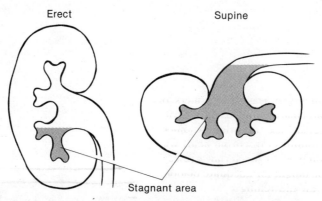

Erect   Supine

Stagnant area

FIGURE 4-3. In the supine person, urine must flow uphill for about 2 inches to escape from the kidney. Changes to the side-lying or erect position help produce normal gravitational drainage. (From Browse NL: The Physiology and Pathology of Bed Rest, 1965. Courtesy of Charles C. Thomas, Publisher, Springfield, IL.)

mineral has been lost. Heterotopic calcification is detectable by X-rays, and may be found in about one out of five spinal cord injured persons (although most have no resulting limitations of mobility).

Early resumption of activity in reversible illness will minimize osteoporosis. In permanent disabilities, the calcium losses cannot be prevented. Standing for weight bearing with braces or on a tilt-table may diminish the rate of calcium loss, but without the added stress of muscle pull, this is not as valuable as was once supposed. Eliminating dairy products from the diet does not prevent calcification in the urinary tract or soft tissues, although excessively large calcium intakes should be avoided during the first year. It is sometimes useful to maintain a high enough fluid intake to ensure at least 1.5–2 liters of urinary output per day. This dilutes the urine and helps prevent stone formation. Osteoporosis should be assumed to be present in paralyzed limbs, and precautions against falls should be taken, such as the use of wheelchair lap belts. Pathologic fractures usually heal uneventually with ordinary management.

For those with temporary periods of bed rest or inactivity, early remobilization is the best protection against osteoporosis. Persons with permanent disabilities should be educated to take the precautions outlined above. Special vocational considerations are rarely needed. Successful vocational rehabilitation produces increased activity and other benefits which outweigh the risks of pathologic fractures.

URINARY TRACT

Inactivity increases the urinary calcium load, which may be three or four times normal within 3 weeks after the onset of complete bedrest. The risk of urinary stone formation is increased further by the recumbent position, which produces the additional problems of stagnation and loss of gravitational emptying of the kidneys (fig. 4-3). Complete emptying of the bladder also may fail to occur when voiding in a supine position on a bedpan or into a urine bottle. This stagnation makes urinary tract infection more likely, especially if a catheter is being used. It is impossible to avoid introducing bacteria with a bladder catheter, and urine containing bacteria (positive urine cultures) can almost always be obtained from persons with indwelling catheters. In men, the catheter can also produce prostate and scrotal infections and erosions from the urethra through the skin at the base of the penis (urethral fistulae), caused by kinking and pressure from the catheter. Without a catheter, any resistance to outflow when the bladder contracts can cause "reflux," the forcing of urine back up into the kidneys under high pressure. Kidney damage from infection (pyelonephritis) and back-pressure (hydronephrosis) is still the major cause of mortality in spinal cord injured persons, where a paralyzed (neurogenic) bladder increases all of the above risks still further.

Stones usually produce severe pain and bloody urine. However, large stones can form gradually and grow to fill the kidney (staghorn calculi) without symptoms. Infections typically cause fever, chills, and burning on urination, often with pain and tenderness over the kidneys or bladder. However, chronic pyelonephritis can also progress silently until eventually the signs of kidney failure (uremia) appear (see chap. 25).

Evaluation and Management

Periodic urine analysis and cultures for the presence of bacteria will detect unsuspected infection. An excretory urogram (EUP) and voiding cystogram are special X-ray procedures needed once or twice yearly by every spinal cord patient to detect silent kidney damage from reflux, infection, or stones (see chap. 5, p. 69, 70, 74).

Most of these urinary tract complications can be prevented by early mobilization, effective patient education, and proper bladder care. Enough fluids should be drunk to maintain at least 1.5-2 liters of urine output daily, particularly for patients with indwelling catheters. Regular use of urine acidifiers like cranberry juice or vitamin C (ascorbic acid) will make the urine inhospitable to bacterial growth. Techniques can usually be taught for adequate bladder emptying without using an indwelling catheter. The recent introduction of intermittent catheterization technique has decreased infection rates significantly. Proper use of external collecting equipment will usually keep persons dry and free from socially objectionable odors which would interfere with employment and acceptance. If bladder catheters are used for men, they should be taped up onto the abdomen to avoid the dangling and kinking that leads to urethral fistula.

Two health professionals are invaluable in the prevention and management of urinary tract problems: a rehabilitation nursing specialist and a urologist who is knowledgeable about the neurogenic bladder. The rehabilitation counselor should see that all spinal cord injured clients are referred for regular followup and training by these two specialists.

HEART

The heart is a muscle, and it undergoes disuse atrophy like other muscles when a patient remains inactive. Being weaker, it can pump less blood per contraction, so it must pump more rapidly to move the same amount of blood per minute. Studies sponsored by the National Aeronautics and Space Administration (NASA) in preparation for manned space flight revealed that after 3 weeks of bed rest, the resting pulse of healthy young men increased by 10 beats per minute, and that their pulse after exertion was 40 beats per minute greater. Exercise tolerance did not return to normal again until after 5 to 10 weeks of vigorous reconditioning. Older or debilitated persons suffer even more cardiac deconditioning after bed rest or inactivity. This is manifested by shortness of breath (dyspnea) on exertion, palpitations, light-headedness, and easy fatigability.

In the past it was believed that lying flat decreased the strain on the heart and was proper after heart attacks. Recent evidence, however, has shown that the cardiac output and workload are 20-30 percent greater when recumbent than when sitting well supported in an easy chair. Defecation and urination are also less stressful in the sitting position.

Evaluation and Management

Rehabilitation counselors should be alert to the possibility that a severely physically disabled person may have unnecessary additional limitations on his physical performance as a result of cardiac deconditioning. Referral to a physician who is familiar with physical disabilities or to a cardiac work evaluation unit, if one is available, can help answer the question.

Exercises and activities of increasing strenuousness, prescribed by a physician and supervised by a physical therapist, will improve cardiac fitness and work tolerance in disabled as in able-bodied persons. Graded athletics and wheelchair sports are very useful here. Once the work tolerance is adequate for entry into employment, the physical demands of the job and related travel exertion will produce additional gains in cardiac fitness. There is no evidence that hard work harms a normal heart. As with the remainder of the body, rest may be a necessary evil in certain heart diseases, but it does not directly benefit the heart.

When permanent heart damage sets limits on the work tolerance, even with optimal cardiac rehabilitation, it may be necessary to reduce the vocational demands for exertion. Abundant data is available to guide the physician, physical therapist, and counselor regarding the energy requirements of various occupations, and the extent to which physical disabilities increase energy demands.

CIRCULATION

A common and potentially lethal complication of bed rest is the clotting of the blood in the deep veins of the lower limbs and lower abdomen, commonly known as *thrombophlebitis.* Studies have shown a direct correlation between the length of bed rest and the likelihood of having thrombophlebitis, which will be found in the large majority of persons after a few weeks of bed rest. Calf pain and tenderness may be present, but deep thigh and pelvic vein thrombosis often presents no symptoms or signs. The real danger of thrombophlebitis results when a blood clot breaks loose and flows rapidly to the lungs (pulmonary embolism) via the great veins and right heart. A clot will become trapped in the lungs, suddenly obstructing all flow through the occluded vessel. Symptoms are chest pain, cough, and bloody sputum. A significant number of pulmonary emboli cause sudden death (often attributed incorrectly to a heart attack).

Another circulatory complication of bed rest is a drop in blood pressure upon sitting or standing up (orthostatic hypotension), due to the pooling of blood in the legs and abdomen. The patient may feel dizzy and weak, or may actually lose consciousness. Lying down promptly restores the blood pressure and consciousness to normal. Orthostatic hypotension is common after even a week or two of bed rest, especially if paralysis is present.

Evaluation and Management

Careful frequent examination of the legs will help detect early thrombophlebitis. A chest X-ray or radioactive isotope scan of the lungs will detect most pulmonary embolism. Prompt use of anticoagulant drugs (heparin, Coumadin) usually controls the clotting and prevents embolization if begun early enough. In high-risk repeat cases, a sieve may have to be surgically placed in the inferior vena cava to strain out large clots which may break loose from the lower extremity.

Elastic stockings help prevent thrombophlebitis. Some centers use anticoagulant drugs prophylactically in high-risk groups such as recent spinal cord injuries. Early mobilization is, of couse, an important preventive measure.

Orthostatic hypotension is managed by use of elastic stockings and a firm corset to prevent pooling of blood in the abdomen and legs. Patients can be elevated in small stages using a tilt-table, and blood pressure can be monitored as they gradually adjust again to the vertical posture.

Clients with a history of thrombophlebitis should be taught to move about frequently and exercise their leg muscles whenever they have to sit for a prolonged period. This is possible in most job situations. Elastic stockings may be needed permanently. Garters and other constricting clothing should not be used. Obesity and pregnancy are also aggravating factors which may obstruct venous return from the legs and pelvis.

LUNGS

Prolonged bed rest produces several changes in the respiratory system which predispose persons to pneumonia and other lung complications. The thin film of mucus which normally lines the air passages (see chap. 3, p. 42) may collect or pool in the dependent portions of the lungs. Sedation and dehydration increase this tendency. The cough reflex is less active and the diameter of the bronchioles decreases during recumbency. The work of breathing is greater when recumbent or slumped than when sitting erect. Fewer deep breaths are taken in. All of these factors tend to obstruct air passages, leading to collapse of small portions of the lung (atelectasis). This favors bacterial growth leading to pneumonia.

Other complications of bed rest include pulmonary embolism (see p. 59) and aspiration of vomitus,

especially likely in a supine patient who is lethargic or sedated.

Evaluation and Management

The "vital capacity," the greatest amount of air that can be moved in a single breath, is easy to measure (see chap. 3, p. 44). This and other more complex pulmonary function tests help indicate the likelihood of lung complications. The physical examination and the chest X-ray help detect atelectasis and pneumonia.

Prevention of respiratory complications takes awareness and teamwork to provide bed activities, frequent position changes, and as much time up in a chair as possible. Adequate fluid intake prevents dehydration. Deep breathing and coughing should be encouraged frequently. High-risk patients such as postoperative patients benefit from chest physiotherapy techniques to mobilize secretions and stimulate coughing and deep breathing. When the vital capacity is limited by paralysis or other diseases, inhalation therapy or regular use of mechanical breathing and coughing devices may be appropriate. Such patients require more aggressive treatment for minor colds and upper respiratory infections.

Over 20 years ago when polio was widespread, respiratory rehabilitation centers possessed the equipment and expertise to maintain an active life even with total respiratory paralysis. Portable, battery-powered respirators mounted on electric wheelchairs allowed a few of these persons to attend school, go to work, and socialize. Today we are again seeing more and more patients with severe respiratory paralysis from high spinal cord injuries, muscular dystrophy, and certain other diseases. As a result, rehabilitation centers are rediscovering the technique for managing chronic respiratory insufficiency. With improved architectural accessibility and vocational rehabilitation services, a productive life can be possible for them.

GASTROINTESTINAL TRACT

Bed rest is often associated with a decreased appetite. Hospital food may be unfamiliar and the surroundings unappealing. The simple mechanics of eating or being fed may be quite cumbersome for the severely disabled person. Swallowing while reclining is more difficult. As a result, malnutrition may develop after prolonged bed rest. Some patients may nibble at "junk food" and mask their malnutrition behind a weight gain.

Constipation is another common problem in bed-bound patients. The lack of gravity assisting elimination, the awkwardness of the bedpan, and inability to hunch over and bear down all conspire to

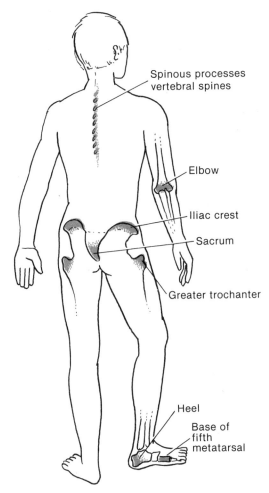

Spinous processes
vertebral spines

Elbow

Iliac crest

Sacrum

Greater trochanter

Heel

Base of
fifth
metatarsal

FIGURE 4-4. These are the common sites of decubitus ulcers in a recumbent patient. A sitting patient may develop pressure sores over the ischial tuberosity, the bones in each buttock upon which we sit.

cause constipation. Hard fecal impactions may form and require removal by the gloved finger of a nurse or physician.

Evaluation and Management

A nutritional history, physical examination, and blood tests will point to malnutrition if present. Abdominal and rectal examination detect constipation. Evaluation by a nutritionist may be extremely helpful.

Early mobilization and eating in a chair at the bedside or group dining in pleasant surroundings are important. Adaptive aids and occupational therapy may allow self-feeding, always more appetizing than being fed. A nutritionist can recommend nutritious foods that are simple for disabled persons to prepare and eat. An active life is the best stimulus to the appetite.

Bowel training is facilitated by use of a bedside

commode chair rather than a bedpan. The guidance of a nurse skilled in rehabilitation is invaluable. The use of suppositories may help regulate the bowel. Dependence on laxatives and enemas can usually be avoided, although oral stool softeners are often helpful. With regular eating habits and experience, most problems with constipation and diarrhea can be avoided.

SKIN

The bedsore, pressure sore, or *decubitus ulcer* (plural: decubiti), is one of the commonest, most expensive, and most misunderstood complications of bed rest. There is nothing mysterious about the cause—simple pressure is the common factor. If the pressure outside a blood vessel exceeds the pressure inside, the vessel will collapse and blood flow will cease. (This can easily be demonstrated by pressing the lens of one's eyeglasses, or any clear glass, against a knuckle. One is surprised at how little pressure causes the skin to blanch. Over a soft, fleshy area, much more pressure is required to produce tissue blanching.) Tissues that lose their blood supply for a few hours will die. This is called *infarction*. A decubitus ulcer, then, is a hole or gap in the skin and underlying soft tissues, caused by their infarction due to prolonged pressure.

The earliest sign of a decubitus ulcer is an area of redness which does not disappear within 15 minutes to an hour after removal of the pressure. Next comes a blister. The dead, or infarcted, tissues decay, liquefy, and separate out, leaving the gap or ulcer. The process may be even more extensive deep down, where bony prominences compress the soft tissues from the inside. Common sites are those places where bony prominences are thinly covered with skin and fat (fig. 4-4). They are totally preventable, yet it is not uncommon to see a neglected decubitus ulcer big enough to put one's fist inside.

Normally, prolonged pressure on skin causes pain, and we shift our position to allow blood to re-enter those tissues. Persons who have lost their protective pain sensation due to neurological injury or disease are the principal candidates for decubiti. Pure motor paralysis without sensory loss (e.g., after polio) rarely leads to bedsores because the protective pain sensation causes the patient to complain and get someone to change his position. Other risk factors are age, anemia, malnutrition, diabetes, urinary or fecal incontinence, immobilization in plaster or traction, use of sedatives or narcotics, habitual alcohol or drug intoxication, senility, and any other brain damage which impairs alertness or awareness. Wet skin, wrinkled sheets, or rough handling during transfers can be additional contributing factors. However, none of these will cause a bedsore if prolonged pressure is avoided.

Evaluation and Management

Physicians and nurses who are experienced in rehabilitation can evaluate a pressure sore or a decubitus-prone client and recommend treatment or preventive measures. Numerous local medications, salves, and powders have been promoted to cure or prevent decubiti. Most of them work, not so much because of any direct effect but because their use focuses attention on the trouble spot and leads to frequent bandage and position changes. The key is the elimination of all pressure once an ulcer has begun to form and the limitation of pressure to not more than 2 hours on intact skin. Large decubiti, like large burns and other skin deficits, may require plastic surgery and skin grafts to close them (see chap. 32). Small decubiti, like any other small skin ulcer or wound, should heal promptly if pressure is eliminated and they are kept clean and dry.

Clients with decubitus ulcer problems require a team approach by a physiatrist, physical therapist, nurse, and equipment dealer. The wheelchair user must develop the habit of frequent pushups and position changes. Special wheelchair cushions help, but none yet developed offers total protection. High quadriplegics who cannot change position unaided may need an electrically reclining wheelchair or arrangements for an able-bodied person to assist them with a position change every 2 hours.

Special mattresses using flotation principles allow longer periods without position changes, but the skin must be kept dry and watched carefully. Paraplegics and quadriplegics should personally inspect their own skin every morning and night using a mirror.

Patient education and motivation are closely related to the incidence of pressure sores. The depressed, idle, poorly trained paraplegic is much more likely to develop decubiti than the optimistic, involved paraplegic who has had proper medical rehabilitation training and is actively pursuing an educational and vocational goal.

Rehabilitation counselors should not hesitate to commit large amounts of client service to prevent decubitus ulcers. A $100 cushion or a $2,500 electrically reclining wheelchair do not seem so expensive when compared with the $5,000 or more that it may cost to heal a decubitus ulcer. Proper equipment and training will permit entry into competitive employment with fewer restrictions on sitting tolerance.

MENTAL STATE

NASA-sponsored studies of eight normal young men who were kept in bed for 5 weeks showed increases in anxiety, hostility, and depression, and altered sleep patterns. Bed rest appears to be a subtle form of sensory deprivation. Bed-bound persons lose environmental stimuli via the five senses, as well as stimuli from their own musculoskeletal systems. It was of interest that exercising during the 5 weeks of bed rest reduced these deleterious effects significantly.

Perhaps even more psychologically disabling is the learned helplessness and dependency caused by medical treatment. The bed-bound patient is expected to play a sick role. The "good" patient is the one who is docile and compliant, taking medications and following professional orders without question. Care-providers are likely to positively reinforce this sick behavior, and react more negatively to those who attempt to manipulate or challenge hospital routine. The bed-bound patient loses control over the most intimate aspects of his own life. Other forces control his diet, sleep hours, money, social contacts, and sexual expression. Medications, appointments, and health records are managed by others.

On the day of discharge from the hospital, the patient is expected to resume independent management and decision making for his own life. If it has been a 10-day stay for appendicitis, he returns to the same niche in the community, with his own capabilities and self-image unaltered. But if it has been a 6-month stay for treatment of spinal cord injury, his self-image may be greatly altered and his niche in the environment inaccessible (see chap. 2). Adults who have grown up with a congenital or pediatric disability may never have learned the skills of social survival.

Evaluation and Management

Psychologists and other rehabilitation professionals with testing and counseling skills can recognize and develop an understanding of the psychological disabilities concomitant with a physical handicap. Individual and group counseling may be needed. Rehabilitation programs should be structured to allow gradual resumption of control by the patient for such things as medications, appointments, and health records. Transitional living programs allow time to learn or relearn the social skills necessary for independent living. It may be helpful to arrange for contacts with older, more experienced disabled persons who are successfully rehabilitated and living independently. Staff expectations should be realistic to allow frequent successes. Every new skill mastered, every small hurdle overcome, will help restore a positive attitude.

As with the other complications of bed rest, the best prevention is early mobilization and as short a hospital stay as possible.

BIBLIOGRAPHY

Browse NL: *The Physiology and Pathology of Bed Rest.* Springfield, Thomas, 1965.
This easily readable monograph reviews the literature on the effects of bed rest. An interesting historical review of attitudes toward rest introduces the book. There are numerous illustrations and references.

Deitrick JE, Whedon GD, Shorr E: Effects of immobilization upon various metabolic and physiologic functions of normal men. Am J Med **4**:3-6, 1948.
A classical article describing the altered calcium and protein metabolism and other physiologic effects in four healthy young men who were immobilized in plaster casts in bed for 6 weeks.

Fisher SV: A literature review: the energy cost of ambulation in health and disability. Arch Phys Med Rehabil **59**:124-133, 1978.
The energy cost of walking and the effects of prosthetics, orthotics, and ambulation aids on energy demands are reviewed.

Fordyce WE: Psychological assesment and management. *In* Krusen FJ, Kottke FJ, Ellwood PM (eds): *Handbook of Physical Medicine and Rehabilitation.* Ed 2, Philadelphia, Saunders, 1971, pp.168-195.
This chapter reviews the psychological reaction to disability and dependency. Strategies for psychological assessment and management are presented, with a discussion of the role of behavior modification techniques in rehabilitation.

Gordon, EE: Energy costs of activities in health and disease. Arch Intern Med **101**:702-713, 1958.
This article reviews the energy requirements of normal and handicapped persons during many ordinary activities and various occupations.

Kottke FJ: Therapeutic exercise. *In* Krusen FH, Kottke FJ, Ellwood PM (eds): *Handbook of Physical Medicine and Rehabilitation.* Ed 2, Philadelphia, Saunders, 1971, pp.385-428.
This chapter reviews the pathology of contracture formation and the clinical assessment and management of contractures. Several helpful diagrams supplement the text.

Muller EA: Influence of training and of inactivity on muscle strength. Arch Phys Med Rehabil **51**:449-462, 1970.
A good review of the data on muscle strengthening exercises and disuse atrophy. The author has been prominent in exercise physiology for many years, and pioneered the concept of isometric exercise.

5 SPINAL CORD INJURY

William H. Donovan, M.D.

DISEASE DESCRIPTION

The vast majority of individuals paralyzed as a result of spinal cord injury are young. Recent studies have shown that while the mean age of spinal cord injured patients is about 30 years, the median age is 25 years, and the age groups most represented lie between 18 and 21. Therefore, most patients are attending or have dropped out of high school, or they have completed high school and have embarked on college education or employment. Because they generally survive the injury with intact cognitive faculties, they still have potential vocational careers ahead of them.

The incidence of spinal cord injury in the United States is about 25–30 new injuries per million population per year. The data on accidents responsible for spinal cord injury show that the automobile has accounted for 35 percent of all spinal cord injuries, falls 15 percent, gunshot wounds 10 percent, and diving accidents 6 percent.

Spinal Cord Anatomy

The spinal cord lies within the vertebral canal formed by the vertebrae of the spinal column (see chap. 3). The spinal cord iteself does not occupy the entire length of the vertebral canal, but rather ends at the level of the L1 vertebra (fig. 5-1). Openings (intervertebral foramina, see fig. 3-21, p. 35) between adjacent vertebrae lie along both sides of the vertebral column, through which motor and sensory spinal nerve roots exit from the spinal cord and course outward to various parts of the body. Nerve roots derived from the cervical and thoracic part of the spinal cord leave the vertebral canal through intervertebral foramina close to their origin. On the other hand, roots exiting the spinal cord around and below L1 travel first down the vertebral canal to their respective intervertebral foramina before exiting. These nerve roots are referred to as the *cauda equina*.

The neural tissue within the spinal cord consists basically of nerve cells and nerve fiber tracts. Fiber tracts, in particular the corticospinal tract, carry motor, or movement, messages down the spinal cord *from* the brain to the gray matter (anterior horns)

within the spinal cord. The anterior horn cells within the spinal cord then transmit impulses out the anterior

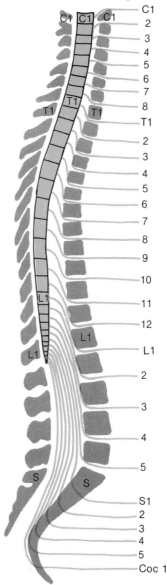

FIGURE 5-1. Relationship of spinal nerve roots to vertebrae. Termination of spinal cord is at the level of the L1-L2 vertebrae.

spinal roots to the muscles. Sensory messages from the skin and other tissues enter the spinal cord via posterior spinal roots and travel up the spinal cord *to the brain* (see chap. 3). When a complete spinal cord injury occurs, impulses cannot be transmitted either down or up fiber tracts past the point of injury. The extent of the resultant paralysis and sensory loss is determined by the level of the injury. Table 5-1 lists the most important muscles and the functions they serve at each of the spinal cord levels.

The first important nerve roots, cervical 3 and 4 (C3 and C4), travel via the phrenic nerve to the diaphragm. The action of this muscle accounts for approximately 75 percent of the lung's breathing capacity and the intercostal muscles between the ribs account for the remaining 25 percent. Injuries below C4, therefore, spare the respiratory function and individuals are able to breathe adequately to sustain life.

The remaining cervical nerve roots and the first thoracic nerve root (T1) innervate the muscles of the upper extremities. Spinal cord injuries affecting any segment between C3 and T1 will produce impairment of function in the upper extremities, a condition called *quadriplegia*. However, the arms do not have to be completely paralyzed for quadriplegia to exist. Rather, quadriplegia is present if any of the segments of the spinal cord (C5–T1) which innervate the arms are involved.

The thoracic nerve roots innervate the upper and lower intercostal, the abdominal, and the middle back muscles. Lumbar nerve roots and the first sacral root innervate the muscles of the lower extremities, and the remaining sacral nerve roots innervate the bowel, bladder, and the muscles controlling continence and sexual function. Injuries to the spinal cord below T1 will therefore spare the upper extremities, and the spinal cord impairment is referred to as *paraplegia*.

Sensory impulses carry information from the skin and other tissues via peripheral nerves and the spinal roots into the spinal cord and then to the brain. Sensory innervation also has a segmental distribution which corresponds to the sensory nerve roots of the spinal cord. The distribution of sensation served by each root is shown in figure 5-2.

Mechanism of Spinal Cord Injury

Considerable force is necessary to disrupt the bones and ligaments of the vertebral column. A bone fracture, a dislocation (caused by the disruption of ligaments between individual vertebrae), or both may result from a severe trauma. When this happens, the normal configuration of the vertebrae, one on top of the other, is altered, and the spinal cord lying within the vertebral canal becomes bruised, crushed, or torn (fig. 5-3). The degree of the disruption of the vertebral column determines how severe the injury to the spinal

cord will be, and whether sensation and voluntary muscle movement below the level of the lesion will be completely or only partially lost.

Following this initial trauma, several things may happen that can increase the severity of the injury. The disruption of the vertebral column may lead to instability at the injury site. Abnormal movement may then be possible in this area, and further damage of the spinal cord can occur if care is not taken to immobilize the patient adequately when he is being rescued. Secondly, the tissues around the spinal cord and within the spinal cord itself react to the injury by swelling. This swelling (edema) reaches a peak at around 48 to 72 hours after injury. The swelling at the injury site may further compromise function in the spinal cord in areas adjacent to the injury. Thus, paralysis may worsen 2 or 3 days after the injury if steps are not taken to reduce the development of edema.

Therefore, proper management of the patient during the acute phase of spinal cord injury is most important, since the spinal cord does not have the ability to regenerate. If the cells and fiber tracts within the spinal cord are completely destroyed at the time of injury, no recovery of function below the level of the lesion can be expected. However, if the same tissue is only partially damaged, then function may still be present below the level of the lesion at the time of injury and some further recovery of function may occur after the stage of spinal shock has passed. Obviously, then, every effort must be made to prevent further damage to the spinal cord as a result of instability, edema, or hemorrhage during the rescue and acute phase of treatment.

Spinal shock is a condition not only of paralysis and sensory loss, but also absence of reflexes below the level of injury. It generally lasts from several days to several weeks. When it has passed, reflexes will return. If the injury is in the region of vertebrae T12, L1, L2, or below, reflexes in the legs cannot return because the afferent and efferent components within the cauda equina are damaged. If reflexes return *before* voluntary function is present, it likely that voluntary function will never develop and the lesion is complete. In such an instance, the spinal cord injury interrupted all tracts to and from the brain. Commands originating in the precentral gyrus of the frontal lobe of the cerebrum cannot be transmitted across the defect, and total paralysis occurs below the level of the lesion. Similarly, sensory information originating from those parts of the body which transmit impulses through nerve roots entering the spinal cord below the level of the lesion will be unable to travel past the injury site to the thalamus for relay to the parietal lobe. Therefore, total loss of sensation (anesthesia) will result.

Frequently, however, a lesion will be referred to as being incomplete. This can mean either of the following:

1. A localized portion of the spinal cord may be

TABLE 5-1
MUSCLES SUPPLIED AND FUNCTIONS SERVED BY SPINAL NERVE MOTOR ROOTS

Root Segment	Representative Muscles	Function Served
C1 & C2	High Neck Muscles	Aid in head control
C3 & C4	Diaphragm	Inspiration (breathing in)
C5 & C6	Deltoid	Shoulder flexion, abduction (arm foward, out to side)
	Biceps	Elbow flexion (elbow bent)
C6 & C7	Extensor Carpi Radialis	Wrist dorsiflexion (back of hand up)
	Pronator Teres	Wrist pronation (palm down)
C7 & C8	Triceps	Elbow extension (elbow straight)
	Extensor Digitorum Communis	Finger extension ("knuckles" straight)
C8 & T1	Flexor Digitorum Superficialis	Finger flexion (fist clenched)
	Opponens Pollicis	Thumb opposition (thumb brought to little finger)
	Interossei (intrinsics)	Spreading and closing the fingers
T2–T6	Intercostals	Forced inspiration (breathing in) Expiration (breathing out, coughing)
T6–T12	Intercostals	Forced inspiration (breathing in)
	Abdominals	Aid in expiration (coughing) Aid in trunk flexion (sitting up)
L1, L2, L3	Iliopsoas	Hip flexion (thigh to chest)
	Adductors	Hip adduction (thigh to midline, legs together)
L3 & L4	Quadriceps	Knee extension (knee straight)
L4, L5, S1	Gluteus Medius	Hip abduction (thigh out to side, legs apart)
	Tibialis Anterior	Foot dorsiflexion (foot up, walk on heels)
L5, S1, S2	Gluteus Maximus	Hip extension (thigh in line with trunk, hips straight, e.g., standing)
	Gastrocneumius	Foot plantar flexion (foot down, walk on toes)
S2, S3, S4	Anal Sphincter	Bowel function (fecal continence)
	Urethral Sphincter	Bladder control (urinary continence)

totally unable to transmit messages in either direction, while the remainder of the cord is near normal. Examples of this include (a) the *Brown-Sequard syndrome,* in which one side of the cord is functional while the opposite side is not; (b) the *anterior spinal artery syndrome,* in which the anterior two-thirds of the spinal cord is nonfunctional while the dorsal one-third is functional; (c) the reverse of this, namely, the *dorsal column syndrome;* and (d) the *central cord syndrome,* which applies to lesions, usually in the cervical region, where the internal or central portion of the cord is nonfunctional but the periphery is functional. Examination of figure 3-10, p. 26, will reveal which tracts and parts of the spinal cord are involved in each type of incomplete lesion. In pure examples of any of the four conditions

listed, tracts in unaffected areas are normal and the sensory or motor functions which they serve are also normal.

2. The cord is diffusely injured. Such a lesion is considered incomplete because certain nerve tracts are still functioning, but in an abnormal way. For example, the part of the corticospinal tract to the lower extremity might be only partially interrupted, producing less than normal strength in the legs.

Spinal cord injuries are also described as upper motor neuron lesions or lower motor neuron lesions. Generally, bone injuries above the T12–L1 vertebrae, where the spinal cord terminates, leave reflexes intact below the lesion. Such lesions are termed *upper motor neuron lesions.* The paralyzed leg muscles still have

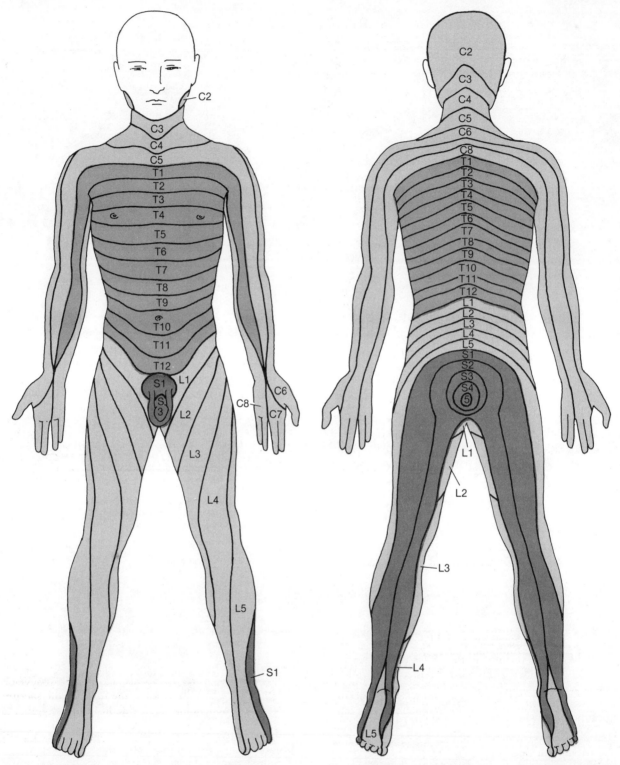

FIGURE 5-2. Main areas of skin sensation served by the sensory components of each spinal nerve. Some overlap into neighboring segments also exists. *(A)* Front view. *(B)* Back view.

reflexes. On the other hand, when the lesion occurs either *around* the T12, L1, L2 vertebrae or below, thereby destroying the lowest portion of the spinal cord (the *conus medullaris*) or the cauda equina, the afferent and efferent components of reflex arcs are interrupted. Therefore, the paralyzed extremities will be without

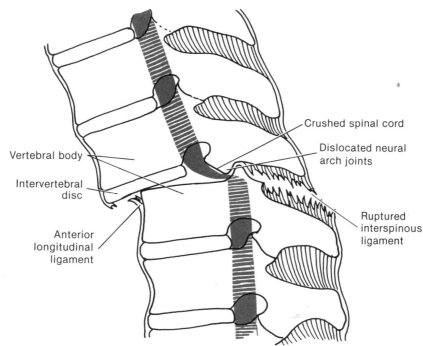

Crushed spinal cord

Dislocated neural
arch joints

Vertebral body

Intervertebral
disc

Ruptured
interspinous
ligament

Anterior
longitudinal
ligament

FIGURE 5-3. Vertebral dislocation with rupture of disc and posterior interspinous ligaments. Neural arch joints are totally dislocated. Spinal cord is crushed and angulated by the displacement.

reflexes. This is referred to as a *lower motor neuron lesion* since the symptoms result from destruction of anterior horn cells or their axons.

Complications

Paralysis and anesthesia, the primary results of spinal cord injury, whether partial or complete, may lead to the development of complications in other areas of the body. These complications are listed below, and some of them will be discussed in more detail later.

Acute phase (first month).

1. *Respiratory*: (a) infection in the lungs (pneumonia); (b) collapse of all or part of a lung (atelectasis); (c) occlusion of the pulmonary artery (pulmonary embolism) from blood clots arising from veins of the legs or pelvis (thrombophlebitis) which break off and float to the lungs (pulmonary embolus); (d) need for tracheostomy for assisted or improved breathing.

2. *Gastrointestinal*: (a) gastrointestinal bleeding, usually caused by ulcers in the stomach which can be related to stress; (b) absence of intestinal movement (paralytic ileus) which accompanies spinal shock and interferes with nutrition.

3. *Genitourinary*: (a) infection of the kidney (pyelonephritis); (b) distention of the bladder, due to plugging of a catheter or inadequate frequency of catheterization; (c) urethral fistulae due to improper positioning of urethral catheter; (d) formation of abnormal solidified masses of mineral salts (calculi),

either in the bladder or in the kidneys, due to the high content of calcium in the urine following paralysis.

4. *Cardiovascular*: (a) sudden increase of blood pressure, with profuse sweating and flushing (autonomic dysreflexia), usually caused by overdistention of the bowel or bladder; (b) lowered blood pressure when changing from a supine to an erect position (orthostatic hypotension), due to the inability of blood vessels to accommodate rapidly to change in posture and maintain an adequate blood pressure; (c) inflammation of veins followed by formation of blood clots (thrombophlebitis).

5. *Skin*: (a) pressure sores (decubitus ulcers), due to an inability of the patient to shift his weight because of paralysis, and the absence of pain appreciation when lying too long without moving. Patients with complete lesions are liable to develop skin breakdown over bony prominences due to sustained pressure on the skin for long periods of time. These ulcers are likely to develop over the buttocks, the sides of the hips, or the sacrum (low back), depending upon whether the individual is spending most of his time sitting, lying on his side, or lying on his back. They are also likely to develop over the heels, knees, and other bony areas (see fig. 4-4, p. 61).

6. *Musculoskeletal*: (a) abnormal formation of calcium in muscles surrounding joints (myositis ossificans); (b) loss of range of motion of joints (contractures), which may occur if the joints are not moved by a therapist or other person; (c) vertebral column instability.

Chronic phase (usually after 1 month).

1. *Respiratory*: (a) pneumonia; (b) lung collapse (atelectasis); (c) pulmonary embolus (less likely to occur beyond 3 months from the date of injury).

2. *Genitourinary*: (a) pyelonephritis, calculi, and urethral fistulae must always be guarded against, even in the chronic phase; (b) infection of the prostate gland (prostatitis) and infection of the epididymis and testis are ever-present possibilities in males, particularly those who have indwelling catheters in their bladders; (c) urine from the bladder flowing back up towards the kidneys (urethral reflux) can develop, particularly in bladders that are infected.

3. *Cardiovascular*: All the complications listed above for the acute phase are likely to develop in the chronic phase.

4. *Skin*: Formation of pressure sores is a persistent source of concern at any time in the chronic phase.

5. *Musculoskeletal*: Fractures of the long bones, particularly of the legs, secondary to osteoporosis; contractures; myositis ossificans; and vertebral column instability with pain are problems that can also occur in the late stages.

6. *Neurologic*: (a) abnormal painful sensations below the level of the lesion (paraesthesia); (b) excessive sweating (diaphoresis), together with autonomic dysreflexia; (c) spasticity, an exaggerated involuntary reflex activity of paralyzed muscles, can be a serous, functionally-limiting complication in upper motor neuron lesions.

FUNCTIONAL DISABILITIES

Physical Disabilities

As one might infer, the physical limitations in a spinal cord injured patient vary greatly depending upon the level of the lesion. Impairment of some or all of the following functions is present: personal hygiene (i.e., bathing, grooming, and socially acceptable bowel and bladder function); ambulation (bipedal or wheelchair); transfers (i.e., movement on and off beds, chairs, and toilets, in and out of cars and tubs); dressing; eating; writing; and automobile driving. The higher the level of the injury, the more extensive the disabilities. In appropriate treatment facilities, many of the disabilities originally present can be completely or partially removed through adaptive techniques and training. The level of performance at any time, either before or after treatment, is characterized by one of the following:

1. *Independence*. The activity can be physically performed with consistency and safety by the patient alone, without anyone else in the near vicinity.

2. *Needs standby assistance*. The patient can physically perform the activity, but not consistently. Therefore, someone needs to be there during the activity to ensure safety.

3. *Needs partial physical assistance*. The patient can perform most of the activity himself consistently and safely, but cannot complete the activity without some physical assistance.

4. *Total dependence*. For the activity to be part of the patient's repertoire, someone else needs to perform nearly all of the task for him.

The following discussion considers these functions for each injury level and indicates what functions are impaired as a result of the injury and to what degree they are removed with appropriate treatment. Table 5-2 summarizes this in more detail.

At all injury levels genital sexual functions are impaired. (Page 78 in Total Treatment details these impairments and chapter 21 discusses approaches to treatment.)

Sacral (S2, S3, S4) levels. Only bowel and bladder function is initially impaired with injuries at these levels. With appropriate treatment, the patient can obtain complete independence in the execution of these functions.

Lumbosacral (L5, S1, S2) levels. Initially, bowel, bladder, and ambulation functions are impaired. Complete independence in bowel and bladder function is achieved through appropriate treatment. Independence in bipedal ambulation is also restored with the assistance of two canes or two crutches and sometimes short leg braces (ankle-foot orthoses, AFO). Prolonged standing may remain impaired. No wheelchair is necessary.

Lumbar (L1, L2, L3, L4) levels. Initially, bowel, bladder, and ambulation functions are impaired. With treatment, bowel and bladder function can become independent. Bipedal ambulation can become independent for short distances. Wheelchairs are also used, in which the patient develops complete independence.

Thoracic (T7–T12) levels. Initially, personal hygiene, ambulation, transfers, dressing, and driving are impaired. Complete independence in bowel and bladder function can be achieved. Independent bipedal ambulation is usually achieved only for exercise, and complete independence in wheelchair ambulation is achieved. With training, transfers, dressing, and driving become independent.

Thoracic (T2–T6) levels. Initially, personal hygiene, ambulation, transfers, dressing, and driving are impaired. With extensive treatment, the patient can become independent in all of these functions. The ambulation achieved is by wheelchair.

Cervical (C7, C8, T1) levels. Initially, personal hygiene, ambulation, transfers, eating, dressing, writing, and driving are impaired. Almost all patients in this group become completely independent, with extensive treatment, in all functions consistent with

TABLE 5-2
FUNCTIONAL EXPECTATIONS AND EQUIPMENT REQUIRED
FOR SPINAL CORD INJURY PATIENTS
(Levels indicate lowest functioning nerve root)

Activities	C5	C6	C7–C8	T1–T5	T6–T12	L1–L3	L4–S1
Self-care:							
Eating	D/P_1	P_2	P_2/I	I	I	I	I
Dressing	D	P/I	P/I	I	I	I	I
Toileting	D	P_2/I	P_2/I	I	I	I	I
Work with hands:							
Writing	D	P_2	P_2	I	I	I	I
Typing	$P_{1,3}$	$I_{2,3}$	I_3	I	I	I	I
Operating telephone	P	I	I	I	I	I	I
Bed Independence:							
Rolling over; sitting up	$P_{4,5}$	P_5/I	I	I	I	I	I
Wheelchair Independence:							
Transfers to/from wheelchair	D	P/I	I	I	I	I	I
Propel wheelchair	I_6	I_7	I	I	I	I	I
Ambulation	O	O	O	D_8	P_8	I_9	I_{10}
Driving with hand controls	P	I	I	I	I	I	I
Public transportation:							
Bus	O	O	O	O	O	O	P/I
Train	D	D/P	P	I	I	I	I
Plane	P	I	I	I	I	I	I
Public toilets	O	P_{11}	P_{11}	P_{11}	P_{11}	$P_{11,9}$	I

LEGEND

I   Complete independence is possible
P   Partial independence is possible with use of special equipment
D   Dependence is to be expected
O   Not possible

1   With electric or CO_2 powered splints
2   With nonpowered hand splint
3   With electric typewriter
4   With loops, balkan frame—electric bed
5   With electric bed
6   With electric wheelchair
7   With adapted hand rims (special lugs or hose wrapped)
8   Not practical
9   With long leg brace and crutches
10   With short leg braces and crutches
11   With zipper-back wheelchair

living alone. Independent ambulation is by wheelchair. For some patients, however, personal hygiene may require partial physical assistance, transfers may require standby assistance, and dressing may require partial physical assistance.

Cervical (C6) level. Initially, all functions are impaired. Only a small number of patients achieve complete independence in all functions, and living alone is not practical even for these patients. The majority require partial physical assistance for personal hygiene. Wheelchair ambulation is independent. Transfers require standby assistance and dressing requires partial physical assistance. Complete independence is achieved in eating, writing (although slower than usual), and driving.

Cervical (C5) level. Initially, all functions are impaired. With extensive treatment, independence in electric wheelchair ambulation is achieved and nearly full eating skills are achieved. Total physical dependence remains for personal hygiene, transfers, dressing, writing, and driving.

Cervical (above C5) level. Initially, all functions are impaired. In addition, the breathing function is severely compromised. Training in the use of special respiratory equipment is required. The patient remains totally physically dependent for all functions, although some self-propulsion in an electric wheelchair is possible.

Psychosocial Disabilities

In addition to their physical disabilities, it is well recognized that spinal cord injured patients usually suffer psychosocial disabilities as well. Patients and their families must make a tremendous adjustment to the sudden changes in their lives. Patients must come to accept their physical disabilities and learn to function as independently as possible as handicapped persons in a world full of normal people who have very little concept of the architectural and attitudinal barriers that the disabled must face.

Both patients and their families are likely to make this major adjustment if they receive the appropriate guidance and continued counseling from all members of the treatment team, beginning as soon as possible after the injury. From the beginning, emphasis is placed upon the positive, i.e., things that patients *can* still do or learn to do rather than the negative, i.e., those activities which are now impossible. If the hospital staff, the family, and the counselor focus their attention on the positive and offer the patient support for every task completed along the rehabilitation pathway, constant brooding over residual deficits is less likely to persist.

Generally speaking, the injury heralds the onset of a crisis phase and a significant reduction in activity caused by the abrupt onset of paralysis. Significant emotional problems are common during the first few days and weeks thereafter. Frequently, they are accompanied by a mixture of disorganization and depression. As time goes on, the emotional crisis state should abate. If this state seems to continue excessively, it usually means that the environment either supports the depression or fails to provide a viable alternative.

Depression at this stage is to be expected. If it does not appear, one should strongly suspect that the patient has not yet accepted the reality of the situation. He may be thinking or verbalizing that ''this really didn't happen to me'' or ''the doctors overemphasize the importance of all this and I'm going to walk out of here regardless of what they say.'' Depression may therefore be considered a ''good sign'' in that it generally means that the patient is no longer denying the reality of the situation. This reactive depression seldom requires pharmacological management unless it interferes with treatment. Intervention of the rehabilitation team generally consists of encouraging the patient to behave in ways that are appropriate to his disability — that is, to acquire behaviors necessary for successfully facing life as a disabled person.

The rate or degree with which an individual incorporates these behaviors and succeeds in increasing his activity during the rehabilitation phase depends to a large extent on his preinjury personality. If he was prudent, careful, and persistent in the past, his chances of success are greater. If he was careless, imprudent, and reckless, as many persons who sustain spinal cord injuries are, the rehabilitation phase will be more difficult. If his personality was primarily motor-manipulative centered and he viewed the world of physical movement and sports as primarily reinforcing, it will be more difficult for him to adapt to a life of relative immobility than for a person who is either symbol centered or interpersonal centered.

For some, persistent use of denial mechanisms may become a significant psychological problem. Such patients are prone to achieve less satisfactory rehabilitation results and less than optimum continuing good health, and are more prone to medical complications through carelessness.

Finally, social and financial problems are common. The costs are high, and the disruption of family and social roles is extensive.

Rehabilitation Potential

As discussed above, capabilities of spinal cord injured patients will vary widely. Their overall ultimate functional ability will depend upon the level of the lesion and residual muscle function, the extent and success of their rehabilitation training, their psychological adjustment to disability, their overall general medical health, their preinjury vocational or educational progress, and their postinjury educational and vocational progress. When these factors are known, a vocational counselor may plan long-term vocational goals for his client. The lesion itself does not become progressively worse and long life can be anticipated.

If a counselor follows the patient's course while he is still in the rehabilitation center, he will understand how these factors are developing. If the client is referred at a later stage, the counselor can still understand the progress of these factors from a careful review of what has occurred. If it appears that mobility training is being impeded by the appearance of medical complications, or the patient is remaining depressed longer than anticipated and is still uninterested in pursuing vocational goals, then short-term contingencies might best be planned. If these short-term goals are met, and a pattern of meeting the short-term goals is established, long-term plans can be made.

STANDARDS OF EVALUATION

Acute Phase

Ideally, when a patient is admitted to a spinal cord injury center with an acute injury he should have the services of at least four medical specialists available to him: the neurosurgeon, the orthopedist, the urologist, and the physiatrist or rehabilitation specialist. Additional consultation may also be needed from a plastic surgeon and an internist, depending upon the patient's initial problems.

If an acutely injured patient is brought directly to the Emergency Room of the spinal cord injury center, the initial attending physician is either the neurosurgeon or the orthopedist, with the others acting as consultants. Either surgeon will determine the extent of paralysis, initiate protective measures for the paralyzed parts of the body, and make decisions regarding surgery.

Attending physician responsibility usually shifts in a spinal cord injury center to the rehabilitation specialists within 4 weeks after injury, with the other physicians assuming consultative roles. During this initial period, evaluations are performed by a social worker, clinical psychologist, rehabilitation nurse, vocational counselor, physical and occupational therapists, and frequently by an orthotist and speech therapist as well. While acute care is sometimes administered away from a rehabilitation center with later transfer to the facility, it is considered less optimum because collective expertise is more likely to exist at the special facility.

Postacute Phase

Following the evaluation, and under the leadership of the physiatrist or rehabilitation specialist, the spinal cord injury team meets collectively and formulates initial treatment goals with respect to medical treatment needs, ultimate bowel and bladder systems, ambulation, transfers, dressing, eating, and personal hygiene skills, emotional, social and family support systems, and initial vocational directions. An initial treatment plan directed toward these goals is formulated and instituted with the patient.

A continuing evaluation of treatment, including goal modification, continues until initial discharge, with collective review by the team members in concert with the patient and his family on a weekly or biweekly basis.

While increasingly less frequent, some spinal cord injured patients receive acute treatment and some rehabilitation care at a community hospital incompletely staffed with the professionals common to a rehabilitation or spinal cord injury treatment center and present themselves to a vocational counselor without the prior benefit of comprehensive rehabilitation treatment. To ensure the achievement of maximum function, the counselor should receive an evaluation at a medical rehabilitation center where a collective review can be performed by a medical rehabilitation physician and his medical consultants and, in addition, at least a clinical psychologist, social worker, and physical and occupational therapists, together with the patient and the counselor. Such a review can be achieved on an outpatient basis or during a short inpatient stay.

Maintenance

During rehabilitation in a spinal cord injury center, the patient should have acquired skills and necessary equipment appropriate for the level and degree of completeness of his lesion so that he is as independent as possible. He should be in excellent general medical health. He should have had a chance to interact with the staff, his peers, and normal individuals outside the hospital in a meaningful way so that he is prepared to meet the world as a disabled person. He should have developed some appropriate mechanisms to cope with the fact that he is different from most people, yet possess the confidence and feeling of self-worth necessary to carry on a meaningful existence. He should have acquired the knowledge and skill necessary to maintain his general health. This includes taking prescribed medications and carrying out vital techniques and routines, such as performing push-ups in the wheelchair to relieve pressure on his skin, performing a bowel program to maintain bowel continence, and following the necessary steps to ensure that his bladder will remain as free of infection as possible. Finally, he should have had a sampling of some work-related experience in order to develop the skills necessary to carry on a work or school routine once discharged.

Maintenance of health and achieved goals and possible further enhancement of goals requires continuing followup evaluation, particularly to abort potential medical or psychosocial complications (see above). This evaluation includes periodic evaluation by knowledgeable rehabilitation physicians and necessary allied health staff at least three to four times the first year, or more often if required. Urological re-evaluation at least twice a year initially and once a year thereafter is essential.

TOTAL TREATMENT

Acute Phase

Important factors in the early medical treatment of the spinal cord injured patient include:

1. Support of respiration. Sometimes a tracheostomy must be performed in quadriplegics or high paraplegics with chest injuries to prevent complications associated with lung collapse (atelectasis), such as pneumonia and lung abscess.

2. Maintenance of blood pressure.

3. Maintenance of adequate urine output and adequate drainage of the urinary bladder, since the inability to void can be predicted with virtual certainty.

4. Protection of the anesthetic skin by adherence to a frequent turning schedule so that pressure sores (decubiti) do not develop over bony prominences.

5. Maintenance of range of motion of all the joints in the paralyzed portions of the extremities so that rigid contractures do not develop and interfere with mobility training.

6. Appropriate attention to the gastrointestinal tract, including close observation and immediate treatment of stomach ulcers and hemorrhages, should they develop, and the institution of an appropriate

bowel program to ensure effective and predictable elimination once bowel activity has resumed.

7. Institution of appropriate measures to prevent pooling of blood in the veins (venous stasis) due to loss of muscle activity in the legs, which may in turn lead to the development of thrombophlebitis and, subsequently, to pulmonary emboli if a clot in a vein should break off, flow through the heart, and lodge in a lung.

In addition to the precautionary measures just given, a physician in charge of the acutely injured patient must decide on the preferred method of treating the spinal cord itself. This will in large part depend upon (a) the nature of the injury and related trauma; (b) the mechanism that produced it; (c) whether it is a complete or an incomplete lesion; and (d) whether the vertebral column is stable or unstable and needs surgery.

An example of an acute treatment regimen for a cervical spinal cord injury might include the insertion into the skull of tongs to which traction can be applied to distract and realign the bony elements of the cervical vertebrae. If distraction in this way does not result in realignment, the physician may try to realign the vertebrae by manipulation under anesthesia. He may decide to keep the patient in tongs in bed on a special frame for at least 6 weeks, or alternatively, to operate and fuse the adjacent injured vertebrae in the area of the spinal cord injury with a piece of the patient's own bone, generally taken from the pelvis. When this bone graft fuses (usually by 6 to 12 weeks), stability of the injured vertebral column is usually assured so that further trauma to the spinal cord will not ensue. If this decision is made, the individual is generally kept in bed for another 2 weeks postoperatively, followed by immobilization in a protective cervical collar. Whether fusion is carried out or the patient is kept in bed on a frame with or without tongs, a collar is generally worn for a period of 6 weeks once mobilization has begun, and usually the patient can gradually be weaned from the external protective device.

Typical management for paraplegia is similar in concept to the above and will differ according to the same variables. Since an injury in the area of the junction of the thoracic and lumbar regions (i.e., at T12–L1) is often unstable, a decision to fuse the adjacent vertebrae may be made. Realignment of the bony fragments is again often attempted either preoperatively or operatively. Injuries within the thoracic region are often stable without surgery because the adjacent vertebrae are attached to each other via the ribs. However, if multiple rib fractures are also present, this stability is often lost and surgery is attempted. Various metal implants such as ''Harrington rods'' and ''Weiss springs'' are often used at surgery to provide internal immobilization of the vertebrae of paraplegics.

Generally speaking, if a lesion is incomplete and the patient is improving, surgical intervention is deferred, since a stabilization procedure can be done electively at a later date, and the patient would have a longer bed rest period. If the patient acutely develops a progressively higher level of paralysis, immediate investigations must be carried out to determine if there is increasing pressure developing on the cord that should be relieved. This can be accomplished by (a) realigning the vertebrae; (b) removing material pressing on the cord, such as disc material, bone chips, or hematoma; or in some instances, (c) removing the roof (lamina) of one or more vertebrae. In addition, steroid medication intended to prevent or reduce swelling of the spinal cord in response to the injury is also given within 72 hours. Change in the neurologic status might occur under circumstances where the spinal cord is compressed further because an unstable lesion developed a progressive bony deformity or a cyst developed within the spinal cord. In most instances this does not occur and the level of paralysis remains unchanged. It should be realized, however, that a patient's general medical condition can deteriorate from complications that may develop in other areas of the body, such as the lungs, kidneys, or skin.

Other than relieving pressure on the cord, controlling edema, and attempting to restore stability, one must await the results of time and natural healing processes to determine the ultimate residual deficits.

Rehabilitation Phase

The postacute treatment or rehabilitation phase is concerned with the specific treatments to achieve the goals established by the staff with the patient and his family in (a) bladder function, (b) bowel function, (c) skin care system, (d) psychological adjustment, (e) social, family, and home planning, (f) vocational planning, (g) ambulation and transportation, (h) transfers, (i) eating, (j) dressing, (k) personal hygiene, and others as may be necessary.

Bladder function. The ideal end result in bladder training is to achieve a sterile urine free of bacteria; a balanced bladder; a system for voiding which is socially acceptable and does not soil clothes; the absence of the need for a catheter; and maintenance of the anatomical integrity of the kidneys, ureters, bladder, and urethra.

The ideal is not always achieved. While bacteria may not be completely eliminated from the urine, excellent control and prevention of actual infection manifested by real sickness is, in almost all instances, possible with appropriate antibiotics. A bladder is said to be balanced when the amount of urine voided at any one time is much larger than the amount of urine left in the bladder (residual urine). The usual requirement is a residual urine that is no more than 25 percent of total bladder capacity.

The current preferred technique of working toward

the goals listed above is the use of intermittent catheterization until urine begins to flow and the bladder empties by itself or with appropriate stimulation by the patient. Electrical and other devices for stimulating the bladder for voiding or for control of the sphincter are likely to be available in the near future. With intermittent catheterization the urine can be maintained sterile. A less desirable technique is the use of the continuous indwelling Foley catheter to drain the urine until such time as the physicians deem trials at voiding are feasible. The catheter is then removed and voiding trials begin in an effort to work toward a balanced bladder. The urine cannot be maintained sterile while the indwelling Foley catheter is in place. With intermittent catheterization about every 4, 6, or 8 hours, the patient can have a nearly normal fluid intake. With an indwelling Foley catheter, the patient must consume large volumes of fluid, up to three liters per day, to dilute the bacteria. In addition, he often must use an irrigant to prevent crusts from attaching to the catheter and must ensure the maintenance of a low urine acidity through appropriate medication. Other factors that contribute to the achievement of a balanced bladder and a socially acceptable voiding system vary at the different levels of injury.

The prevention of the complication of autonomic dysreflexia, particularly in lesions above T6, deserves special mention. Autonomic dysreflexia is often induced by an overly distended bladder which triggers off the sympathetic nervous system, causes the blood pressure to increase to dangerous levels, and is associated with a pounding headache. Educating the patient in the control and prevention of this potentially dangerous complication is necessary.

Determination of the best bladder emptying system depends upon the neurological exam, the character of the bladder reflexes as assessed by cystometrogram (CMG) tests, the character of the urethral sphincter, and the general health of the urinary tract. The latter is assessed by urinanalysis, bacterial culture of the urine, and an excretory urinary (intravenous) pyelogram (IVP or EUP). An EUP is a special X-ray test to visualize the kidneys, ureters, and bladder, and a cystogram is another special X-ray test to visualize the bladder. Very often a movie-type X-ray film of the actual process of the emptying of a dye instilled in the bladder is also performed.

Bowel function. The development of socially acceptable regular bowel elimination is often easily achieved as long as the patient maintains proper diet and fluid intake, and avoids foods and infections that are productive of diarrhea. If diarrhea occurs, soiling is inevitable. Control of the anal sphincter is affected by spinal cord injury, but the reflexes for bowel function are not particularly disturbed. The patient controls the timing of elimination through the use of special suppositories (e.g., Dulcolax) and digital distention of his anal sphincter, coupled with the ingestion of food shortly before the elimination. Stool softening medications (e.g., Colace) can also help.

Skin care system. In areas where the skin is anesthetic, particularly over bony prominences, the patient is unable to appreciate when too much pressure has been sustained for too long. Unrelieved pressure for a length of time sufficient to squeeze blood out of the skin will cause skin breakdown. Ulcers produced in this way must be studiously avoided because they severely interfere with the patient's independence and often confine him to bed for extended periods. They may even require surgical closure. Initially, the patient must be periodically turned and moved by the staff and nurses to relieve pressure on skin areas susceptible to breakdown. Later, the patient is trained how to do this himself or to have others assist him, so that periodic relief over pressure areas is achieved.

Psychological adjustment. Psychological treatment consists of assisting the patient through a depression phase and helping him to curtail the use of denial mechanisms to handle the stress of the illness, particularly if such mechanisms are interfering with his ability to learn how to care for himself and move actively toward achieving rehabilitation goals. Therapeutic tools available are those dealing with operant behavior modification techniques, individual counseling with patient and family members where appropriate, and group therapy techniques. These and often other methods, coupled with increasingly intense forays into the public, help the patient to make a satisfactory social and vocational adjustment.

Social, family, and home planning. The patient and his family are actively involved with a social service worker who assists in the maintenance of stable interpersonal relationships and the family's relocation. (Psychological, social, and sexual issues are further discussed in chapters 2, 16, and 21.)

Vocational planning. Vocational planning builds on the patient's prior educational and vocational experience, his current interests and aptitudes, his ultimate levels of function and mobility after treatment of his spinal cord injury, and the nature of the labor market. While initially vocational explorations start at a low key, they build up to a crescendo as rehabilitation and functional goals are achieved.

Spasticity. Although control of spasticity is often not a specific goal in itself, spasticity is an issue that greatly interferes with functions such as ambulation, transfers, dressing, bladder function, and skin care. If the reflexes in the lower extremities below the level of the lesion become so hyperactive that they are difficult to control and therefore interfere with the above functions, specific treatment to reduce the intensity of these spasms is necessary. Current medications are Valium (diazepam) and Dantrium (dantrolene sodium). Other medications will certainly be developed in the future. If control by medication is insufficent, a so-called motor point block is performed, in which a dilute solution of phenol is injected into the small motor nerves close to the motor end plates of muscles. Sometimes it is even necessary to actually cut a nerve or a nerve root. In the most severe cases, a surgical procedure called a Bischoff myelotomy (a longitudinal section of the middle portion of the spinal cord on both sides) may be performed by a neurosurgeon. This operation is performed in the part of the spinal cord where there is paralysis, hence no additional weakness results. Maintenance of good general health is essential in the control of spasticity since it can be aggravated by any infection in the lower extremities (such as in the toenails), bladder infections, or skin sores of any sort.

Functional goals. The achievement of functional goals in ambulation, transportation, transfers, eating, dressing, and personal hygiene have as their basis the maximum strengthening of the muscles that are unaffected by the paralysis, the prevention of contracture in the parts of the body that are paralyzed, and the teaching of special techniques to utilize the remaining functional parts to assist the achievement of these skills.

Generally speaking, physical therapists assist in the development of ambulation and transfer skills, while occupational therapists ordinarily deal with the development of eating, dressing, personal hygiene, and transportation skills. Table 5-2 presents the ultimate optimum expectation for independence and the necessary aids in these main functional areas. Certain additonal comments with relation to the different levels of injuries are given below. In table 5-2 and in all of the following comments, the assumption is that the spinal cord injury is complete. If the spinal cord injury is incomplete, then achievable goals are greater than those listed. The level of spinal cord injury given refers to the lowest level that is still functioning and under voluntary control. This level, which is the more significant factor to consider, is not always synonymous with the actual level of the bone injury.

1. *Levels L5, S1, S2.* Ultimate bladder function is usually excellent in these patients. No catheters are needed. Elimination is usually accomplished by increasing abdominal pressure (bearing down). Residual urines close to zero are generally achievable. Since at these levels the sphincter might be weak, some dribbling may occur. If dribbling is significant, males may use an external collecting system consisting of a condom, a tube, and a collecting bag, and females might wear absorbent pads. In some instances, artificial sphincters can be surgically implanted. They are still relatively experimental and require the patient to inflate and deflate the artificial sphincter by squeezing hydraulic fluid through tubes and valves implanted under the skin. Bowel function results are quite good. Again, since sphincters may be lax, some

leakage may occur, and hence the patient generally might prefer a more constipated stool.

To circumvent the male patient's inability or difficulty in obtaining an erection, plastic devices such as dildos can be worn, or a prosthesis can be surgically implanted within the penis. Further, the erection mechanism can be influenced by surgery performed on the arterial and venous supply of the penis. Competent sexual counseling should be offered before any such procedures or devices are recommended so that the patients and their partners can assess their present attitudes and feelings toward each other.

Transfers, eating, dressing, and personal hygiene pose no problem.

The patient's ambulation is quite good, usually with two short leg braces (ankle-foot orthoses, AFO) that essentially "lock" the ankle joint. Two canes or crutches are usually required, although at the lower level one cane may be sufficient. Wheelchairs may be totally discarded in many cases. At the lower levels, automobile driving without special hand controls can be achieved, although hand controls may be preferred by some patients. No attendant care is necessary.

The rehabilitation phase of hospitalized treatment is about 1 month, usually no more than 2 months.

2. *Levels L1, L2, L3, L4.* At these levels urethral and anal sphincters are inclined to be spastic and tight. Bladder elimination is still usually accomplished by abdominal pressure, perhaps accompanied by dilatation of the anal sphincter, which also relaxes the urethral sphincter and permits complete emptying. External collecting systems for the male and absorbent pads for the female are less necessary. Bowel leakage is less of an issue, although diarrhea would still be a problem. Transfers, eating, dressing, and personal hygiene are independent after training.

Bipedal ambulation may now require above-knee orthoses (knee-ankle-foot orthoses, KAFO) and two crutches or perhaps even a walker. The gait pattern used may be the so-called four-point, swing-through, or swing-to gait. Wheelchairs at these levels are usually not discarded, particularly not at the higher level. Automobile driving requires the use of hand controls. No attendant is necessary.

The rehabilitation phase of hospitalized treatment is about 3 months, usually no more than 4 months.

3. *Levels T7-T12.* Bladder and bowel function is as above for the higher lumbar levels. However, bladder reflexes at these levels might be more active. External collecting systems for males and pads for females may therefore become necessary. If the sphincters are too tight, they may have to be surgically weakened with a sphincterotomy, particularly in males.

The higher the level between T7 and T12, the greater the loss of control over the abdominal and back musculature. Since these muscles are used for coughing, the higher the lesion, the less effective the cough. Therefore, these patients are at greater risk from respiratory infections.

Transfers, eating, dressing, and personal hygiene are easily achieved through training. Bipedal ambulation at these levels is less and less functional, and may only be used for exercise. Long leg orthoses(KAFO) and crutches are definitely required, but the wheelchair is the main mode of ambulation. Therefore, use of public toilets is restricted to those that are wheelchair accessible. Hand controls are required for automobile driving.

The rehabilitation phase of hospitalized treatment is about 3 months, usually no more than 4 months.

4. *Levels T2–T6.* Bladder elimination involves more direct triggering of the bladder reflexes as well as efforts at anal dilation. Control of leakage is generally more difficult and most patients wear external collecting systems all the time. Females may find that leakage is not controlled sufficiently by pads, and hence use of a continuous indwelling catheter with drainage to a leg bag may be required. Bowel function control is as above. Transfers, eating, dressing, and personal hygiene, while achievable, require much training.

Bipedal ambulation is no longer practical even for exercise, though some patients might choose it. The wheelchair is the main mode of ambulation. Hand controls and sometimes external trunk support are required for automobile driving. No attendant is necessary, although a roommate could be helpful.

The rehabilitation phase of hospitalized treatment is about 3 months, usually no more than 4 months.

5. *Levels C7, C8, T1.* At these levels, the hands and the wrists are beginning to become involved. Training now takes much longer because special adaptive equipment is needed and techniques need to be learned.

Bladder elimination is accomplished by stimulating the bladder reflex. Sphincterotomies are often necessary in males. External collecting systems in males are mandatory, and almost all females use a continuous indwelling Foley catheter. Autonomic dysreflexia may be a significant problem. Bowel function, particularly the insertion of suppositories and the use of digital stimulation of the anus, becomes more difficult, but can be achieved with a finger splint.

Modifications of the wheelchair to make propulsion easier may be required, such as applying friction tape, tubing, or projections on the hand wheel rims. Transfers usually require a sliding board, and double-width electric beds are helpful. Clothing modifications such as the use of snaps or Velcro will circumvent the difficulty these patients have with buttons. Dressing and personal hygiene may require partial use of an attendant for pants and total body bathing. Special adaptations of bathroom systems are required. Hand controls and sometimes steering wheel attachments are necessary for automobile driving.

The C7 level is the highest level compatible with no attendant whatsoever, although not all achieve this goal.

The rehabilitation phase of hospitalized treatment is about 4 months, usually no more than 5 months.

6. *Level C6.* The only remaining hand and wrist function at this level is extension or dorsiflexion of the wrist. The patient cannot forcibly extend his elbow. Preservation of full range of elbow motion is essential.

Bladder and bowel function is the same as for the C7, C8, and T1 levels. Eating skills are achieved with adaptive equipment applied to the hands, such as a wrist-driven flexor hinge splint that creates opposition of the second and third fingers by dorsiflexing the wrist, or a cuff worn over the hand with a slot for a spoon or fork.

Ambulation is still by manually operated wheelchair with modifications of the wheel rims as above, although in certain situations electric wheelchairs may be appropriate.

The completion of total dressing and personal hygiene usually requires an attendant. Some patients can achieve this independently with the aid of loops sewn onto the clothes into which they can hook a finger, but this may be too time consuming. Pull-over garments for the upper torso are usually preferable to buttoned shirts because of the difficulty with manipulation of buttons, snaps, and the like. If the arms are long enough, a sliding board is used for transfers. Transfers in and out of bed and on and off a toilet can be achieved, and car transfers can also be achieved by certain patients without assistance. C6 is the highest level compatible with automobile driving with hand controls at the current time. The use of special vans enhances this function. An attendant or at least a helpful roommate is usually required to assist with dressing, personal hygiene, and some of the bladder and bowel care functions. Such patients are not likely to be successful living absolutely alone.

The rehabilitation phase of hospitalized treatment is about 6 months, usually no more than 7 months.

7. *Level C5.* At this level the patient has shoulder and elbow flexion function but no wrist and hand function.

Bladder elimination is achievable if automatic reflex emptying can be developed. If automatic emptying does not occur, an attendant is required because the patient cannot assist in stimulating reflexes. For bowel function, an attendant must provide a suppository, and digital and cleanup function. Eating, except perhaps for cutting, can be developed with set up (i.e., food already cut, cartons opened and straws inserted), but transfers, dressing, and personal hygiene are literally totally dependent on an attendant.

Ambulation is by electric wheelchair which the patient controls by placing his hand on a stick mounted on the control box of the wheelchair on the same side as his stronger arm. Automobile driving is generally unlikely, but more specialized vans and operating techniques might allow this to be achieved. A full-time attendant is necessary to assist with the functions but need not be at the patient's side at all times. With appropriate seat cushions, these patients can sit for 8 to 10 hours a day with perhaps some pressure relief provided by the attendant.

Other adaptive equipment used by some patients with lesions at C5 includes battery-powered and cable-operated wrist-driven hinge splints, and ballbearing feeders (mobile arm supports) anchored to the wheelchair which allow the patient to feed himself and do some facial grooming. To operate the mobile arm supports, the patient places his arms in special troughs attached to movable hinged bars. By using the shoulder muscles, the patient can make the troughs swivel to bring his arms toward his body and move them out again, and also to tip the troughs downward at the elbow to raise his hands.

The rehabilitation phase of hospitalized treatment is about 3 months, usually no more than 4 months.

8. *Levels C2, C3, C4.* The C4 level is the last compatible with life, unless at the time of the accident assisted respiration was provided by someone in the vicinity. The C2 and C3 patients invariably require permanent assisted ventilation, as do some of the C4's. A battery-powered portable respirator can, for some, be fitted to the wheelchair. The C2 and C3 patients usually require a permanent tracheostomy and special techniques to control lung and throat secretions.

C2, C3, and C4 patients may be able to use a chin, mouth, or breath control device and perhaps a voice-controlled device to operate electric reclining wheelchairs. They may have greater control of their environment thorough so-called environmental control systems. In these systems, the patient can control a telephone, radio, television, lights, buzzer, and the like from one place. Selection of one of these options is made by using breath, mouth, sound, or residual muscle power to activate the system. A full-time highly skilled attendant is required for the patient, and probably should always be available near him.

The rehabilitation phase of hospitalized treatment is as long as 6 to 8 months or longer because of the need to develop a rather complex physical and social environmental support system.

Sexual Function

Sexual functioning is another area that is affected by spinal cord injury. While many aspects of sexuality, including sexual libido, production of sex hormones, feelings of sexual attraction to potential partners, and the ability to be sexually attractive to others are essentially undisturbed by spinal cord injury, certain areas of sexual behavior will be disrupted. As with other functions disrupted by a spinal cord injury, modifications will be needed in the spinal cord injured

person's techniques of behaving sexually. Nonetheless, the psychic, hormonal, and many of the physical aspects of a love relationship are still present and available to the spinal cord injured person.

Physical aspects of the love relationship such as the involvement of the senses of vision, smell, and touch via oral or manual contact still exist for spinal cord injured persons. Areas in which sensation is preserved that were previously erogenous to the person will remain so. Such areas might, in fact, have heightened erotic meaning to the person after his injury. Very often, the transition area between normal sensation and no sensation acquires a heightened erotic feeling, and if the lesion is incomplete, some sensory areas below the main level of paralysis may also have heightened erotic feeling. Sensation in the genital area itself requires an intactness of the second, third, and fourth sacral nerves. Thus, almost no spinal cord injured person will have direct appreciation of touch or contact in these areas. Some of the higher lumbar nerves around the upper thigh approach the genital area and might convey genital-like sensations. Spinal cord injury does alter physical mobility, and therefore will alter the "gymnastic" aspects of sexual interactions and will necessitate modification of technique.

Genital sexual functions of the male may be broken down into erection, seminal emission into the urethra, and forceful ejaculation of the semen. Erection is controlled by the parasympathetic nerves, emission by the sympathetic nerves, and ejaculation by the regular motor nerves. The achievement of a full orgasmic experience requires a coordination and integration of these three nervous system functions. This coordination occurs in the spinal cord and is dependent upon higher centers. The coordination of these nervous systems is thus very much reduced in high spinal cord injuries, but becomes more and more possible with lower injuries. Therefore, the fertility rate for males with lumbar lesions is higher than for males with cervical lesions, but in both cases it is well under 10 percent.

Reflex erection is usually possible for all spinal cord injured males with lesions at about T12 and above. Mechanical stimulation can produce and sustain an erection. In some males with lower thoracic and upper lumbar level lesions, physically produced weak erections can occur. Lumbar lesions, particularly if they involve the cauda equina, will interfere with the development of a full reflex erection, but may allow for a less intense psychic erection which may or may not be strong enough to allow for vaginal intromission. Since emission depends upon sympathetic nerve function, it may appear without intense ejaculation in males with lumbar lesions. Ejaculation does not appear in males with lesions at any level, although some techniques have evolved which, although somewhat dangerous, have been successful in producing ejaculation. Despite the absence of ejaculation, some sexually active spinal cord injured males do report an orgasmic-like experience associated with a certain amount of sexual tension release.

As with spinal cord injured males, females with spinal cord injures may develop sensory areas that convey heightened erotic meaning. Lubrication of the vaginal area will be inconsistent and may necessitate the use of additional lubrication. While females will reflexly exhibit engorgement of the clitoris (equivalent to erection in males), they will not exhibit the spasmodic contractions of the perineal and vaginal musculature (equivalent to ejaculation). The absence of the latter orgasmic experience is sometimes replaced, as in the male, by an orgasm-like experience associated with a release of sexual tension. Female fertility is generally undisturbed by spinal cord injury. Immediately after an injury, menstruation may cease temporarily, but then return in a regular pattern. Thus, spinal cord injured females can conceive and carry a fetus to term. A spinal cord injured female who chooses to do this needs careful medical attention during pregnancy, since there is an increased risk of certain complications during pregnancy and delivery. For females who do not wish to conceive, birth control methods must be considered carefully, as the problems associated with some of them may be increased in spinal cord injured women.

It should be obvious that a spinal cord injured person can develop a long-term interpersonal relationship including love, respect, affection, and a mutually satisfying sexual relationship with another person. As with able-bodied persons, the development of such a relationship requires communication and mutual understanding between the partners involved. Counseling by informed professionals may be helpful to facilitate communication between partners, to help them consider exploring alternative sexual behaviors, to provide accurate information regarding sexual functioning, and to give specific suggestions for modifying sexual techniques.

Post-Rehabilitation Followup

Regular medical outpatient followup is essential for spinal cord injured persons for the remainder of their lives in order to ensure that they have a long life-span. The purpose of the regular medical followup is to maintain good general medical health and, in particular, to avoid the complications discussed above, especially skin ulceration and kidney disease. Maintenance and modification of drugs is also a regular part of the followup. A complete evaluation of the urological system must be done at least once a year, if not more often. Attained rehabilitation goals need to be monitored and upgraded and new techniques developed for further functional improvement. Attention to psychological and social aspects of the person's life can anticipate problems or correct those that have developed. Furthermore, followup keeps the person abreast of the development of new adaptive devices that can continually enhance and upgrade his vocational potential.

VOCATIONAL IMPLICATIONS

Because the effect of spinal cord injury is so pervasive, a counselor must look carefully at education, interests, and aptitudes, as well as physical requirements.

Education

Plans for long-term vocational goals requiring further education should include consideration of the client's general health, his level of functional independence, his adjustment to disability, and his interest, aptitudes, and intelligence. Since spinal cord injury itself in no way affects the cognitive processes, the counselor must decide whether to support a training or educational program on the basis of factors that would be important in vocational planning for any individual, handicapped or not. Some of these, such as emotional stability and medical conditions, have already been discussed. If intellectual and vocational testing disclose candidacy for further schooling, and other considerations are favorable, every effort should be made to encourage the client in this direction, because the more education he has, the more employable he becomes. However, no rules that would apply to all situations can be given. Each case must be weighed individually.

Aptitudes

Impairments of intellect, learning ability, verbal skills, numerical skills, form and space perception, or motor coordination, which one would expect to encounter in diseases involving the brain, are not seen unless the client sustained head injuries in addition to the spinal cord injury.

Factors to be considered regarding a client's ability to perform in a given work situation include (a) his ability to sit for long periods of time, which in turn depends on his skin tolerance, the stability of his vertebral column, the fit of his wheelchair, and his general strength and endurance; and (b) the appropriateness of his equipment. Since quadriplegic clients have difficulty using their arms, their ability to function at a desk will critically depend upon the segmental level of their lesions and the adaptive equipment which is available, including splints, special handles or holders, tape recording equipment (dictating equipment), and the like. For example, a complete C6 quadriplegic would have difficulty lifting a telephone because flexors of the fingers are absent. However, if an L-shaped attachment were placed on the telephone receiver under which he could slide his hand, he could support the attachment between the index finger and the thumb and be able to use the receiver. Similarly if he had a "dialing stick," held with the aid of a wrist-driven flexor hinge splint, he would be able to dial the telephone using the muscle power remaining at the shoulder.

Interests

In addition to factors discussed earlier, the counselor should be cognizant of the client's likes and dislikes in vocational and avocational areas, his ability to learn and perform new tasks, his ability to interact with people pleasantly, and his ability to handle stress. Ideally, the vocational counselor should have a chance to observe the client at a spinal cord injury center during a simulated work experience, or at least in several occupational therapy sessions, to determine how well he functions in carrying out activities which are well mastered compared with those just learned or still unlearned.

From his own knowledge of the client acquired through testing and interview, as well as first-hand information about performance, the counselor will be in an ideal position to form plans and construct some long- or short-term goals with the client. The counselor should also be aware of the fact that interests do change. Quite often, for example, a turbulent emotional reaction to disability will gradually crystallize into acceptance, and new interests in work or school will appear. A client may agree to use adaptive equipment to permit performance of a work-related task although he had previously rejected such equipment. If he succeeds in this effort, further interest in work experience may follow. Interests incompatible with the client's physical function because of the paralysis cannot be developed.

Physical Demands

In attempting to match a client to the physical demands of a job, the counselor must first consider the segmental level of the injury and whether the lesion is complete or incomplete. Clients with low-level spinal cord injuries who require only AFO's may easily be able to work in situations that require walking from place to place on level ground or negotiating a few steps. However, activities that require stooping, bending, climbing, or standing for a long time would be inadvisable.

Clients with lesions at higher levels who are able to ambulate with KAFO's should generally be considered for work that can be carried out from a wheelchair, since they will probably not be able to remain standing for long periods. Their ability to tolerate the upright position will depend upon the stability of the vertebral column around the fracture site, the presence or absence of deformities in the lower extremities, the amount of standing balance, the fit of the braces, and the condition of the skin (especially around the feet and knees), as well as general strength and endurance. Since these factors will vary widely among individuals, one should generally plan for the majority of the work to be done from the sitting position with standing permitted as tolerated. Occasionally, a strap attached to the work bench at both sides and placed behind the client's buttocks aids standing balance. It should also be borne in mind that even though a client with long leg braces may be able to walk, he may actually prefer not to because of the energy required and the demand on the heart and lungs. Further, any walking requires crutches and the hands are not free to carry objects.

Clients with lesion levels from T12 up through T6 may also be able to walk with long leg braces for short distances but will not be able to walk functional distances because of cardiovascular demands. Therefore, they also must be considered only for activities that can be performed primarily from the wheelchair. Counselors should be aware of the architectural barriers that may exist in many work situations and should ascertain the accessibility and location of elevators, toilets, cafeteria, and parking lot. For males with external urine collection devices and females who remain odor free with the use of absorbent pads, lack of access to public toilets or toilets in the place of employment is not catastrophic, since males can empty the collection bags and females can change the absorbent pads in any area which offers privacy. However, for those individuals who are continent even though they may not have control of urination, and who therefore are able to get along without catheters or collection devices, it is important that at least one toilet be wheelchair accessible where they are working or attending school. Lacking this, a commode can be placed in a room where privacy is afforded so the individual can empty his bladder.

The same considerations apply to clients with lesion levels higher than T6, i.e., T6 through C3, who will rely solely on a wheelchair. If an attendant or other person can provide the C4 quadriplegic with transportation, work outside the home certainly is possible. All activities must be handled from a wheelchair and the amount of activity will be limited. Schooling is certainly within the realm of possibility, providing a tape recorder is available for preserving notes. Since use of the hands is not possible in any work-related activity, special adaptive equipment will be needed to operate a telephone or electric typewriter or any other tool in conjunction with the job.

C4 or C3 quadriplegics can be expected to have diminished vital capacity and may require ventilatory assistance administered through a mechanical respirator mounted on the wheelchair. Clients with lesions at C4 and above will not be able to use their hands and will require telemetric equipment and probably the presence of an attendant in the work or school environment. Any work or school situation, therefore, must be considered in terms of its wheelchair accessibility.

Clients with lesions below C7 can be considered for some outside work if their wheelchairs are equipped with air-filled, treaded tires rather than solid rubber ones. Paraplegics, in general, can handle a wheelchair adequately outdoors, although rough ground, gravel, or grass may pose insurmountable problems. Clients who ambulate with AFO's and crutches can work even longer times outdoors, occasionally even in inclement weather.

Quadriplegic and high paraplegic clients have difficulty with body heat regulation, and therefore the temperature of the work environment should be considered. These clients have difficulty conserving heat in a cold climate because the blood vessels of the skin do not constrict normally. Similarly, they have difficulty losing heat in a hot environment because they are unable to perspire normally.

The circulation and the cleanliness of the air should also be considered, since clients with quadriplegia and high paraplegia have difficulty with forceful expiration and coughing. In a dusty work environment, more mucus than normal is secreted in the bronchial passages. Because they will have difficulty raising this sputum, quadriplegics will be more liable to develop respiratory infections if they must work in these conditions.

In most instances, consideration of a sheltered workshop will not be necessary except for a client with high quadriplegia for whom a job in the competitive market commensurate with his physical limitations cannot be found. It must be borne in mind that if workshop activity is considered, the client should be informed and assured in advance that, even though many of those about him might be mentally retarded or brain damaged, he will not be compared with them from an intellectual point of view, he will be adequately protected from individuals who may be subject to uncontrolled outbursts, and there will be adequate supervision and attention to his particular needs. Utilization of quadriplegics in some administration activities of the sheltered workshop or other charitable organizations might prove advantageous in some instances.

BIBLIOGRAPHY

Fordyce WE: A behavioral perspective on rehabilitation. *In* Albrecht, GL (ed): *The Sociology of Physical Disabiltiy and Rehabilitation.* Pittsburgh, University of Pittsburgh Press, 1976, pp. 73–95.

The principles of psychologic approaches to the disabled patient, including the spinal cord injured patient, are explained very clearly and concisely. This is an excellent chapter for individuals who have had only limited exposure to the rehabilitation of the physically disabled.

Fordyce WE: Behavioral science and rehabilitation. Rehabil Psychol 21:82–85, 1974.

This reference will provide the reader with an overview of psychologic principles and how they can be specifically applied to the spinal cord injured. Research horizons in psychologic management methods are also explained.

Glenn, JW, Miller KH: Voice terminal may offer opportunities for employment to the disabled. Am J Occup Ther 30:309–312, 1976.

Discussion of the feasibility of employing the severely disabled in the information industry. Description of a computer terminal that has been developed which is operated entirely by voice, obviating the necessity of using the hands.

Goldberg RT, Freed MM: Vocational adjustment, interests, work values, and career plans of persons with spinal cord injuries. Scand J Rehabil Med 5:3–11, 1973.

Twenty-one spinal cord injured patients (ages 18–60) were assessed for their vocational development through interviews both pre- and postinjury. The interview also included diagnosis, severity of disability, age, education, level of function, months since injury, and level of verbalization. The best predictors of vocational adjustment are discussed and ranked.

Hohmann GW: Psychological aspects of treatment and rehabilitation of the spinal cord injured person. Clin Orthop 112:81–88, 1975.

Discusses the stages a spinal cord injured person goes through in accepting disability, namely, denial, depression, withdrawal and internalized hostility, externalized hostility, and reaction against dependence. Also discusses pain, sexual function, family, and the importance of using Spinal Cord Injury Centers for treatment.

Long C II: Congenital and traumatic lesions of the spinal cord. *In* Krusen FH, Kottke FJ, Ellwood PM (eds): *Handbook of Physical Medicine and Rehabilitation.* Ed 2, Philadelphia, Saunders, 1971, pp. 566–578.

An excellent introduction to the medical problems encountered by spinal cord injured patients. It deals further with treatment methods discussed in this text and with functional expectations. Problems faced by patients with congenital spinal cord dysfunction are also discussed.

Long C II, Lawton EB: Functional significance of spinal cord lesion level. Arch Phys Med Rehabil 36:249–255, 1955.

This reference describes in further detail the functional capabilities of spinal cord injured patients and the muscles needed to perform various tasks. It is a bit outdated as far as the functional performance of quadriplegics is concerned, but principles discussed and therapeutic goals given for paraplegics are still valid.

Miller DK, Wolfe M, Spiegel MH: Therapeutic groups for patients with spinal cord injuries. Arch Phys Med Rehabil 56:130–135, 1975.

Spinal cord injured patients were given the option of attending a short-term therapeutic group designed to help them adjust to their disability by receiving information and discussing experiences and feelings. Knowledge and attitude before and after the group experience were measured and compared with those of non-group members. The value of group therapy as an effective means of disseminating information and aiding patients' adjustment is assessed.

Romano MD, Lassiter RE: Sexual counseling with the spinal cord injured. Arch Phys Med Rehabil 53:568–572, 1972.

Description of a sex education and counseling program for both male and female spinal cord injured patients. Both sensory and motor changes as a result of injury, common problems and concerns, and some helpful adaptations are discussed.

Symington DC, Boyd E, Vasa J: Rotating table for the high level quadriplegic. Arch Phys Med Rehabil 55:481–483, 1974.

Description of a table with a rotating top on which several pieces of eqiupment can be mounted. A high-level quadriplegic can use a mouth wand to rotate the table and operate the equipment independently.

Symington DC, McKay DW: A study of functional independence in the quadriplegic patient. Arch Phys Med Rehabil 47:378–392, 1966.

This is a more up-to-date representation of the performance capabilities of quadriplegics than is provided in the article by Long and Lawson cited above. It is well written and the tables are quite useful.

Talbot HS: Management of neurogenic dysfunction of the bladder and bowel. *In* Krusen FH, Kottke FJ, Ellwood PM (eds): *Handbook of Physical Medicine and Rehabilitation.* Ed 2, Philadelphia, Saunders, 1971, pp. 634–642.

Problems of bowel and bladder management in the spinal cord injured patient and how to overcome them are discussed. This chapter will give the reader a clear understanding of how elimination techniques are performed and what and how equipment is used to make these tasks easier or possible. The physiology of micturition is also discussed.

6 NEUROMUSCULAR DISEASES

Paul J. Corcoran, M.D.

INTRODUCTION

Included in this chapter is discussion of a group of diseases that affect the motor system at one of several points (fig. 6-1). The reader should review the basic anatomy and physiology of the nervous system in chapter 3 for a better understanding of these disease mechanisms. This somewhat arbitrary grouping includes the following neuromuscular diseases:

1. Huntington's disease
2. Parkinson's disease
3. Spinocerebellar degeneration
4. Friedreich's ataxia
5. Amyotrophic lateral sclerosis
6. Spinal muscular atrophy
7. Poliomyelitis
8. Guillain-Barré syndrome
9. Myasthenia gravis
10. Muscular dystrophy

The impairments produced by this group of disorders are limited mainly to the motor system, causing weakness or clumsiness on voluntary motion, as well as troublesome involuntary movements in some cases. Except perhaps in the later stages of the first five diseases discussed, communication is generally unaffected. In all the diseases, sensation is generally not affected and pain is not a major problem. With the exception of poliomyelitis and Guillain-Barré syndrome, these are progressive diseases whose causes are unknown.

Six other neurological diseases that affect movement are of sufficient medical complexity and vocational importance that they are treated in separate chapters: spinal cord injury (chap. 5), peripheral neuropathy (chap. 7), multiple sclerosis (chap. 8), stroke and cerebral trauma (chaps. 9 and 10), cerebral palsy (chap. 11), and epilepsy (chap. 12). These six disorders produce a variety of other neurological limitations in addition to the motor system impairments described in this chapter. There are, however, a number of areas of similarity or overlap.

It should be kept in mind that many persons with neuromuscular diseases do not fit neatly into any of the classical disease categories to be described in this chapter. Physicians often use the suffix "-opathy" to help describe, as best they can, those diseases which cannot be more precisely labeled. Thus the rehabilitation counselor will meet expressions such as "myopathy associated with neoplasm" or "encephalomyelopathy related to vasculitis." An understanding of the classical patterns, however, will provide a framework for dealing with those clients who fall into these "gray areas."

Specific evaluation and treatment measures are discussed under each disease category and a general philosophy of management is presented in the summary at the end of the chapter.

HUNTINGTON'S DISEASE

Disease Description

Huntington's disease is also called Huntington's chorea or chronic progressive chorea. It is a hereditary disease of the brain with onset usually in adult life, characterized by jerky involuntary movements (chorea) and mental deterioration. Most cases begin between ages 30 and 50, although occasional cases have begun in childhood or old age. It is quite rare in the general population (3 to 6 cases per 100,000 population), but it may be more common in certain communities where families affected with the disease happen to live. It persists in these communities because of its strong hereditary tendencies and the fact that it does not usually become severely disabling until after child-bearing age. For example, over 1,000 cases have been traced to 2 brothers who emigrated to Long Island from England about 200 years ago.

The direct cause is unknown. Autopsies show widespread degeneration throughout the brain, with shrinkage of the brain tissue and enlargement of the fluid-filled cavities (ventricles) inside the brain. Severe degenerative changes are found in the basal ganglia, the deeply lying relay stations for nerve tracts that control movement (see p. 21).

The first clinical signs of the disease are usually the jerky involuntary "choreiform" movements. These abrupt, sudden, jerky movements can occur in any of the muscles of the trunk or limbs, as well as the head

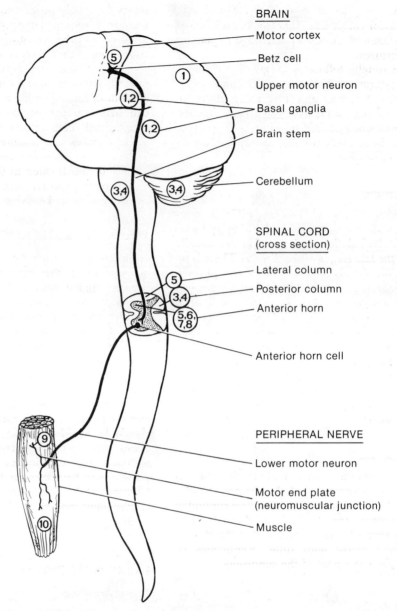

FIGURE 6-1. Major components of the motor system. Numbers refer to the sites of pathology associated with the 10 diseases covered in this chapter: 1. Huntington's disease; 2. Parkinson's disease; 3. Spinocerebellar degeneration; 4. Friedreich's ataxia; 5. Amyotrophic lateral sclerosis; 6. Spinal muscular atrophy; 7. Poliomyelitis; 8. Guillain-Barré syndrome; 9. Myasthenia gravis; 10. Muscular dystrophy.

ation, usually begins later but sometimes appears years before the involuntary movements start. There is progressive impairment of memory and intellectual functioning, impulsive behavior, and personality changes with neglect of business affairs and personal hygiene. Fits of violence sometimes occur, and suicide is much more common than in the general public or in unaffected siblings. This suggests that

and face muscles. They are increased in intensity by emotional stress or concentration on performance of physical tasks; they diminish when the person is sitting quietly, and disappear during sleep. In the early stages of the disease, the patients are often able to mask the involuntary movements as mannerisms or "the fidgets."

The other major manifestation, mental deterior-

suicide is due to the mental deterioration and impulsive behavior rather than to a fear of the disease, as was once suggested. A small percentage of patients will develop seizures.

The disease usually follows a progressive downhill course. The duration between onset and death averages 15 years but may be considerably shorter or longer. Death seldom results from the disease directly, but is more commonly caused by injuries, infections, overindulgence in alcohol, suicide, or other results of the mental deterioration.

Functional Disabilities

Highly skilled functions become difficult after several years, and help is needed in dressing and self-care activities. Ambulation and transfers are usually retained until the late stages of the disease. There is no true paralysis, but the involuntary movements plus the mental deterioration impair physical performance. The ability to go out alone and use public transportation is eventually lost. The speech becomes thick and hard to understand, but hearing and vision are retained intact. The social consequences of the bizarre involuntary movements and organic mental deterioration result in greater and greater dependence on family members. Lacking a social support system, patients are commonly institutionalized in the later stages of the disease.

Rehabilitation Potential

Short-term rehabilitation potential may be good, in view of the slow progression of the disease. Skillful redirection of the vocational path may allow continued productivity within the limitations that develop. However, the counselor may assume that the disease will get steadily worse with time. Remissions or improvement are not a part of the syndrome.

Standards of Evaluation

A neurologist should see patients, and can usually make the diagnosis without much difficulty from the family history and the characteristic involuntary movements. Extensive neurological tests are usually not necessary. A psychologist should assess the presence or degree of organic mental deterioration. A social worker can evaluate the family and social support system. An occupational therapist is helpful to assess whether the performance of activities of daily living could be facilitated by training of the patient or family members.

Total Treatment

There is no known treatment that will halt or slow down the steady progression of Huntington's disease. Certain tranquilizing drugs sometimes decrease the severity of the involuntary movements. Genetic counseling of the family is of great importance to allow the patient and any as-yet-unaffected children or other relatives to make an informed decision about the wisdom of having children. An occupational therapist can help the patient or family with techniques to simplify self-care activities. Counseling support and social services are usually needed by the families. Psychiatric intervention directly with the patient is not usually of much value in organic mental syndromes, except perhaps to recommend drugs that might help control antisocial behavior.

Vocational Implications

Short-term training or education may be appropriate in the early stages, where evidence of organic mental deterioration is absent. It should be remembered that many years may go by before the client becomes incapacitated or unable to continue work. Clients can be expected to gradually lose their aptitude for intellectual work or fine manual dexterity. The client's interests should probably be encouraged in the direction of routine, structured tasks without excessive emotional stress or job tension. Physical demands may be medium to heavy, but jobs involving climbing, balancing, or handling dangerous materials should be avoided. There is no particular reason to avoid extremes of temperature, humidity, noise, or air pollution. Clients with more advanced stages of the disease may have obvious limitations in verbal skills, learning ability, memory, or dexterity. Sheltered employment may be the highest practical goal at this stage.

PARKINSON'S DISEASE

Disease Description

Parkinson's disease ("paralysis agitans," "parkinsonism," or "shaking palsy") is a progressive disease of older adults characterized by muscle rigidity, slowness of movements, and a unique type of tremor. There is no actual paralysis, and the word "paralysis" or "palsy" in the names of the disease are misnomers. The usual age of onset is 50 to 70; the disease is rare prior to age 40. It is a relatively common disease, having a prevalence of about 187 cases per 100,000 population. It is estimated that 1 in 40 persons alive today will contract the disease. Since it affects an older age group, its prevalence increases as the population ages. There is a slight familial tendency.

Pathological findings in advanced cases include extensive degenerative changes in the basal ganglia. Degenerative changes are also found in the cerebral cortex and often in the brain stem.

The cause is unknown. Many cases in the past occurred in persons who survived the encephalitis epidemic of 1918 through 1923. This type of "encephalitis lethargica" is rare today, and is not likely to be a cause of current cases. Arteriosclerotic changes in the cerebral blood vessels are related to the disease, but the two conditions do not always coexist. Occasional cases follow poisoning with carbon monoxide, heavy metals such as manganese, or overdoses of certain tranquilizers and drugs. There is some experimental evidence of a deficiency in the neurotransmitter chemical dopamine in affected areas of the brain, a finding which led to the successful trial of the drug levodopa in treatment of Parkinson's disease.

The most prominent and disabling physical sign of Parkinson's disease is muscle rigidity. On passive movements, the muscles resist elongation, alternately yielding and tightening up to give a "cogwheel" sensation. Voluntary movements are impeded by the muscle rigidity, which leads to slowness of movement and greater effort, causing fatigue. Even the abilities to speak and write are impaired by muscle rigidity. The voice volume becomes low and handwriting becomes much smaller than normal.

A second group of physical signs is related to lack of spontaneous movements or difficulty initiating movements. Patients sit very still in their chairs, with few spontaneous changes in position or movements of the trunk or limbs. They blink less frequently and tend to have a mask-like, expressionless face. Intense concentration may be required to perform ordinary voluntary activities such as standing up or beginning to walk.

The tremor is the obvious sign that gave rise to the common names for Parkinson's disease, but is not as disabling as the rigidity and diminished movements. There is a characteristic to-and-fro tremor at a frequency of about three or four per second, often affecting only one extremity and later spreading to other extremities or the opposite side. The tremor can be suppressed for several seconds by concentration and voluntary effort, so that performance of fine activities of brief duration remains possible. There is no true paralysis, although some disuse atrophy results from the impeded movements. Sensation, vision, and hearing are unaffected. The speech may become faint and hard to understand due to low volume and stiffness of the speech muscles. There is no pain directly caused by the disease, but patients may complain of muscle aching and stiffness secondary to the rigidity.

The complications of the late stages of Parkinson's disease are complications of inactivity. The disease itself does not cause death, but patients may become immobilized, develop contractures, and become bedridden. Flexion contractures of the trunk and limbs

are a special hazard in patients with Parkinson's disease who do not exercise properly. Other complications are related to poor nutrition caused by the patient's difficulty feeding himself, or slowness of chewing and swallowing if being fed by another person. Institutionalized patients with Parkinson's disease may literally starve to death if overworked staff members do not have time to sit long enough to feed them.

The disease generally follows a rather slow course, with an interval of 10 to 20 years between the onset and severe disability. Remissions or spontaneous improvement do not occur. The progression may be temporarily slowed by surgical procedures or the new drug levodopa, but it is too soon to know whether the overall course of the disease will be affected.

Functional Disabilities

In the early stages of the disease, most functions can be performed independently. After several years, gait becomes slow and frequent falls may occur. Patients tend to stand and walk with a characteristic flexed, stooped posture. The ability to initiate transfer activities may be severely impaired. The muscle stiffness causes fatigue after minor exertion and limits work tolerance. The jerking and swaying of public transportation vehicles may make them unsafe for patients with poor balance or difficulty making sudden movements. Because each physical act requires concentration, patients find difficulty performing more than one physical task at a time. Self-care activities such as dressing and grooming may require a prolonged time, making it hard for some patients to arrive at work on time in the morning. Chewing and swallowing may be quite slow, requiring prolonged lunch hours. There is an increased rate of saliva formation which, together with the swallowing difficulty and the tendency to hold the head forward, may lead to drooling of saliva. Communication may be difficult due to the slowness of speech and low volume. The slow writing with tiny letters may cause handwriting to be hard to read.

Emotional changes, chiefly depression, commonly occur as one might expect with a major physical impairment. Occasionally there is mental deterioration or confusion, or personality changes with decreased drive and impaired judgment. Patients who become more and more dependent on others for self-care create stresses on their social support sytems, which may break down, leading to institutionalization in the later stage of the disease.

Rehabilitation Potential

Because of the gradual onset and slow progression of the disease, persons with Parkinson's disease have a good potential for rehabilitation. The counselor's expectation should be for a slow but steady progression of symptoms and deficits and he should plan in anticipation of further involvement. The future rate of progression is likely to be predicted by the past rate of progression.

Standards of Evaluation

The diagnosis can be made by any physician from the characteristic history and physical exam. There are no specific diagnostic tests that are helpful in Parkinson's disease. A neurologist can recommend the most appropriate medical treatment. A physiatrist may be useful to evaluate functional deficits such as gait and self-care, to assist the rehabilitation counselor with vocational recommendations, and to prescribe and oversee the physical management of the patient. A physical therapist can be helpful in evaluating limitations of gait and range of motion. An occupational therapist can assess self-care limitations. A psychologist may be helpful to assess the presence and degree of organic mental deficit or personality change. A social worker can provide valuable information about the family and support system.

Total Treatment

Optimal treatment of Parkinson's disease requires manipulation of several drugs and is ordinarily best done by a neurologist who should monitor the patient at intervals of no more than 3 to 6 months. The drugs levodopa and carbidopa are the mainstay of treatment at the present time. It may take several months to achieve the optimum therapeutic effect and to regulate the dosage. The symptoms of rigidity and decreased movements are benefited the most, while the tremor may persist. Many patients experience troublesome side effects, the commonest being nausea and vomiting, loss of appetite, a drop of blood pressure on standing up (postural hypotension), and development of involuntary movements of the limbs. These side effects usually are controlled by lowering the dosage and rarely require that the drugs be discontinued.

Another useful group of drugs, widely used prior to the introduction of levodopa and carbidopa, is the belladonna family of drugs. Their therapeutic effect is less powerful, and they too cause a number of side effects, such as hot flashes, dry mouth, blurred vision, and dizziness. A combination of a belladonna-type drug and levodopa in reduced dosage is effective for many patients. Antidepressant drugs may also be useful in despondent patients with a low energy level.

Surgical intervention was commonly practiced in the past, and included various neurosurgical procedures to destroy small areas within the basal ganglia to interrupt the pathways associated with the rigidity and tremor. These have been largely rendered obsolete by the success of levodopa.

The physical management of the patient is no less important than the pharmacologic management. A physical therapist should see the patient at regular intervals to supervise a daily routine of home exercises. These exercises are designed to maintain the range of motion in the joints and prevent contractures; to prevent deterioration of the muscle strength and gait; and to encourage normal speaking, writing, and deep breathing. Exercises do not alter the basic course of the disease, but they do maintain function and prevent the unnecessary additional complications of immobility. If contractures occur, particularly at the ankle, surgical correction is sometimes helpful in maintaining ambulation.

An occupational therapist can assist patients and family members to use simplified energy-saving methods of performing daily activities or employment activities, and can also suggest modifications for home and work environments. Short-term individual or group psychotherapy may be helpful, and psychoactive drugs may be needed from time to time. A social worker can help support the family and arrange for specific services as they are needed.

Vocational Implications

White collar jobs may be continued until the disease is relatively far advanced unless a large amount of speaking is required. Transportation to and from the office may be the greatest obstacle. Jobs requiring short-duration manual dexterity may also be continued. Heavy physical labor with a large amount of walking, carrying, and climbing may have to be changed earlier in the course of the disease. Since mental functioning is not usually affected, it may be feasible to retrain a physical worker to do a less strenuous and perhaps more skilled occupation. The major obstacles to learning are related to the age at which the disease usually appears, rather than directly due to the disease itself.

It should be remembered that the client will have diminished aptitudes for prolonged fine rapid movements of the hands or feet and is likely to develop diminished speaking abilities eventually.

Most interests may be encouraged. Interpersonal contacts of a sophisticated nature, such as those of a salesman, should perhaps not be promoted, since the low voice, mask-like face, and occasional drooling may interfere with this. Highly stressful occupations should probably be avoided, since emotional stress often increases the severity of the tremor.

The physical demands of an occupation may become limited to sedentary or light work levels. The slow movements and gait difficulty make it undesirable to have jobs involving climbing, kneeling, or working in dangerous environments. The muscle rigidity causes fatigue after moderate exertion, but frequent short rests will increase the total amount of work that can be done in a day. However, prolonged sitting in one position is to be avoided because it increases the stiffness and may promote contracture.

Certain environmental factors should be avoided. Cold working environments increase the stiffness of persons with Parkinson's disease. Heavy metal pollution in the air should be avoided, since this may be a contributing factor in the disease. Similarly, areas of concentrated vehicular traffic should be avoided because of the relationship between carbon monoxide poisoning and Parkinson's disease. Those clients who are troubled by excessive sweating should avoid working in a hot or humid environment.

SPINOCEREBELLAR DEGENERATION

Disease Description

The spinocerebellar degenerations are a family of hereditary diseases that affect, to varying degrees, the cerebellum, the brain stem, and the long tracts of the spinal cord. Those that affect predominantly the cerebellum and brain stem tend to begin in late middle life, progress more slowly, and have less of a familial tendency. The commonest are *olivopontocerebellar degeneration* and *cerebellar atrophy*. Certain other diseases in this family tend to affect the spinal cord to a greater degree than the cerebellum. These have an earlier age of onset (teenagers or young adults), a more rapid rate of progression, and a strong familial tendency. Common examples are *Marie's ataxia*, *Roussy-Levy syndrome*, and *Friedreich's ataxia*. The latter has sufficient individual characteristics and vocational implications to be considered separately (see p. 89).

The spinocerebellar degenerations are relatively uncommon. Degenerative changes and shrinkage involving the cerebellum, brain stem, and certain tracts of the spinal cord occur. Damage to these areas is associated with clumsiness and poor coordination. The spinal cord tracts most commonly affected are the posterior columns, which carry position and movement sensation up to the parietal lobe, and the lateral corticospinal (pyramidal) tracts, which carry the signals for voluntary movement from the frontal lobe (see p. 21).

The cause of the spinocerebellar degenerations is unknown. Symptoms usually include unsteady gait, clumsiness of the hands, thick slurred speech (dysarthria), weakness and easy fatigability of the limbs, and sometimes a tremor of the head or limbs. The tremor is usually brought on or increased by voluntary effort (intention tremor), and is usually absent when the individual is at rest. There is steady progression at a variable rate, but 10 to 30 years are usually required before the patient is severely incapacitated. Remissions or spontaneous improvement are rare.

Functional Disabilities

The ability to walk may be progressively impaired due to clumsiness and unsteadiness with frequent falls. After several years, patients may begin to use canes or crutches. In later stages, they use walkers or hold on to the walls or furniture. A wheelchair may be required for safe mobility in late stages.

Self-care and other hand functions become slow, laborious, and clumsy and may eventually require the assistance of another person. Speech may become difficult or impossible to understand, especially to those not acquainted with the patient. Handwriting also becomes less legible with increasing hand clumsiness. Vision and hearing are generally unaffected.

There are no specific mental or psychological changes. A certain amount of anxiety or depression may be seen, usually related to the extent of interference with ordinary activities and functional abilities. Intelligence and personality are unaffected. Family relationships may undergo strain as the patient becomes more dependent on others.

Rehabilitation Potential

These diseases tend to begin during the productive years of employment and have good rehabilitation potential because of their slow progression. They can be expected to worsen steadily over time, however, and the counselor should be aware of the deficits to be anticipated.

Standards of Evaluation

The diagnosis of spinocerebellar degeneration requires a skilled neurologist. It is important to rule out other diseases, such as tumors of the cerebellum, which may respond to appropriate treatment. The diagnosis is made from the characteristic history and physical findings, but more extensive neurological and laboratory tests may be required to rule out other, more easily treatable diseases.

A physiatrist should evaluate the patient to assess residual abilities and complications of inactivity, and to prescribe and supervise a physical restoration or maintenance program. A physical therapist can help evaluate gait, muscle strength, and use of ambulation skills, hand function, and the need for adaptive equipment. A social worker is important to assess the need for family counseling or outside agency intervention to maintain satisfactory social function of the family unit.

Total Treatment

There is no known medical or surgical treatment that has any effect on the course of spinocerebellar degeneration. A supportive family physician or physiatrist may be very helpful. Physical and occupational therapy will be needed from time to time to maintain function at the optimum level, or to train patients in the use of adaptive equipment that may become needed. The patient should have access to a social worker when specific needs for support arise. A genetic counselor may be helpful to inform the family about the risks of occurrence in the children of affected families.

Vocational Implications

Spinocerebellar degenerations do not affect intelligence, making these clients good candidates for appropriate retraining or education. Aptitudes for verbal skills and manual dexterity may be expected to deteriorate as the disease progresses. A variety of different interests are compatible with these diseases. Physical demands for medium to heavy work may be tolerated by most clients, as long as coordination is not essential. Jobs involving prolonged walking, climbing, balancing, and crawling should be avoided, as these skills may be expected to deteriorate. Similarly, jobs involving sophisticated verbal communication or fine hand function may not be appropriate. There are no particular environmental factors that need to be avoided.

FRIEDREICH'S ATAXIA

Disease Description

Friedreich's ataxia is a hereditary disease of unknown cause, usually beginnning in children or teenagers with signs of spinal cord and cerebellar degeneration. The average age of onset is 13, with a range from 5 to 25 years of age. There is steady deterioration, and many patients are severely incapacitated by the time they reach their middle twenties. Although the condition is relatively rare, it has important vocational implications because of the age group affected. With improved management and rehabilitation measures, patients are living longer than was previously supposed possible.

Friedreich's ataxia probably belongs in the family of spinocerebellar degenerations. The first signs are usually clumsiness and incoordination (ataxia), affecting the lower extremities first with unsteady gait and frequent falls. There is easy fatigability, and the muscles of the limbs may atrophy. A high arch may develop in the feet due to muscle imbalance. Hand clumsiness and thick, slurred speech (dysarthria)

develop. Muscle imbalance in the trunk may lead to curvature of the spine (scoliosis).

Some patients with Friedreich's ataxia develop progressive heart failure due to degenerative changes and scar tissue formation in the heart muscle. About 10 percent of patients also have diabetes mellitus. Occasionally there are disturbances of respiration and difficulties in swallowing. These medical complications or the affects of inactivity and bed rest are the causes of eventual death. The disease itself does not ordinarily cause death directly.

Functional Disabilities

Ambulation becomes progressively more unsafe and laborious. The use of crutches helps for a while, but a wheelchair is generally needed for ambulation within 5 to 10 years after onset. Self-care skills become progressively more difficult as hand clumsiness increases. The speech may become slurred and hard to understand. Psychological and social impairments as already discussed above for the other diseases are commonly seen.

Rehabilitation Potential

Short-term rehabilitation potential is good. Long-term potential is hard to predict because of the steady progression. The past rate of deterioration is the best predictor of the future course. Intelligence may be assumed to remain constant. With proper management, many patients can be expected to have 10 to 20 years of productivity ahead of them.

Standards of Evaluation

The diagnosis should be made by a neurologist who is skilled in differentiating other, treatable diseases which may present similar symptoms. A careful medical evaluation is also appropriate to detect associated heart disease or diabetes. A physiatrist can evaluate residual function and prescribe and oversee a program to correct unnecessary additional disabilities and maintain function at the optimum level. A physical therapist should evaluate muscle strength, joint range, and use of ambulation aids. An occupational therapist should evaluate self-care skills and adaptive equipment. Where pyschological or social impairments are prominent, evaluation by a psychologist or social worker is important.

Total Treatment

There is no specific medical or surgical treatment that is effective in altering the course of Friedreich's ataxia. Associated medical problems listed above may require appropriate treatment. A physiatrist can manage the restorative treatment, and physical and occupational therapy are important to maintain mobility and hand function. A social worker is usually a necessary member of the treatment team.

Vocational Implications

Intelligence and learning ability are unimpaired, but lengthy educational plans should be considered in light of the probable rate of progression. Aptitudes for fine hand skills, motor coordination, and verbal activities may be assumed to deteriorate steadily. A variety of interests is compatible with the limitations of the disease. Unlike the predominantly cerebellar members of this disease family, in Friedreich's ataxia muscle strength and exercise tolerance may diminish with time, limiting clients to light physical demands. Occupations demanding good balance or dangerous surroundings are probably inadvisable. The ordinary range of temperature, humidity, and air quality should be well tolerated.

AMYOTROPHIC LATERAL SCLEROSIS

Disease Description

Amyotrophic lateral sclerosis (ALS) is a progressive disease of adults causing degeneration of motor nerve cells and their axons, leading to replacement of corticospinal tracts by scar tissue (sclerosis). The disease attacks both the lower motor neuron—the anterior horn cell of the spinal cord and the motor cells of the brain stem and cranial nerve nuclei—and the upper motor neuron—the Betz cells of the precentral gyrus. For this reason the British call the disease "motor neuron disease." The corticospinal (pyramidal) tract runs down the lateral columns of the spinal cord, where its damage causes the so-called "lateral sclerosis" seen in cross sections of the cord.

The cause of the disease is unknown. Occasionally there is a familial tendency, but most cases are sporadic. The prevalance is about 5 cases per 100,000 population. The usual age of onset is between 30 and 60, and males are affected three times as often as females.

Initial symptoms and signs depend on whether upper or lower motor neurons are involved first and where the damage first strikes. Lower motor neuron involvement leads to weakness and atrophy, frequently presenting in one upper or lower extremity and later spreading to the other limbs or the facial and tongue musculature. If upper motor neuron damage predominates, there is spasticity and exaggeration of the tendon reflexes. Eventually, the spasticity disappears as the lower motor neurons are lost and the muscles undergo denervation atrophy. Difficulty speaking and swallowing commonly result from damage to the motor nuclei in the brain stem which control the tongue, face, and throat muscles. Affected muscles exhibit a constant fine twitching (fasiculations) due to spontaneous contraction of individual motor units. Sensation is unaffected by the disease and vision, hearing, and intellectual functioning remain normal. There is usually no disturbance of bowel or bladder function.

The disease pursues a steady, fairly rapid downhill course. The average duration from onset to death is about 4 years, with a range of 1 to 10 years. Death usually results from the complications of inactivity or from paralysis of the muscles of respiration.

Functional Disabilities

Functional disabilities depend on which muscles are affected at a given point in the disease. The pattern of involvement tends to be randomly scattered. Lower extremity involvement may cause weakness and easy fatigability, leading to the need for ambulation aids and eventually a wheelchair for mobility. Transfer activities become increasingly difficult. Upper extremity involvement leads to weakness of the arms and hands, but fine hand coordination for light activities remains intact until the late stages. The patients may need increasing help with self-care activities. Communication skills are unaffected except for speech, which may become somewhat thick and low in volume if the speech or breathing muscles are affected. There are the expected psychological and social problems resulting from increasing dependency, but there are no specific intellectual or personality changes that can be attributed directly to the disease.

Rehabilitation Potential

Long-term potential is very poor due to the steady progression of the disease. It is uncommon for patients to survive more than 6 to 8 years. Short-term rehabilitation potential may be considerably more favorable if the patient can be redirected into an occupation that is consistent with his functional limitations and a minimum of time is required for the training.

Standards of Evaluation

A neurologist should make the diagnosis and rule out treatable diseases that may resemble ALS. Electromyography and nerve conduction studies are very helpful in establishing the diagnosis. Myelography and other neurological tests may be necessary to distinguish ALS from other directly treatable diseases causing similar symptoms.

A physiatrist can evaluate residual abilities, correctable complications of inactivity, and the need for therapy or assistive equipment. A physical therapist can assess muscle strength and joint range of motion, and an occupational therapist can assess hand skills and self-care abilities. An assessment of the social situation is important, since the patient will become increasingly dependent on others for mobility and self-care.

Total Treatment

There is no medical or surgical treatment that has any effect on the course of ALS. A physical therapist should monitor the patient at regular intervals to detect contracture formation and to supervise a daily home range-of-motion exercise routine. The patient may also need training in the use of orthotics, ambulation aids, or wheelchairs as time goes on. In the later stages, as arm strength and endurance wanes, an electric wheelchair may substantially improve independent mobility, and mobile arm supports can assist upper extremity function (see p. 78).

An occupational therapist can train the patient or his family in the use of self-help equipment and energy-saving techniques for activities of daily living. Some patients require psychological counseling, and most patients and their families need the support of a social worker to adapt to the increasing physical deficits.

Vocational Implications

Short-term retraining into more appropriate occupations is often feasible, since intelligence and communication skills are unaffected by the disease. Adaptation at the current place of employment may be more feasible. Even in the early stages of the disease, however, no more than 6 to 12 months of retraining will ordinarily be appropriate, due to the short life expectancy. The clients may retain their aptitudes for fine hand and finger dexterity with lightweight objects, since sensation and coordination are unaffected. However, grip strength and lifting abilities may be expected to deteriorate steadily. A variety of interests may be encouraged, as long as these physical limitations are understood. Physical demands of any future occupation should be light and sedentary, without the requirement for much, if any, lifting, carrying, pulling, or pushing. Even in an ambulatory client, a wheelchair-accessible occupation should be selected, since the ability to walk will be lost within a few years. Ordinary environmental extremes are tolerated normally, except in late stages when respiratory involvement may make dusty or polluted air hazardous.

SPINAL MUSCULAR ATROPHY

Disease Description

Spinal muscular atrophy is a hereditary childhood disease of unknown cause with progressive degeneration of the anterior horn cells. The weakness and flaccidity of the trunk and limb muscles may develop during infancy or even be present at birth, causing the so-called "floppy infant" picture. The disease is relatively rare, and was originally described under several different names, which are now felt to be variations of the same disease. When the onset is at birth or in the first year of life, it may be called *Werdnig-Hoffman disease* or *infantile muscular atrophy*. If the onset is between ages 1 and 3, it is sometimes referred to as *Kugelberg-Welander disease* or *juvenile muscular atrophy*.

Infants with the disease usually lie quietly with little spontaneous movement. They are slow to develop the mobility milestones of rolling over, sitting up, and walking. These skills, once present, may be lost if the disease appears in the second or third year, leading to progressive weakness and increasing limitations of muscular function. Wheelchair use becomes more difficult as trunk control is progressively lost. Many children die within the first decade of life, usually of pulmonary complications or other results of inactivity. A few affected children, however, progress more slowly and may survive into the second or even third decade of life and come to the attention of the rehabilitation community.

Functional Disabilities

The wheelchair is the usual mode of ambulation, and older children may use electric wheelchairs if arm endurance becomes low. Transfers require the assistance of another person. Self-care skills and eventually eating require another person's help. Vision and hearing are unaffected, but speech may be hard to understand due to low voice volume and weak facial or tongue muscles. The extensive disability during the early formative years usually leads to significant social retardation due to the lack of normal learning opportunities during childhood. Children who survive into the teens are usually quite dependent psychologically upon their parents.

Rehabilitation Potential

The few children who survive into the teenage years and come to the attention of a rehabilitation counselor have poor long-term potential due to the low longevity. Short-term potential may be somewhat more favorable, since intelligence is unimpaired. However, social retardation and extreme physical dependency sharply limit the potential for gainful employment. Rehabilitation goals are generally more concerned with developing meaningful interests and opportunities for socialization.

Standards of Evaluation

Until the availability of electromyography 20 years

ago, children with spinal muscular atrophy were often mistakenly diagnosed as having muscular dystrophy. Electrical testing of the nerves and muscles, enzyme tests of the blood, and muscle biopsy can all help establish the diagnosis and differentiate other causes of weakness in infants. A neurologist is the appropriate specialist for diagnosis.

A physiatrist can evaluate residual abilities and recommend a physical and maintenance program. Physical and occupational therapists should assess mobility and self-care skills. Clearly, a social worker can help delineate the family relationships and the likelihood of reduced social skills. Educational background also needs careful review for adequacy.

Total Treatment

As for any child in a wheelchair, frequent monitoring by a physical therapist and changes in the size and components of the wheelchair will maximize residual abilities of children with spinal muscular atrophy. Older children should be given electric wheelchairs as soon as they are unable to propel a manual chair for significant distances. This will provide independent mobility in school settings and encourage social growth. The family must be taught a simple daily routine of range-of-motion exercises to prevent contractures. Self-help devices and training in activities of daily living may reduce dependency on parents. Corsets or spinal orthotics may be necessary to provide trunk support or to control scoliosis. Sometimes an adapted wheelchair with a semireclining back or trunk and head supports will accomplish the same thing with greater comfort. Surgical correction of deformities or contractures is hardly ever appropriate, since any useful function of the limbs is likely to have been lost due to the progressive muscle weakness. Family counseling and social services are usually helpful. A genetic counselor should be available to parents and relatives.

Vocational Implications

Education is important, especially for the older child with a slow progression, since the mind and the voice are the only factors left with which to perform any rewarding activities. Educational plans should be short-term in nature. It should be understood that aptitudes for hand function will be severely limited. Interests should be encouraged that lead to emotional and social development and counteract the dependency. Physical demands of any occupation or activity must be very slight. These clients will not be able to handle extremes of weather except during brief outdoor period for transportation or avocational pursuits.

POLIOMYELITIS

Disease Description

Poliomyelitis is an acute virus infection of the spinal cord often followed by residual paralysis of muscles. It was the major cause of physical disabilities in this country until 20 years ago. It is also known as *acute anterior poliomyelitis*, *infantile paralysis*, or *Heine-Medin's disease*; it is most commonly referred to simply as "polio." Unlike the other diseases described in this chapter, poliomyelitis has a known cause, is preventable, and is not progressive after the acute phase.

Before the development of effective vaccines, poliomyelitis was the most common virus infection of the nervous system. The disease occurred most often in children under age 10. Because of its widespread prevalence, most people after this age had had enough random exposures to develop immunity. Major epidemics of poliomyelitis occurred in 1946, 1949, 1952, and 1954. Until 1954, 25,000 to 50,000 cases per year occurred in the United States. The introduction of the Salk vaccine in 1955 and of Sabin's vaccine in 1961 has practically eliminated poliomyelitis in the United States. Thus, it is rare to see residual paralysis from poliomyelitis in persons under 20, and the major group still bearing residual deficits from poliomyelitis as this book is published are adults in the 30 to 50 year age group, the prime years for gainful employment. This makes polio a disease that is still of major importance for rehabilitation counselors.

The polio virus has a predilection for the anterior horn cells of the spinal cord. Other areas of the central nervous system may be affected to a lesser extent, but usually recover completely. Damage to the anterior horn cells leads to flaccid paralysis of the muscles they supply. Some anterior horn cells recover, but many do not, leading to degeneration of their axons extending down the peripheral nerves to the muscles, which in turn may undergo atrophy due to denervation. A characteristic of poliomyelitis is the scattered involvement of anterior horn cells at many different locations in the spinal cord. The result is that affected muscles may retain a few motor units, which during the recovery phase may enlarge to produce weak, but functionally useful, contractions of these muscles. For the same reason, limb involvement is usually asymmetrical. It is not uncommon for one extremity to have major paralysis while the opposite one remains largely unaffected. In a given limb, muscle groups may be affected to differing degrees, leading to muscle imbalance and deformities. Uneven involvement of trunk muscles may lead to curvature of the spine (scoliosis). If an entire limb is extensively paralyzed during the growing years, its rate of growth decreases, resulting in a small, shortened limb in the adult.

The cause of poliomyelitis is any of several strains of polio virus. The virus enters through the mouth from breath droplets of another affected person or through contaminated water. The virus spreads via the lymphatics or blood stream. Initial symptoms are those of an upper respiratory or gastrointestinal infection, with flu-like symptoms. There may be an interval of recovery lasting a few days, followed by a recurrence of fever with headache, stiff neck, and muscle soreness. Two to five days later, paralysis begins, and increases in severity for another three to five days. Paralysis of the respiratory muscles may create the need for mechanical respiratory maintenance using devices such as the Emerson tank respirator, or "iron lung." Tracheostomy is usually needed when there is respiratory paralysis. The need for mechanical respiratory maintenance may continue for weeks or months, and in a few cases where no respiratory muscle recovery occurs, this need may be permanent.

About 5 percent of acute cases are fatal, usually due to respiratory paralysis or pulmonary infections. In nonfatal cases, control of facial and neck muscles is almost always recovered. Improvement of the paralysis begins 1 to 2 weeks after onset, and is usually complete or well along toward recovery within 2 to 3 months. Continued improvement after this time is usually related to hypertrophy of surviving muscle cells, and sprouting of surviving motor nerves to reinnervate other muscles cells that have lost their original nerve supply.

Functional Diasbilities

A wide variety of functional disabilities can be seen after poliomyelitis, depending on the highly variable pattern of residual muscle paralysis. Major deficits in the lower extremities may impair ambulation and transfers and necessitate the use of orthotics, ambulation aids, or wheelchairs. If the upper extremities are also involved, cane or crutch use may not be possible. Occasionally the upper extremities are severely or totally paralyzed in a person who remains able to walk normally, due to recovery in the lower extremities. Self-care skills and hand functions may be impaired to varying degrees. Slight remaining function in affected muscles allows poliomyelitis patients to develop a variety of substitutions or "trick movements" to facilitate hand functions. Intellectual functioning, personality, and communication skills are unaffected. Psychosocial impairments are variable, depending mainly on the pre-existing personal and social strengths.

Rehabilitation Potential

Short- and long-term rehabilitation is excellent in poliomyelitis patients. The deficits are stable and recurrences are almost nonexistent.

Standards of Evaluation

A physiatrist is the medical specialist best suited to evaluate functional deficits and residual abilities in a person who has had poliomyelitis at an earlier age. The physiatrist can advise on the need for the variety of therapeutic interventions that may be helpful. Physical and occupational therapy evaluations are often useful, depending on the location and extent of residual paralysis.

Total Treatment

During the acute phase of poliomyelitis, treatment is supportive in nature, with care to maintain hydration, nutrition, and ventilation, and precautions to avoid the complications of bed rest. As soon as recovery begins, muscle re-education and skill training is started. A variety of orthotics, ambulation aids, and self-help devices must be provided and the patient trained in their use. Occasionally muscle transplantation and other orthopedic procedures can help improve hand function and ambulation.

Postpoliomyelitis patients who are entering middle age must guard against deterioration due to obesity, deconditioning from inactivity, degenerative joint disease (see chap. 14), and associated injuries. Whenever a period of bed rest is required for some unrelated medical problem, it is essential to begin vigorous therapy to maintain muscle strength and joint range until normal activities can be resumed.

More specifically, fractures secondary to osteoporosis of a paralyzed limb can occur after minimal trauma. The treatment of these fractures requires careful assessment by the orthopedic surgeon of the patient's individual methods of compensating for his specific impairments. Degenerative joint disease may occur in the large joints of the legs (hip and knee) or in the lumbar spine because muscle weakness may have left them relatively unprotected over the years. Leg length discrepancies, in particular, may result in late-onset back pain in need of careful attention. Further, as the patient gets older, heavier, and less athletic, modification in whatever braces, canes, or crutches he is using may be required. Joint ligament laxity may also develop, particularly at the knee where hyperextension (genu recurvatum) can occur. For a reason often not clear, muscles that are known to be weak may develop further weakness through use and require brace protection that might not have been needed earlier.

Finally, patients with mild respiratory difficulty may find greater respiratory difficulty with age as their lungs and thoracic cage lose some of their elasticity.

Patients permanently on respirators should be periodically reviewed, for more portable new equipment may become available and allow greater mobility. In later years, more frequent medical evaluation is useful in anticipating, aborting, or treating these late-onset problems.

Vocational Implications

Education and training may be considered without limitations in poliomyelitis clients. Life expectancy for these persons should be the same as for nondisabled persons of the same age. There may be some limitations in aptitudes for hand or leg activities, depending on the paralysis. However, the muscles which continue to function should have normal coordination and skill. Any of a variety of vocational interests may be encouraged, depending more on the underlying make-up of the individual than on the poliomyelitis residuals. The physical demands of the job should not tax the client's strength excessively, as there is some evidence that muscles weakened by past poliomyelitis may deteriorate if the load imposed upon them is heavy relative to their residual strength. However, ordinary levels of activity within the remaining strength of muscles is important to maintain their function. No special environmental factors need to be considered beyond the obvious limits imposed by the residual paralysis.

GUILLAIN-BARRÉ SYNDROME

Disease Description

A disease with many similarities to poliomyelitis is Guillain-Barré syndrome, also known as *infectious polyneuritis* or *Landry's ascending paralysis*. About two-thirds of the cases give a history of a preceding infection of the upper respiratory or gastrointestinal tracts, but no virus has yet been identified. There is some experimental evidence that suggests allergic or autoimmune factors, but no definite cause has yet been established. The disease causes segments of the myelin sheath of peripheral nerve axons to be progressively destroyed (demyelination), causing the conduction of nerve impulses to slow down. In very severe cases, the axon itself degenerates.

In those cases preceded by a respiratory or gastrointestinal infection, there is usually an interval of 5 to 12 days before weakness begins. The lower limbs are often affected first, with weakness ascending within a few days to involve the trunk, upper limbs, and the muscles supplied by the cranial nerves. Maximum paralysis is usually reached within 1 to 3 weeks. Facial and respiratory muscle paralysis is rather common, and patients may need mechanical respiratory support during the acute phase. Like poliomyelitis, flaccid

paralysis with denervation atrophy may be found in affected muscles. The deficits are usually bilateral and symmetrical, unlike those caused by poliomyelitis. About 85 percent of patients recover completely with no neurological residuals. The myelin sheath slowly regenerates, and full muscle strength returns after many months.

The remaining 15 percent are those patients with axonal degeneration. Although the axons do slowly regenerate (1 mm per day; 1 cm per week; 1 inch per month), there is no full recovery of muscle function. The rehabilitation problems of these patients depend on their residual disabilities.

Functional Disabilities

Residual weakness or complete flaccid paralysis may remain. The hands and feet are most commonly affected. Deficits are usually uniform and symmetrical, and the deformities common after polio are not usually a problem in Guillain-Barré syndrome. Respiratory paralysis may persist for months or be permanent, requiring mechanical respiratory support. There is rarely any sensory loss or cerebral damage.

Rehabilitation Potential

Since the deficits are confined to motor neurons, without sensory or cerebral damage, rehabilitation potential is good. Recurrences are very rare.

Standards of Evaluation

A neurologist usually manages the patient during the acute phase. The diagnosis is made from the typical history and course and from a spinal tap showing a characteristic elevation of the protein level of the fluid without the associated elevation of white cells found in the cerebrospinal fluid of acute poliomyelitis patients. An electromyogram may be helpful.

A physiatrist can assess residual functional abilities and the need for equipment and therapy. An occupational therapist evaluates hand function and self-care skills. A physical therapist can assess muscle strength, joint range, and gait. When the severity of the paralysis necessitates major changes in occupation or life style, assessments by a psychologist, social worker, and rehabilitation counselor are important.

Total Treatment

Acute management for Guillain-Barré syndrome is similar to that for poliomyelitis. Long-term care depends on the degree of residual weakness, and may include self-help devices, orthotics, ambulation aids, or wheelchairs, and training in their use. Extensive permanent paralysis may require an electric wheelchair and sometimes mechanical respiratory support.

Vocational Implications

The guidelines for poliomyelitis also apply to Guillain-Barre syndrome. Education and retraining are usually feasible since intelligence and communication are unimpaired by the disease. If paralysis is severe, clients may need retraining for occupations having fewer physical requirements, especially for hand and wrist function and foot and ankle function. Occupations requiring fine finger dexterity or pushing, pulling, and gripping would be contraindicated. Short leg braces or a cane restrict walking, stooping, and bending.

MYASTHENIA GRAVIS

Disease Description

Myasthenia gravis is a disease that causes weakness and fatigability of the muscles. There may be remissions and exacerbations, but the disease is generally progressive. It can begin at any age, but is commonest in young adults, where female cases outnumber males 3 to 1; after age 40, males and females are affected equally. The prevalence is about 3 cases per 100,000 population.

While the cause is unknown, the symptoms are known to be caused by a decrease in the amount of acetylcholine at the neuromuscular junction (see p. 31). There may also be an increased amount of acetylcholinesterase, the chemical that inactivates acetylcholine.) Acetylcholine is the neurotransmitter chemical at the motor end plate which, when triggered by a motor nerve impulse, initiates the contraction of the muscle. The reasons for its deficiency are unknown, but it is probably a form of autoimmune disorder. The disease is frequently associated with tumors of the thymus gland, and may improve after removal of the thymus. It may also occur in association with a number of other conditions, including pregnancy, increased or decreased thyroid function, rheumatoid arthritis, lupus erythematosus, or malignant tumors of the lung or pancreas.

The disease usually begins with weakness of the eyelids, throat muscles, or trunk or limb muscles. The weakness is greater after exercise or at the end of the day and improves with rest. A common sign is drooping (ptosis) of the eyelids. There is often fatigue after chewing and difficulty swallowing. In late stages of the disease, respiratory muscles may be involved, leading to pneumonia and other pulmonary complications. Except for cardiac deconditioning, the complications of inactivity are not usually seen, since patients are usually able to continue with ordinary light activities of short duration.

The disease usually worsens progressively, although remissions are common. In untreated patients, death may result within a few years. Life expectancies are somewhat longer in recent years, due primarily to the introduction of neostigmine and related drugs of the "anticholinesterase" family. These drugs inactivate the acetylcholinesterase which breaks down acetycholine, thus prolonging and enhancing the effect of the diminished supply of acetylcholine at the neuromuscular junction. They are ordinarily taken by mouth on a long-term basis to maintain exercise tolerance, but may be given intramuscularly or intravenously in severe attacks. Some patients with severe flare-ups become refractory to neostigmine treatment (myasthenic crisis) and require tracheostomy and mechanical respiratory assistance. With changes in medication, improvement may occur and allow resumption of ordinary activities. With careful management, many patients may remain relatively active for many years with the disease.

Functional Disabilities

In general, the disabilities caused by myasthenia gravis affect strenuous and repetitive activities of the muscles. Light activities of short duration or few repetitions can usually be performed satisfactorily. Thus, patients may have difficulty with prolonged standing, stair climbing, or long-distance walking, but can usually walk for short distances without difficulty. Self-care activities are usually performed independently, but they may take longer than normal. Even light activities that are prolonged in duration may be impaired, such as writing or typing. With careful medical treatment, many of the impairments can be diminished.

Social disabilities are usually not as severe as with other neuromuscular diseases, since a limited amount of normal activity can be continued. The usual psychological reactions to disability may be seen (see chap. 2), but there are no special personality or intellectual changes associated with the disease. Young men or women who present the symptoms of myasthenia gravis are frequently misdiagnosed as "hysterics," which often results in their losing the emotional support of family and friends when they need it the most.

Rehabilitation Potential

Short-term rehabilitation potential is generally quite good, since most patients respond well to medical management. Long-term potential is also good, except in those patients who have rapidly progressive severe symptoms that do not respond to treatment. In general, the rehabilitation counselor may anticipate 5 to 20 years of productive life. The somewhat unpredictable nature of the disease, with inexplicable remissions, should also be kept in mind. Patients may be done a serious injustice if vocational rehabilitation services are withheld on the assumption that all patients necessarily deteriorate.

Standards of Evaluation

If myasthenia gravis is suspected, the diagnosis can usually be made without difficulty from characteristic history and physical findings. A neurologist should confirm the diagnosis and rule out related diseases. The neostigmine or Tensilon test is usually diagnostic of the disease: an injection of one of these drugs should be followed within a short time by significant improvement of weakness. Characteristic findings on electromyography and repetitive nerve stimulation will confirm the diagnosis.

A careful and thorough general medical examination is important to identify the several related diseases that may coexist with myasthenia gravis (see above). There is generally no need for examination by a physical or occupational therapist unless associated physical disabilities are present. The treating physician or a nurse should take the time to explain the nature of the disease and the organic cause of the symptoms, especially with patients who have been misdiagnosed.

Total Treatment

Three related drugs in the anticholinesterase family are the mainstays of treatment: neostigmine (Prostigmin); pyrostigmine (Mestinon); and ambenonium (Mytelase). Patients generally take these drugs orally in several daily doses. In severe cases they may be given by injection. These drugs may produce some troublesome gastrointestinal side effects including diarrhea, abdominal cramps, or excessive salivation. The side effects can usually be controlled with atropine, belladonna, or related drugs.

In recent years, surgical removal of the thymus gland (thymectomy) has been used with success in over half of the patients so treated. Benefits may not appear for several months or a few years after the surgery. Some permanent remissions have been reported after thymectomy.

Psychological or social counseling may be necessary in situations where the disease has produced serious disruption of the social structure or major psychological complications.

Vocational Implications

Clients with myasthenia gravis are good candidates for re-education to less physically demanding occupations. In cases under good medical control, a 2 to 4 year educational plan may not be inappropriate.

In unresponsive or rapidly progressive cases, shorter-term education might be more suitable. Intellect, learning ability, and motor coordination and dexterity should all remain intact. A variety of interests may be encouraged if they do not involve prolonged or repetitive performance of muscular activities. Physical demands should be those of sedentary or light activities with frequent rest periods possible. Prolonged lifting, carrying, or pulling should be avoided in an occupational choice. Continuous writing or typing may be troublesome, although their intermittent performance may present no problems. Speech, hearing, and vision will all remain unimpaired. The job site should be accessible by motor vehicle or public transportation, without long walks or multiple flights of stairs. Unusually cold working environments should be avoided, but other ordinary environmental or weather conditions should be well tolerated.

MUSCULAR DYSTROPHY

Disease Description

Muscular dystrophy refers to a family of hereditary diseases that cause degenerative changes in the muscles, leading to progressive weakness and disability. The cause of muscular dystrophy is unknown. It is known that there is abnormal function of a number of enzymes found in muscles, but the underlying cause for this is not well understood. There are about 4 cases per 100,000 population. Since the disease affects children and young adults, it has major vocational implications.

There are several major types of muscular dystrophy, each affecting different ages with different patterns of involvement and rates of progression. The commonest, Duchenne, or childhood muscular dystrophy, accounts for about 85 percent of all cases. It is carried by a sex-linked recessive gene and occurs only in boys. Symptoms and signs are usually present before the age of 5, and within one decade patients usually require a wheelchair for mobility.

Duchenne dystrophy occurs first in the hip muscles, where weakness in young children leads to clumsiness, difficulty running and later walking, and weakness, particularly when arising from the floor or going up curbs or stairs. Later the shoulder muscles become weakened, with difficulty reaching over the head or lifting heavy objects. The small muscles, such as those of the face and hand, usually retain their function until late stages of the disease. The respiratory muscles weaken progressively, and the vital capacity falls steadily. In some cases the heart muscle is involved, leading to heart failure. About one-third of affected children have some degree of mental retardation. Most of the physical findings are related to weakness of the affected muscles. Shoulder involvement causes difficulty with reaching or heavy lifting and a drooping of the shoulder or protrusion ("winging") of the scapula. There may be a waddling gait and an increase in lumbar lordosis (see p. 207) due to weakness in the abdominal and hip muscles. Contractures may be present in affected joints. Since the disease is confined to muscle cells, there are no sensory changes.

Most of the remaining 15 percent of muscular dystrophy cases fall into the categories of limb-girdle dystrophy or facioscapulohumeral dystrophy. These forms begin in teenagers or young adults, affect mainly the shoulder and hip muscles, and progress more slowly, usually requiring two decades or more before patients are severely incapacitated. They differ from one another primarily in the involvement of the facial musculature in the latter.

Two relatively rare forms of dystrophy are myotonic dystrophy, and ocular or ophthalmoplegic dystrophy. Typically, these forms begin in young adults, progress quite slowly, and do not cause severe disability for several decades or longer. Myotonic dystrophy, unlike the other forms, affects distal muscles first, particularly the muscles of the hand. The characteristic myotonia is a cramp-like inability to relax muscles for several seconds after a forceful contraction. Typically, patients with myotonic dystrophy also exhibit cataracts, frontal baldness, and testicular atrophy, presumably due to associated genetic abnormalities. Facial muscle paralysis and drooping of the eyelids are common. There is a high degree of associated mental retardation and other congenital physical defects. Ocular dystrophy is usually limited to the eye and throat muscles, causing double vision, drooping of the eyelids, and difficulty swallowing.

The pathological findings in early phases of muscular dystrophy may include swelling of the muscle cells, leading to enlargement of the weakened muscles (pseudohypertrophy). In later stages, there is degeneration of muscle cells, which are replaced with collagen fibers and fat.

Complications of muscular dystrophy are related to inactivity and bed rest. Injudicious use of the wheelchair or prolonged bed rest after routine illnesses often leads to premature loss of the ability to walk. Contractures of the joints are common, particularly when daily home range-of-motion exercises are not administered faithfully. Trunk muscle imbalance often leads to scoliosis. Pulmonary complications are common in late stages when the breathing and coughing ability is limited.

The muscular dystrophies pursue a variable course. Most patients with Duchenne dystrophy are severely disabled by the middle teens and few survive past their twenties. There are exceptions, however; a variation called Becker's dystrophy begins like other Duchenne cases but progresses more slowly. Limb-girdle, facioscapulohumeral, or late-onset Duchenne dystrophy patients may progress slowly and remain functional well into middle life. In general, the later the age of onset, the slower the progression. Many patients who die of respiratory failure could continue to live with mechanical respiratory assistance, although their physical abilities would be severely limited. Mechanical respiratory assistance is not usually introduced to end-stage muscular dystrophy patients unless their intellectual and social skill levels are sufficiently high to permit self-directed independent living after their parents become unable to care for them.

Functional Disabilities

The major functional disabilities result from weakness of the proximal muscles of the shoulders and hips. Ambulation skills diminish steadily, leading to wheelchair mobility. Because of the difficulty in rising from a sitting position, wheelchair transfers usually require assistance. Eating, dressing, and personal hygiene become more and more limited. The ability to use public transportation is lost because of the inability to mount bus steps or subway stairs. Many of these disabilities can be diminished with appropriate rehabilitation therapy. Communication skills are usually unaffected. Vision and hearing are not involved, and speech should be normal except for low voice volume in late stages.

As expected in a severe disability, there are often major psychological and social disabilities. In many cases, social retardation with dependence on parents and lack of normal school and play experience leads to a syndrome which may be hard to distinguish from mental retardation. Mainstreaming of these children and appropriate parental counseling should diminish the psychosocial disabilities in these children.

Rehabilitation Potential

Short-term rehabilitation potential is usually good except in the end stages of muscular dystrophy. This is especially true if intelligence is normal. Educational or training programs to develop mental or verbal vocational skills may be quite appropriate. Hand and finger function for light activity is usually preserved until the end stages. Some forms of muscular dystrophy progress quite slowly, as outlined above.

Long-term rehabilitation for Duchenne muscular dystrophy is quite limited, unless intelligence is normal or above normal and social growth is possible. On the other hand, even a highly intelligent or verbally skillful teenager with muscular dystrophy has very little rehabilitation potential if he has been allowed to remain totally dependent on his parents and siblings and has not had access to the normal social opportunities that go with peer contact in school, playgrounds, and community settings. The total patient, rather than the extensiveness of the muscular weakness, is what determines long-term rehabilitation potential.

Standards of Evaluation

A neurologist or physiatrist who is experienced with muscle diseases should make the diagnosis of muscular dystrophy. The Muscular Dystrophy Association sponsors clinics in most parts of the United States where diagnostic services are available. The characteristic medical history and physical findings point to the proper diagnosis in most cases. Several laboratory studies help confirm the diagnosis. The level of various muscle enzymes in the blood, such as creatine phosphokinase (CPK), may be elevated in the early stages of rapidly progressive dystrophy such as Duchenne dystrophy, but is normal in the later stages or the more slowly progressive forms. Electromyography is very useful in ruling out diseases with similar clinical pictures. A muscle biopsy is helpful, but must be done with caution to prevent temporary bed rest or disuse of the biopsied area, since the patient may never regain function after a little disuse atrophy or joint contracture has been allowed to form. Electrocardiography should be done to detect associated cardiac muscle involvement.

A physical therapist can evaluate muscle strength, joint range, and gait skills. The occupational therapist can evaluate self-care abilities and the use of adaptive equipment and energy-saving techniques by affected patients or the care providers in their families.

A psychological assessment is useful to identify and quantitate mental retardation. Evaluation by a skilled psychologist is also required to distinguish organic mental retardation from the equally common social-emotional retardation resulting from severe dependency in childhood. A social evaluation of the family's strengths is also important.

Total Treatment

There is no drug treatment that is effective against the primary symptom, the weakness of muscular dystrophy. In the small percentage with myotonia, this symptom can be alleviated by oral drugs to relax muscular tension, such as quinine, procaine amide, or Dilantin. Surgery is only necessary when contractures have been allowed to develop through failure to do range-of-motion exercises regularly. Contractures, once formed, should be surgically corrected only if they interfere with some specific function that is important enough to justify the surgery. The postoperative immobilization and bed rest must be as short as possible, and vigorous bedside physical therapy is essential to maintain muscle strength and joint range during any postoperative period of immobility. The same is true after muscle biopsy. It is common in muscular dystrophy clinics to see patients who lost the ability to walk after "successful" surgical correction of a contracture or biopsy of a muscle for diagnostic purposes.

Physical therapy is essential to maintain the range of motion of affected joints. However, muscle strengthening exercises are usually not helpful, as the patient is usually using his weakened muscles to the maximum of their ability already. The physical therapist also instructs patients in the use of ambulation aids and wheelchairs. Occupational therapy may be needed for training in self-care skills and the use of assistive devices, such as arm slings or balanced forearm orthoses, to preserve hand function if shoulder weakness is severe. Orthotics may be needed to provide ankle stability and prolong the period of walking. When scoliosis is present, corsets or trunk orthotics, such as body jackets, may provide better trunk control or sitting balance. In a patient who already uses a wheelchair, special trunk-support attachments or a slightly reclining wheelchair back may accomplish the same thing without the need for a body jacket.

Several types of counseling are important at various stages in the disease. Genetic counseling has obvious value to assist unaffected relatives in their family planning. Psychological and social service counseling helps patients overcome various hurdles and accept their limitations. Nutritional counseling and special care to avoid obesity will prolong ambulatory or transfer independence, and ease the burden of care for family members after the patient has become dependent in mobility and self-care.

The medical management of muscular dystrophy, then, revolves around the maintenance of good health and nutrition, the treatment of routine intercurrent illnesses and injuries, and the counseling and guidance of the patient and his family so that proper decisions are made at the proper time regarding rehabilitation.

Vocational Implications

Educational planning should take into account the anticipated remaining life expectancy. The past rate of deterioration is the best predictor of future progression. When intellectual and social skills make independent self-direction still possible even after extensive physical impairment has developed, the option of mechanical respiratory maintenance should not be ruled out. Connecting the end-stage muscular dystrophy patient to a respirator will probably prolong his life by 10 to 20 years. Most clinicians feel that this is inappropriate for the mentally, socially, or educationally retarded teenager or adult who is dependent upon aging parents. On the other hand, it may be highly appropriate for the intelligent and independent-minded teenager or adult with advanced muscular dystrophy who is running out of lung capacity, but is independent or has the potential for continued education leading to independent living.

Aptitudes for intellectual functioning and learning may be limited where mental retardation is associated with the muscle weakness. Verbal and communication skills are usually intact. Hand and finger dexterity may be well preserved, although grip strength is usually diminished. If myotonia is present and cannot be medically controlled, hand and finger skills may be markedly limited. A variety of interests may be encouraged as long as the progressive physical impairments are kept in mind.

Physical demands for sedentary or light activity may be well tolerated. In the earlier or more slowly progressive forms of muscular dystrophy, fairly heavy work may remain possible. Shoulder involvement may prohibit heavy lifting, pulling, or pushing. Hip involvement will limit stooping, kneeling, and crawling. However, standing and walking may remain possible in the more slowly progressive forms of the disease. Eye muscle involvement may interfere with reading or fine work due to double vision or drooping of the eyelids. Associated cataracts or cardiac impairments may add further limitation. The advanced-stage client in a wheelchair will have difficulty protecting himself from extremes of weather outdoors, but otherwise no special environmental factors need to be considered.

SUMMARY

This chapter has reviewed some rather mysterious and frightening diseases which have tended to be misunderstood by the general public and sometimes mismanaged by the health professions. Studying or managing them may produce some strong personal reactions in the counselor or student. In order to best serve the needs of clients and avoid some common pitfalls, several caveats are in order concerning the management of neuromuscular diseases.

Do not be a slave to statistics. One should avoid a blind over-reliance on mean survival times and similar statistical data. For an individual client, his own survival time is what matters, and this may not be easy to predict. A great disservice is done to the client who is told such things as, "You have 3 years to live," only to find 10 to 15 years later that he fell at the long end of the range of survival times, and wasted his life waiting to die. A more constructive approach is to try to maximize the available functional abilities at the point in time when the client is encountered.

Do not overlook the complications of inactivity. Few of these diseases are the direct causes of death; clients die of the complications of inactivity or bed rest (see chap. 4). Some of these complications may be present when the client is first encountered and may even be the major causes of the functional disabilities he presents. Common examples are joint contractures, disuse

atrophy of muscles, cardiovascular deconditioning, and psychological depression or social retardation. These can all be prevented, detected, and corrected. To overlook them is to condemn the client to unnecessary additional disability on top of the unavoidable burden of his basic neurological deficit.

Do not overestimate functional limitations. Health professionals have a tendency to exaggerate the degree to which a physical deficit produces a functional impairment. Experience with disabled persons will teach the open-minded professional to appreciate the sometimes amazing feats of independent performance which are possible even with extensive physical deficits. The task is not to constrict the horizons of clients, but to make available all of the training, equipment, and motivational supports that can be mustered to maximize their functional potential.

Do not personalize the emotional response of the client. Some health professionals conclude that they would feel overwhelmed or devastated if they had the client's problem, and then assume that the client shares their feelings. Assuming that the client must be terribly depressed, they may respond with excessive empathy or patronizing pity. It turns out, however, that persons disabled by chronic progressive diseases are often less depressed than those previously able-bodied persons who are suddenly struck down with an acute disability. These persons have the psychological advantage of having had time to adapt to gradually progressive deficits. In addition, those with a family history of the same disorder may have had an opportunity to develop an appreciation of the residual abilities.

Hope is a stronger human urge than despair. Even those clients who have been given a grimly specific prognosis by some well-meaning physician will usually choose to hope for recovery or improvement. This is a healthy reaction which should be directed into constructive, realistic action plans and not extinguished by the professional's own personal notions of how he might feel under the same circumstances.

Do not use pejorative or negative terms. This is a corollary of the preceding precaution. The client is not a polio "victim" or a muscular dystrophy "sufferer," nor is he "afflicted" with Parkinson's disease. Persons are not "confined" to crutches or wheelchair "bound." The client is a *person* who happens to have a disability due to polio, muscular dystrophy, or Parkinson's disease. His crutches do not confine, but rather free him from the chair or bed. The wheelchair does not bind, but liberates its user, so that he may go to school or work or travel around the world. Our language reflects our attitudes, and these pejorative terms have no place in the jargon of rehabilitation.

In progressive neuromuscular diseases, as with other categories of disabilities, the counselor should develop a positive philosophy of management based on an appreciation of the constructive medical and physical treatment measures available and the realistic rehabilitation potential of this group of disabled persons.

BIBLIOGRAPHY

Anderson AD, Levine SA, Gellert H: Loss of ambulatory ability in patients with old anterior poliomyelitis. Lancet 2(7786): 1061–1063, 1972.
A brief report of several cases, this article discusses the possible causes and strategies for prevention of late deterioration in patients who had poliomyelitis in the past.

Cailliet R: Rehabilitation in parkinsonism. *In* Licht S (ed): *Rehabilitation and Medicine*. Baltimore, Waverly Press, 1968, pp. 435–445.
This chapter reviews the pathology and clinical picture of parkinsonism in nontechnical terms with helpful diagrams. The management and physical rehabilitation are well covered.

Chusid JG: *Correlative Neuroanatomy and Functional Neurology*. Ed 16, Los Altos, CA, Lange Medical Publications, 1976.
This paperback guide provides simple explanations of the anatomy and physiology underlying the disorders of the neuromuscular system.

Downey JA, Low NL (eds): *The Child with Disabling Illness: Principles of Rehabilitation*. Philadelphia, Saunders, 1974.
This textbook discusses all types of childhood disabilities with special emphasis on rehabilitation considerations. The section on the neuromuscular system has an excellent chapter on muscular dystrophy.

Greenfield JG: *The Spino-Cerebellar Degenerations*. Springfield, Ill., Thomas, 1954.
This short monograph presents an excellent summary of the family of spinocerebellar degenerations, including Friedreich's ataxia. An interesting historical review is presented, and the range of symptoms, signs, and rates of progression are described.

Martin RD, Flegenheimer WV: Psychiatric aspects of the management of the myasthenic patient. Mt Sinai J Med NY 38:594–601, 1971.
This article describes the need for psychiatric care in the management of myasthenic patients. Because strong emotions often precede symptoms, and emotional disturbances can exacerbate the condition, ways of releasing emotions or handling anger need to be taught. Mild depression is also a common problem.

Merritt HH: *A Textbook of Neurology*. Ed 5, Philadelphia, Lea and Febiger, 1973.
A basic neurology textbook. Good sections on the diseases covered in this chapter.

Singer E: Premature social aging: the social-psychological consequences of a chronic illness. Soc Sci Med 8:143–151, 1974.
A group of Parkinson patients 65+ years of age and a group of younger Parkinson patients were compared with normal populations of the same age groups. The younger Parkinson patients appeared to be more affected by restriction of social and vocational activities than the older patients as compared to the normal population.

Taft LT: The care and management of the child with muscular dystrophy. Dev Med Child Neurol 15(4):510–518, 1973.
A pediatrician discusses problems likely to occur in the initial stages of counseling and treating a child with muscular dystrophy and also those likely to occur as the child gets older. Written for physicians but general enough for counselors, this text provides useful background and evaluation guides.

7 PERIPHERAL NEUROPATHIES

Joseph Goodgold, M.D.

DISEASE DESCRIPTION

A precise statement concerning the incidence of peripheral neuropathy is not readily formulated because of the wide variety of causes of this condition. According to one report, of a total of 130,922,500 disabled United States citizens, over 11 percent had problems which included lifting, reaching, handling, and fingering, and an inability to use the lower extremities. About 1.5 million individuals in this group suffered from paralysis of various types. While not all of the paralyses are peripheral neuropathies, their contribution is large and there appears to be little dispute that the numbers are increasing. In one neuromuscular center (New York University), it is estimated that more than 1,500 peripheral neuropathies are examined annually in the electrodiagnostic section, while at least twice that number are identified solely by clinical examination. Multiplying these figures over the many major medical centers throughout the country suggests the magnitude of the problems likely to come to the attention of the rehabilitation counselor.

Peripheral neuropathies are diseases of the peripheral nervous system, i.e., those nerves that are located outside the brain and the spinal cord (see chap. 3 for a review of the nervous system). Included, therefore, are the cranial nerves, all the spinal nerves and their associated plexuses and distal nerve divisions, and also the nerves of the autonomic nervous system. All three systems carry information between the central nervous system and the periphery. Involvement of the somatic nervous system is generally of greater importance in peripheral neuropathy than involvement of the involuntary autonomic nervous system. The terms "peripheral neuritis" and "polyneuritis" are sometimes used as synonyms of peripheral neuropathy and polyneuropathy. The "itis" suffix means inflammation. Since inflammation is not always present, these terms are best avoided.

Figure 3-1 (p. 19) depicts the basic unit of the peripheral nervous system and the structures that can be diseased in peripheral neuropathies. Since the cell body is essentially a central nervous system structure, peripheral neuropathies will involve the axon, or the myelin, or both. Thus, in a peripheral neuropathy, the disease may primarily affect the axon (axonal disease) or cause loss of myelin (demyelinating disease), or the disease may be axonal and secondarily demyelinating. In some situations, axonal disease and demyelinization occur simultaneously. In the primary demyelinating diseases, the process may be distributed along the entire nerve fiber, or it may occur segmentally.

The speed with which an electrical impulse travels in a peripheral nerve depends on several factors: the health of the axon membrane; the diameter of the axon; and, if the fiber is myelinated, the thickness of the myelin and the distance between the nodes of Ranvier.

In the resting state, a nerve axon is polarized, with a layer of positive electrical charges on the outside surface of the membrane and a layer of negative electrical charges on the inside. Thus, the voltage is negative inside compared to outside. The amount of this polarization depends predominantly on the differences in the concentration of potassium (K+) and sodium (Na+) ions between the inside and the outside.

The concentration of sodium is greater on the outside and the concentration of potassium is greater on the inside. The magnitude of these concentration differences is governed by the ability of the membrane to allow or prevent the passage of these ions (membrane permeability).

When an impulse begins, either at the cell body or, if induced from the outside, by an electrical current shock, the amount of the polarization (i.e., membrane voltage, membrane potential) is reduced at the point of stimulation. When the polarization is reduced to a certain level (threshold), the membrane suddenly becomes very permeable to Na+ ions, which rapidly diffuse into the axon from the outside. The polarization then become negative on the outside and positive on the inside (fig. 7-1).

An unstable situation is created when the polarity of one region of the axon membrane is reversed and the polarity of adjacent regions is normal. Local electrical currents result, which make the neighboring regions also less polarized, and therefore more permeable to Na+ ions. In this way, a wave of depolarization travels down the length of the axon. The speed of propagation of this "action potential" (electrical impulse) is termed the conduction velocity of the nerve.

The more rapid the permeability change in the membrane, the greater the magnitude of the local currents, and the faster the speed of conduction. The larger the axon diameter, the faster the speed of conduction. If the fiber is also myelinated, the thicker the myelin, the faster the propagation speed. In addition, for myelinated fibers, the longer the distance between the nodes of Ranvier, the faster the conduction speed, because depolarization "jumps" from node to node. Myelinated fibers therefore conduct impulses much more rapidly than unmyelinated fibers do.

In a demyelinating peripheral neuropathy, the myelin thickness diminishes, and the speed of conduction is reduced. If the demyelination is diffuse, the speed is reduced along the entire length of the fiber. If the demyelination is segmental, the speed may be reduced only in those demyelinated sections and be normal in other sections. If the demyelination is severe, the fiber may not conduct at all, and strength and sensation will be reduced.

In an axonal peripheral neuropathy, axon diameter may decrease and cause a decrease in conduction velocity. The decrease in conduction velocity in axonal disease is much less than in demyelinating disease. The more usual effect of axonal disease, however, is a cessation of impulse conduction. Axonal disease therefore causes weakness and a reduction in sensation, usually more than in demyelinating disease.

Peripheral neuropathies can be mostly sensory, mostly motor, or a combination of both. In addition, a peripheral neuropathy may only involve one nerve (mononeuritis or mononeuropathy); several nerves, with complete sparing of the others (mononeuritis or mononeuropathy multiplex); or all of the nerves usually in a somewhat symmetrical manner (polyneuritis or polyneuropathy). The disturbances associated with autonomic system neuropathy, often referred to as trophic changes, include dryness and thinning of skin and subcutaneous tissue, brittleness and slowing of growth of nails, loss of hair, and other phenomena associated with the peripheral vascular system, such as swelling and discoloration. Sweating may also be impaired where skin sensation is reduced.

When an axon dies in axonal disease because of death of the cell body, the segment distal to the cell body undergoes what is referred to as *Wallerian degeneration*. If an axon is interrupted, as it may be in acute trauma, the axon distal to the interruption also undergoes Wallerian degeneration. The axon may lose its ability to conduct an externally applied electric current immediately after interruption or it may take a few days before conduction ceases.

Recovery requires regeneration of the axon down the residual tube which previously contained the healthy fiber. Growth rates are about a millimeter per

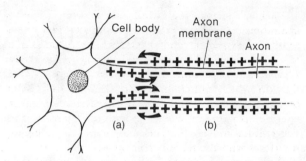

FIGURE 7-1. Schematic representation of the depolarization wave beginning at the cell body of an unmyelinated nerve. The region of depolarization, *(A)*, is close to the cell body. The normal resting polarization is at *(B)*. The arrows indicate the local currents, which cause neighboring regions to become successively depolarized toward the right. After a very short period of depolarization, the membrane restores the polarization to its normal resting condition.

day. Therefore, if the location of the axon death is known, as is usually the case when it is caused by external injury, the recovery time can be estimated. It is rare in such regeneration processes for recovery to be complete. The longer the path over which regeneration must occur, the less complete the recovery will be. Regenerating axons are of smaller diameter, have less mature membranes, and, if they are myelinated, a thinner layer of myelin and perhaps also a reduced distance between the nodes of Ranvier. A regenerating axon therefore has a much slower conduction velocity than a normal axon. Even when the regenerating axon is fully mature, its conduction velocity may still be less than normal.

Another interesting form of recovery or partial recovery, which results particularly in the case of motor nerves, is the ability of unaffected motor nerves to begin to "take over" for a dead nerve fiber. A residual motor nerve fiber can send out additional branches to make connections with muscle fibers that have lost their nerve connections. This branching process may take up to 2 years to be fully complete, and again, recovery via this technique is never a total return to normal.

There is a broad range of severity in peripheral neuropathies. The effects of motor nerve involvement may vary from only very mild and barely perceptible weakness to profound and total paralysis. Sensory involvement may range from mild feelings of numbness to complete loss of sensation. Usually in peripheral neuropathy, the further away part of an extremity is from the central nervous system, the more severe the disorder. Thus, sensory changes and weakness may be major in the hands, but less marked at the elbows and shoulders, and similarly, major in the feet and ankles, but mild at the knees and hips. The latter is not entirely true in the case of mononeuritis and mononeuritis multiplex.

Various terms are used to describe sensory symptoms. *Anesthesia* refers to complete loss of all sensation. *Hypalgesia* and *hypesthesia* are reductions in the sensations of pain and touch, respectively. *Hyperesthesia* is an abnormally increased sensitivity of the skin, which is often annoying. *Paresthesia* is a feeling of tingling, or "pins and needles." Further, continuous pain can occur, ranging in intensity from very minor to very excruciating pain which greatly interferes with the patient's behavior.

With regard to motor symptoms, weakness is the subjective complaint made by the patient. Partial loss of strength (*paresis*) or total loss (*paralysis*) are the signs detected by examination. *Atrophy*, a reduction in the mass of muscle, may also be an associated sign.

For discussion purposes, the remainder of the chapter groups the peripheral neuropathies into two classes: polyneuropathy and traumatic neuropathy. Under polyneuropathy, the peripheral neuropathies associated with hereditary causes and various acquired diseases, and those induced by toxins, are included. Under traumatic neuropathy, the peripheral neuropathies due to nerve injury from external trauma or from internal mechanical trauma are included. Internal mechanical trauma includes nerve constriction by such things as ligaments, bone overgrowth, extra ribs, or ruptured discs.

Polyneuropathy

Classification. The polyneuropathies may be hereditary, toxic, associated with other known diseases, or idiopathic (i.e., primary, but of unknown cause).

A sampling of the major *hereditary neuropathies* includes:

1. Charcot-Marie-Tooth disease
2. Dejerine-Sottas disease
3. Hereditary sensory neuropathy
4. Friedreich's ataxia
5. Spinocerebellar degenerations of adulthood
6. Familial spastic paraplegia
7. Refsum's disease
8. Acute intermittent porphyria

Since the diagnosis may simply list these names and not actually say "peripheral neuropathy," the counselor should be aware that when such diagnoses are given, possible disabling consequences of peripheral neuropathy should be anticipated.

Table 7-1 lists the *toxic causes of peripheral neuropathy:* the heavy metals, drugs (including, in addition to the prescription type, two of the "street drugs"), and those organic compounds (some of which are used in industry) capable of inducing peripheral neuropathy.

There are a number of *diseases associated with peripheral neuropathy.* These include:

1. Diabetes mellitus
2. Alcoholism
3. Chronic renal insufficiency
4. Cancer
5. Rheumatoid arthritis
6. Sjögren's syndrome
7. Scleroderma
8. Systemic lupus erythematosus
9. Hypothyroidism
10. Polyarteritis nodosa
11. Sarcoidosis
12. Chronic liver disease
13. Thermal burns
14. Diphtheria
15. Leprosy
16. Herpes zoster
17. Vitamin B1, B2, B6, and B12 deficiency
18. Postgastrectomy state

Several of these diseases, namely, rheumatoid arthritis, alcoholism, diabetes, and cancer are discussed in chapters 14, 17, 24, and 28, respectively.

TABLE 7-1
TOXIC CAUSES OF PERIPHERAL NEUROPATHIES

Heavy Metals	Organic Compounds	Drugs
Lead	N-Hexane	Nitrofurantoin (Furadantin)
Arsenic	Acrylamide	Diphenylhydantoin (Dilantin)
Thallium	Tri-ortho-cresyl phosphate	Vincristine
Mercury	Methyl-butyl-ketone	Isoniazide
Antimony	Carbon disulfide	Dapsone
Gold	Carbon monoxide	Corticosteroids
	Dichlorophenoxyacetic acid	Sodium cyanate
		Halogenated oxyquinoline derivatives
		Hydralazine
		Chloramphenicol
		Disulfiram (Antabuse)
		Sulfonamides
		Heroin
		LSD

Familiarity with this list of diseases associated with peripheral neuropathy will alert the counselor to the fact that clients with these diseases may also have peripheral neuropathy as one of the complications.

The four *idiopathic neuropathies* are:

1. Guillain-Barré *syndrome*
2. Chronic polyradiculoneuropathy
3. Fisher's syndrome
4. Shoulder girdle neuritis

Of these, Guillain-Barré syndrome (see chap. 6) and shoulder girdle neuritis are the most important.

Peripheral neuropathy of unknown cause may later be found to be associated with cancer. Cancer apparently may produce derangement in the biochemistry of the nerves. The neuropathy may appear before the cancer itself becomes obvious. Cancer can, however, more directly and on a mechanical basis produce a mononeuropathy or mononeuropathy multiplex. Tumors growing near nerves may compress them directly and thus block the conduction of impulses, or the tumors might interefere with the blood supply to the nerves, causing nerve damage. In some instances, invasion into nerves by malignant cells can occur.

While primary tumors of the axon are rare, tumors arising from myelin sheaths do occur and can produce neuropathies by compressing the axons. Neurofibromatosis, or von Recklinghausen's disease, is an example of a tumor arising from myelin sheaths. It is a congenital disorder characterized by the presence of multiple tumors, which can appear in almost all nerves or segments of nerves and produce neuropathy if the tumors are not removed. The disease is associated with other signs and symptoms affecting, for example, skin and bone.

Prognosis. The hereditary neuropathies generally get progressively worse with time, but the time course of these diseases is very slow, and the counselor should be aware of the expected progression when planning with his client. Acute intermittent porphyria, however, is not relentlessly progressive, but is rather inclined to be stationary once it occurs, or to improve with time. Central nervous system impairment is associated with some of the hereditary neuropathies. When a client has a hereditary neuropathy, the counselor may need to find out if brain damage is part of the syndrome to determine whether any intellectual and behavioral changes are to be expected.

The toxic neuropathies usually have very good prognoses after the offending agent has been removed. As already indicated, however, it is rare to have total regeneration of nerves back to normal, and hence some disability may remain.

The prognosis for the peripheral neuropathies associated with the diseases listed on page 103 depends in great part on the success of the primary disease treatment. This is particularly true for diabetes, alcoholism, chronic renal disease, and the vitamin deficiencies. To assist planning, the counselor should obtain advice regarding prognosis of the disease-related peripheral neuropathies from the client's physician.

The prognosis of the idiopathic neuropathies varies. In Guillain-Barré syndrome, if normalcy does not return within 3 to 4 months after onset, patients will not fully recover and will have residual disability but no progression. In shoulder girdle neuritis, the neuropathy will not progress, but at the same time will not necessarily improve. The prognosis of chronic polyradiculoneuropathy varies greatly and must be considered on an individual basis.

Traumatic Neuropathy

Classification. Three types of injuries make up the traumatic neuropathies: compressions, tractions (stretching), and transections, as may occur in a knife wound. The symptoms are determined by the site and severity of the injury. They may be minor, as in the case of a mild compression, or major, as in the case of a severe traction or complete transection.

In the traumatic neuropathies, the condition of the nerve is described in any one of three ways depending upon the severity of the injury. The least serious lesion is *neurapraxia.* The nerve axon is still anatomically intact but there is a block to the conduction of impulses. Removal of the pressure causing the neurapraxia will result in a return of conduction in 1 to 2 months with complete recovery. *Axonotmesis* refers to the condition of a nerve which, while still anatomically intact, has profound axonal degeneration. Removal of the compression inducing the degeneration will result in partial recovery as regeneration of the axon occurs. A traumatized nerve may initially show a neurapraxia, but if the lesion is not treated soon enough, progression to axonotmesis may occur. In *neurotmesis,* a complete severance of the nerve has occurred. Repair and recovery requires first suturing the nerve ends together. Regeneration past the suture down the distal portion of the nerve then follows.

Compression or entrapment neuropathies may occur in any region where nerves pass through apertures formed by bone, tendon, muscle, and other soft tissue. For example, entrapment of a portion of the brachial plexus (see p. 27) may take place as the nerves forming the brachial plexus descend at the base of the neck into the upper extremity. The nerves here pass through a narrow outlet (the thoracic outlet) in the region of the first rib and the clavicle where they may be compressed. Accessory congenital ribs or malformed cervical vertebrae may reduce the volume of this outlet and also result in compression.

The most well-known compression or entrapment neuropathy involves the median nerve at the wrist where it passes through a tight tunnel to serve the muscles of the thumb, and skin of the thumb, index, and middle fingers. This tunnel is referred to as the carpal tunnel, and when the median nerve is compressed, the term "carpal tunnel syndrome" is used. The incidence of carpal tunnel syndrome with minimal obstruction in the tunnel is associated with other diseases which apparently make the nerves more susceptible to damage. For example, roughly 20 percent of the patients with hypothyroidism are prone to developing carpal tunnel syndrome.

An exhaustive review of each of the signs and symptoms associated with the various different nerve damages that can occur in compression, traction, or transection is beyond the scope of this discussion. The reader may refer to tables 3-1 (p. 19), 3-2 (p. 20), 3-3 (p. 20), and 5-1 (p. 65) for additional information regarding specific nerves and the sensory and motor consequences of their injury. A brief overview of the sites of damage (spinal nerves, plexuses, and distal nerve trunks) is useful, however.

If a nerve lesion involves the spinal nerve roots, a *radiculopathy* is said to be present. A herniated intervertebral disc, spondylolisthesis, and some forms of degenerative disc disease (see chap. 15) may give rise to characteristic symptoms, depending upon the spinal nerve involved.

Plexuses are formed by combinations of spinal nerve roots in the upper and lower extremity. The brachial plexus in the upper extremity and the lumbosacral plexus in the lower extremity are the two major combinations. Traumatic neuropathy involving a plexus causes multiple muscle and sensory symptoms corresponding to the part of the plexus damaged. The plexuses redivide to the final distal nerve trunks, the major ones being the median, ulnar, and radial nerves in the upper extremity, and the sciatic, femoral, peroneal, and tibial nerves in the lower extremity. The specific disabilities that result depend upon which of the distal nerves are involved.

Prognosis. Compression injuries have the best prognosis, for if the compression is recognized and removed early, recovery may be practically complete. It is rare for compressions to produce total paralysis or total loss of sensation because the patient will usually consult his physician before the problem has gone that far.

Traction injuries do not have a good prognosis. Severe stretching can disrupt the nerve and cause it to become quite scarred and greatly inhibit the likelihood of regeneration. Further, traction injuries are associated with chronic pain more than the others.

Cleanly sectioned nerves have a better chance for recovery if the nerve is sutured together, although recovery is never complete. The longer the segments through which the regenerating nerve must grow after suture, the less complete the recovery.

Complications

The major potential complications of peripheral neuropathy are contractures, causalgia (reflex sympathetic dystrophy), and osteoporosis.

Contractures. In peripheral neuropathy, contractures are secondary to profound weakness and paralysis. If the joints associated with the involved muscles do not receive appropriate range-of-motion exercises, muscle and ligament shortening may occur, leading to a limitation of joint motion and added disability. Prevention of contractures and measures for treating them when they have occurred are discussed in chapter 4.

Causalgia. The disabling condition in causalgia is pain, which is generally intense, severe, burning, and paroxysmal. It is precipitated by minor stimuli, including even the pressure of clothing or a slight breeze. The intensity may range from extremely disturbing to frankly intolerable and can precipitate drug abuse. The process is generally confined to the extremities, most commonly only one. Causalgia is more likely to occur in the traumatic neuropathies, particularly in those caused by traction. The limb is usually swollen, cold, and sweaty. The skin may be shiny, the joints contracted, and the bones osteoporotic. Exquisite tenderness of the limb may be present, causing the patient to avoid minimal contact. Severe fear and emotional anxiety are generally associated.

The cause of causalgia is frequently a severe intial trauma to a major nerve. This event triggers a massive outflow of impulses from the sympathetic nervous system to produce most of the signs and symptoms. Treatment is difficult and consists of interruption of the sympathetic outflow with local anesthesia, certain drugs, and sometimes surgical excision of the sympathetic ganglia associated with the limb. In addition, the original lesion is treated, and the limb is remobilized through physical therapy.

Osteoporosis. In peripheral neuropathy, osteoporosis may develop if there has been a profound paralysis of the muscles of the extremity. The paralysis results in reduced tension on the bones, which in turn causes calcium to dissolve out of the bone. Chapter 4 deals with some of the secondary problems that can result from osteoporosis.

FUNCTIONAL DISABILITIES

Physical Disabilities

A peripheral neuropathy involving the nerves of the lower extremities, with the production of weakness and sensory loss, will cause ambulation impairments. Level ambulation, stair climbing, and rough-ground negotiation may be affected. Sensory losses will affect balance, for the patient will not receive adequate messages concerning the location and position of his limbs. Negotiation is particularly difficult in the dark, since the patient has no visual input to guide him.

Peripheral neuropathic involvement in the upper extremities, with weakness and sensory loss in the hands, may interfere with dressing and eating skills, and, if sufficiently severe, with personal hygiene and writing skills as well. Fortunately, rehabilitation techniques can reverse these physical disabilities, even if the peripheral neuropathy is unchanged, through appropriate training, technique instruction, and adaptive equipment.

Psychosocial Disabilities

Patients with peripheral neuropathies are relatively free of psychosocial disabilities unless the neuropathies are associated with some of the diseases listed on page 103. Chapters 14, 17, 24, and 28 discuss the psychosocial impairments that may be associated with four of these primary diseases.

Pellagra (vitamin B2 deficiency), porphyria, and some of the hereditary peripheral neuropathies also affect brain function. Variable cognitive and personality problems may therefore appear and be in need of evaluation. Further, in severe peripheral neuropathy with extensive nonreversible sensory and muscle function loss, problems of dependency and depression, and family, social, and financial upheaval may also be present, similar to those associated with spinal cord injury (see chap. 5).

Rehabilitation Potential

As a general rule, rehabilitation potential is very good for persons with peripheral neuropathies, and long-term planning in most instances can be considered. Except for those associated with the major diseases, peripheral neuropathies are inclined to be stable or to improve, rather than progressively worsen. Hereditary neuropathies may progress, but slowly enough to allow for planning programs of 2 or more years in duration.

STANDARDS OF EVALUATION

Peripheral neuropathies are best evaluated by a neurologist and/or a physiatrist, although internists with special interest in nerve disease may also perform the evaluation. If any of the diseases listed on page 103 are present, evaluation by an internist would be essential.

The evaluation includes a search for hereditary factors, a search for exposure to toxic substances, and specific examination of the nervous system. Careful testing of muscle strength, sensory function, and reflexes is included. Special instruments are sometimes used to quantify the sensations of touch and pain. Von Frey hairs, of various thicknesses, can record the pressures required for touch to be perceived. An algesimeter measures pain sensation by recording the force, when applied to a fine steel needle directed at the skin, that results in the perception of pain.

Since peripheral neuropathy may be the first manifestation of some of the diseases listed on page 103, certain basic tests may also be done to search for the primary disease entity. Muscle and nerve biopsies may be required if the diagnosis is unclear. In the traumatic neuropathies, consultation by a neurosurgeon or orthopedic surgeon is usual.

In the detailed diagnosis of the nerve involvement in peripheral neuropathy, electromyography and nerve-conduction studies, usually performed by a physiatrist or a neurologist, are important. In electromyography, a needle electrode is placed in the various muscles whose nerves are suspected of involvement and the electromyographer looks at the nature of the electrical activity when the muscle is at rest and when it is actively contracting. Axonal disease is suspected if special electrical potentials are present when the muscles are at rest and there is abnormal electrical activity during motion. Nerve-conduction studies examine the speed with which messages travel in nerves. The examiner electrically stimulates the nerve and records how fast the electrical impulse travels down the length of the nerve. For the long nerves, the examiner can determine the speed of conduction in different segments. If the speed of conduction is markedly reduced, demyelinating disease is suspected. If it is reduced only in segments, segmental demyelinization is suspected. Electrical stimulation of nerves can also help evaluate the reflexes and hence the character of the spinal nerve roots (see p. 26). So-called H-reflex and F-wave studies are helpful in this regard. Electromyographic and nerve-conduction studies are not only helpful in establishing the definitive diagnosis with regard to the location, nature, and site of the disease, but they are also useful in following the course of treatment and in determining prognosis.

In addition to these medical evaluations, evaluations by a physical therapist and an occupational therapist are helpful. The physical therapist can assess ambulation and transfer skills and the occupational therapist can assess whether eating, dressing, and personal hygiene difficulties are present and, if so, how they might be reversed. Where weakness, particularly in the legs and the hands, interferes with certain skills, an orthotist may assist by fabricating braces to restore function.

Since most peripheral neuropathies are likely to be self-limiting and not very progressive, psychological evaluation and family and social service review may not be necessary. However, in conditions that might affect central nervous system function, review of intellect and personality by a psychologist may help the counselor with planning. Certainly, severe disability, with its potential family, financial, and social disturbances, may warrant social service review. Finally, patients with disease-related peripheral neuropathies may require psychosocial review for problems associated with the disease, rather than with the peripheral neuropathy itself.

TOTAL TREATMENT

Polyneuropathy

There is no specific treatment that reverses the neuropathy in the hereditary disorders. Exposure to toxic agents and trauma must be avoided, and nutrition and vitamin B intake must be adequate, since patients with hereditary neuropathies may be more susceptible to insults from toxins, trauma, and vitamin deficiencies.

In addition to removing the patient from exposure to the agent, specific therapy for the toxic neuropathies includes the administration of detoxifying substances designed to remove the poison from the system. Examples are penicillamine for lead and mercury, and the chemical British anti-lewisite (BAL) for arsenic. In addition, specific antidotes also exist for the organic compounds.

Specific therapy for the peripheral neuropathies associated with the diseases listed on page 103 is basically the primary treatment of the disease itself. Thus, the best treatment for diabetic neuropathy is good diabetic control; for chronic renal insufficiency, appropriate dialysis or kidney transplantation; and for hypothyroidism, treatment with thyroid medication.

For the idiopathic neuropathies, in particular Guillain-Barré syndrome and chronic polyradiculo-neuropathy, corticosteroid treatment has been introduced and is considered helpful. Hospitalization, bed rest, and analgesics for pain control usually are required for the severe acute-onset neuropathies.

Traumatic Neuropathy

Surgery is the specific treatment for the traumatic neuropathies, particularly those associated with compression. *Neurolysis* refers to the surgical freeing of a nerve from encapsulating and constricting neighboring ligaments or adhesive bands. Suturing cut nerve ends together is called *neurorrhaphy*. If a nerve is moved to a less constricting location, it is referred to as a *translocation*.

Rehabilitation Treatment

Rehabilitation measures include prevention of unnecessary additional disabilities. Contractures are prevented by appropriate range-of-motion exercises performed for and by the patient. Exercise activities to strengthen both weak and uninvolved muscles, and training in the appropriate use of canes and crutches help restore ambulation and transfer functions. In severe lower extremity paralysis, short or long leg braces might be prescribed to improve standing endurance and walking. Treatment by an occupational therapist usually eliminates any impairments in eating, dressing, and personal hygiene skills through appropriate techniques and adaptive equipment. In most instances, writing and driving difficulties can also be overcome. Orthoses and splints may also be used when there is profound paralysis to maintain a joint in its functional position in order to prevent deformity. If joint deformity has already occurred, certain orthoses may need to be prescribed to correct it. In addition, there are orthoses that can assist function when weakness is present. They are designed to be used while the function is being performed, and are referred to as dynamic or kinetic devices.

Electrical stimulation of paralyzed muscles on a regular basis can retard atrophy, although it cannot accelerate recovery. If recovery is expected in a reasonably short time (e.g., within 4 to 6 months), an electrical stimulation program to be carried out by the patient at home may be prescribed. Trancutaneous electrical stimulation is also sometimes helpful in the control and alleviation of pain, especially in herpes zoster and in some cases of causalgia.

The need for psychosocial treatment, such as ongoing care by a psychologist or social worker, is usually only required for patients with the more profound paralyses, as discussed in chapter 5.

Followup Treatment

Medical followup after the initial treatment is generally dictated by the condition involved, and usually includes monitoring changes in status, and perhaps modifying treatment. The hereditary neuropathies might not need followup more than once or twice a year. The followup required for disease-related peripherial neuropathies is dictated by the primary disease, rather than the peripheral neuropathy. In the toxic neuropathies, once the offending agent is removed and specific treatment is instituted, followup is usually not required after 1 year unless there is persistent paralysis and observation is required to avoid complications. The idiopathic neuropathies require closer followup during the period of active treatment. Some patients may be seen once a month, or more often, until full stabilization occurs, after which followup can be less frequent.

VOCATIONAL IMPLICATIONS

Since residual physical impairments in muscle and sensory function may vary so widely in location, quality, and degree, the rehabilitation counselor needs to obtain rather detailed and accurate information from the client's physician, and perhaps from the counselor's medical consultant, regarding etiology, the extent of functional disabilities, the efficacy of various treatments, and the prognosis. Further, the counselor should verify that his client has had access to all possibilities for improving function, such as surgery and the various treatment modalities of physical rehabilitation.

Although the extent of disease in peripheral neuropathies varies greatly, the following general statements may serve as a useful baseline.

Education

Peripheral neuropathy does not generally limit long-term planning, such as extended education or specific vocational training for 2 or more years. Education planning may have to be modified if the client has a peripheral neuropathy secondary to one of the diseases listed on page 103. In this case, the primary disease will determine whether short-term goals will be more appropriate.

Aptitudes

Intellect, learning ability, and verbal and numerical skills may be partially impoverished in those conditions with central nervous system effects, such as pellagra, alcoholism, and porphyria. In these situations, careful aptitude and intellectual testing may be necessary. Finger and hand dexterity, eye-hand coordination, and eye-hand-foot coordination difficulties may result from a sensory impairment in the hands and feet or from weakness in the hands and lower extremities. A client with sensory impairment may need to have his hands in constant view during manipulation. This may prevent activities that require direct observation of the object being manipulated, as well as hand activities that are out of sight. Jobs that may involve hand dexterity and eye-hand-foot coordination should be carefully reviewed to ensure that performance is possible for the client.

Interests

In peripheral neuropathy, a clash between the client's interests and his level of physical function is unlikely, except when interests are in activities within the medium and heavy work categories. Such tasks may exceed the strength and endurance of the client who may, however, handle light and sedentary activities quite well.

Physical Demands

Peripheral neuropathy in the legs, with or without obvious weakness, may mean that the client will have difficulties with jobs requiring extensive ambulation, standing, lifting, and carrying. Balancing, stooping, and kneeling may also have to be avoided. For some, sensory impairments in the legs may require sedentary and indoor work. Indoor work may also be required if the client's ambulation is impaired on uneven, rough, or hilly ground. Even if leg function is normal and neuropathy is confined to the upper extremities, the client may be unable to handle more than light work because pushing, pulling, and carrying requirements may exceed his upper extremity limits. Motor or sensory leg and arm impairments will interefere with climbing. For some clients, relatively minor sensory deficits in the upper extremities, even with good muscle function, may impair fine manipulation sufficiently to require occupational adjustment.

Environment

A client with reduced sensation may be unable to appreciate excessive heat, with the result that accidental burns may be possible if he works near flames or hot objects. Employment environments containing any of the toxic agents that can contribute to neuropathy, such as lead, arsenic, or organic compounds, should be avoided.

Hot and cold climatic extremes may aggravate the pain of causalgia, and should be avoided by clients with this complication.

In general, the rehabilitation counselor should find relatively easy success and rewarding outcomes when working with the client with peripheral neuropathy. The nature of the disability is rather clear and distinct, the condition is relatively stable, physical restoration possibilities are good, and complicating psychological and social problems are generally minimal. These factors, coupled with careful communication with the treating physicians involved, should allow the counselor to effectively plan with his client.

BIBLIOGRAPHY

Brain, Lord: *Brain's Diseases of the Nervous System.* Ed.8, revised by Walton JN. Oxford, Oxford University Press, 1977.
Complete text on the nervous system, with a well-written section on peripheral nerve diseases.

Dyck PJ, Thomas PK, Lambert EH (eds): *Peripheral Neuropathy.* Philadelphia, Saunders, 1975.
Most recent exhaustive two-volume consideration of almost every aspect of peripheral nerves, e.g., anatomy, physiology, pathology, and therapy.

Haymaker W, Woodhall B: *Peripheral Nerve Injury.* Ed.2, Philadelphia, Saunders, 1953.
Relatively old but excellent book based on extensive experience with traumatic lesions. Easily understood, with simple review of clinical diagnostic features.

Kopell HP, Thompson WAL: *Peripheral Entrapment Neuropathies*. Ed.2, Huntington, NY, Krieger, 1976.
Brief but concise review of peripheral neuropathies due to compressive lesions.

8 MULTIPLE SCLEROSIS

George H. Kraft, M.D.

DISEASE DESCRIPTION

Multiple sclerosis (MS) is one of the most common neurological diseases in North America and Europe, affecting as many as 500,000 persons in the United States alone. The disease is two to three times more common in the northern half of the United States than in the southern half. MS can affect any age, but most commonly has its onset between the ages of 20 and 40, with a peak incidence occurring around age 30, and is more common in females (F:M = 60:40). Because MS occurs during the most significant periods of one's vocational life, rehabilitation and vocational services are particularly necessary.

Etiology

The cause of MS is unknown and there are many theories as to its cause. A series of new discoveries during the past few years suggests that MS may be the result of a complex interaction of infection, immune, and genetic factors. One such theory suggests that a viral infection may precipitate an attack by the body's antibody (immune) system on the myelin, the fatty substance that sheaths nerve axons (see p. 19). In the last few years, many scientists have been studying measles (rubeola) and other viruses as triggering agents. Other investigators feel that the attack on myelin is mediated by different mechanisms. Some evidence suggests that there are certain genetic predispositions to the disease.

Pathology

The lesions of MS may occur in various places in the central nervous system (brain and spinal cord), and can therefore cause almost any type of central nervous system symptom, depending on the location of the lesions. It only minimally affects the nerves in the arms and legs (peripheral nervous system). The myelin sheaths are attacked and destroyed in localized areas within the brain and spinal cord. Patches of destroyed myelin are later replaced by scar tissue, producing lesions known as *plaques*. These plaques interrupt or distort the flow of nerve impulses in much the same way that breaks in the insulation on electrical wires can cause a malfunction of an electrical system. There is evidence that alterations of the nerve impulses may also occur before the myelin has been destroyed.

The symptoms that any one patient with MS may develop depend on the location of his specific lesions. The lesions may be distributed widely over the cerebrum, cerebellum, brain stem, or fiber tracts of the spinal cord. When located in the frontal or parietal lobes, symptoms of mental and psychological deterioration may occur. If corticospinal tracts in the cerebrum, brain stem, or spinal cord are involved, a spastic paralysis of the extremities may result. Similarly, involvement of sensory axons anywhere in the spinal cord, brain stem, or cerebrum along their path to the parietal lobe may produce numbness. Visual disturbances may result from direct involvement of the optic nerves or in the optic radiations in the occipital lobe. Plaques in the cerebellum may produce loss of coordination (ataxia), loss of balance, and tremors, particularly in the upper extremity when a person moves to grasp a specific object. Lesions in the cerebellum and the cerebrum can also cause speech and language disturbances. Bladder dysfunction may result from lesions distributed anywhere within the central nervous system. Not all of these symptoms are seen in each MS patient.

Transiently impaired vision is an early sign in about 20 percent of patients, and the most common problems are double vision (diplopia) or blurring. When these symptoms first appear, the physical and ophthalmologic examinations may still be normal.

As the disease progresses, many patients show a combination of weakness, spasticity, ataxia, and tremor. An inability to normally control bladder function is one of the most common, frustrating, and difficult problems encountered. Both a difficulty in initiating urination and incomplete emptying of the bladder (urinary retention) and dribbling (incontinence) can occur. Many patients with MS also need to urinate often (frequency), are unable to hold urine once the sensation to urinate has occurred (urgency), and have frequent urinary tract infections. Speech problems often occur, with dysarthria much more common that aphasia (see p. 129). Confusion, because it also can affect language performance, is often misjudged as aphasia.

Late in the disease, the mental abilities of some patients with MS may be affected. Of the various mental changes which can occur, euphoria is the most common and occurs in 31 percent of patients. Intellectual deterioration occurs in 26 percent, lability of mood (see p. 133) in 16 percent, depression in 7 percent, and psychotic episodes in 4 percent.

One of the characteristics of MS patients in general is that they are intolerant of heat and generally feel weaker in hot weather or in warm environments. Fatigability is another common symptom; patients may have good strength to begin a task but fatigue rapidly.

The classical pattern of MS is one of general overall progression of symptoms in a pattern of exacerbations and remissions. Symptoms become worse (exacerbation), then partially resolve (remission), only to become worse again in a continuing cycle. An exacerbation may be an exaggeration of prior symptoms or the appearance of new symptoms due to additional lesions in previously unaffected neurologic areas. An exacerbation typically lasts 2 to 3 weeks, although it can last longer. The average interval between exacerbations early in the disease is about 5 years. Some patients exhibit a continuous progression without remission.

Complications

The major complications that can occur include (a) contractures, which result in limitations of joint range of motion; (b) skin breakdown (decubitus ulcers) over bony prominences, particularly over back, hips, and buttocks; (c) chronic urinary tract infections, resulting in compromised renal function; and (d) seizures in a small percentage of patients. Although more of an exaggerated common MS symptom, excessive spasticity may also be considered a complication, for if it exists, it makes the prevention of contractures, skin breakdown, and urinary tract infection extremely difficult.

The development of *contractures* may be due to weakness or spasticity. Weakened muscles result in a joint not receiving its normal range of motion. Muscles with spasticity actually prevent the joint from being put through a normal range of motion. Contractures aggravate the physical disability beyond that caused by the lesions themselves.

Decubitus ulcers develop when numbness or reduced sensation is part of a patient's symptom complex. The patient is unable to tell when he has been lying or sitting for too long without shifting his weight. Weakness also contributes to the development of decubitus ulcers because it reduces the ability to shift weight off the pressure area. With sufficient time, continuous pressure on the skin over bony prominences reduces the blood supply to the skin. The skin then dies and a localized ulcer results. The bony prominences over which these ulcers are likely to occur are the low back (sacrum), the hips (trochanters), and the sitting bones (ischial tuberosities). Ulcers left unattended can progress and involve the underlying bone to produce osteomyelitis. The infection can also enter the bloodstream and create a widespread acute infection.

Urinary tract infections are basically secondary to bladder dysfunction, particularly chronic retention of urine and incomplete emptying of the bladder. Difficulty with perineal hygiene contributes to infection due to contamination from the anal area.

A complete discussion of *seizures* may be found in chapter 12.

Severe *spasticity*, particularly in the lower extremities, can be devastating. The slightest stimulation may cause the legs to involuntarily move into postures of flexion of the hip and knee. Severe adduction forces can also develop so that separation of the legs is difficult to accomplish. The limbs may actually cross over (scissoring). Flexion can be severe enough to maintain the heels drawn up against the buttocks. The resultant inability to sit or lie contributes to the possibility of decubitus ulcer development and aggravation of bladder, bowel, and perineal hygiene problems.

Prognosis

MS is an unstable and unpredictable disease. Early prognostic indicators that can determine which patients are likely to show rapid disease progression and which will show only slow progression have yet to be determined. However, it should be noted that many more patients have a mildly progressive form of MS than previously recognized. The vocational counselor will see persons who can function relatively normally for many years. Severe, rapidly progressive disease occurs in fewer than 10 percent of patients and 5- and 10-year periods between exacerbations are common. A significant number of patients are never seriously incapacitated.

MS itself does not produce mortality. Mortality is due rather to pneumonia or widespread infection secondary to decubitus ulcers in advanced disease where general debilitation is present.

FUNCTIONAL DISABILITIES

Physical Disabilities

The most common symptom preventing patients with MS from working is spasticity. This was demonstrated by a comprehensive vocational study of over 1,200 patients with MS in Germany. Two-thirds of the patients who were not working considered spasticity of the legs or arms to be the main reason they had to drop out of the employment market.

The combination of weakness, spasticity, ataxia, and tremor may interfere with walking and ultimately necessitate a wheelchair for mobility.

The use of a cane illustrates the functional problem encountered in the rehabilitation of a patient with both weakness and tremor. A cane might be very helpful to a patient with generalized weakness alone. However, a patient with MS might have great difficulty in placing a cane properly because of tremor, and consequently the cane might not be an effective ambulation aid. It might actually impair walking. A patient with coordination problems might need more time to ambulate a given distance than a patient with weakness alone. Curbs, stairs, and other barriers may present severe problems for a patient with both weakness and ataxia. Ambulation ouside the home will become increasingly difficult and time consuming as the disease progresses. Transfer skills are impaired because of incoordination. With ataxia, a patient may not have the balance required to get from a wheelchair to a bed or a toilet, or in and out of a car. With ataxia, a patient may not have the balance required to get from a wheelchair to a bed or a toilet, or in and out of a car.

With severe intention tremor, eating skills may diminish considerably and the patient may have difficulty in getting his hand to his mouth. Similarly, personal hygiene, bathing, and grooming may be very difficult for a patient with severe incoordination.

Speech slurring may reduce the patient's ability to communicate effectively. If the patient needs to communicate well in his job, this becomes a functional impairment as well as a "cosmetic" impairment. Because of tremor, handwriting also may be very difficult. Visual symptoms may have a deleterious effect on reading and driving.

In some patients, the loss of normal bladder control is the main reason for not being able to function vocationally, socially, or as a homemaker. Symptoms such as urgency and incontinence produce much embarrassment and perceived loss of social acceptability. It is important to specifically ask a client whether bladder problems occur, since the client may simply withdraw from the vocational environment. Withdrawal from work because of this is unfortunate, since most bladder dysfunction can be improved sufficiently with appropriate treatment to achieve a socially acceptable system.

Psychosocial Disabilities

The specific configuration of intellectual or cognitive deficits associated with MS varies with the individual case. As in other forms of cerebral insult, the single most likely interference will be in the ability to learn and retain new information, skills, or procedures; i.e., learning rate is impaired, though not necessarily the ability to learn. The contours of the intellectual impairments are likely to be scattered and diffuse, rather than discrete and focal, as often happens with stroke (see chap. 10).

Because of the pattern of exacerbations and remissions, the psychological stresses associated with MS are variable and unpredictable, rather than occurring in a single episode as in a stable disability. The MS patient needs to adjust to each new disability associated with an exacerbation, and must also adjust to the uncertainty inherent in his disease. This uncertainty, together with the psychological and intellectual effects of the cerebral plaques (emotional lability, intellectual deterioration, euphoria, depression, and, occasionally, frank psychosis), may produce disruption of the patient's social and family life and his vocational capabilities. Therefore, the disease can have an impact not only on the patient, but on family members and job colleagues as well.

Rehabilitation Potential

The major problem in determining the rehabilitation potential of patients with MS is the uncertainty of the future course of the disease. Some patients may have a very slowly progressive disease, while others may have a very rapidly progressive course. Fortunately, in the majority of MS patients, the disease progresses slowly and the patient has only a slightly shortened life expectancy. Yet, the combination of weakness, spasticity, and ataxia may significantly shorten the period of employability.

Studies are currently underway to determine early vocational prognostic indicators, but they are not yet available. At the present time, probably the most useful indicator is the past course of the disease. A patient who has had only very mild and infrequent exacerbations may be expected to continue this pattern for a number of years in the future. On the other hand, a patient with a rapidly progressive disease course could be expected to continue this pattern. Some clinicians feel that patients with primarily sensory symptoms (such as numbness or tingling) have a better future course than those with weakness or ataxia. Consequently, it would not be appropriate to plan a program requiring prolonged education and training for a young client with rapidly progressive MS. The appropriate plan would be a short training course to prepare the client for a vocation with minimal physical demands.

A certain degree of optimism must be retained by the vocational counselor when working with a client with MS. In a recent vocational study of MS in Israel based upon a country-wide survey of patients, only 24 percent of patients under 50 years of age were considered to be completely handicapped with no rehabilitation potential. Fifty-five percent were still working, without the aid of vocational rehabilitation services, and 21 percent were in need of these services. As might be expected, patients who were working in occupations that did not require much physical effort were better able to keep their jobs than those in occupations requiring physical effort.

Other studies have shown that the percentage of patients still able to work 10 years after the onset of MS ranges from 12 to 60 percent. In the comprehensive German study mentioned earlier, the overall percentage of employment dropped from 71 percent after 5 years of disease, to 50 percent after 10 years, and 31 percent after 15 years, with no further subsequent drop.

STANDARDS OF EVALUATION

Medical Evaluation

The diagnosis of multiple sclerosis is difficult. Several different experimental chemical laboratory tests have been reported from various medical centers as able to diagnose MS, but as yet none is conclusive. Currently, therefore, there is no diagnostic laboratory test specific for MS, although in the future there may be.

The diagnosis of MS must therefore be made from the history. A history of diffuse neurologic symptoms (multiple lesions) occurring over a period of time with physical examination signs of disease in more than one part of the central nervous system are required. Therefore, a long interval, usually 5 years, is common between the first symptoms and a diagnosis. The diagnosis can rarely be made with any degree of assurance at the time of the first attack. Even when the symptoms have been present for many months or years, considerable diagnostic skill is necessary to exclude the many conditions that may be simulated by MS.

Diagnostic errors are not uncommon, and it has been estimated that approximately 10 percent of the patients studied in a major epidemiologic survey were misdiagnosed and actually had other neurologic diseases. The extensive hospital and laboratory testing that may be performed are therefore not done to diagnose MS, but to eliminate similar-appearing and perhaps treatable diseases. It should be emphasized that this is an important undertaking since, at the present time, there is no cure for MS. Therefore, treatable conditions that mimic MS should be sought.

The only significant, but nondiagnostic, abnormalities among the usual laboratory tests are changes in the cerebrospinal fluid. Examination of the fluid usually shows an elevation of a certain type of protein (gamma globulin) and an absence of an increase in blood cells, as well as an abnormality of the colloidal gold curve test. In this test, cerebrospinal fluid dissolved in varying concentrations of salt solutions is mixed with a colloidal suspension. When the fluid has increased protein, generally in the gamma globulin fraction, there is a change in color of the suspension. The dilutions in which this change is noted define a positive test. This test is often positive in MS. Other types of neurologic conditions may produce similar findings, and some MS patients show no spinal fluid abnormalities. Therefore, spinal fluid tests are helpful but not infallible in confirming the diagnosis of MS.

MS is so variable that it is not possible to set forth in detail tests which should be authorized to rule out the possible presence of treatable disease. As a minimum, a 2- to 3-day hospitalization is appropriate for the spinal fluid examination and other tests, such as X-rays of the spine, a myelogram, and an electromyogram. In some cases, depending on the types of symptoms, other tests must also be done. For some patients, such an evaluation may be conducted in a number of outpatient clinic visits. These decisions should be based on the judgement and experience of a competent neurologist.

Very recently, several new electrophysiologic techniques, such as visually evoked cerebral potential, auditory evoked cerebral potential, the blink reflex, and electrospinogram, have been developed. They appear to be positive in the 75-95 percent range when used to test portions of the central nervous system affected by MS. These tests can be obtained in only a few research institutions and are not available in most hospitals at the present time. At their current stage of development, they would not be appropriate for making a diagnosis of MS. In the future, however, these tests may be developed sufficiently to be very useful.

If a visual disturbance is present, evaluation by an ophthalmologist may be necessary. Speech disturbances should be evaluated by a speech pathologist who will determine the type of dysarthria and recommend suitable therapy. A urologist may be necessary to evaluate bladder dysfunction. Consultation by a neurosurgeon may be suggested to determine whether mechanical pressure on the spinal cord exists rather than MS.

When impairment in ambulation and perhaps other physical disabilities occur, evaluation by a physiatrist and a comprehensive rehabilitation team is appropriate. Such an evaluation is particularly appropriate when speech, vision, and the urinary system are also involved and psychosocial problems are present or impending. In a comprehensive rehabilitation setting, physical and occupational therapy assessment and multidisciplinary review can produce the best evaluation for total treatment and vocational planning.

Psychosocial Evaluation

Administration of the Reitan test battery by an

appropriately trained psychologist to determine the patient's intellectual abilities, learning abilities, verbal skills, numerical skills, form and space perception, eye-hand coordination, and color discrimination may be useful to the counselor, both to identify subtle higher level intellectual impairments otherwise overlooked and to help him and others working with the patient to direct their rehabilitation efforts in light of cognitive/intellectual impairment. It should be remembered, however, that these tests will determine present dysfunction and, in a progressive disease such as MS, future performance must be couched in probabilities.

A psychiatrist or qualified psychologist should also evaluate the patient to detect the presence of emotional lability, euphoria, depression, or the possibility of psychosis. In addition, the patient's adjustment to his disabilities and to the uncertainty inherent in MS should be assessed.

Evaluation of the family unit by a social worker is important to detect problems caused by the patient's disability and by the recurring stress associated with the pattern of exacerbations and remissions.

TOTAL TREATMENT

Medical Treatment

There is no treatment to prevent MS, to prevent progression of the central nervous system lesions, or to prevent new lesions from developing. Furthermore, there is no conclusive proof that any medicine can alter the plaques. However, some physicians believe that ACTH (adrenocorticotrophic hormone) or corticosteroids (e.g., prednisone) can reduce the severity of exacerbations. Many patients receive such treatment. ACTH must be given by injection into a muscle at intervals up to twice daily or by continuous infusion into the veins. Long-acting preparations are also available which can be injected every few days. Intramuscular injection of ACTH must be given by a nurse or physician, and consequently require many clinic visits. Medicine given into the veins requires hospitalization. Other treatments, such as fat-free diets, sunflower seed oil, and vitamin supplements are not considered to be efficacious.

Some of the disabling symptoms can be reduced in intensity. For example, an intention tremor that seriously complicates the rehabilitation of a patient with MS may be managed by a neurological procedure. Surgical removal of an area of the brain (the ventrolateral thalamus) has been effective in some MS patients in reducing this tremor. This is a major operation carrying serious potential risks (e.g., hemiplegia) of its own. The risks must therefore be carefully weighed against the potential benefit before it is performed. To date, success has been variable.

Profound fatigue may be especially marked in the early afternoon. Mild central nervous system stimulants such as caffeine, Ritalin, or dextroamphetamine may be tried with occasional beneficial results.

Double vision can often be managed by patching one eye.

Treatment of Complications

Contractures. The joints associated with weakened and spastic muscles need to be carried through a passive range of motion daily to prevent or delay the development of contractures. In the early stages of the disease, the patient may be able to do this himself, but in later stages he may require the assistance of a family member. If the weakness or spasticity is severe, the assistance of a physical therapist will be needed.

The best physical therapy technique for treating mild contractures is deep heat combined with prolonged static stretch. When contractures are severe, they are disabling and cannot be controlled by conservative physical therapy treatment. In such cases, surgical correction by an orthopedic surgeon may be indicated.

Decubitus ulcers. Patients should shift their weight at least every hour when sitting and every 2 to 4 hours when lying to help prevent the development of decubitus ulcers. For wheelchair patients, special cushions, particularly those of a gel consistency, are helpful. They may not, however, prevent ulcer development if weight shifting does not occur. When ulcers are impending or have developed, removal of all pressure over the site and meticulous cleaning of the wound until it is healed are required. If the ulcer is extensive, surgical repair is necessary (see p. 417). When infection is present in the wound, antibiotics may be needed.

Bladder dysfunction and urinary tract infection. Management of bladder dysfunction and urinary tract infection requires the careful assistance of a urologist. Bladder dysfunction, particularly retention, is the precipitating event that allows infection to develop in the urinary tract.

Urinary frequency and urinary urgency are often effectively treated with the drug Probanthine or other agents blocking the parasympathetic nervous system to the bladder. For retention, agents such a Urecholine that increase the force of the bladder contraction and agents or techniques that reduce the resistance at the sphincter can be helpful. Medication that reduces spasticity (see below) may also affect and help the urinary sphincter if it too is spastic. Urological surgical procedures such as sphincterotomy, which cuts the sphincter muscle, or transurethral bladder neck resection (TUR) in male patients may be effective to provide a successful bladder. Where urgency is severe but retention is minimal in the male, a condom collecting system (see p. 76) may help produce a socially acceptable system. When severe urgency and minimal retention occur in females, there may be no option but a permanent indwelling catheter.

When urinary tract infections occur, the offending organism is identified and an appropriate antibiotic given. Simultaneous treatment of the bladder dysfunction is necessary to prevent recurrence.

Seizures. The drug management of seizures is discussed in chapter 12.

Spasticity. Oral medications, in particular Valium, Dantrium, and, more recently, Lioresal, are useful in the management of spasticity. These must be taken on a regular basis to control the spasms. Possible liver toxicity with Dantrium requires ongoing monitoring with liver function tests. Where one or a few offending muscles can be identified, spasms in these muscles may be managed by phenol motor point blocks (see p. 75), usually performed by a physiatrist or anesthesiologist.

If such measures are not effective, more major surgical procedures, such as injecting chemicals like alcohol or phenol directly into the spinal cord, cutting of spinal cord roots, or cutting the muscles from their points of attachment or insertion, can be dramatically effective. Recently, surgical implantation of electrical stimulators in the posterior columns of the spinal cord has been advocated as effective in the control of spasticity, but as yet the experience with this technique is limited. These procedures are only considered after the more conservative, less destructive procedures have been tried, and are usually performed by a neurosurgeon or an orthopedic surgeon.

Rehabilitation Treatment

A rehabilitation program must maximize ambulation and transfer skills in particular. As a general guideline, any patient falling more than twice a month needs an ambulation aid. In a patient who has severe ankle spasticity unrelieved by treatment with medications or motor point block, immobilization of the ankle with a brace may be the treatment of choice to maintain walking. This can be accomplished with either a metal or plastic brace, and may also require a special type of shoe incorporating a lateral "T-strap" to prevent the ankle from turning in. Knee instability can be treated by the use of two canes or, if hand function is poor, forearm crutches. Long leg braces are less desirable since they lock the knee and make walking difficult.

In patients with weakness, ataxia, and tremor, a weighted walker may be the only device that will provide sufficient stability for walking. A wheelchair might also be needed to provide functional ambulation. Often a patient will need a wheelchair for prolonged periods of mobilization and a cane for short periods. Skill in the use of a cane in a patient who can only ambulate over limited distances without a wheelchair improves his ability to be mobile in areas that are not wheelchair accessible.

In late stages of the disease when weakness is more pronounced, the patient may need devices to assist in eating and dressing. An occupational therapist may be needed to help the patient learn techniques for dressing, reading, writing, and personal hygiene. In general, the patient can be taught strategies to carry out these activities, although they may take considerably longer than normal to perform.

Management by a speech pathologist may be necessary for patients with swallowing difficulty and problems of articulation, including the common slurred speech. The speech pathologist will assist the patient in the use of compensatory systems for communication.

Psychological management may be required to help the patient deal with depression or denial. In addition, there may be a need for social case work with the patient and his family during various periods in the course of the disease to deal with the continued or recurring psychological stress associated with the severe problems occurring over a long period of time.

Patients with a number of physical impairments and associated psychosocial or speech problems are best managed in a comprehensive rehabilitation setting where various professionals work together to identify treatment goals. In such a setting, vocational planning is likely to be more appropriate because the counselor may be able to gain insight into what further progression may occur and be able to plan accordingly.

If a specific physical function has been lost within the prior 6 months and no active rehabilitation treatment for it has occurred, rehabilitation techniques and adaptive aids and equipment might allow the function to be regained. While some patients may require inpatient treatment for 3 to 6 weeks, others may be able to attain their goals in an outpatient program. Strenuous exercise, per se, is not useful because of the easy fatigability associated with MS.

Followup Management

Because of the remissions and exacerbations that occur in MS, continued medical followup is necessary even though such visits are not likely to influence the central nervous system lesions. Visits to a neurologist, a physiatrist, or a rehabilitation center every 1 to 2 months can help abort a potential loss of functional skills, or restore a functional skill recently lost through an exacerbation. Adaptive equipment, environmental manipulation, and utilization of residual function plus technique training can help restore independence or at least minimize dependency. In addition, regular followup is important to detect and/or treat any complications that may occur. A counselor may therefore wish to incorporate such a followup system in his vocational planning.

VOCATIONAL IMPLICATIONS

As shown in the Israeli study discussed earlier, more than one in five MS patients are in need of vocational rehabilitation services. Because the disease is so variable, the length of time spent in a retraining process should be based on the physician's judgment of the expected future course of the disease. A patient with a rapidly progressive form of MS should not be enrolled in a long-term training program, but a short training course to allow such a client to learn a less physically demanding task might be highly appropriate. On the other hand, if retraining is needed to teach the client with a slowly progressive form of MS a less physically demanding skill, it might be reasonable to enroll the client in a 1- to 2-year, but probably not a 4-year, program.

The vocational counselor should give major consideration to the physical demands of the client's occupation. Vocational interests of the client with MS which require heavy physical work should not be encouraged because of the fatigue factor in particular. The ultimate goal of vocational rehabilitation of a client with MS should be to provide services that lead to light rather than heavy work. All things being equal, the client should be trained and directed toward sedentary work, since the ability to work from a wheelchair, should it later become necessary, would prolong the period during which a client can be vocationally productive.

Even in the late stages, the client might be quite mentally capable of a vocational pursuit that does not demand physical strength. The Israeli study cited earlier found that fewer persons with sedentary jobs had to change their occupation as a result of their disease than persons with nonsedentary jobs. The sedentary work chosen, though, should not require fine hand movements, since tremor and ataxia are likely to develop. With tremor and ataxia, even writing might become difficult.

Fatigability is a major component of MS, and consequently occupations requiring repetitive physical tasks may need to be avoided. Some patients may actually need to lie down and rest for a short period of time in the afternoon, and vocational considerations may need to center around this.

Persons with MS tend to do less well at high temperatures, and therefore the temperature of the environment in which the client works is very important, and should not be excessively high.

Finally, persons with MS are thought to function less well outdoors and, if possible, should be placed on inside jobs protected from the extremes of temperature. Also, because ambulation may be a problem in late stages, a minimum of physical movement from place to place within a vocational area is desirable.

A vocational plan should also take into consideration the bladder needs of a client. Clients with catheters need to be able to empty the collection bags in an area affording privacy. Toilets need to be close to the work area for clients with frequency and urgency, and they must be wheelchair accessible if the client is in a wheelchair.

MS should have no effect on whether the client functions better dealing with things and objects rather than people and ideas, except that the client with advanced MS who has slurred speech and bladder incontinence might function less well with people than with objects. It has been the feeling of many physicians that stress should be avoided by clients with MS and, in the absence of contrary findings, it is appropriate that the less emotionally stressful the occupation, the better.

In the late stages of MS, the mental abilities of some clients may be affected. These disturbances may be the major reason why the client must finally stop working.

In view of the unstable nature of MS, a vocational counselor should provide continuous intermittent contact with the client. This may salvage the vocational situation when an exacerbation develops. The counselor also needs to be alert to new functional losses associated with an exacerbation which may interfere with a client's vocational activity. When an exacerbation occurs, it is important to consider rehabilitation treatment or environmental adaptations in the job to re-establish a function that the exacerbation may have caused to be lost or impaired.

In conclusion, an indoors, sedentary, physically nondemanding job requiring minimal hand dexterity may be optimal for a client with MS. Trained in such an occupation by vocational rehabilitation services, a client with MS may have many more productive years than if vocational rehabilitation services had not been provided.

BIBLIOGRAPHY

Bauer, HJ, Firnhaber W, Winkler W: Prognostic criteria in multiple sclerosis. Annals NY Acad Sciences 122:543–551, 1965.
This is an excellent review of the working capacity of patients with multiple sclerosis. The study was done in Germany for the German Ministry of Labor to determine the feasibility of rehabilitating MS patients who were receiving compensation. The study sample is large, involving over 1,200 patients with MS.
Brown JR: Recent studies in multiple sclerosis: Inferences on rehabilitation and employability. Proc Mayo Clinic 44:758–765, 1969.
This article discusses the rehabilitation potential of MS pa-

tients with reference to four major areas: the neurological systems involved; the course of the disease; the severity of the disease; and the patient's personal and vocational adjustment.

Kelly R: Management of MS. Nurs Mirror 143(6):48–59, 1976.
This is an up-to-date, very brief, and easy-to-read review of the management of MS.

Matson RR, Brooks NA: Adjusting to multiple sclerosis: An exploratory study. Soc Sci & Med 11:245–250, 1977.
In this study of 174 MS patients, a measure of self-concept was used as the key indicator of adjustment to the disease, and a four-stage process of adjustment to MS is proposed. The authors contend that a successful adjustment to MS is often misinterpreted as euphoria.

Maugh TH II: Multiple sclerosis: Genetic link, viruses suspected. Science 195:667–669, 1977.
_____: Multiple sclerosis: Two or more viruses may be involved. Science 195:768–771, 1977.
_____: The EAE model: A tentative connection to multiple sclerosis. Science 195:969–971, 1977.
This is a comprehensive and thoughtful analysis of the multiple sclerosis problem, with an emphasis on basic scientific investigation. It is not written for physicians but for the intelligent layman with an in-depth interest in multiple sclerosis.

Mei-Tal V, Meyerowitz S, Engle GL: The role of psychological process in a somatic disorder: Multiple sclerosis. Psychosom Med 32:67–80, 1970.
Twenty-eight of thirty-two patients studied were found to have had psychological stress prior to the onset of MS and/or exacerbations. The kinds of stress found and case studies illustrating the stress situations are included.

Poser CM: Diseases of the myelin sheath. In Merritt HH (ed): A Textbook of Neurology. Ed 5, Philadelphia, Lea & Febiger, 1973. p.566–727.
This is a comprehensive, medically oriented review of accepted medical information on multiple sclerosis and related neurologic diseases. Although most of the information in the chapter is beyond the scope of interest of the vocational counselor, it will be useful for two purposes: (a) to suggest as a guide to the counselor's medical consultant, and (b) to look up the accepted relevance of a variety of diagnostic tests.

Pulton TW: Multiple sclerosis: A social psychological perspective. Phys Ther 57:170–173, 1977.
This article includes a brief description of MS, mention of the relation between stress and the onset of MS and/or exacerbations, and the personal, familial, and social problems the MS patient may have.

Rozin R, Schiff Y, Kahana E, Soffer D: Vocational status of multiple sclerosis patients in Israel. Arch Phys Med Rehabil, 56:300–304, 1975.
This highly recommended article for vocational counselors surveys the problem of multiple sclerosis and its vocational implications in Israel. Although the study was not done in the United States, the data can be extrapolated to patients with MS in the United States. The article is very readable.

Tourtellotte WW: Multiple sclerosis. In Conn HF (ed): Current Therapy. Philadelphia, Saunders, 1968, p.664–673.
This is an easy-to-read review of a variety of common treatments for the common complications of MS. It is well written and concise.

9 STROKE AND CEREBRAL TRAUMA: MEDICAL ASPECTS

Thomas P. Anderson, M.D.

DISEASE DESCRIPTION

Stroke is the term given to the condition often referred to by the medical profession as cerebral vascular accident (CVA). Stroke can be defined as a sudden onset of weakness or other neurologic symptoms as a result of injury to a blood vessel in the brain (cerebrum, cerebellum, or brain stem). Approximately 50 percent of strokes are transient ischemic attacks (TIA's). These produce only temporary or transient neurologic deficits, from which a patient recovers within hours. The remaining strokes leave some permanent neurological damage and are termed *completed strokes*. In this chapter, the term "stroke" refers to completed stroke.

Cerebral trauma, or injury, which can occur anywhere in the brain, may differ from stroke in the mechanism of insult to the brain tissue, but the results and effects on the person are sufficiently similar that they can be discussed together. To avoid confusion in the discussion of cerebral damage, one should always keep in mind that damage to one side of the brain generally affects the opposite side of the body. A patient, therefore, who receives an insult to the right hemisphere will have a left hemiparesis and vice versa. Strokes and head injuries can also occur which are largely confined to the brain stem and cerebellum. Such insults, even if largely one-sided, are likely to influence the action of both sides of the body because of the smaller size of the brain stem and cerebellum compared to the cerebrum.

Because our culture is deeply involved with the automobile and motorcycle, the prevalence of cerebral trauma is steadily increasing. In some rehabilitation centers, brain trauma is more common than stroke. While the average age of patients with cerebral trauma is younger than the average age of stroke patients (45 to 55 years), stroke can also occur in children, adolescents, and young adults. Stroke has received much attention because it ranks third as a fatal disease in the U.S. Of greater significance to the vocational counselor, who deals with patients who survive completed stroke or cerebral trauma, is that stroke is second only to arthritis as a crippling disease and, as indicated, many patients fall within the working age group.

Stroke is often accompanied by one or more other medical problems associated with diseases of blood vessels, such as hypertension, heart disease, diabetes mellitus, atherosclerosis, elevated blood cholesterol, and peripheral vascular disease. Similarly, patients who have suffered an injury severe enough to result in cerebral trauma have often sustained injuries to other parts of the body as well, and these injuries may cause symptoms unrelated to the area of the brain damaged. Hence, when dealing with patients with cerebral trauma and/or stroke, it is important to remember that other related conditions often must be taken into consideration (see chaps. 22 and 24).

Pathology

The response of brain tissue to injury is similar whether the injury results from direct trauma or from a vascular accident. In either case, function in the area of the brain affected either stops altogether or is impaired. There are three main causes of stroke:

1. *Thrombosis* is the most common cause. A blood clot (thrombus) forms in a blood vessel and reduces or blocks the blood flow past that point. The part of the brain served by the blood vessel dies within minutes through lack of nourishment. The size of the area of brain death partly depends on how much of the area might also receive a partial blood supply from a blood vessel not involved in the stroke. In the older patient, the area will be larger because blood vessels are generally smaller and the collateral circulation is poor. In the younger patient, the area is apt to be smaller because of a good collateral circulation.

2. *Hemorrhage* is caused by a rupture of a blood vessel resulting in bleeding into the brain tissue. Damage from hemorrhage is likely to be twofold. In addition to brain death associated with lost nourishment from the vessel, damage to involved brain tissue can also occur from the pressure produced by the blood. Hemorrhagic stroke is often associated with high blood pressure, a factor in causing the blood vessel to

rupture. In the younger patient, hemorrhage can occur from rupture of an *aneurysm*. An aneurysm is a ballooning out of a vessel because of weaknesss in the vessel wall. Aneurysms are usually on the surface of the brain; hence when bleeding occurs, the blood fills the subarachnoid space, and the term *subarachnoid hemorrhage* is used to describe the situation.

3. *Embolism* occurs when a blood clot that has formed elsewhere (thrombus), such as in the heart or in the great vessels leading off from the heart, breaks off (embolus) and travels up the blood stream until it reaches an artery that is too small for it to pass and thereby blocks the artery.

The way brain tissue responds to interference with its blood supply is called an *infarct*. The infarcted area has two components: the tissues that have died as a result of blood supply loss, and the peripheral area in which there may be temporary dysfunction due to swelling (edema) or ischemia. If a part of the brain does not function for a period of time after cerebral trauma or stroke, but function gradually begins to reappear within 4 to 5 months, it is assumed that the period of nonfunctioning or altered functioning was due to swelling that was slow and gradual in subsiding.

Different portions of the brain are highly specialized in their functions, and therefore the effects on the whole person as a result of a vascular accident in the brain depend on several factors: (a) the side of the brain damaged (particularly for cerebral lesions); (b) the location of the infarct (cerebrum, cerebellum, or brain stem); (c) the size of the infarct; (d) the general character of the blood vessels and collateral circulation; and (e) the recovery of the involved tissue.

It is often said that no two patients are ever alike who have suffered brain damage. Although this is quite true, some generalizations can be made. The stereotypical stroke that is referred to in most of this chapter is the cerebral lesion produced when the middle cerebral artery (MCA) or one of its branches (see p. 25) is involved, because this is the most common artery involved in cerebrovascular accidents. Unless otherwise specified, "stroke" refers to this stereotype.

Anterior and posterior cerebral arteries and arteries in the brain stem may also suffer stroke syndromes, and areas served by these arteries (see p. 25) can be damaged by brain trauma. Brief summaries of the particular characteristics of these lesions as they may differ from the middle cerebral artery lesion will be considered later.

Signs and Symptoms

The outward signs and symptoms of stroke or cerebral trauma depend on whether the right or left cerebral hemisphere is affected. Patients with lesions in the dominant left cerebral hemisphere may have impairment in communication (speaking, understanding, reading, writing, and judgment), along with paralysis of the right arm and leg. Patients with lesions in the right cerebral hemisphere generally have perceptual (visuospatial) and judgment deficits, along with paralysis of the left arm and leg. The left hemisphere is dominant not only in right-handed persons, but in most left-handed persons as well. The right hemisphere controls communication functions in only 15 percent of left-handed individuals.

The most obvious finding in completed MCA stroke or one-sided cerebral trauma is paralysis or weakness of the opposite side. Soon after the onset of completed stroke, the paralysis of the involved side may appear to be complete. As edema resolves within a few days or weeks, some muscles may begin to show return of functioning and are classified as weak, or *paretic*.

More disabling are the sensory deficits produced by the brain damage. All sensations may be involved (light touch, pain, temperature, deep pressure, vibratory, visual, and position sense) or only one or two may be affected. Impairment of the sense of verticality and loss of the ability to maintain sitting and standing balance are also seen early after the onset of brain damage. When all modalities of sensation are affected but not totally paralyzed, there appears to be a dominance of pain sensation, such that any kind of stimulus to the patient's involved side is recognized as pain, even though it might have been only light touch. Sometimes lesions in the parietal lobe of the cerebrum (see p. 20) produce a total neglect by the patient of all sensory signals from his impaired side (anasognosia; see p. 130).

Visual deficits include a failure to recognize and respond to input from the visual field (see p. 48) on the side opposite the lesion because fibers to the occipital cortex crossing over the midline are interrupted. Most commonly, one-half of the visual field in both eyes is involved. Persons with left cerebral damage tend to have right visual field involvement and persons with right cerebral damage tend to have left visual field involvement. The effect on vision is rather like wearing goggles with either the right or left half of both lenses taped over, making it difficult to see objects positioned on the taped side. This condition is referred to by a variety of terms, such as visual field cut, visual field defect, visual field impairment, or homonymous hemianopsia. The most common manifestation of this symptom is the patient's failure to see the food on his tray on his involved side.

In anterior cerebral artery strokes, sensory deficits are usually absent and motor deficits usually involve the leg more than the arm. In posterior cerebral artery strokes, both sensation and motor impairment may be minimal, but visual impairments and balance and coordination problems may be significant. In brain stem strokes, weakness and sensory deficits are usually bilateral, although one side may dominate. Furthermore, brain stem strokes may produce paralysis of the cranial nerves, in particular those that control eye movement (cranial nerves III, IV, and VI; see p. 24) and those dealing with swallowing and tongue movement (cranial nerves IX, X, and XII; see p. 24). One of the more disabling symptoms in brain stem strokes is a swallowing difficulty severe enough that feeding may initially require utilization of a tube through the nose into the stomach. Brain stem strokes are often also associated with an initial period of coma because of the damage to the areas in the brain stem associated with alertness and wakefulness.

Brain trauma, more often than stroke, will produce bilateral effects even though one side may dominate. Thus, brain trauma affecting the cerebrum may produce communication as well as perceptual difficulties. Cerebral trauma and even brain stem trauma are also often associated with initial periods of coma. *Pure brain stem strokes and pure trauma episodes affecting the brain stem alone, by sparing the cerebrum, are not associated with intellectual, communication, or perceptual dysfunction.*

Complications

In addition to the communication or perceptual dysfunction and the motor and sensory deficits discussed above, which are the primary consequence of stroke or cerebral trauma, there are several secondary conditions which may occur and affect the patient's recovery and rehabilitation.

Depression. By far the most common complication is depression. However, it should not be considered a part of the natural history of these disorders. The depression can often be avoided or at least minimized.

Contractures. If a joint is not moved through its full range of motion several times a day, the surrounding muscles, tendons, ligaments, and joint capsule tighten and shorten, causing joint motion to become limited. The most common sites of these contractures are in the shoulders, the muscles that flex the hips, and the calf muscles that point the foot downward.

Contractures develop much more readily in the presence of spasticity. In fact, spasticity and contracture have a special relationship which can become a vicious cycle. When the contracture becomes severe enough to cause pain, the pain causes increased spasticity, and this in turn enhances the development of more contracture.

Now that contractures are better understood and preventive measures are more commonly practiced, they are not nearly as frequent a complication of brain damage as they were in the past.

Spasticity. As much (or more) disability can be caused by spasticity as by paralysis or weakness. An involved extremity is usually flaccid in its paralysis right after

the onset of a stroke. Loss of moderating influence from higher brain centers then causes reflexes to become hyperactive. Spasticity is a state of very hyperactive reflexes. The muscles may contract rhythmically, particularly at the ankle (ankle clonus). Spasticity can also appear in flexors of the fingers, extensors of the knee, and other muscle groups. It is often enhanced by any condition that causes pain, such as corns and bunions, or by tension, emotional upset, or trying to hurry. In some cases, spasticity may enhance the patient's functional abilities. This is particularly true if it occurs in the lower extremity where the spastic contractions of muscles may help stabilize the hip or knee for standing or walking.

Bowel and bladder dysfunction. Soiling or incontinence may occur and is usually due to a temporary loss of control of the sphincters. In the male, the problem can be further complicated by an enlarged prostate which was no problem prior to the stroke. Bowel and bladder dysfunction is usually temporary and can be corrected except in patients with the most severe strokes and head injuries.

Urinary tract infections. Chronic or recurring urinary tract infections may appear in patients who have had an indwelling urinary catheter during the acute phase of treatment. These infections, while usually treatable, can continue to be a problem long after the catheter has been removed and urinary function has apparently returned to normal.

Pneumonia. Pneumonia may occur as a complication of brain stem stroke or trauma because of the interference with the swallowing mechanism. Food particles may pass into the lungs and cause pneumonia.

Seizures. Seizures may also occur after brain damage, particularly after cerebral trauma. The damage and resultant scar may irritate the cortex and cause a spontaneous discharge of nerve impulses which may generalize to a full grand mal convulsion (see chap. 12).

Shoulder problems. Two shoulder problems may occur in stroke patients, particularly when the shoulder is not completely paralyzed. The shoulder joint (glenohumeral joint) may nearly dislocate (sublux). The weight of the arm simply draws the head of the humerus from the socket of the scapula (see p. 35). This condition may be painful, but can be controlled. Further, a chronically painful shoulder can lead to a shoulder-hand syndrome, a complex condition producing severe pain, swelling, contracture, and edema of the hand and shoulder on the involved side.

Others. Complications of the primary diseases associated with and partially contributory to the stroke may also exist. Thus, complications associated with hypertension, myocardial infarction, generalized atherosclerosis, peripheral vascular disease (see chap.

22), diabetes (see chap. 24), and sickle cell disease (see chap. 26) may also be present in patients with stroke.

Course and Prognosis

There are generally two types of functional improvement that occur after the onset of cerebral trauma or stroke. The first type is *spontaneous recovery* from the neurologic deficits that have occurred. The second type of functional improvement is due to *adaptation and/or training.*

Spontaneous recovery usually occurs as edema in the brain tissues subsides or the impaired circulation begins to improve. At present, usually very little can be done to influence this with medication, although agents may be developed in the future. Spontaneous recovery usually takes place within the first 3 to 6 months, although some smaller changes may be seen during the rest of the first year.

In general, a person with the typical middle cerebral artery stroke shows spontaneous recovery in the lower extremity before the upper extremity, and in muscles in the proximal part of an extremity before those at the distal end of the extremity. Therefore, the hand is often the last part to show return of function, if it occurs at all. Only 10 percent of stroke patients develop good hand function. Recovery of hand function beginning before the third week usually means useful function in the hand will develop. A person who has gone over 3 weeks with no evidence of returning hand function is not likely to have useful function of the hand. In contrast, the prognosis for lower extremity function is quite different; approximately 90 percent of stroke patients can learn to walk again.

While most spontaneous recovery has finished by the end of 3 months after onset, patients and their families do not like to give up hope at that time. Maintaining hope should be encouraged if it motivates a person's efforts for rehabilitation. However, if hope is associated with denial and postponement of rehabilitation efforts, progress is impeded (see p. 15).

Improvement in functioning through training and adaptation is a result of the person making use of his remaining abilities, coupled with technique development. This may consist of his learning to do things with one hand and even changing hand dominance. A few individuals may be able to devise their own adaptations, but often persons with brain damage are sufficiently depressed to have poor motivation to try new ways of carrying on former activities without guidance and direction. Hence, rehabilitation training helps the patient adapt and adjust to decreased neurologic function in the limbs on the involved side. The loss of the use of one hand does not necessarily mean loss of independence in self-care and most activities of daily living.

Once a person has survived the first week or two

of brain damage from cerebral trauma or stroke, it is more often not the brain damage that limits his survival, but rather the accompanying conditions such as diabetes, hypertension, or heart disease. However, it is true that elderly persons who have once had a stroke are more likely to have a second stroke than the rest of the population. Young patients who have suffered strokes from obscure causes and without underlying disease can expect a long life. Even in older persons, survival after stroke may be as long as 7 or 8 years after onset.

FUNCTIONAL DISABILITIES

Physical Disabilities

Almost all patients with cerebral or brain stem strokes or trauma initially develop physical disability affecting skills in eating, dressing, personal hygiene, transfers, and ambulation. In left cerebral lesions, verbal communication is impaired but nonverbal communication may remain unimpaired. In right cerebral lesions, verbal communication is unimpaired but nonverbal (perceptual) interpretation is impaired.

Visual field defects may impair reading even in the absence of language dysfunction. Reading may also be impaired by right cerebral lesions because the visuospatial deficits result in poor tracking across the printed page.

Finally, driving skills may also become impaired, not only because of arm and leg paralysis, but also because of the communication and reading deficits and possible perceptual deficits.

Psychosocial Disabilities

The cognitive functions of learning, memory, and judgment are usually involved. Emotional lability may also appear mostly through a release of inhibition, although a true reactive depression may occur as a result of the insult. Denial of disability can also occur. These disabilities are discussed in more detail in chapter 10.

Stroke or brain trauma can also have a significant effect on the family unit. Removal of homemaker, breadwinner, or young adult can seriously disrupt the entire family.

Rehabilitation Potential

When planning for the vocational rehabilitation of a person with stroke or cerebral trauma, several factors should be considered.

The damage produced by a stroke or head injury is not progressive. Improvement occurs after the acute period. Furthermore, the patient's adaptation to the various disability components appears to improve over the long term.

Particularly for insults occurring in the under-40 age group, a long life can be expected because there are usually no underlying diseases. Even for the older age group, a certain amount of long-term planning can be considered, since the average life expectancy after stroke is 7–12 years.

Most of the impairments listed above can be removed through effective treatment, instruction, and training.

Planning may have to be monitored if any underlying diseases are present which produce complications or other impairments that need to be considered. The limits of the ultimate vocational rehabilitation may be dictated not so much by the degree of paralysis but rather by the total residual verbal and nonverbal intellectual function with regard to learning, memory retention, and judgment.

Although no single factor in the early stage of stroke or cerebral trauma can positively or negatively predict the ultimate functional outcome, some generalizations can be made.

1. The shorter the coma (or absence of coma), the better the person's chances for functional recovery.
2. The earlier the beginning of return of function in the involved limbs, the greater the overall return of function.
3. If some return of function shows up only 2 months after the onset, the likelihood of ultimate functional use of this return is low.
4. Persons with higher socioeconomic and educational backgrounds tend to make greater use of their potentials.
5. Persons with significant family members who are capable of providing emotional support and meeting some of the person's minimal residual dependency needs not only avoid institutionalization, but are more apt to succeed vocationally.

STANDARDS OF EVALUATION

Diagnosis

In many cases, the diagnosis of stroke or cerebral trauma is not difficult to make. However, there are some conditions which can easily be mistaken for stroke initially. These are tumors (neoplasms), either primary in the brain or spread to the brain from other areas of the body; subdural hematomas; multiple sclerosis; and toxic conditions due to drugs, such as barbiturates, alcohol, or bromides, or to metabolic conditions, such as myxedema and diabetes. Infections such as meningitis, encephalitis, or brain abscess may occasionally have an abrupt onset that simulates stroke. Sometimes persons with epilepsy can have a stroke-like paralysis for a short period after a severe

seizure. Suspicion that the diagnosis of stroke or cerebral trauma may be incorrect should be aroused whenever it is observed that the neurologic deficits are progressively becoming worse.

The essentials of medical diagnosis of stroke and cerebral trauma include history and general physical examination, neurologic examination, skull X-rays, and lumbar puncture, if indicated. Sometimes cerebral arteriography or angiography and other procedures such as brain scan, computerized axial tomography (CAT scan), echoencephalography, and ophthalmodynamometry are indicated. This last group of procedures are not standard evaluations but are done in some special cases, particularly when there is a question about the diagnosis. If the counselor encounters a patient who has had some or all of these special procedures performed, he can feel more certain that the diagnosis is unquestionable.

Patients with conditions related to stroke (e.g., hypertension) should have appropriate evaluation and treatment to keep these conditions under good control, particularly during and after rehabilitation treatment.

Evaluation of Function

Neurologists, neurosurgeons, and some internists are the specialists most involved with the diagnosis and immediate acute treatment of cerebral trauma and stroke. Evaluation of the severely involved brain-damaged person's ability to function is optimally handled by a physiatrist. The physiatrist is familiar with all the various impairments of function in the brain-damaged person, and most of them work with a full interdisciplinary allied health team to carry out such evaluations and subsequent treatment.

Often, but not always, the impairments of ambulation and transfers are evaluated by the physical therapist working with the physiatrist. A rehabilitation nurse or an occupational therapist assists in evaluation of eating, dressing, and personal hygiene skills, as well as homemaking.

A master's level speech pathologist experienced in working with brain-damaged persons is needed to evaluate communication deficits in patients with aphasia or dysphasia. He can describe the level of verbal communication the patient can handle and properly interpret to the family and staff the patient's level of verbal communication. A speech pathologist can be helpful to patients with brain stem strokes or trauma in which involvement of cranial nerves interferes with the peripheral speech mechanism and swallowing. Evaluation by a speech pathologist can also assist in developing techniques likely to allow successful reading for patients with right cerebral lesions who have dysfunctions in visual perception that interfere with tracking across the printed page.

Clinical psychological assessment, particularly of patients with strokes or brain damage involving the cerebrum, allows for a more precise understanding of memory functions, learning potential, and personality patterns. The psychologist can determine whether the patient is best approached through pantomime, verbal communication, or both.

Early in the course of stroke or brain damage, evaluation of the patient and the family unit by a social worker can help detect problems brought on by the patient's deficits that can possibly be alleviated by various traditional social case work interventions.

Simultaneously, review by the vocational counselor of prior education and work experience, specific requirements of the patient's pre-onset job, and current job possibilities can encourage positive efforts not only toward physical restoration, but toward vocational readjustment as well.

TOTAL TREATMENT

Acute Phase

Diagnosis determination is the first part of acute treatment. This is followed by control of hypertension if present, maintenance of adequate nutrition, and maintenance of respiration. Direct treatment of any underlying heart disease or heart rhythm irregularities, such as atrial fibrillation, may be necessary if embolism is suspected. Anticoagulants, such as Coumadin for TIA's and sometimes for slowly progressive thrombotic strokes, may be used. Anticoagulants are not used for completed strokes, although some patients may be put on aspirin and Persantine. These medications may prevent or delay future additional thrombotic strokes by reducing the speed with which arterial walls narrow. Anticoagulants are never used acutely in cerebral trauma or in strokes in which hemorrhage has occurred.

Bed location and position are part of acute treatment. The bed should be positioned in such a way that when the patient is supine, personnel and family approach toward his strongest side, the side not likely to show a defect in visual field.

Neurosurgical procedures are sometimes indicated. Surgery on the carotid arteries in the neck (see p. 25) may be indicated for thrombosis which occurs in these arteries or if such arteries are a source of emboli. As a preventive measure, such surgery may be performed on patients who suffer TIA's and who demonstrate partial obstruction in the carotid arteries. Neurosurgical procedures may be performed on patients who suffer hemorrhages from rupture of aneurysm walls. The surgery removes the aneurysm and prevents additional bleeds in the future. Similarly, surgery may be performed on malformed arteries or veins if bleeding from them can be demonstrated. Hemorrhage into or around the brain which appears to aggravate the situation might also lead to neurosurgical procedures to decrease pressure. Finally,

paralytic episodes that might be induced by tumors mimicking strokes usually also require surgical removal.

Acute treatment also includes measures to prevent pneumonia, standard methods to ensure adequate bladder function, the prevention and treatment of urinary tract infection, and the initiation of bowel regularity, sometimes assisted by suppositories and oral medications.

From the start, contractures are prevented by regular daily performance of passive range-of-motion exercises of paralytic parts by a nurse or physical therapist.

Early participation by the patient in self-care activities, even if only eating skills and face hygiene are attempted initially, will usually prevent a reactive depression. Further, depression may be aborted if the patient and his family learn the nature of the functional improvement to be expected from a rehabilitation program.

Rehabilitation Phase

Specialists in internal medicine and neurology usually attend the patient during the acute stage and are able to manage the rehabilitation of patients with less complicated and less severe strokes. However, physicians specializing in physical medicine and rehabilitation and the team associated with them in rehabilitation centers are generally more experienced and better prepared to deal with the more severe strokes.

The rehabilitation phase usually begins within the first week of the acute episode and is best not delayed, for delay is inclined to aggravate complications. During the evaluation phase, the rehabilitation team identifies the problems of dependency in ambulation, transfers, eating, dressing, personal hygiene, cognitive functions, communication, social and family function, homemaking skills, and vocational function. They then simultaneously approach these problems in a systematic way and communicate with one another throughout the rehabilitation program. Using techniques that work around whatever residual sensory, paralytic, and communication deficits the patient may have, they help him achieve maximum independence in all of these activities.

Under the direction of the physiatrist, the rehabilitation phase includes activity by several professionals. The *speech pathologist* works daily with the patient with communication deficits, particularly aphasia. Verbal reading and writing skills, as appropriate, are developed, as well as additional means of communication through gesture, alphabet (word) boards, and other techniques. As skill training progresses, the speech pathologist analyses the patient's communication strengths and instructs the family and staff in the best techniques of communicating with the patient.

The *occupational therapist* develops the patient's independence in personal hygiene, dressing, writing, eating skills, and, as necessary and appropriate, homemaking and possibly driving skills as well. The occupational therapist assists in the utilization of whatever adaptive equipment may be necessary to allow even a one-handed individual to be independent and suggests home modifications to encourage independence.

The *physical therapist* initially provides range-of-motion exercises to paralytic parts and attempts to stimulate function in the paralyzed extremities. Strength development in the uninvolved extremities so they can begin to "take over" for lost functions also proceeds. These activities are associated with training in sitting balance, wheelchair ambulation, transfers, standing balance, and ultimately ambulation. Walking then follows and includes, as necessary, stairs, ramps, rough ground, and public transportation. Ambulation may require the use of a cane in the uninvolved hand and a short leg brace (ankle-foot orthosis) on the involved leg.

The *clinical psychologist* may be able to recommend approaches by staff and family that may be useful if depression or denial mechanisms are troublesome and how best to work around certain intellectual deficits. Intervention may be indicated if there are severe emotional reactions by any family members to the patient's disability.

The *vocational rehabilitation counselor* begins early to assess prior educational and employment background and to receive information on current function and ultimate goals. The counselor begins to plan with the patient, attempting to draw on prior background and current strengths which, coupled with goals of treatment, suggest vocational rehabilitation plans.

The length of hospitalization is usually no more than 4 to 6 weeks, although for severely and multiple handicapped patients and in certain cerebral trauma situations, hospital treatment may be as long as 3 months.

Treatment of Complications

Spasticity. When severe spasticity exists, particularly in the shoulder, forearm, hand, and ankle, to the extent that gains in function are impeded, specific treatment may be necessary. Medications, such as Valium and Dantrium, and certain special physical therapy techniques may help. Rigorous attention to ensuring full range of motion of involved parts is usually the mainstay of treatment. Injections of phenol into the muscle often lessen spasticity. In severe cases, cutting the tendons of the involved muscles may be necessary.

Shoulder subluxation. The use of an arm sling is indicated when shoulder subluxation occurs in a patient with no voluntary motor function in the involved shoulder. In order to inhibit the weight of the arm simply pulling the humerus away from the scapula, a sling fashioned to support the weight of the arm is usually helpful.

Shoulder-hand syndrome. The shoulder-hand syndrome usually requires special injections in the sympathetic nerves of the neck to block sympathetic nerve innervation in the involved extremity, coupled with specific physical therapy treatment to the hand and shoulder, and sometimes shoulder joint injections.

Seizures. Usually all patients who have had subarachnoid hemorrhages or cerebral trauma are placed on seizure medication as a preventive measure. Patients with vascular strokes who develop seizures several months after their strokes are placed on seizure medication after the first episode and this usually prevents any further seizures. The likelihood of seizures is small and need not be considered when making vocational plans.

Followup

Following discharge from the hospital, the patient with stroke or cerebral trauma should initially be seen monthly, progressing to perhaps no less than two to four times per year. Initially after discharge, physical therapy as often as three to five times a week might be part of the treatment program to develop further ambulatory skills.

The patient needs regular followup by his physician to ensure that he has an adequate system of maintaining range of motion in his involved side and that he maintains skills achieved during his rehabilitation. Further, management of any underlying disease (e.g., hypertension, seizures, heart rhythm irregularities) is necessary. The counselor should encourage the patient to protect himself against future problems by maintaining his outpatient visits. During the followup phase, it is appropriate for the counselor working actively with the patient on vocational objectives to maintain some measure of contact with the patient's physician to ensure that vocational plans are compatible with health status.

BIBLIOGRAPHY

American Heart Association: *Strokes: A Guide for the Family.* Dallas, TX, 1969.
  This booklet is written for easy understanding of the complexities of stroke. It defines stroke and covers the blood supply of the brain, the various mechanisms of stroke, and how the affected area repairs itself. It also briefly but accurately deals with prevention, treatment, and rehabilitation for stroke, and includes three keys to successful rehabilitation.

Anderson E, Anderson TP, Kottke FJ: Maintenance

of gains achieved during stroke rehabilitation. Arch Phys Med Rehabil **58**:245–352, 1977.

Patients with completed stroke maintained the gains in function achieved during stroke rehabilitation throughout their long survival time, averaging 7 to 8 years. This article describes the factors that influence the maintenance of functional gains.

Dresser AC, Meirowsky AM, Weiss GH, McNeel ML, Simon GA, Caveness WF: Gainful employment following head injury: Prognostic factors. Arch Neurol **29**(2):111–116, 1973.

Over eight hundred Korean conflict veterans who received head injuries were evaluated 15 years later to determine employment status. The factors contributing to unemployment or lower employment are discussed.

Espmark S: Stroke before 50: A follow-up study of vocational and psychological adjustment. Scand J Rehabil Med Suppl 2: 1973.

This study evaluated the readjustment to work and the psychological adjustment of the younger age stroke patients. Some patients were followed for several months to obtain an indepth psychiatric evaluation to learn more about the factors influencing the adjustment to stroke.

Gresham GE, Fitzpatrick TE, Wolf PA, McNamara PM, Kannel WB, Dawber TR: Residual disability in survivors of stroke—the Framingham study. N Engl J Med **293**(19):954–956, 1975.

Of the 123 survivors of the original 5,209 persons in the 1952 Framingham study, 119 were successfully evaluated. This article discusses the mean age of onset and the percent of persons who were living at home, who were institutionalized, who were independent in mobility, who were independent in activities of daily living, who resumed normal vocational function, and who showed no decrease in social activity outside of the home.

Lehmann JF, DeLateur BJ, Fowler RS, et al: Stroke: Does rehabilitation affect outcome? Arch Phys Med Rehabil **56**:375–382, 1975.

A sample of 114 consecutive stroke admissions to a rehabilitation center was studied statistically to determine functional gains achieved and retained after rehabilitation. A functional profile was developed that evaluates seven activities, each according to a five-point scale.

McHenry LC, Anderson TP, Raskind R, et al: *Essentials of Stroke Diagnosis and Management*. Philadelphia, Smith, Kline and French Laboratories, 1974.

This brief booklet, designed for use by the medical profession, covers all important aspects of stroke. After classifying strokes according to both temporal and causal aspects, it lists symptoms of various types of stroke. The schematic drawings are excellent. The diagnostic work-up is outlined and treatment is described in three parts.

Sarno JE, Sarno MT: *Stroke: The Condition and the Patient*. New York, McGraw-Hill, 1969.

This book on completed stroke for those ouside the health profession is written in the form of pertinent questions and answers covering such aspects of stroke as cause, physical consequences, associated speech disorders, intellectual and emotional aspects, rehabilitation, and prognosis. The index facilitates the book's use as a quick reference for specific questions about stroke.

Waite NS: Social problems and the social work role. *In* Licht S (ed): *Stroke and its Rehabilitation*. New Haven, Licht, 1975.

This chapter deals with the adjustments the stroke patient and his family must make, including changes in image and role, communication, work, and living arrangements. Social work roles are briefly explained.

Weisbroth S, Esibill N, Zuger RR: Factors in the vocational success in hemiplegic patients. Arch Phys Med Rehabil **52**: 441–446 and 486, 1971.

This article describes a study of patients with hemiplegia resulting from CVA, tumor, or trauma. The results indicated that one third of the patients returned to work, with more women returning than men. The factors influencing return to work for both left and right hemiplegics are delineated.

10 STROKE AND CEREBRAL TRAUMA: PSYCHOSOCIAL AND VOCATIONAL ASPECTS

Roy S. Fowler, Jr., Ph.D.

INTRODUCTION

There is a continuing tendency to regard human behavior and brain function with prejudice, awe, and misunderstanding. The brain-damaged person may receive inadequate or ineffective services because his behavioral deficits are misdiagnosed as psychiatric illness. Because it is commonly known that the central nervous system does not repair itself, the brain-damaged person may be regarded as permanently and hopelessly disabled. At best, he may be viewed as unpredictable and as a continuing source of puzzlement.

This chapter is designed to help clarify some of the intellectual, behavioral, and emotional changes that occur as consequences of stroke and cerebral trauma. It is hoped that the chapter will help the counselor understand why the brain-damaged person behaves the way he does, as an understanding of a person's abilities in these areas is required for effective services. Vocational considerations and some guidelines for evaluation are also included.

Cerebral vascular accident (CVA), stroke, and cerebral trauma are all synonymous with brain damage. These terms imply that an individual has had a normally functioning brain, consistent with his age, which was acutely damaged in some fashion, either by a disruption in blood flow or by tissue damage caused by a blow or a lesion of any sort (see chap. 9). Such damage will almost always result in behavioral deficits, which may include decreases in physical abilities, intellectual performance, social functioning, emotional control, or any combination of the four. Even very mild injuries, which may not give observable evidence of damage, can show up as behavioral deficits later.

Prognosis

Almost without exception, a person who has experienced brain damage has lost some cognitive ability and behavioral function. Rarely, if ever, is a patient behaviorally better off following brain damage than he was when his brain was functioning normally. The extent of deficits, the course of recovery of function, and the individual's level of maximum performance will all depend upon a variety of issues.

Age. The effect of brain damage is closely related to the age of the individual at the time of the injury. The younger the person, the better the prognosis. Given the same magnitude of injury, a child will have fewer long-term deficits than the adolescent. The adolescent, in turn, will do much better in the long run than the person over age 30. The aging process seems to be associated with a decrease in plasticity and a tendency to be less able to compensate for deficits. These tendencies are expected in all of us but are especially noticeable in the brain-damaged person.

Severity and magnitude of the lesion. There is a positive relationship between the severity of deficit and the amount of brain tissue damaged: the more tissue lost, the higher the probability of significant deficits. There is also a relationship between the length of coma and prognosis: the longer the period of coma, the greater the probability of permanent deficits and the greater the severity of impairment. A possible exception is coma secondary to pure brain stem injuries that spare the cerebrum. If even a relatively young person is in a coma longer than 13 weeks, there is a significantly reduced probability that he will achieve independent living, whereas a person who is in a coma less than 13 weeks has a much higher probability of being able to function independently, although it is very unlikely that he will be totally deficit free.

Premorbid function. Prognosis following a brain injury is largely affected by the patient's previous abilities, personality, milieu, and life style. The brighter, better educated, productive person with excellent family support will tend to perform at a higher functional level, given the same injuries, than his duller, less well educated, less productive, more lonely counterpart. This is, however, a potentially dangerous generalization, because there are many factors that influence ultimate level of function. Premorbid personality patterns will also play a role. Generally, personality characteristics are not so much changed by cerebral damage as they are exaggerated.

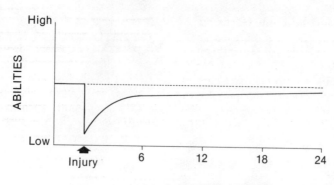

FIGURE 10-1. Time course of spontaneous recovery of intellectual function following brain injury. Most of the functional improvement occurs in the first 3 months, with smaller gains in the next 3 months. Thereafter recovery tends to stabilize.

The so-called "well-adjusted" person who suffers brain damage has a much greater probability of maintaining an "appropriate" repertoire of social skills, and also is more likely to have supportive friends and family who are of much value in helping achieve maximum performance levels, than a less "well-adjusted" person.

The demands of the environment in which the person has lived or will live are also very important. The bright person living in a low-demand environment may be able to resume his roles even after fairly significant deficits have occurred. The less bright "over achiever," functioning in a high-demand setting, cannot afford to have even minor impairments if he is still to perform adequately. Persons whose premorbid behaviors were characterized by impulsivity, poor judgment, and carelessness may demonstrate more of the same characteristics after brain damage.

Course of Recovery

The typical course of recovery is illustrated in figure 10-1. An individual may be characterized by a particular level of function prior to injury. After stroke or brain injury, an immediate precipitous decrease in his total breadth of function occurs. With time, there is a spontaneous recovery of many abilities, the extent of which will depend upon the variables described above and the treatment the patient receives. Most spontaneous recovery will have occurred, however, by the sixth month following the insult (fig. 10-1). Recovery of function and improvement in abilities may, for some, occur for several years after injury, but the rate of recovery slows considerably after the initial, more rapid gains and is usually well stabilized at 12 months.

The following generalizations are helpful: (a) the more closely an individual's abilities immediately following an injury resemble his premorbid abilities, the greater the probability that his future function will approximate his premorbid function; (b) the greater the loss immediately after injury, the lower the probability that, even with time, the individual will come close to approximating his premorbid level; (c) the longer the period of time that the deficits persist, the greater the probability that they will be permanent.

Data on the level of performance in stroke patients following discharge from a rehabilitation program suggests that more than 60 percent and as many as 90 percent of all patients, including the most severely damaged, will walk, dress themselves independently, feed themselves, and have bowel and bladder control. They may need some adaptive devices, such as short leg braces, crutches, or special fasteners on their clothing, but the vast majority of patients will be independent in most activities of normal daily living.

Between 50 and 70 percent of all stroke patients with language problems will be able to communicate at a functional level sufficient for the mechanics of living. This does not mean that they will not have deficits, but it does mean they will have useful communication skills.

Area of Cerebrum Affected

The area of the cerebrum damaged, namely, right or left, largely determines the nature of the deficits the individual will experience, although variations are seen. Thus, while a person may appear at times as capable as ever when confronted with some intellectual tasks, he may at another time be totally unable to perform seemingly comparable or less taxing intellectual tasks. In spite of these apparent inconsistencies, there are patterns in the behavior of brain-damaged persons which can be identified, and which tend to be related to the side of the cerebrum damaged. The following sections describe these behavior clusters and are useful as general guidelines. They are usually true but not always correct, as there are inevitably exceptions. Patients with strokes affecting the cerebrum usually have one or the other side affected (unless, of course, they had more than one stroke). Cerebral trauma may well affect both sides and produce mixed behavior patterns. This may hold true for patients with multiple emboli that lodge in both sides. Stroke or trauma patients with pure brain stem or cerebellar damage may not show either of the following behavior patterns.

LEFT CEREBRAL DAMAGE

Deficits

Typically, the most visible sign of left cerebral damage will be a motor and sensory paralysis of the right side of the body (*right hemiplegia*). Because the left cerebral hemisphere is associated with language function (the processing and coding of data into verbal symbols), individuals with left hemisphere damage may be unable to understand spoken or written language or even produce it. Thus, when teaching such a patient a task like dressing, spoken instructions may need to be supplemented by pantomime.

Communication deficits may involve any or all of the four language modalities (auditory comprehension, speaking, reading, and writing). The term *aphasia* is most commonly used in the United States and Europe to refer to disorders of the language processing centers in the brain. The term *dysphasia* is sometimes used interchangeably with aphasia, although literally aphasia means totally affected and dysphasia means partially affected. Usually aphasic symptoms are present in all of the language modalities; however, all of the modalities usually are not equally involved.

The counselor will encounter numerous terms associated with various patterns of aphasic disorder. The terms *expressive, nonfluent,* or *Broca's aphasia* refer to a language disorder characterized by effortful, halting speech with reduced grammar and relatively good comprehension. Reading ability is usually better than writing ability. Lesions producing such language disorders are usually located in Broca's area (see fig. 3-4, p. 21). The terms *receptive, fluent,* or *Wernicke's aphasia* refer to a language disorder characterized by fluent speech with reduced information content, impaired auditory comprehension, and impaired reading and writing. Lesions associated with this type of aphasia are usually located in Wernicke's area (see fig 3-4, p. 21). Care must be taken *not* to assume that receptive functions are normal if the label is "expressive aphasia," and vice versa. The impairment of sound production accuracy often accompanying a lesion in Broca's area is known as *apraxia of speech*.

Other communication deficits may be caused by brain damage. *Dysarthria* is an impairment of the speed, accuracy and coordination of movement of the vocal cords, lips, tongue, and palate (speech mechanism), which results in reduced speech intelligibility. Lesions causing dysarthria can occur in several areas of the brain. For example, lesions of the cerebellum result in incoordination of speech-mechanism movement, while lesions of the cranial nerve nuclei in the medulla result in weakness and thus reduced speed of speech-mechanism movement.

Alexia or *dyslexia*, almost exclusively a reading disturbance, and *agraphia* or *dysgraphia*, almost exclusively a writing disturbance, are considered by some to be specific forms of aphasia.

Resulting Behavior

When confronted with a new problem, persons with damage to the left cerebral hemisphere tend to respond in a slow, scattered, disorganized, anxious fashion, regardless of whether the problem is presented verbally or by demonstration. They may exhibit an extreme and disruptive transient emotional disturbance. This may appear as an acute, often disorganizing agitation or anxiety that may completely disrupt ongoing activity, and very frequently appears if the new problem highlights the person's limitations. As the person becomes familiar with the new problem and begins to handle it, anxiety disappears.

Depression can be a very common overall emotional response because the person with left cerebral damage tends to be overly sensitive to his disabilities. However, with time and experience, these persons frequently are capable of compensating rather well and making a satisfactory adjustment to their disability and living situation, which in turn resolves the depression.

Therapeutic Techniques

When dealing with persons with left cerebral damage, it is essential to have a clear understanding of the nature of their language problems. For this reason, it is advisable to obtain an accurate and current speech assessment from a certified speech pathologist. The speech pathologist should be able to provide an accurate estimate of the person's current level of language functioning, an estimate of his future language potential, and an operational appraisal of what level of function can be achieved and in what period of time. In addition, the speech pathologist can recommend the most appropriate techniques for maximizing communication with the person, and ways of structuring the environment to increase communication effectiveness and minimize those deficits in performance which are due to communication problems.

While the specifics for each person with left cerebral damage will differ, some generalizations can be made for helping them deal with their communication problems. It is important to understand that speech and language are different. Language refers to the symbols (words, sounds, signs, noises, movements, gestures, and expressions)—which people use to communicate with each other. Speech, on the other hand, refers only to the sounds made with the mouth. A deaf person, for example, may have no speech but have excellent language function with hand symbols. A great deal of normal day-to-day communication is carried on without speech through the use of a variety of nonverbal techniques. Therefore, a person who cannot speak and be understood or listen and understand may still be able to use and understand considerable "body" language. Often the use of demonstration or pantomime, rather than words, is very effective in teaching right hemiplegics a task. Demonstrating how to put on a shirt may achieve immediate learning, while verbally describing the process may produce no learning.

Persons with language problems may be able to understand a short and simple message, but miss a long or complicated one. For example, asking the person, "Open the door, let the cat out, pick up the newspaper, and bring in the mail," may yield only one of these actions, or perhaps none of them, because the stream of words is overwhelming. Delivering the request one stage at a time and awaiting the response before presenting the next stage may yield full performance.

Aphasic persons should be addressed with normal voice volume and inflection. Since shouted messages tend to be short and concise and are usually associated with a body posture whose meaning is quite clear, it appears that shouting to an aphasic person is more effective than speaking at normal volume. However, it is the brevity and the gesture, not the volume, that is effective.

Because right hemiplegics tend to be very cautious and anxious about performing any new tasks, they are likely to need reassurance and frequent indications that they are performing correctly. Smiles, nods, or pats on the back after successful completion of each stage of a task will reassure the person and encourage him to proceed to the next step.

Cautions

1. Do not overestimate the ability of a patient with left cerebral damage to understand spoken speech. Sometimes a person becomes so adept at understanding nonverbal communication that it is possible to mistake it for verbal understanding. A right hemiplegic may seem uncooperative, cross, senile, or irrational if his understanding is overestimated. Verify his level of comprehension.
2. The fewer words the better. Keep messages simple and concise.
3. Normal voice volume is preferred.
4. Use your ordinary voice. Avoid slipping into the affected voice one might use with a child.

RIGHT CEREBRAL DAMAGE

Deficits

The most visible sign of right cerebral damage will usually be a motor and sensory paralysis of the left side of the body (left hemiplegia). Of often greater importance is the loss of the intellectual functions governed by the right cerebral hemisphere. The intellectual functions concerned are depth perception, appreciation of the concept of wholes from incomplete or fragmentary data, intuition, critical imagination, and nonverbal perception. The primary deficit of right cerebral hemisphere damage is the inability to accurately interpret visual information and properly orient oneself with respect to the environment. The terms visuospatial deficits or perceptual deficits are often used to describe this condition. Minor visuospatial failures (e.g., attempting to put down a coffee cup and missing the table while reading) are experienced by many normal persons when they are very tired or concentrating on something else. Persons with right cerebral lesions may have deficits that are more major and pervasive.

Visuospatial deficits, although equally as important as speech and language deficits, are easily overlooked. Consequently, the abilities of the left hemiplegic may be overestimated. These deficits may cause the person to be mislabeled by disappointed observers as uncooperative, unmotivated, overly dependent, or confused when he unexpectedly encounters difficulties with what appear to be simple daily routine activities.

Persons with severe visuospatial deficits have more difficulty learning to care for themselves than persons with speech deficits. Even with concentration, they might be unable to steer a wheelchair through a large doorway without bumping the frame. They might confuse the inside and the outside of their clothes, or they may miss buttons and not get their clothes on correctly. They may have difficulty knowing whether they are sitting upright or tilting, and they may have difficulty estimating their distance from objects. They may be unable to read a newspaper or add a column of figures, not because they lack the ability to read or add, but because they lose their place on the paper. A person with even minor visuospatial deficits will probably not be safe driving a car.

In addition, persons with right cerebral damage have more problems with visual field deficits (see p. 48) and with one-sided neglect (anosognosia) than those with left cerebral damage. The problem of neglect cannot be explained solely by sensory loss, nor is it due to a visual field deficit. A person with a serious neglect problem behaves as if he were selectively ignoring everything that happens on his involved side, even if he might be able to see it. He may ignore a person approaching from his left side, or he may not recognize his left arm or leg as parts of his own body.

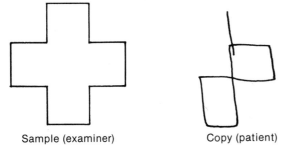

Sample (examiner)   Copy (patient)

FIGURE 10-2. Attempt at copying a cross by a left hemiplegic patient with a left neglect problem. While the patient's reproduction of the right portion of the cross is not complete, the larger error is in his reproduction of the left portion.

A person with a neglect problem can easily become confused when traveling. If he is wheeled down an unfamiliar corridor and back again, he may think he has been in two different corridors because he saw only one side of the corridor going one way and only the opposite side when returning.

Some persons with severe neglect problems divide the things they see at the midline (e.g., read the word "woman" as "man"). A useful test for neglect is to ask a person to reproduce a drawing of a Greek cross. If he has a neglect problem, he will often only draw the right half of the cross (fig. 10-2).

Resulting Behavior

Persons with right cerebral hemisphere damage tend to behave in ways that promote overestimation of their abilities. They are often completely unaware of their deficits or may deny or ignore them. They tend to be quite satisfied with even a poor performance, are often unable to profit from experience, and sometimes seem to be complacent or euphoric. They tend to set unrealistic goals for themselves which they frequently fail to achieve because they do not take their deficits into consideration. This tendency toward diminished self-awareness often makes them insensitive to the needs and desires of others and may result in their being rejected by family and friends.

The left hemiplegic will frequently attempt to do things that are not within his limits or abilities and thereby endanger himself. He may fall when he tries to walk across the room without putting on his brace, or he may attempt to drive his automobile and injure himself or others.

Unlike persons with left cerebral damage, persons with right hemispheric lesions do not usually become depressed following stroke or cerebral trauma. If depression does occur, it frequently develops over a long period of time and is associated with repeated inability to achieve unrealistic goals. It tends to be more chronic and debilitating than the depression of persons with left cerebral damage and is often fairly resistant to intervention techniques.

Therapeutic Techniques

It is important to remember that the verbal abilities of persons with right cerebral damage remain intact. Because of this, and because they are so often poor judges of their own abilities, they can often describe in detail a task they are about to attempt but which they cannot, in fact, perform safely. Their verbal skills, however, can be used to supplement faltering visuospatial skills. In teaching these persons to perform a task, it is often helpful to talk them through the steps to be mastered or for them to talk their own way through the task. Demonstration is frequently quite ineffective because of faulty interpretation of visual information. Persons with right cerebral damage need a great deal of verbal feedback when they are attempting to learn a new task, and they need to be encouraged to slow down and check each step carefully as it is completed.

Since left hemiplegics have difficulty processing visual cues, it is important to consider the clutter of the environment. A poorly lit or cluttered room with vividly patterned wallpaper or rapid movements of people and objects around the person may be very distracting and hinder his performance. A well-lighted room and clearly marked reference points, such as door frames or mirrors, are helpful. Removal of unnecessary equipment and furniture is advisable.

In general, it is helpful to give the person with a severe neglect problem as much information as possible about his neglected environment. Important items that have been neglected can be pointed out in a calm, informative manner. When traveling with the person, it is helpful to point out landmarks to the right and left along the way and to give frequent reminders of destination.

If neglect is particularly persistent and disabling, the left hemiplegic may perform better when the environment is modified to compensate for his deficit. Furniture or equipment can be moved to the nonneglected (i.e., right) side of his bed, wheelchair, or desk. His clothes can be hung on the right side of his closet, and commonly used items can be arranged on the right side of his dresser drawers. His place at the table can be arranged so that he receives food from the right and passes to the left. This same model may be used for arranging work-related items.

Cautions

1. A person with right cerebral damage is likely to overestimate his abilities. Ask him to demonstrate skills he attributes to himself.
2. Words are more effective than demonstration with left hemiplegics. Do not use gestures or other nonverbal instruction techniques.
3. Simplify the environment to minimize visual distractions.

BRAIN DAMAGE IN GENERAL

We have discussed intellectual problems which are typically associated with damage to the right or left cerebral hemisphere. Some patients will give no evidence of paralysis and yet they may show many of the signs of intellectual deficits discussed so far. Others will show paralysis but little or no evidence of the problems mentioned. If, however, the patient has experienced brain damage, it is very likely that his behavior will give some evidence of decreased ability. Some functions of intelligence are so complicated that they need virtually a totally functioning brain. Even minor damage may interfere with these complicated functions.

Quality Control

Quality control refers to the ability to guide and check one's own behavior. This means doing the "right" thing at the "right" time. Frequently, a quality control problem is first identified by those closest to the patient. They see changes in behavior that are missed by someone less familiar with the patient's premorbid abilities. The once fastidious person may become sloppy and seem to care little about his appearance. He may say the wrong thing at the wrong time. He may perform inconsistently, making errors today on a task he performed quite well yesterday. A person formerly described as shy may become immodest and aggressive, or the quiet person, noisy.

Because quality control problems annoy others and are not well understood, it is easy to incorrectly infer an emotional or psychological problem. While it is possible that a brain-damaged person may have significant emotional problems which may or may not need professional help, it is important that his problems not be made more severe by failure to recognize intellectual deficits.

The person with quality control problems due to brain damage needs special assistance from his environment. He needs to learn to analyze his behavior and respond appropriately to the situation. It is more likely that his need is for more cues, feedback, and information than for psychotherapy.

Memory

Almost any injury to the brain, however minimal, produces memory problems. Even a healthy person will develop memory problems as he grows older. Memory has both visuospatial and language components, and memory problems can therefore be related to the side of the brain that has been injured. The person with left cerebral damage tends to have more memory deficits associated with language, and the person with right cerebral damage will have more memory problems associated with visuospatial information. It is also possible to have neither obvious language nor visuospatial deficits and still have significant memory problems. The effect of brain damage on memory has many components. Three of the most important components will be considered here.

Old versus new learning. There is a tendency for information to be remembered selectively according to whether it involves new information or old learning. Old learning refers to information acquired prior to the brain injury, and new learning refers to information acquired since the injury. Brain-damaged persons tend to have difficulty with new learning even when they have very little difficulty recalling previously learned material. For example, a person may be able to describe in great detail friends, events, or situations that occurred many years in the past but may be unable to remember what he had for breakfast, the name of a new person recently introduced, or the task to be performed at this time.

Sometimes the forgetful patient can improve his level of function if he uses a "prosthetic memory." Typically, this involves the systematic use of such memory aids as lists, appointment calendars, schedules, or written notes. The patient records the activity he plans to accomplish over a given interval (minutes, hours, days, or weeks, depending upon the severity of the memory problem). When in doubt as to appropriate action, the patient learns to consult his list. He then carries out the recorded activity for that interval, checks the task off as it is completed, and goes on to the next step on the list. More elaborate systems involving tape-recorded messages and timers have been devised for patients who cannot read. Many patients spontaneously discover that a small weekly appointment book carried in a pocket can help them avoid embarrassment. It is typically used to record names, appointments, addresses, and other bits of data that can be retrieved later to bolster a faulty memory.

Retention span. Retention span refers to the number of pieces of information in a given message which can be retained and used. A brain-damaged person frequently has a limited retention span; that is, he can remember only a few parts of a complicated message. For example, if he were asked to stand up, take off his coat, put it on a chair, pick up a magazine, and hand it to another person, a person with a short retention span might assimilate only the part concerning the magazine. He might also simply look puzzled and not act at all, being overwhelmed by the complexity of the instruction.

A person with a short retention span may perform very well if he is given only brief, simple messages. Instructions should be broken into small components and the components presented one at a time.

Generalization. Persons with memory problems also frequently have a decrease in their ability to generalize. In its simplest form, generalization means applying what has been learned in one setting to another setting. A person with a generalization problem will therefore have difficulty carrying over learning from one setting to another. It has been found that in a rehabilitation setting, a patient may perform less well on a task he has done day after day if he is confronted with a new physical therapist rather than his usual therapist. The patient who learns to perform a task in a hospital or workshop setting may or may not be able to perform that identical task when he goes home or into a competitive employment situation. Transfer of learning from one setting to another is by no means automatic when the brain has been damaged.

Many rehabilitation programs include home visits by therapy personnel to facilitate the transfer of learning and the carry-over of skills. It is also reasonable to attempt to mock up, in a sheltered work setting, those kinds of activities that are to be performed in a competitive setting, and to give the person an opportunity to participate in a work-station program.

A reliable and consistent daily routine is usually helpful for persons with generalization deficits. As they are very sensitive to any minor changes in their environment, they will frequently respond to change by becoming irritable and confused because change is frightening. When there is a need for change, a deterioration in the person's abilities should be expected. It is helpful to warn him in advance and discuss the events that are likely to occur so he can anticipate and rehearse behaviors in his mind. If a new routine is quickly and effectively established, the person is likely to improve rapidly.

Some patients, particularly in the early periods following the onset of brain injury, will demonstrate a problem called *perseveration*. The patient becomes "stuck" in a pattern of repeated responses. For example, he may say the same word over and over or, when asked to draw a circle on a piece of paper, he may continue making circles until someone stops him. As an analogy, it is very much like a faulty record player, which fails to track properly and plays a record groove over and over until it is nudged into continuing to play the remainder of the record. Many perseverating patients will have to be "nudged" in order to break up their pattern of perseveration. Generally, asking the patient a new question, calling him by name, or touching him lightly will be sufficient to distract him and break up the perseveration.

Emotional Lability

Brain-damaged persons very frequently show partial loss of emotional control. They may switch from laughing to crying without apparent reason. Feelings and the overt expression of emotion are not always linked as cause and effect. Excessive crying is the most common problem and is frequently due to the insult to brain tissue (organic emotional lability), rather than to depression or sadness over perceived losses. Organic emotional lability is characterized by little or no obvious relation between the start of emotional expression and what is happening around the person. The emotional behavior (crying, unexpected laughter, flares of anger, or moaning) is typically easily interrupted by diverting the person's attention by saying his name or asking him a question. Crying caused by depression is not so easily interrupted.

An effective therapeutic approach is to interrupt the emotional behavior of a person with organic lability, if possible. If the emotional expression is due to brain damage, the person himself has little control over it. Interrupting the behavior may help him to avoid embarrassing and fatiguing activity.

STANDARDS OF EVALUATION

It is highly advisable to have an adequate assessment of a patient's deficits and abilities performed by the appropriate professionals when stroke or head trauma has occurred. In the case of emotional, intellectual, and behavioral problems, the minimum workup should include an evaluation by a clinical psychologist with a Ph.D. or equivalent who is well trained in evaluation of brain damage and behavior.

Evaluations are equally necessary for patients with minimal problems and those with severe deficits. The patient with severe deficits needs to be evaluated not so much from the point of view of what he cannot do, but for what he can do. Much too frequently, the patient with obvious deficits is simply deemed hopeless. An analysis of his abilities as opposed to his disabilities can be highly enlightening.

Significant deficits which can influence behavior and emotion often exist without noticeable physical evidence. The patient may only be aware of decreased energy and efficiency, accompanied by a prevailing depression. Often such a patient is experiencing emotional difficulties because he is working very hard to compensate for unrecognized minor deficits. These deficits may only show up on standardized tests of intellectual function when evaluated by a knowledgeable and skilled professional. An accurate assessment may allow the patient to adjust his goals or develop compensating approaches to the problem and thereby reduce his energy expenditure.

The following guidelines may be useful in selecting a consultant.

Select a psychologist with experience in rehabilitation medicine. Ideally, this psychologist's frame of reference will be the restoration of function. He is likely to be working within the context of a rehabilitation treatment team whose members will be able to contribute significant observations of the client's behavior and abilities from several points of view.

If a psychologist working within a rehabilitation program is not available, select a consultant who identifies himself as a neuropsychologist. An increasing number of psychologists are trained in the assessment and evaluation of the neurological basis of behavior. Typically, these professionals work in medical contexts, such as departments of neurology or neurosurgery, and specialize in the diagnosis of brain damage and its behavioral consequences.

If neither of the above is available, select a clinical psychologist who completed his training after 1960. Most of the advances in neuropsychological assessment have occurred since 1960. It is expected that at least some training in neuropsychological assessment procedures will be included in any current, competent graduate training program for clinical psychologists. Persons trained before 1960 may be fully competent if they have remained knowledgeable of the neuropsychological literature.

Finally, a counselor is much more likely to receive the kind of information he desires if he learns how to use his consultants. Simply requesting "an evaluation" of a client will in no way guarantee that the consultant will provide the kinds of information the counselor needs. If the referral is vague, the consultant may simply perform a routine evaluation, which may or may not include useful, vocationally oriented information. Typically, the counselor will be more concerned about the prognosis than the diagnosis. The consultant should be asked the following questions: (a) What are the client's current deficits and strengths? (b) What is the projected course of recovery and estimate of maximum abilities? (c) When will the client be ready for rehabilitation and vocational endeavors? (d) What kind of remedial or modification techniques are needed and how can they be implemented most effectively?

It may well be advisable and necessary to obtain evaluations of a client several times throughout his course of recovery. An initial evaluation should probably be performed within 6 to 8 weeks after the stroke or injury. Followup testing should be accomplished between the fourth and sixth month. It may be desirable to evaluate the client again following the first year or year and a half. This repeated evaluation will allow for the development of a curve of recovery and estimation of function.

VOCATIONAL IMPLICATIONS

Returning a person to work following brain injury will demand a very careful evaluation of (a) the individual's job or school setting; (b) the nature of his deficits; (c) the severity and kind of brain damage; and (d) the type of job and its location, physical demands, complexity, interpersonal requirements, language or visual perceptual requirements, and degree of new learning required. Each person's situation will be different, but the following general guidelines may be helpful.

Brain-damaged clients may have the use of only one hand and are thereby limited in their ability to perform lifting, carrying, pushing, and pulling, especially if they use a cane. The majority will need to be confined to sedentary or light work, though a few may be able to perform medium work. Generally, they should be limited in the amount of walking they are required to do, but may tolerate standing for a long period. Climbing, balancing, stooping, and kneeling also generally have to be limited for these clients.

Lack of speed is a critical vocational implication. The majority of these clients do not function as rapidly as they did prior to their stroke or brain injury. Some of them work so slowly that it is preferable for them to be employed in a sheltered setting. Others can produce high quality work as long as they do not feel they need to hurry. The pressure of trying to hurry may itself decrease quality. Hence, the competitive workshop is often less than ideal for some of these clients.

Some brain-damaged persons have good tolerance for outside work, such as farmwork, but the majority probably do better on inside work where they are protected from the weather. There are no general limitations with regard to climate, noise, vibration, gases, fumes, dust, and ventilation. Clients with right cerebral damage will perform best in an uncluttered environment with good light and a minimum of distracting movement around them.

Special consideration needs to be given to impairments in speaking, hearing, writing, and seeing, all of which are often seen in these clients. Vocationally, these impairments are often more limiting than physical impairments.

The ideal place setting is one in which it is possible to arrange job or academic challenges that will vary directly with demonstrated ability. Such an ideal program will have a job sampling possibility ranging from a fully sheltered workshop setting, through semisheltered job settings, on to full competitive employment. Where such facilities exist, it is possible to return the brain-damaged client to some type of vocational activity quite early in the course of recovery and then adjust his activity to his needs as he improves. This type of setting will maximize the probability of appropriate vocational disposition.

If such an ideal setting is not available and the rehabilitation plan is to return the client directly to the competitive labor market or to an academic program where remedial education is not possible, it is important to wait until maximum recovery has been reached or there is a very clear leveling off in return of function. This usually means waiting at least 6 months following brain injury or stroke. It is very important to maximize the probabilities of success for a client entering a competitive setting. If the client returns to such a setting too early, the probability that he will fail increases.

Early failure holds many risks. The client and his family may become so discouraged that they may give up. The client's employer may be so upset by his errors that he may prematurely terminate employment. An even greater problem is that the reputation the client may gain through such failure may prejudice future opportunities in similar settings.

The young student returning too early to school may find himself placed in a special education program which may not be flexible enough to adjust to his changing status. In many school settings it is not easy to make the transition from special educational programs into normal competitive academic programs. The student who waits until his condition has stabilized usually only runs the risk of falling behind his peers in the chronology of the educational process. While delay may be very distressing to adolescents, the long-term potential problems of returning to school too early must be considered and weighed very carefully.

Statistics gathered here and abroad suggest that in the under-50 age group a rather high percentage of stroke patients will be able to return to work. The data from Scandinavia and England indicate that between 32 and 70 percent of all "young" stroke patients will be able to return to employment. Some of this employment may be part-time or sheltered workshop activities. In the United States, the estimates run as low as 17 percent to a high of 40 percent.

In this country, males are more likely to return to work than females. Persons with a high school education or greater are more likely to return to work than blue collar workers. It would appear, however, that we do not return as many brain-injured persons to work as we might. The knowledge and treatment techniques exist and we should be doing a better job. Brain-damaged individuals in our society should be more active and productive. The counselor may not be able to "cure" the client of his deficits, but he can be a major agent for change in the quality of services received.

BIBLIOGRAPHY

Bond MR: Assessment of the psychosocial outcome of severe head injury. Acta Neurochir (Wien) 34:57-70, 1976.
Fifty-six patients with severe head injury and post-traumatic amnesia exceeding 24 hours were studied to evaluate the neurophysical, mental, and social results of their brain injuries, and the relation of duration of amnesia to degree of disability.

Darley FL: A retrospective view: Aphasia. J Speech Hear Disord 42:161-169, 1977.
This article presents the current status of research on the nature of aphasia and related disorders, the location of brain lesions causing aphasia, language dissolution in aphasia, and aphasia therapy.

Diller L: Cognitive and motor aspects of handicapping conditions in the neurologically impaired. In Neff WS (ed): Rehabilitation Psychology. Washington, D.C., American Psychological Association, 1971, p.1-32.
This chapter is an overview of what is known about the sensory, cognitive, and motor functions of neurologically impaired adults and children, with special attention devoted to the assessment and treatment techniques of aphasics, hemiplegics, children with minimal brain injury, and children with learning deficits.

Fugl-Meyer AR, Jaasko L, Norlin V: The post-stroke hemiplegic patient II. Incidence, mortality, and vocational return in Goteborg, Sweden, with a review of the literature. Scand J Rehabil Med 7:73-83, 1975.
A thorough review of the literature on incidence, mortality, and prevalence of stroke worldwide is presented in this article. It contains a review of the probabilities of return to work following a stroke.

Geschwind N: Language and the brain. Sci Am 226:76-83, 1972.
This article describes some of the research on language disorders and brain function that has led to a model of how the language areas of the brain are interconnected and what each area does. It provides useful background for understanding language dysfunction.

Lezak MD: Neuropsychological Assessment. New York, Oxford University Press, 1976.
This excellent textbook covering adult neuropsychological assessment provides a detailed overview of the current state of knowledge regarding the relationship between brain and behavior. It also contains a comprehensive description of current neuropsychological testing techniques.

Sheridan J: Restoring speech and language skills. Geriatrics 31:83-86, 1976.
This article describes some common speech problems in geriatric patients and the role of the speech pathologist in treating them. The common speech disorders are described in nonmedical terms.

Smolkin C, Cohen BS: Socioeconmic factors affecting the vocational success of stroke patients. Arch Phys Med Rehabil 55:269-271, 1974.
Seventy-four stroke patients were evaluated for vocational outcome after rehabilitation services. The major factors determining successful return to work after stroke were found to be: (a) level of education; (b) prior occupation; and (c) sex.

Vignolo LA: Evolution of aphasia and language rehabilitation: A retrospective exploratory study. In Sarno MT (ed): Aphasia: Selected Readings. Englewood Cliffs, NJ, 1972, P. 370-384.
An evaluation of the effects of speech therapy on the course and outcome of aphasia following stroke.

11 CEREBRAL PALSY

Jessie K.M. Easton, M.D.
Daniel Halpern, M.D.

DISEASE DESCRIPTION

The term "cerebral palsy" refers to disorders of movement resulting from damage to the brain. By convention, the term is used to describe individuals who have suffered damage to the brain at some time during its period of growth and development. This period is generally considered to continue to 8 years of age, though some authorities extend it to 12 years. The neurological condition itself is not progressive, but manifestations vary in expression with the maturity of the brain and body, the activity and experiences of the individual, and the quality of management. By the time the person has reached vocational counseling age, however, the condition is stable.

The incidence of cerebral palsy is difficult to determine, since many cases of congenital origin are not diagnosed until after 6 to 12 months of age or older. Also, many secondary complications associated with cerebral palsy have their onset somewhat later in life. While some statistics indicate the incidence of cerebral palsy is declining with improved neonatal and perinatal care, other considerations indicate that as pediatric or neonatal intensive care units save the lives of more seriously ill and involved infants, the incidence of cerebral palsy is increasing. Undoubtedly both trends are present.

The prevalance of cerebral palsy, at a conservative estimate, is about 900,000 clinical cases in the United States, or 4.5 cases per 1,000 in the general population. The prevalence is increasing because more children with cerebral palsy are surviving into adulthood, including the more severely involved. Thus, the total number of individuals with cerebral palsy is gradually increasing. They will come to the attention of vocational counselors in greater numbers than heretofore.

A diagnosis of cerebral palsy requires the presence of a motor disorder. It is based on the clincial finding of abnormal neurological function regardless of the ability to identify anatomic or histologic pathology. The array of problems is not confined to those associated with control of movement. Other deficits in function due to damage to parts of the brain other than the motor cortex also occur. (The reader will find a review of the nervous system and musculoskeletal system sections of chapter 3 helpful in understanding the following discussion.)

Since areas within the brain in addition to the cerebral cortex may be involved, the diagnosis of cerebral palsy does not have the precision or accuracy of most other medical diseases. For this reason, some authorities feel uncomfortable with the term, since it does not truly describe a discrete entity, its etiology, or its anatomical location. It is useful as an administrative term, however, since all the conditions included require a comprehensive understanding, continuous management, and similar facilities for proper care.

The manifestations of cerebral palsy depend upon the location and severity of the brain damage. Although the locations are not precisely known, they can be inferred from the symptom complex seen. Typical patterns of dysfunction are produced when the damage is limited to one area of the brain, when it is scattered throughout the brain, when it is unilateral, and when it is bilateral. The manifestations also depend upon the cause of the damage, the relative sensitivity of different structures to these causal factors, and the state of development of the brain at the time of the injury.

Basically, the motor or movement problem in cerebral palsy is lack of control of the muscles rather than muscle weakness. This lack of control is often expressed by a failure of inhibition of some specific central nervous system reflexes. These reflexes involving muscle movement, in increasing order of complexity, are:

1. Stretch
2. Crossed extension
3. Long spinal
4. Symmetrical tonic neck
5. Asymmetrical tonic neck
6. Vestibular
7. Startle

The stretch reflex (see p. 27) is the simplest, and its center is located at the level of the spinal cord appropriate to the muscle being considered. The startle reflex, which is much more complex, is centered at the midbrain (see fig. 3-6, p. 22). In table 11-1, the muscle movements associated with each reflex, in

TABLE 11-1
REFLEXES LIKELY TO BE UNINHIBITED IN CEREBRAL PALSY

Reflex	Definition	Usual Site of Pathology	Functional Ability Likely To Be Disturbed When Uninhibited
Stretch	Stretch of a muscle resulting in contraction of the muscle. Hyperactivity of these reflexes is referred to as spasticity.	Central nervous system above the level in the spinal cord of the innervation of the muscle being considered	Ambulation when lower extremities involved; dexterity, fine manipulation, complex motor skills when upper extremities involved; speed and strength
Crossed extension	Extension of one arm or leg produces flexion of the opposite arm or leg.	Same as stretch reflex	Transfers, dressing, writing, standing with both legs straight; activities requiring bimanual control
Long spinal	Flexion of one leg results in extension of the arm on the same side. Extension of the leg results in flexion of the arm on the same side.	Central nervous system above the level of innervation of the muscles involved	Sitting balance, standing with both legs straight, ambulation, transfers, standing balance, eating, dressing
Symmetrical tonic neck	Flexion of the neck results in flexion of the arms and extension of the legs. Extension of the neck results in extension of the arms and flexion of the legs.	In or above the midbrain or upper medulla	Sitting balance, ambulation, transfers, eating, dressing
Asymmetrical tonic neck	Turning or tilting the head to one side results in extension of the arm and flexion of the leg on that and the opposite side.	Central nervous system above level of midbrain; usually considered to be in basal ganglia, cerebral cortex, or both	Writing, sitting balance, transfers, standing balance, eating, dressing

essence their definitions, are described. The usual location of the damage (pathology) and the functional skills likely to be disturbed when these reflexes are uninhibited are given.

These reflexes exist in all people and are normally well controlled (inhibited) and effectively utilized. In cerebral palsy, control is incomplete, and the reflexes are said to be uninhibited and hence exaggerated. For example, uninhibited long spinal and vestibular reflexes are shown in figures 11-1 and 11-2, respectively. Voluntary motion therefore becomes impaired or impossible. Persons with cerebral palsy may be able to inhibit the reflexes when they are relaxed, but if they are excited or anxious, they can no longer exert this voluntary inhibition and the reflexes override any attempt they may make to perform voluntary or controlled actions.

Etiology

Most cases of cerebral palsy are acquired, either congenitally or postnatally, although a few show evidence of being hereditary (hereditary spastic diplegia and hereditary tremors). In some cases, no

TABLE 11-1—*Continued*—

Reflex	Definition	Usual Site of Pathology	Functional Ability Likely To Be Disturbed When Uninhibited
Vestibular	A series of complex responses to the position and movement of the head. Tipping the head back or upward results in flexion or abduction of the arms and extension of the legs. Tipping head downward may result in extension and adduction of the arms and flexion of the legs. Tilting head to the left may result in extension of the left arm and flexion of the left leg with opposite actions on the right side.	Above the vestibular nuclei and midbrain	Writing, ambulation, standing balance, tranfers
Startle	A quick generalized flexion, usually of all four extremities. Head and back often extend at the same time. Head extension occurring together with upper extremity flexion often resembles a vestibular reflex, but differs in that it is elicited by loud noises, frightening or sudden occurrences. Even nonthreatening and mild stimuli may be sufficient to trigger the startle reflex.	Midbrain or above	Sitting balance, ambulation, transfers, standing balance, dressing, eating

etiology can be established. Any agent or event that causes damage to the brain during its development can cause the syndrome of cerebral palsy. Table 11-2 summarizes the causes seemingly responsible during pregnancy (prenatal), at labor and delivery (natal), and after birth (postnatal). The type of damage (e.g., infections, toxins, or trauma) is also summarized.

Prenatal causes. Among the more common prenatal causes are bacterial, protozoan, or viral infections in the mother. Different clinical syndromes result, depending on whether the infection occurs early, when the basic structure of the brain is initially developing, or later, when more specific functional interactions are maturing. Infectious agents definitely identified are rubella, toxoplasmosis, and congenital syphilis. Occasionally, other infections are implicated, such as influenza or kidney infections, but the cause and effect relationship is not as well documented.

Toxic causes of brain damage in the developing fetus usually relate to certain pathologic conditions in the mother, such as eclampsia, toxemia of pregnancy, and maternal "poisoning" by drugs and heavy metals. There are no clear-cut relations between narcotic ingestion by the mother and brain damage. Some infants born to chemically dependent mothers, however, do have cerebral palsy and many have overt evidence of addiction at birth and suffer from unrecognized withdrawal. Rh factor incompatibility is also technically a toxic cause, the toxin being the antibodies developed by the Rh negative mother to the child's Rh positive blood.

Trauma is not a very common prenatal cause of cerebral palsy. A premature birth, either spontaneous or associated with trauma to the mother, can result in poor fetal nutrition and oxygenation, with possible damage to the fetal brain. Other events in the mother, such as asphyxia, severe anemia, or hypotension, may interfere with the oxygen delivery to the fetus. Further,

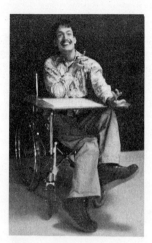

FIGURE 11-1. This patient's long spinal reflexes are poorly inhibited. An attempt to perform an activity with the right upper extremity results in purposeless patterned positioning of all other limbs, and is characteristic of athetosis.

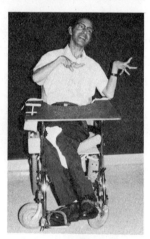

FIGURE 11-2. Uninhibited vestibular reflexes cause this man's arms to lift up as he raises his head, making it difficult for him to use his hands at table level. The severe hyperextension of the fingers, coupled with wrist and elbow flexion, is a characteristic dystonic posture elicited when reaching is attempted. This patient's particular condition is called tension athetosis with spasticity.

a bleeding tendency in the mother (hemophilia) may induce bleeding in the fetus. If the bleeding occurs in the brain, damage will result, which can give rise to cerebral palsy.

Natal causes. Most cases of cerebral palsy occurring around the time of birth are associated with difficulty during labor and delivery, resulting in hemorrhage or anoxia and subsequent loss of functioning brain tissue. Premature infants are particularly susceptible, but prematurity alone is not felt to cause cerebral palsy unless these other factors are present.

Postnatal causes. In the period immediately after birth, infections such as meningitis or encephalitis may affect the brain directly, pneumonia may cause anoxia,

and any kind of trauma to the head in the neonatal period may cause brain damage. When the blood sugar is temporarily very low (hypoglycemia), the child may suffer convulsions. Either direct brain damage from the hypoglycemia or anoxic damage during convulsions may occur.

Rarely, a child may have a congenital aneurysm, which will cause brain damage if it bleeds. Occasionally, an X-ray will show an empty space within the brain substance (porencephalic cyst). Most often, this is due to severe damage, with disappearance of the brain tissue. Cerebrospinal fluid fills the empty space, which gives it the appearance of a cyst.

Classification

The movement disorders in cerebral palsy are classified both by the area of the body affected (topography) and by the symptom complex exhibited.

Topography. The topographic classification of cerebral palsy describes six areas of the body or limbs affected by the brain damage.

1. *Quadriplegia* describes the involvement of all four extremities relatively equally.
2. *Diplegia* describes involvement of the lower extremities predominantly, with only mildly affected upper extremities.
3. *Paraplegia* refers to involvement of the lower extremities alone, with apparently normal upper extremities.
4. *Monoplegia* describes involvement of only one extremity, either upper or lower.
5. *Hemiplegia* describes involvement of both limbs on one side.
6. *Triplegia* describes involvement of three extremities, with only one extremity unimpaired.

Symptom complex. The motor problems associated with brain damage in cerebral palsy may occur alone or in conjunction with others and may affect one or more body parts. Nine symptoms are included in the concurrent symptomatolgic classification accepted by the American Academy for Cerebral Palsy and Developmental Medicine. These include: (a) spasticity, (b) athetosis (nontension and tension), (c) dystonia, (d) atonia, (e) rigidity, (f) ataxia, (g) tremor, (h) mixed, (i) undetermined. Of the above, spasticity, ataxia, and athetosis are the main movement disorders and are discussed first.

Spasticity occurs when the stretch reflex (see table 11-1) is not inhibited, and is manifested in three ways: (a) an excessive response to rapid stretch of the involved muscles when the tendons are tapped by a reflex hammer during a clinical examination; (b) one or more "bouncing" contractions (clonus) occurring spontaneously when the muscle is stretched and held by a force; and (c) stereotyped postures assumed as a result of persistent excessive muscle contraction (tone)

TABLE 11-2
ETIOLOGY OF CEREBRAL PALSY

Prenatal Factors *(Conception to onset of labor)*	Natal Factors *(Onset of labor to birth)*	Postnatal Factors *(After birth of viable fetus)*
Hereditary Genetically transmitted, often sex-linked, symptoms present at birth or soon after, does not progress (e.g., hereditary athetosis, familial tremors)	*Anoxia* Mechanical respiratory obstruction	*Traumatic* Contusions of the brain Skull fractures
Acquired in utero Prenatal infection (e.g., toxoplasmosis, syphilis, rubella, or other maternal infection)	Atelectasis Narcotism Placenta previa or abruptio	*Infections* Acute (e.g., meningitis, encephalitis) Chronic (e.g., syphilis, brain abscess, granulomas)
Prenatal anoxia Maternal anoxia, anemia, or hypotension Placental pathology (e.g., abruptio, infarcts, premature atrophy)	Maternal anoxia or hypotension (e.g., spinal anesthesia) Breech deliveries, with delay of aftercoming head Prolapse of cord	*Vascular* Hemorrhage Embolus Thrombosis
Prenatal cerebral hemmorrhage Toxemia Trauma Maternal bleeding diathesis	*Cerebral hemorrhage & contusion* Trauma Physiologic (e.g., disproportion, dystocia) Obstetrical (e.g., inaccurate forceps application)	*Anoxia* Carbon monoxide poisoning High altitude & low pressure anoxias Respiratory distress syndrome
Rh factor *Metabolic disturbances* (e.g., maternal diabetes)	*Constitutional factors* Prematurity, congenital anemias of the newborn Hypoprothrombinemia	Respiratory obstruction (e.g., croup, foreign bodies, drowning) *Metabolic abnormalities* Insulin reaction *Postneoplastic*

in certain muscles, associated with persistent reduced tone in their opposites (antagonists). Typical postures are flexion of the wrists, elbows, and knees; flexion, adduction, and internal rotation of the hips, and plantar flexion of the feet.

Together with these abnormalities of tone, spastic patients also demonstrate a very reduced ability to perform complex varied movements. Movements available may be quite stereotyped, regardless of what movement may be attempted. A loss of dexterity and reduced ability to learn motor skills results. Spasticity may occur in conjunction with athetosis or, less often, with ataxia.

Ataxia is defined as difficulty in controlling the accuracy of a needed muscle length or limb position. It may result from a loss or reduction of sensory input from joints or, more frequently, from an inability to appropriately activate or inhibit muscles with sufficient rapidity and accuracy, usually associated with cerebellar dysfunction. The patient exhibits an uncertain aim in reaching, grasping, or transferring objects, manifested as a "hunting" movement, or dysmetria. There is repetitive overshooting and overcorrection of each motion, giving rise to a continuous tremor during each attempted motion (intention tremor). In walking, the gait is staggering, with uncertain and inaccurate foot placement, poor balance, and constant readjustment of position that has the appearance of alcohol intoxication.

Athetosis refers to the involuntary occurrence of purposeless movement when the patient attempts purposeful motion. The abnormal movements may occur not only in the limb that is being purposefully moved, but may also involve an "overflow" of activity to all the other limbs (fig. 11-1). Most often, the motor activity can be identified as an exaggeration of one or more of the reflexes described in table 11-1. Athetosis varies from patient to patient and from time to time, but is usually characterized either by flailing or writhing movements of the trunk or extremities that are not voluntarily initiated. The patient may be able to learn, with training, to inhibit athetotic movements so that purposeful movements can be performed with improved accuracy and diminished overflow to the other limbs. Emotional excitation above a certain level can cause the patient's voluntary control or ability to inhibit the movements to weaken, with resultant return of the involuntary (overflow) motor activity and loss of control.

Dystonia, an expression of abnormal increased muscle tone occurring simultaneously in both muscles and their antagonists, may be a component of athetosis. The symptom complex is then described as dystonic or *tension athetosis* (fig. 11-2). Impairment of function of the extrapyramidal system is associated with athetosis or certain forms of dystonia. Dystonia is exaggerated by central nervous system excitation or stimulation, and it may be induced even by the simple activation required for an attempt at voluntary movement. Characteristic dystonic postures are often elicited during certain motor activities. In figure 11-2, the dystonic component of tension athetosis is evident in the posture assumed by the patient's hands. Dystonia may also occur in association with uninhibited stretch reflexes, when it is recognized as a component of spasticity. It also often occurs alone.

Rigidity exists when severe excessive muscle tone, such that no passive motion is possible, appears simultaneously in both flexors and extensors. The rigidity may mask underlying spasticity and/or athetosis.

Atonia or *hypotonia*, a condition where muscle tone is decreased or practically absent, occurs only in a small number of patients with cerebral palsy.

Although not part of the list of symptoms used for classification by the American Academy for Cerebral Palsy and Developmental Medicine, other symptoms of brain damage occur in cerebral palsy and affect the patient's ability to function. One such motor symptom is *apraxia*, the inability to organize movement of body parts consistently in appropriate sequence and coordination to perform a useful activity. The key factor here is sequencing the muscles in appropriate order. When arm movements are involved, the term "constructional apraxia" is used, and when the muscles of speech are involved, the term "verbal apraxia" is used.

Other symptoms are not related to movement, such as certain behavioral deficits, which can also be directly attributed to specific brain damage. A prototype of a behavioral abnormality is the hyperkinetic, distractible individual with a short attention span. A behavior pattern of this type is primarily due to a defect in the ability to regulate a response to a stimulus on the basis of its relevance or significance to ongoing situations or problems. Thus, a characteristic of this behavior may be a response made to stimuli on the basis of loudness, brightness, or suddenness, rather than social importance. The person cannot inhibit either the influence of the stimuli on the central nervous system or his responses to them.

Another form of behavior deficit almost the opposite of the above is *perseveration* of an ongoing activity. The individual is unable to identify the need to stop one activity and attend to other stimuli clearly more important.

Complications

In describing the symptom complexes, only those concerned with the basic movement disorder were elaborated. Others, such as visual and auditory deficits, are also primarily due to brain damage. They are discussed in this section, however, because they compound the vocational rehabilitation problem, as do the true complications resulting from a primary symptom.

Contractures. Limitation of passive and active joint range of motion (contracture) arises from a shortening of the muscles or the capsules around the joints (see fig. 3-13, p. 30). The cause of contractures in cerebral palsy is the hyperactive stretch reflexes in spasticity. Activation of the stretch reflex at an increasingly earlier point in the range of motion makes full motion progressively more difficult to achieve. Capsular shortening usually follows muscle shortening. After a prolonged period of time, relief of the contracture may require an attack on the capsule as well as the muscle.

The joints most commonly affected by contractures are the ankles, feet, hips, knees, elbows, wrists, thumbs, and sometimes shoulders. Contractures can interfere with walking, self-care, bed position, sitting posture, and perineal hygiene.

Bowel and bladder incontinence. In cerebral palsy, bowel and bladder incontinence arises most frequently from inability to attend or respond to sensory signals indicating a need to void or evacuate. This is especially difficult when the response requires interruption of an ongoing activity. The person may ignore sensory signals but not on any deliberate or conscious basis. Rather, appreciation of the stimulus is inhibited by the ongoing activity. Perseveration in the ongoing task, even when the stimulus is perceived, may also be present. Discrimination amongst stimuli is a function of the limbic system of the brain.

Constipation. Insufficient fluid or bulk in the diet and/or failure to establish and maintain a regular schedule for bowel movements may result in constipation. If the patient requires assistance, problems may arise from inability to attract the attention of the attendant or to communicate the need to evacuate.

Dental problems. The same factors that caused the brain damage may also have affected developing tooth enamel. If the noxious event occurred at the time of tooth formation, the teeth will be less resistant to decay. Further, the patient's motor problems may make it very difficult to brush the teeth adequately and the diet may be insufficient to keep the teeth clean through chewing. Chewing and the ability to manipulate food with the tongue may also be impaired.

In addition to problems of tooth decay, cerebral palsy patients often have overbites as a result of persistent tongue thrust against the upper incisors. Patients who receive phenylhydantoin for seizure control commonly have hypertrophic gums that are prone to infection and inflammation. Preventive gum care requires careful frequent brushing, which may be very difficult if the patient has poor hand function. Regular, frequent dental prophylaxis is important.

Osteoporosis. The formation of insufficiently mineralized bone sometimes results from inadequate diet, but more often from deficient muscle activity, especially after a patient has been immobilized in plaster for surgical procedures. Osteoporosis may cause pain in the feet and legs when weight bearing is attempted, or the bones may become fragile and fracture on attempts to stretch the joints with excessive force. Sometimes simply transferring the patient may break a bone.

Degenerative joint disease. Abnormal wear and tear on poorly aligned joints may cause dejenerative joint disease (see chap. 14). It occurs frequently in the cervical spine in athetoid patients with poor head control and dystonic neck muscles. It may also affect hips, knees, and ankles in the ambulatory spastic athetoid patient.

Scoliosis. Usually an abnormally curved spine is the result of poorly supported sitting posture with asymmetrical muscle pull on some portion of the spine. It may also occur in bedridden patients who are allowed to lie in one position consistently. Severe scoliosis that is associated with limited respiratory function may be a life-shortening factor. Pneumonia aggravated by inefficient cough is generally the cause of death.

Malnutrition. Several factors may cause malnutrition: the patient's inability to chew or swallow effectively; the patient's inability to feed himself within the time available; "food fads;" and restricted diets. Further, the patient with athetosis or spasticity who expends relatively more than average energy to perform activities may receive inadequate amounts of food for his energy needs.

Respiratory infections. Many patients with cerebral palsy, particularly those more severely involved, have frequent and severe respiratory infections. These infections are due to poor coughing ability and inefficient swallowing. Because of the inability to coordinate the larynx and muscles of respiration and poor muscle control generally, the patient cannot obtain the explosive movement of air which is necessary to move mucus or foreign matter up the bronchial tree. Aspiration of food or fluids may be caused by inefficient swallowing. Food may enter the trachea instead of the esophagus, and the patient may be unable to cough it up before it has acted as a foreign body and produced infection. Patients with cerebral palsy may take longer than normal to recover from an infection.

Visual impairment. Severe specific damage to the occipital cortex results in the total loss of the ability to process visual information (cortical blindness). Partial or unilateral lesions of the occipital cortex give rise to visual field defects in which one side of the visual field is not seen and is therefore ignored (see p. 48).

Less severe involvement results in impaired visual perception or attention. Visual perceptual difficulties may affect appreciation of objects in space, the ability to sort figures from background, the ability to attend to one part of a page preferentially, and the ability to establish directionality. All of these difficulties may interfere with performing the activities of daily living. Occasionally, a patient with good physical ability will have such severe perceptual or perceptual-motor problems that he is much more handicapped than a severely physically involved patient. In all of these deficits, the problem is not in the eye itself but in the processing of the impulses leaving the retina.

Auditory impairment. Hearing losses, as described in chapter 30, may occur incidental to the cerebral palsy. In addition, brain damage may also produce a *central deafness*. In this disorder, brain damage blocks the auditory pathways from the brain stem to the temporal lobe.

Deafness of some type has been reported in about 25 percent of cerebral palsy patients and severe loss in 6 to 16 percent. Hearing loss may be especially important if the person also has some visual deficit. Even if he can hear well, the cerebral palsied person may have difficulty in interpreting auditory input due to central deafness. Poor head control also interferes with localization of sounds.

Seizures. Seizure disorders occur in perhaps 50 to 60 percent of patients with cerebral palsy. Seizures may be typical grand mal, Jacksonian, psychomotor, or petit mal (see chap. 12). They may be more disabling than the physical aspects of cerebral palsy if control by medication is incomplete or impossible. Control of seizures to a reasonable degree is therefore extremely necessary before other management can be successful.

Petit mal and minor seizures may present a serious diagnostic problem. Seizures may be seen by the teacher or other professionals as inattentiveness and may be interpreted as willful behavior. Seizures causing strange behavior are especially prone to misinterpretation. Only good teamwork and interaction among medical, rehabilitation, and educational personnel can succeed in identifying the behavior correctly and referring the patient for appropriate treatment.

Fatigue. Due to the motor control and coordination deficits, performance that is normally relatively automatic requires conscious effort by the cerebral palsy patient. This effort, combined with involuntary movement or excessive tension, results in the expenditure of an enormous amount of physical and mental energy to perform relatively ordinary tasks. Cerebral palsy patients are therefore subject to fatigue, which occurs sooner and is more profound than in normal persons performing the same task. Fatigue also tends to accumulate during the week, and if there is not adequate rest at night or on the weekends, the person may lose efficiency in school or on a job.

FUNCTIONAL DISABILITIES

Functional ability is dependent upon the interaction of joint movement and muscle strength; perceptual function; cognitive and intellectual function; memory function; attention and response abilities; and personal and social attitudes and skills. Any one of these areas can be so deficient or aberrant that satisfactory physical independence and vocational function may be impossible. Training and provision of assistance by aides and/or mechanical and electronic devices can, however, improve the cerebral palsy patient's functional level.

Physical Disabilities

Ambulation. Walking depends upon an ability to appreciate position in space; to balance the body segments above the feet and support them; and to shift weight and to move one foot in front of the other in sequence. Deficits in motor control and/or visuospatial deficits will therefore impair walking ability. Figures 11-3, 11-4, 11-5, and 11-6 demonstrate various types of ambulation.

Most hemiplegics learn to walk, as do diplegics if their spasticity and impairment of control are not too severe. Both may require one of the various canes (figs. 11-3 and 11-4), crutches (fig. 11-5), and/or long or short leg braces. Quadriplegics, depending upon severity and type, more rarely learn to walk. They may be able to walk in sheltered conditions, but often a startle reflex, vestibular reflexes, or an insufficient voluntary motor repertoire interfere with ability to perform.

Wheelchair ambulation requires the ability to sit with fair stability in the chair and to either reach and move the wheels with the hands, or to reach the floor and move the feet to push the chair. A poorly fitted wheelchair can even exaggerate abnormal movements, as shown in figure 11-7. Wheelchair adaptations, such as the specially fabricated contour seat in figure 11-8, can improve sitting posture and the ability to move the wheelchair. Figure 11-9 illustrates a more formidable approach to achieving truncal balance and wheelchair control. Hemiplegics may be able to propel the chair using one hand and one foot, or they may use a wheelchair with both hand rails on one side. The very

severely involved athetoid or spastic quadriplegic patient is unlikely to be able to use a wheelchair independently. Electric wheelchairs have proven practical for many of these patients, though the chairs and the controls may have to be adapted (fig. 11-10). Patients with perceptual deficits will have difficulty steering a wheelchair properly, regardless of their motor ability.

The presence of ataxia alone or, more frequently, in combination with athetosis or spasticity, severely limits the functional possibilities and prospects for walking or wheelchair travel.

Transfers. For patients who can walk, transfers may be totally independent except transfers in and out of the bathtub; in situations where balance depends on specific muscle groups that are under poor control; or where contractures prevent clearing of a leg or arm

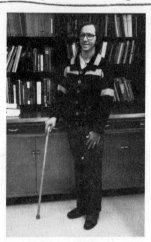

FIGURE 11-3. This man with left hemiparesis and some moderate spasticity is able to walk with a cane in his right hand and no leg braces.

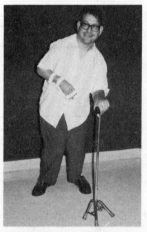

FIGURE 11-4. Even with a broad-base cane, this man with right hemiparesis, spasticity, and apraxia has poor balance because he has trouble learning the appropriate motions to maintain equilibrium. He requires a wheelchair for more than a few steps across the room.

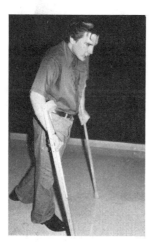

FIGURE 11-5. This man with spastic diplegia can walk independently, using a four-point gait and Kenny crutches. His gait deteriorates to swing-through when he hurries.

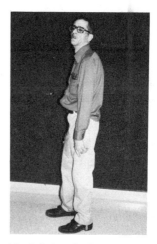

FIGURE 11-6. With a left short leg brace, this man with athetosis and abnormal appearance has good standing balance and is able to walk long distances independently.

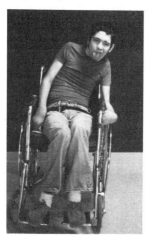

FIGURE 11-7. In a poorly fitting wheelchair, this man has poor trunk control. Note his exaggerated facial grimace as he attempts to use his arm to right himself.

across an obstacle. Patients with visuomotor problems will have difficulty orienting supports properly to aid in transfers. Generally, the spastic diplegic patient who is unable to walk has sufficient upper extremity function to allow independent sliding-board or pivot transfers. Moderately involved individuals who are able to support some weight on the lower extremities and to balance a little can be transferred by a pivot transfer and can be managed by one assistant with ease unless ataxia is extreme. The most severely involved patients will require two-person lift transfers, being unable to assist at all.

Eating. Eating independence is achieved by most mildly and moderately affected individuals. The more severely involved may develop some abilities to feed themselves but require adapted equipment. Those patients who have difficulty with the manual components of motor control in self-feeding activities

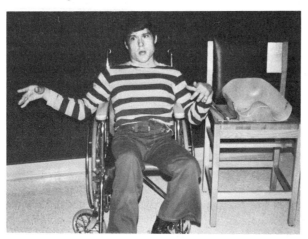
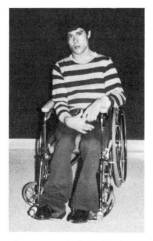

FIGURE 11-8. *(Left)* Without adequate seat support, this man is unable to maintain erect posture in his wheelchair because of poor truncal balance. *(Right)* A specially fabricated contour seat, which is shown on the regular chair, *(Left)*, provides adequate support and improves the man's posture, function, and appearance.

will not be able to feed themselves.

Some eating difficulties are due to poor lip, tongue, and throat control, resulting in slow eating and poor chewing and swallowing ability. Careful technique in assisted feeding is required to prevent the patient from either aspirating the food or pushing it back out of the mouth by tongue thrust. Visuomotor problems often interfere with self-feeding by making the purposefully coordinated sequence of motions for scooping and carrying the food without spilling extremely difficult to achieve, even though the specific hand motions are within the capability of the person. Self-feeding problems due to visual acuity deficits can often be overcome with training.

Dressing. Independent dressing will be possible for mildly and moderately involved patients, regardless of disability type. Moderately involved patients will require more time and more adapted clothing and will function less well with tension or hurrying. A patient may be able to dress himself in most circumstances but prefer assistance, rather than expending the necessary time and effort in dressing himself, if he must get to a job at a certain time.

Contractures, particularly at the shoulder, knee, and hip, can make dressing more difficult. Also, an impairment of visual perception might make it difficult for the person to orient a shirt properly, front to back and right side out, even though the physical ability is adequate.

Personal hygiene. Most hemiplegics without severe sensory disturbance will be independent in personal hygiene activities. Some patients may be independent except for certain transfers, such as in and out of the bathtub, but may become completely independent with minor modifications or adapted equipment.

Impaired upper extremity dexterity and poor sitting balance interfere with the ability to maintain satisfactory perineal hygiene, and hip, shoulder, or elbow contractures may make this quite impossible. The more severely involved patients will be totally dependent in this area.

Language and Communication Disabilities

The development of language and communication skills from infancy depends upon an intact hearing mechanism, an intact brain, an environment of peers and adults in a series of interactions of ever-increasing breadth and depth, and sufficient motor skills to allow the person to be present in many different settings. The person with cerebral palsy may be deficient in all four areas from birth. In cerebral palsy, the speech output may range from normal or nearly normal to complete lack of speech. The average incidence of oral communication disorders among cerebral palsied individuals has been estimated at 70–80 percent.

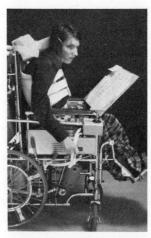

FIGURE 11-9. With a molded plastic body jacket, this patient is comfortable, able to run her wheelchair, and use her communication board (she is nonverbal).

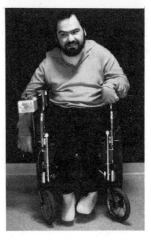

FIGURE 11-10. This patient with spastic triplegia has reasonably good function only in his right arm. In an electric wheelchair, he is fully mobile.

Identification of the causes of the disabilities is not an easy task. The first level is determining whether the person has a hearing impairment (see chap. 30). Then it must be determined whether the brain damage may be so severe that the person does not recognize the social need to communicate. Assuming some recognition of this need exists, the next determination is whether there is capacity for symbolic language, either nonverbal (e.g., pantomime) or verbal. In some, the retardation is such that no symbolic communication is possible and only more concrete responses are present (e.g., pointing at a desired object). Of course, both concrete and symbolic communication require some motor ability to point, look, or vocalize in order to attract sufficient attention.

Verbal communication requires the capacity for symbolic language plus the complex motor skills necessary to vocalize sounds and words with appropriate clarity. Nonverbal communication similarly requires the capacity for symbolic language, but an alternate means of expression is used. Verbal and nonverbal communication in cerebral palsy are not necessarily equally impaired. When verbal skills are impaired but nonverbal skills are not, manual or visual language systems may be used. Communication substitutes, such as the Bliss and Rebus systems, require intact visual perceptual skills, and the manual sign language used by the deaf requires motor skills.

When a verbal person who is not trained in nonverbal methods communicates with those who have only nonverbal skills, there is a tendency to take shortcuts, to restrict communication to concrete immediacies, and hence to limit the verbal exposure of the developing child. Thus, basic language, social, and intellectual development is more limited than it could be under more optimum management.

The breadth of the potential communication problems in the adult with cerebral palsy seem, therefore, to include:
1. Hearing disorders
2. Auditory comprehension problems
3. Visual comprehension problems for verbal and nonverbal input
4. Insufficient experiences
5. Distractability
6. Limited intelligence
7. Weakness, slowness, and/or incoordination of speech mechanism movements

Psychosocial Disabilities

Brain damage may result in deficiencies in one or more of the four basic cognitive abilities: verbal receptive, verbal expressive, visual perceptual, and visual motor. Visual motor skills are not identical with the movement disorder but refer rather to creative construction. Visual perceptual functions include such activities as figure-background discrimination and spatial orientation. The verbal abilities and associated communication impairments have already been discussed.

Behavior deficits, such as the stimulus-bound response and inadequate discrimination among stimuli, are reviewed above. Task preservation and rigidity in approach to problem solving may also mark the behavior of a person with cerebral palsy. Easy distractibility, dependency, and manipulative behavior can further compound the disability. Short attention span and short- and long-term memory impairments may also be present.

The combination of cognitive and behavioral deficits may be viewed as components of the learning disabilities present in cerebral palsy. Deficits in acquisition, retention, interpretation, and application of information, coupled with inadequate training, lead to relatively low levels of achievement.

By the time they reach adulthood, cerebral palsied persons generally still have inadequate social skills. Reduced experiences and fewer interpersonal contacts are consequences of diminished mobility and social isolation. Contact with nondisabled peers will have been very restricted, especially if the person attended a school for handicapped children.

Another general consequence of an individual growing up with a disability is the *qualitative* difference in the kind of social relationships experienced. Other persons, in relating to the cerebral palsy patient, are inclined to present a fairly consistent pattern of support, assistance, and reduced expectations. The patient may actually develop the attitude that he is the "center of the universe." Consequently, basic principles of interaction, such as giving as well as receiving, are not within his developmental experience. He may not recognize the need to take some responsibility personally in social relationships, but rather expect the world to come to him regardless of how he responds. Relationships are often perceived in only two dimensions, as directed either toward or away from himself. Persons who direct themselves toward him are perceived as helpful, and those who direct themselves away from him are perceived as hostile. This egocentricity is often manifested as excessive dependency and self-centered behavior. These behaviors, often acceptable in a child, are objectionable in an adult. Because these social behaviors have developed and have been reinforced for 15 to 20 years for many handicapped adults, they are strongly entrenched and resistant to change.

In addition to these general deficiencies in social relations, cerebral palsied persons also have specific difficulties in developing sexual relationships. They experience normal desires, but lack the skills or training to satisfy those desires. They also have limited access to and opportunity for sexual experience. The person with cerebral palsy has many barriers to overcome in the development of a sexual relationship: physical barriers due to physical disabilities; social barriers due to society's mores and conventions of sexual preferences (e.g., physique and cosmesis); and personal barriers due to the inadequate knowledge of both biological facts relating to sexuality and the accepted social concepts of relationships to peers of the opposite sex.

Rehabilitation Potential

The person with cerebral palsy has a stable lesion. Brain damage does not increase with age, and therefore long-term planning is appropriate. As the cerebral palsied person reaches adulthood, his total physical, psychosocial, and language abilities will be maximal only if prior total treatment was exemplary. The counselor may well find this not to be the case for his client, and full realization of a client's rehabilitation potential may not be present. Treatment intervention may be necessary.

Preservation of skills and abilities is dependent upon repeated regular practice, avoidance of enumerated complications, and effective followup. In middle age, the client may not have as much endurance as his nondisabled peers for the performance of the demanding kinds of work that were performed at a younger age because of a relatively greater decrease in total available energy.

A realistic appreciation of the status of the disability, while important for all diseases, is particularly important in rehabilitation planning with cerebral palsy clients. The inexperienced background and learning disabilities of individuals with cerebral palsy may have interfered with their own appraisal and recognition of their abilities. Expectations may not match abilities. Further, the client may not appreciate the breadth of skills needed for a particular occupation. It may be necessary to assist the client's comparison of his special repertory of skills with those skills required by a potential occupation.

Rehabilitation potential for the person with cerebral palsy is affected by a number of factors in addition to the physical, communication, and psychosocial problems present. These factors include maintenance therapy required, living arrangements required, and the client's desires and attitude toward employment. Rehabilitation potential may be further hindered by an unattractive appearance or the physical need for attendants to assist with personal care. These problems must be taken into account in preparing a rehabilitation plan.

In addition to treatment of physical problems, mature social skills may need to be learned from the beginning. The sexual frustrations of the young person may often need to be addressed before it is possible to deal with other emotional problems and begin training for a job. Negative attitudes toward employment and dependent attitudes toward the world need to be overcome before employers can be satisfied with an applicant with cerebral palsy.

An important element in the successful realization of potential is the availability of an adequate range of placement and support opportunities. The greater the spectrum of possibilities within the community, the better the potential. The existence of sheltered workshops, modified work opportunities, selective job placement, day activity centers, supported residential facilities, group homes with community recreational and educational facilities, and foster homes all enhance the client's potential.

Despite the many obstacles to successful rehabilitation of the client with cerebral palsy, it is worthwhile working with even the most severely involved persons to try to establish some kind of vocational or avocational activity leading toward a goal of maximal functioning and life satisfaction.

STANDARDS OF EVALUATION

Depending on the nature and severity of his problems, evaluation of the person with cerebral palsy may require more disciplines working at a more sophisticated level than is required in most other disabilities. It can also take more time than average to get an accurate evaluation of the individual's abilities. A complete assessment of functional status requires medical evaluation and evaluation of physical function, communication, and psychosocial development.

Medical Evaluation

A neurologist should assess neurological status including, where appropriate, the identification of seizure activity. The latter may require brain wave analysis (EEG). Nutritional requirements and adequacy of diet should be reviewed by a nutritionist. Examination by a dentist is essential to identify dental problems. Not every dentist will have the capacity, interest, and physical facilities to provide evaluation and treatment. A search may have to be made. Orthodontic evaluation for overbite should also be performed. Visual impairments should be evaluated by an ophthalmologist (see chap. 29), and hearing impairments should be evaluated by an otologist and an audiologist (see chap. 30). Evaluation of other organ systems should be done by an internist, with special attention given to problems of recurrent infections. The achievement of the above, while perhaps possible sequentially, may best be performed in a central setting where interest in cerebral palsy exists.

Functional Evaluation

The physiatrist, physical therapist, and occupational therapist working together can evaluate the patient's motor repertory and identify the voluntary, involuntary, and accuracy control aspects of his movement characteristics. They will also assess contractures and skeletal deformities and, where appropriate, refer the patient to an orthopedic surgeon for further evaluation and possible recommendations for surgery. Language and swallowing ability should be evaluated by a speech pathologist, who can identify problems and recommend therapeutic approaches.

Psychosocial Evaluation

Cognition. Intellectual evaluation is a particularly difficult area in cerebral palsy. Ideally, intelligence testing should provide as specific a profile as possible of strengths and deficiencies in the four major areas of intellectual functioning: visual perception, visual-motor performance, verbal reception, and verbal expression. For this purpose, the standard intelligence tests require analysis, modification, and adaptation in their application and interpretation by a psychologist particularly experienced in working with cerebral palsy clients. Standard IQ testing may not be particularly rewarding or useful.

To separate cognitive function from motor function, time-dependent criteria may have to be ignored or other means of ascertaining a response may be advisable. Multiple tests may be required to answer specific questions, since tests differ in the relative emphasis on certain cognitive functional abilities. It is most important to make a distinction between the ability to process visually mediated information and verbally mediated information. Further, if performance is impaired, it is important to make a distinction between difficulty in understanding or carrying out the perceptual and conceptual elements of a task and difficulty in executing the response. Finally, a distinction should be made between the creative constructional aspects of the response and the strictly motor abilities required.

Behavior. Certain generalized difficulties in attentive skills exist in cerebral palsy which contribute strongly to learning disabilities. Therefore, careful observation and analysis of performance should be carried out to identify attention duration, short auditory memory, distractibility, perseveration, or inability to select and respond to stimuli on the basis of their relevance rather than their physical characteristics. Impairment of these functions is often responsible for failures otherwise attributed to cognitive, intellectual deficit. Appropriate analysis will identify a remediation strategy likely to produce improvement.

Personality assessment to identify the patient's behavior patterns, personal attitudes, problem-solving strategies, and level of self-esteem may be critical. The patient's interactions with peers, authority figures, family members, groups, and individuals should also be evaluated. The psychologist and/or social worker can identify problem areas and recommend appropriate remediation approaches.

Evaluation of a condition with all the complexities of cerebral palsy can be carried out effectively only in a context of total management. Since evaluation is an intrinsic component of management in cerebral palsy, it will be appreciated best by the discussion in the following section.

TOTAL TREATMENT

Medical Treatment

Drugs. A number of medications are in use for the control of excessive muscle tone and to induce muscle relaxation. The most common are diazepam (Valium) and dantrolene sodium (Dantrium). Occasionally, some of the phenothiazines (see p. 255) or other tranquilizers are used to assist in management of the excessive muscle tone that may be related to generalized central nervous system hyperactivity. Levodopa (see p. 87) is also in use for the control of excessive muscle tone with some suggestive evidence that it may be of value in cerebral palsy in certain instances. Other medications are very likely to become available. Baclofen, for example, is a new drug for excess muscle tone that has not yet been fully evaluated for use in cerebral palsy.

These drugs have a number of side effects. An unfortunate side effect of diazepam and the tranquilizers, in some cases, is not only lethargy but a true affective depression which will limit their usefulness. Affective depression is occasionally a disturbing side effect of levodopa as well. Dantrolene sodium is often associated with a feeling of lassitude and other subjective signs of discomfort, such as nausea and fatigability. In addition, there are unusual but serious occurrences of liver damage, which require careful medical followup as long as the patient receives the medication. Drugs likely to be prescribed are for use indefinitely. Regular medical attention to monitor side effects, ensure compliance, adjust dosages, and consider newer preparations must be assured.

Neurolytic procedures. For spasticity, in particular, interruption of reflex pathways by blocking nerve impulses is helpful to achieve improved ambulation, upper extremity function, and posture. They are usually done at the point where nerves enter the muscles (intramuscular neurolysis). Phenol or alcohol injections may be used and repeated if necessary.

Surgery. Orthopedic surgery is relatively effective in reducing muscle spasticity. Usually a muscle or tendon lengthening procedure is performed, which effectively decreases stimulation of the stretch reflexes. This form of surgery is not as consistently effective for the excessive tone of athetoid dystonic patients. Various other orthopedic procedures are done to correct deformities in the feet, hips, and wrists.

Recently, the implantation of an electrical stimulator in the cerebellum has been introduced to achieve muscle relaxation. While some dramatic results have been claimed and demonstrated, the evidence is insufficient to define the specific types of problems for which successful results can be consistently expected. Neurosurgical procedures to produce destructive lesions in precisely determined locations in the basal ganglia or thalamus regions of the brain (see chap. 3) have also been advocated to control undesired movements or rigidity. Results vary, and dependable criteria have not yet been established which will predict a reasonable rate of success for any special neurosurgical procedure. With drugs, neurolysis, or surgery, motor skill and balance training are often required to develop improved function with the altered neurological mechanism.

Treatment of Complications

Contractures. Management of contractures is best applied preventively, rather than after deformities have developed. The techniques available for control of contractures are passive stretching, orthopedic surgical procedures, intramuscular neurolysis, and bracing. Where passive stretching cannot be done or is ineffective because tone is too persistent and too strong, surgical tendon or muscle lengthening procedures at an early stage should be performed. This is particularly important around the hips to prevent dislocation and to facilitate perineal hygiene and toileting.

Bowel and bladder incontinence. Bowel incontinence may be managed by a regular evacuation schedule, dietary control, and, on occasion, medications. Training the individual to become more aware of toileting needs must proceed concurrently. Bladder incontinence caused by the inability to pay attention to bladder stimuli may respond to training in attention to significant stimuli. Incontinence may also often be controlled through training of attendants and development of a communication system between them and the patient.

Constipation. Adequate bulk and liquid in the diet and a regular evacuation schedule are essential to prevent constipation. Given the problems in responsiveness and physical difficulties in accomplishing self-care tasks, sufficient time needs to be allowed to evacuate the bowel completely. Often a morning time is not really practical, and an evening before-bed routine will allow adequate time and attention for successful management. Harsh, irritant laxatives are not advisable since they tend to make the bowel more spastic and add to the problem by causing dehydration. Further, they ultimately diminish the sensitivity of the bowel to stimulation.

Dental problems. Careful training in oral hygiene measures is required. If the patient is unable to assume full responsibility for oral care, assistance must be provided. Inaccessibility of dental care is often a serious problem. This may be the result of the patient's inability to cooperate, his inability to get to an upstairs dentist's office, or the inability of the dental office to master specific techniques of managing the hyperresponsiveness of patients with cerebral palsy. For some situations, it may be necessary to admit the patient to the hospital and do the dental work under anesthesia in order to have time and ideal conditions to perform needed work.

Osteoporosis. Osteoporosis may be minimized by maintaining weight bearing and encouraging muscle activity, and maintaining a normal dietary intake of calcium, vitamin D, and protein. Complications of osteoporosis, such as fractures, may be avoided by awareness of its presence, care in handling, and careful graduated restoration of muscular activity to the osteoporotic bone.

Degenerative joint disease. Cervical degenerative joint disease can be minimized by posture control lessening the amount of neck movement and tension. This can sometimes be accomplished by head support and training, assisted by a physical therapist. Otherwise, traction or sometimes a supportive or restrictive neck collar is used. Aspirin and other pain relievers may be indicated, but should be used with care so they do not lead to more stress on the joints as pain is relieved. Obesity may contribute to degenerative joint disease, and a reducing diet successfully lessens pain and improves function.

Scoliosis. Bracing and splinting are used to prevent persistent abnormal postures tending to deformities. Spine deformities can be delayed by appropriate bracing, use of a body jacket, or wheelchair modifications. Corrective orthopedic surgery may be necessary to stabilize the posture of these patients to improve both their function and appearance.

Respiratory infections. Respiratory infections may be prevented to some degree by having the patient sleep on his face so that saliva drains outward at night rather than pooling in his throat. Careful feeding technique will avoid choking or leakage of food into the lungs (aspiration). This may require the combined skills of the rehabilitation nurse, speech pathologist, and occupational therapist, working with the help of the physiatrist. In extreme cases, the use of a feeding tube directly inserted into the stomach (gastrostomy) to bypass swallowing may dramatically lessen repeated respiratory infections. Occasionally, tonsils become inflamed and chronically infected and need to be removed, even in the adult, to reduce a source of continuing infection and a hindrance to swallowing. A speech pathologist or a physical or respiratory therapist can assist in the development of improved breathing patterns, coughing, and lung expansion. Where a poor cough is a problem, respiratory assistance and suction may be needed to avoid the pneumonia resulting from otherwise simple upper respiratory infections.

Seizures. Where seizures have been identified, a neurologist will prescribe seizure-control medications appropriate to their type. Chapter 12 reviews the medication approaches used for the different seizure types.

Fatigue. Management of fatigue will include adequate nutrition, minimized emotional components on the job, and assessment of the total demands on the client in order to set priorities with the client for the use of the total available energy. The client's physician can assist in setting up a disciplined program of activity which includes a period of rest during the day. Avocational as well as vocational activities should be monitored so that the client gets enough rest on the weekends and in the evenings. Part-time rather than full-time work may be necessary to achieve a balanced total life.

Where attentiveness is a problem in controlling fatigue, additional medication, such as dextro-amphetamine, Methylphenidate, or the tricyclic antidepressants, may improve the client's total energy level and make it possible for him to attend more readily to his work. Factors in fatigue, such as the need to concentrate, the need to pay attention, the need to do things the hard way (i.e., unassisted) where an easy way might be possible, must all be considered when managing the client's total energy output in a training or work situation.

Rehabilitation Treatment

Rehabilitation in cerebral palsy covers a wide range of activities. Treatment and training are required to improve motor control and physical function, language, communication, learning abilities, and social skills. This total rehabilitation program requires interaction among many rehabilitation specialists and is best performed in a comprehensive rehabilitation setting. Depending on the breadth or complexity of disabilities, an initial inpatient treatment phase may be required.

Physical function. Close collaboration is required among the physiatrist, physical therapist, and occupational therapist in establishing and executing a motor training program. In addition to their analysis of the patient's motor repertoire, information gathered from other disciplines is incorporated into planning the program. Information from the psychologist regarding the patient's sensory, perceptual, and cognitive processing abilities is required to plan the most appropriate and useful feedback modalities by which the patient can be made aware of the consequences of his performance efforts. Behavioral information from the psychologist, school teacher, rehabilitation nurse, and others on the patient's attention span, distractibility, memory characteristics, and communication abilities is also required to plan the

details of the management and training techniques. On the basis of this information, decisions can be made regarding the extent to which situational structure can be used to enhance attentiveness and learning, and to what extent medication is required to improve attentiveness, diminish stimulus-bound behavior and perseveration, and increase the patient's ability to respond to stimuli from within.

In practice, training of motor skills is carried out by breaking up a desired voluntary motion into small component kinesiological segments, according to the individual's ability to attend, observe, and control the activity. At the same time, undesirable involuntary or reflex activities are brought to the attention of the patient, and he is trained to inhibit these motions. Criteria are set to determine success within the observed ability of the patient. Verbal, visual, tactile, and proprioceptive feedback, as appropriate, is given to identify clearly to the patient the character or quality of his performance.

Improvement of ambulation may have several components. Prescription of diazepam or dantrolene sodium may help relieve dystonia. The surgeon may help in improving mechanics, the physiatrist may help in performing intramuscular neurolysis, and adequate training by the physical therapist in walking techniques may make walking practical.

Where walking is not feasible and wheelchair ambulation must be considered, a joint decision to obtain a wheelchair must be made by the physiatrist, physical therapist, occupational therapist, and rehabilitation counselor working together. Each may have recommendations for special adaptations or equipment for optimum usefulness. Often the social case worker and the rehabilitation nurse who observes the patient's daily self-care functions may have important contributions to the decision. Once the chair is obtained, it must fit, provide the patient with adequate lateral support, have a seat belt for safety, and be suited to the patient's abilities to propel the chair and transfer himself into and out of it (see fig. 11-5). A period of training by the physical therapist, occupational therapist, and nurse in use of the wheelchair is indicated to be certain of optimum utilization and to verify its appropriateness in practice.

Improvement of the ability to accomplish transfers may begin with the surgeon correcting contractures or the physiatrist prescribing braces to allow accurate foot placement and ankle stability. The physical therapist and nurse then cooperate in working out the most useful method for the patient's special needs and assisting the patient in learning the method. They may also recommend adapted equipment, such as a steady seat in the bathtub and handrail or a commode in the shower. Nonslip surfaces are extremely important in reducing danger and anxiety. If the abilities of the patient necessitate a goal that is less than independent, this goal needs to be defined and clearly established and stated, with all disciplines working along parallel lines.

For improving function in eating, a whole-team approach is required. The speech pathologist can provide oral training, the occupational therapist can provide adaptive motor-skill training and adaptive devices (such as a special spoon with a built-up handle or holding strap, or a splint to stabilize the wrist to facilitate scooping of food and bringing it to the mouth), the physical therapist can provide training in balance and coordination, and the nurse can assist with practice in practical application of techniques.

For independence in dressing, team cooperation may again be required. Assistance from the orthopedic surgeon may be necessary to achieve optimum motor function by eliminating contractures. The occupational therapist can provide adaptive devices to assist where hand function is deficient and can recommend clothing modifications to facilitate independence. A physical therapist may be required to assist with the development of sitting balance and moving ability. The nurse may be involved in the teaching and practice of dressing techniques.

Training in personal hygiene is usually carried out by the nurse, although it may be necessary to enlist the aid of the occupational therapist for assistance with manual skills, adaptive techniques, and assistive devices, and the physical therapist for such needed skills as balance, transfers, hand and arm control, and standing. Further, it may be necessary to treat hip adduction contractures to allow adequate perineal hygiene.

It should be emphasized that the patient with cerebral palsy may need to adapt a personal hygiene system to his own particular needs. For those who perspire heavily during the night, it may be advisable to schedule the bath time in the morning so that offensive body odors are not a problem in a work situation; for others, a morning schedule may be too brief to enable them to arrive at work on time. In general, the more time-consuming elements of personal care are best scheduled in the evenings.

Language, communication, and learning. Again, a combined approach is needed to help the person with communication disabilities to function optimally. Where language concepts are inadequate, remedial work with a teacher and language therapist is necessary. The basic concepts may need to be taught and later elaborated with emphasis on grammar, syntax, and accurate expression. It may be necessary, for purposes of communication with fellow workers, to teach the cerebral palsied individual some "street language" and the meaning of certain colloquial expressions, since these have often not been part of his past experiences.

Nonvocal patients may have difficulty utilizing adaptive equipment in order to communicate. The assistance of an engineer familiar with communications technology is often invaluable to adapt available equipment for special needs, to suggest new techniques in a rapidly changing field, or to help in maintenance of the specialized equipment. A teacher, speech therapist, and occupational therapist working together may be needed to determine the best means of communication, to train the person in its use, and to help him practice it until, with improved communication, his language skills also improve up to a practical level. Because these are such skilled activities, daily practice is necessary if they are to be maintained. All members of the team, both professional and nonprofessional, including the family, need to be fully informed of the current level of language being employed, so that daily application of communication skills in a meaningful context is assured.

Some individuals have a severe verbal language problem rather than, or in addition to, a physical inability to vocalize or speak. These persons will not be able to use either manual or electronic spelling boards, word boards, or devices that utilize the written or printed word. Some can develop a visually mediated language, and a pictorial system like the Rebus or a symbolic ideographic system like Bliss symbolics may be most useful and rewarding.

Medication may help alleviate difficulties in attentiveness which contribute to learning disabilities, at least on a temporary basis until skills in attending are learned or the necessary structured environment is established.

The teacher, occupational therapist, psychologist, and behavior analyst will cooperate in working on a patient's perception of spatial orientation. Ways of compensating for visual-perceptual problems may be worked out, or auditory methods of learning may be substituted. If the patient's auditory memory is short, instructions and information must be given in small units, thus allowing digestion and filing before proceeding further to the next unit.

Most of these problems should have been dealt with fairly adequately by the school system prior to the person's entering vocational training. If they have not, it is still not too late to give them some attention and at least try to improve function in these areas, since they are necessary skills if the person is to be successful vocationally. In any case, an accurate knowledge of the specific cognitive abilities and weaknesses is important for appropriate vocational training and placement.

Social function. The management of problems in social functioning involves assessment of what the patient is doing that is unacceptable; determination, if possible, of the reason for the behavior; making the patient aware of what he is doing and perhaps why he does it; removing rewards for unacceptable behavior; and finally, training in ways of interacting that are acceptable and desirable. For a time, this process may involve the whole environment in the treatment process. There is need for a social therapist, who may be a recreational therapist, a social worker, a psychologist, or simply a lay person who is able to accept the handicapped person's disabilities, to be honest with him in informing him when he is being unacceptable, and to be willing to help him learn appropriate social skills. Teaching the person to take responsibility for his own actions and for his own social and emotional life within his capability level is an essential part of developing social adaptability.

When social problems result from the patient's short attention span and/or problems of perseveration and rigidity in approach to problem solving, it is necessary to recognize the organic component of the problem. Medications may be necessary for management in many instances. In all cases, strong, consistent social structuring is required to maintain circumstances within the capability of the individual to respond, to provide the requirement to respond appropriately, and to guarantee appropriate reinforcement to modify the behavior. Simple verbal counseling or instruction is not adequate to cope with these strong behavioral characteristics.

It is necessary for the patient to learn social skills before sexual information can be effectively utilized. Simple training in conventional manners often may be needed. The patient may lack rapid, easy communication and he may not use the conventions like "please" and "thank you" which make the world a little easier for people to live in. Certain individuals may need adapted concrete formulas for such social routines in order to function satisfactorily in the community. These attitudes and skills are learned through experience and effort. The experience necessary to acquire appropriate social skills must be introduced by careful structuring into the daily life of the individual, with adequate, appropriate, and timely reinforcement. Supportive counseling for the individual can then be useful. The significant other individuals in his life must be included as well.

Careful structured experience and counseling are required to alter the egocentric outlook common to cerebral palsy patients. This outlook may not be amenable to treatment if approached too late in life, or if family and peer relations cannot be modified. With careful situational management and teaching, even the mature patient may still be able to acquire a veneer of sociability that allows him to function satisfactorily, in spite of still considering himself the center of the universe.

VOCATIONAL IMPLICATIONS

Some clients with cerebral palsy will be able to enter competitive employment with very little special help. Others, in spite of maximum help, will not really be vocational candidates, but will need assistance to achieve avocational interests and adequate living arrangements. Where seizures are present, the vocational factors discussed in chapter 12 apply. Attention to the detailed requirements for optimum vocational function can suggest those physical adaptations, equipment modifications, and assistance required for a balance between client abilities and performance requirements.

Vocational considerations should begin with a realistic appraisal by the client and the vocational counselor of the client's actual physical, mental, social, and psychological abilities, as developed by appropriate evaluation and total treatment. It is, of course, axiomatic that each individual's personal interests and aspirations need to be taken into account. It is the task of the counseling psychologist to match the client's interests and abilities. Because of the limitations and distortions in life experiences of cerebral palsy clients, their interests may not be mature and are likely to be inappropriate. An organized experiential plan may be required for certain individuals to arrive at an appropriate articulation of their abilities and interests. To accomplish this goal, the fullest resources of the entire rehabilitation team, including the educational system, vocational training centers, or other available community resources, may be required.

Where lack of motivation makes constant supervision necessary, occupations where the client must provide most of his own discipline or initiative will not be appropriate, regardless of physical ability. A person with a hearing disability, receptive language deficit, or short auditory memory will not succeed in an occupation where he must take messages from other people or where long, complicated instructions must be absorbed quickly. On the other hand, if visual-perceptual and visual-motor skills are intact, the client may be successful in work utilizing graphic representational skills, such as preparing and maintaining blueprints. The client with a good deal of spasticity or who requires intense concentration to perform a carefully trained activity may not be able to work full time, may need to take a rest in the middle of the day, or may not be able to continue with a very demanding full-time occupation as long as a normal person and may have to consider a midlife career change.

Work environment may be very important. For example, a distractible person may be able to perform a task quite well if provided with equipment set in a corner rather than out in the middle of a busy office. In general, the cerebral palsy client is most likely to be successful in indoor settings with a minimum of architectural barriers. Temperature extremes may aggravate spasticity. Jobs involving interactions primarily with regular employees, rather than always with new people, will be less stressful.

A period of extended work evaluation may be the

best initial "job placement" after a study of the client's abilities has been achieved in treatment and initial counseling. Extended work evaluation can assist the client in developing work habits and a realistic appreciation of skills prior to actual job placement. Following the initial placement, care must be taken to ensure that the client has the opportunity to progress up the employment ladder as job experiences may allow. Employment below developing abilities should not be allowed to continue indefinitely. Even though the brain damage is present, growth in vocational potential with increasing success should be expected.

Clients with cerebral palsy present the rehabilitation counselor with some of his most difficult challenges. However, once the myriad of problems have been dealt with and adequate support given during the first months or even years of vocational experience, the effort will usually have been very worthwhile.

BIBLIOGRAPHY

Allen RM, Jefferson TW: *Psychological Evaluation of the Cerebral Palsied Person: Intellectual, Personality, and Vocational Applications*. Springfield, IL, Thomas, 1962.
This is a list of tests suited to the assessment of intellectual and perceptual function of individuals with cerebral palsy. Includes some suggestions for adaptation of the tests for individual handicaps and modifications of interpretations.

Denhoff E, Robinault IP: *Cerebral Palsy and Related Disorders: A Developmental Approach to Dysfunction*. New York, McGraw-Hill, 1960.
A survey of cerebral palsy, with emphasis on the intellectual and perceptual handicaps. Also includes evaluations of physical functioning and a review of the basic literature relating to cerebral palsy.

Floor L, Rosen M: New criteria of adjustment for the cerebral palsied. Rehab Lit 37:268-274, 1976.
Report of a study conducted to determine the effectiveness of traditional rehabilitation services for cerebral palsied persons. The results suggest that the traditional vocational criteria of successful rehabilitation should be revised to include improvements in "quality of life."

Guthrie JT: Educational assessment of the handicapped child. Pediatr Clin North Am 20:89-103, 1973.
A discussion of adult expectations for trainable and educable mentally retarded children, cerebral palsied children, and children with learning disabilities; general learning characteristics of each group; a review of available educational tests; and a short review of findings on placement in regular vs. special classrooms, and home vs. institution.

Heisler V: Dynamic group psychotherapy with parents of cerebral palsied children. Rehab Lit 35:329-330, 1974.
The author advocates group therapy for parents of cerebral palsied children on the grounds that parents involved in a process of inner growth themselves will be better able to respond to the inner life of their child. Because handicapped children's greatest resources are in their inner worlds, they need parental support and understanding to develop these resources.

Lekemo U: Technical educational aids for motor handicapped schoolchildren with severe speech disorders. Scan J Rehabil Med 8:67-81, 1976.
A short report on various technical aids to permit schoolchildren with cerebral palsy and allied disorders, combined with lack of speech or severe speech disorders, to communicate with individuals and groups.

Richardson SA: People with cerebral palsy talk for themselves. Dev med Child Neurol 14:524-535, 1972.
This is a transcript of statements by individuals with cerebral palsy. Their personal needs, desires, and perspectives are verbalized. In particular, social and sexual problems faced by individuals with cerebral palsy are highlighted in a frank and open personal discussion.

Samilson RL (ed): Orthopedic aspects of cerebral palsy. *In* Clinics in Dev Med 52/53, Spastics International Medical Publications. Philadelphia, Lippincott, 1975.
A review of the orthopedic procedures and their indications and contraindications, advantages and disadvantages, is presented concisely from the vantage point of expertise and experience in cerebral palsy management. The discussion is largely confined to the operative and postoperative management of the surgical procedure, with little emphasis on any necessary training for improvement of function after the surgery has been accomplished.

Wooldridge CP, Russell G: Head position training with the cerebral palsied child: An application of biofeedback techniques. Arch Phys Med Rehabil 57:407-414, 1976.
Discussion of an effective biofeedback training program which employs a mercury switch device called a head position trainer to provide cerebral palsied children with visual and auditory information regarding their head positions. Equipment, training methods, and data collection and analysis are described.

12 EPILEPSY

Arthur A. Ward, Jr., M.D.
Robert T. Fraser, Ph.D.
Allan S. Troupin, M.D.

DISEASE DESCRIPTION

Epilepsy is the most common of the chronic neurological disorders. A meaningful simple definition of epilepsy is difficult because of its wide variability. A simple epileptic attack may consist of only a brief suspension of activity, as in a brief petit mal absence seizure. In other persons, the attack may consist of automatic motor activity or complex alterations of behavior, as in temporal lobe or psychomotor epilepsy. In still other cases, a full-blown generalized tonic-clonic (grand mal) motor seizure may occur.

The incidence of epilepsy is difficult to determine with accuracy. In practical terms, probably 1 person in 15 has a seizure of some sort during his life, and between 0.5 and 1.5 percent of the general population have chronic, recurring seizures.

As Hughlings Jackson described it some 100 years ago, the seizure consists of "an occasional, an excessive and a disorderly discharge of nervous tissue." This explosive discharge often starts in one area of the brain, the *focus*. It then spreads through the circuits of the brain "like an electrical storm." The pattern of the seizure will be determined by the location of the focus and the pathways of spread. If the focus is located in the motor cortex on the surface of the brain, the first evidence of the seizure would be twitching of the appropriate muscles on the opposite side of the body. If it starts in the visual cortex of the occipital lobe, the first event would be flashing lights, which appear to the patient to come from his opposite visual field. (See chap. 3 for a review of the nervous system.)

Thus, the seizure discharge activates the circuits in which it is involved and the function of these circuits will determine the clinical pattern of the seizure. Since the brain is a very complex communication network, in which many functions are localized in different circuits, it should come as no surprise that the clinical patterns of epilepsy can vary widely from person to person.

Except at those times when this electrical storm is sweeping through it, the brain is working perfectly well in the person with epilepsy. Thus, there is no alteration of brain function except for those few seconds which may come only once a day, once a month, or once a year. At other times, there is no physical disability due directly to the epilepsy itself.

Some persons with epilepsy have a headache, feel nauseous, or experience some other predictable symptom on the day a seizure will occur. About half experience premonitory symptoms just before a seizure occurs. These symptoms are various, consisting perhaps of a sensation of dizziness, discomfort in the abdomen, numbness, or spasm. These *auras* correspond to the first gust before the storm. The time interval between aura and seizure onset may or may not be too brief to allow the patient to sit or lie down. Each person's aura, if he has one, is different.

The International League Against Epilepsy has published a detailed classification of the many types of seizures. Discussion of all seizure types is beyond the scope of this chapter, but five representative seizure types will be briefly described here.

Focal Seizures

The nature of a focal seizure depends on the area of the cortex in which it begins. For example, a seizure beginning in the parietal lobe cortex will cause sensory symptoms, such as numbness or tingling, in the affected extremity. Difficulty in speaking (dysphasia) results from a seizure originating in the speech area of the left cerebral hemisphere.

In focal seizures, the electrical discharge may remain localized and its effects will thus be limited to the areas of the body controlled by the focus. The discharge may, however, spread to other areas of the brain and cause a generalized (grand mal) seizure secondary to the focal seizure.

Jacksonian Seizures

A Jacksonian seizure is a focal seizure originating in the motor cortex. One part of the face, arm, or leg on the opposite side of the body begins to jerk. These convulsive movements then spread in an orderly fashion (Jacksonian march) and may involve the entire side of the body. The person usually remains conscious during the seizure.

Grand Mal Seizures

If the discharge spreads widely through the brain circuits, a seizure will result which has few localizing features and is usually characterized as a generalized tonic-clonic grand mal seizure. An individual first endures a *tonic* state, characterized by body rigidity, and then undergoes a *clonic* state, characterized by convulsive, jerking movements. The person may also salivate excessively, vomit, or lose control of bladder and bowel function. Even when the spread of the seizure discharge is more restricted, the patient is usually amnesic for the seizure because the discharge commonly will spread to at least some deeper relay circuits. Since these deeper circuits are concerned with consciousness, the person loses consciousness during the seizure. Thus, the seizure discharge evokes a crude parody of the function of the circuits involved. For this reason, a careful description of the initial events in a seizure can often serve to localize the part of the brain in which the seizure originates with great accuracy.

After the seizure is over, the nerve cells involved in the "excessive discharge" are metabolically fatigued. It is therefore common, particularly after major seizures, for the person to feel tired and want to sleep for some minutes or even several hours. This fatigue is obviously most marked at the very end of the seizure, and at this time not all the circuits are going to recover equally fast. Thus, for a few minutes, the person may be confused, may have difficulty speaking clearly, or may have some weakness of one arm or leg. These symptoms almost always clear in a matter of minutes, although the person may continue to feel tired.

Individuals may fear a grand mal seizure because of the practical risk of falling or incurring bodily injury, such as burns, chipped teeth, or broken bones. However, it should be recognized that the actual seizure does not cause the person any direct discomfort, regardless of the pattern of the seizure. Nevertheless, the seizure does interfere with performance to varying degrees.

Psychomotor Seizures

If the electrical discharge starts in one temporal lobe, the clinical manifestation would be automatic motor activity and alterations of behavior which may occasionally be rather bizarre. This type of seizure has been called psychomotor epilepsy and represents approximately one-half of all adult epilepsy. The pattern of the seizure varies rather widely from patient to patient. In some, it consists only of a blank stare,

rhythmic picking at the clothes, and often smacking of the lips. In other instances, the psychomotor seizure may be more complex and the person may wander aimlessly, continue to wash the same dish over and over, or perform other semipurposeful but irrelevant behavior. These episodes may last from a short period of time to many minutes. There is always complete loss of memory for the events during the seizure. Attempts to restrain or interfere with the automatic behavior of a patient during a seizure may evoke resentment and strong reaction, but the violence or aggression is poorly directed toward a goal and is usually carried out in a purposeless fashion. A structured violent attack is almost unknown in epilepsy.

Psychomotor epilepsy is sometimes confused with psychiatric illness. This is not surprising, for many of the symptoms of a temporal lobe seizure are those of panic or emotional behavior, both of which occur as primary events in psychiatrically disturbed patients.

Petit Mal Seizures

Petit mal epilepsy occurs almost exclusively in children and they often "outgrow" it as they go through puberty. It is the most common type of epilepsy in children and appears to be set apart from the rest of the epilepsies. It occurs in the young, maturing brain. Petit mal or absence seizures do not arise from a focus on the surface of the brain, but rather arise deep within the core of the brain. They are characterized by a rather typical EEG, and respond to a special category of anticonvulsant drugs.

The seizures themselves consist of very brief lapses of consciousness or "staring spells." There may be a slow rhythmic blinking of the eyes or occasionally other very subtle motor manifestations, but no significant motor component. There may be no loss of motor tone, although in "drop attacks" there may be a sudden slump to the floor with prompt return of consciousness within a very few seconds.

If the petit mal seizures occur *very frequently*, the disruptions of the stream of consciousness may be sufficient to significantly affect performance. Very often it is in the school classroom where frequent absence seizures are first noticed.

In approximately 40 percent of patients with petit mal, major motor seizures (grand mal) develop. It is important to realize that anticonvulsant medication that may benefit petit mal seizures usually has no effect on the grand mal seizures and vice versa.

The most glaring diagnostic errors result from confusing petit mal epilepsy with other types of epilepsy. It must be emphasized that *true* petit mal seizures occur in children and that not all relatively short seizures characterized by a loss of contact are petit mal seizures. When short absence seizures occur in adults, they almost invariably are of focal origin and respond to a different group of drugs than the petit mal seizures. Furthermore, many other types of relatively short seizures are erroneously called petit mal in order to distinguish them from grand mal seizures, which are more dramatic displays of the phenomena of epilepsy. For example, since there are often no twitching movements in psychomotor epilepsy, small psychomotor seizures are often confused with petit mal epilepsy. However, these are very different kinds of seizures and should not be confused because the treatment and prognosis are very different.

Complications

The only cause for major concern is when another seizure follows the first within the next half hour or so, or when a seizure state persists for a prolonged period of time (½ hour for grand mal seizures, ¾ hour for other types). This condition is called *status epilepticus* and requires prompt and aggressive medical treatment. Status epilepticus can occur in petit mal seizures but is relatively uncommon. The major problem occurs in adults with grand mal seizures or, less commonly, with psychomotor epilepsy. When status epilepticus occurs, the patient should be promptly transported (preferably by ambulance) to the emergency room of the nearest hospital. However, a single seizure, lasting a few minutes, is no reason to seek immediate medical care.

Etiology

The causes of some types of epilepsy are well known, but in other instances the causes are poorly understood. One of the least understood and most controversial areas of epilepsy is the question of whether genetic predisposition plays a part. In general, those who study epilepsy in children find a high genetic causality, and those who study epilepsy in adults find the opposite. This is related to the fact that the most common type of epilepsy in children is petit mal and it has been proposed that this type of epilepsy is an expression of an autosomal dominant gene with unusual characteristics. Expression of this gene is very low at birth but it is nearly completely expressed between ages 4½ and 16½ years. Expressivity gradually declines to almost zero after the age of 40.

The practical problem lies with genetic counseling. On the basis of present knowledge, if one parent has epilepsy, the overall risk to a child of developing epilepsy is between 2 and 3 percent. This is comparable to the random risk of having a mentally handicapped child or one with a congenital abnormality. This risk is certainly not great enough to advise limitation of family. However, if both parents have epilepsy, the risk may rise to as high as 25 percent, and in such instances medical advice might be helpful.

For types of epilepsy other than petit mal, the causes are better understood. In the majority of temporal lobe epilepsy cases, the cause of the seizures is scarring of the medial side of the temporal lobe of the brain. In most instances, such scarring appears to be the result of the birth process, a normal part of which is a molding of the skull so it can fit through the birth canal. This molding of the skull compresses the brain and is thought to result in the observed scarring of portions of the brain in a small number of normal births. It appears that, in some instances, this scarring irritates the nerve cells around the scar, resulting in the abnormal electrical discharges.

Scar-induced epilepsy can be the result of trauma, stroke (see chaps. 9 and 10), or even the presence of a tumor. Penetrating wounds of the central regions of the cortex (such as some depressed fractures or gunshot wounds) will result in the development of seizures in about 50 percent of patients, while penetrating wounds of the occipital region are followed by seizures in less than 20 percent of cases. The most common trauma is, of course, closed head injury, and this results in epilepsy in about 5 percent of cases.

Precipitation of Seizures

One of the mysteries of epilepsy is why the brain may function perfectly normally for several months and then produce a seizure, which is again followed by weeks or months of normal brain function before the next seizure. Although the occurrence of a seizure can rarely be predicted, certain factors have been identified which increase the probability of seizure occurrence in a person with epilepsy.

Seizures can be precipitated by excessive alcohol intake and tend to occur during the withdrawal phase. Emotional stress makes it easier for a seizure to occur. Some women tend to have seizures that cluster around the time of menstrual periods. In some patients, seizures may be rare during waking periods, particularly when they are busy, but occur when the brain is "idling." It has been repeatedly demonstrated that patients with frequent seizures who are leading protected, nonproductive lives (such as in an institution) will undergo a dramatic reduction in seizure frequency when they are put into a sheltered workshop where they are kept busy, active, and productive. Thus, many of the factors which are known to influence seizure frequency are amenable to modification, and the therapeutic results may be as useful as with medical treatment.

Prognosis

The outcome of epilepsy depends on many factors: type of seizures, age, underlying cause, and finally, quality of treatment. An overall picture which emerges from the literature is that complete seizure control is achieved for 2 years in 30 to 37 percent of patients, but this statistic reduces to approximately 20 percent at 5 years and 10 percent at 10 years. It is clear that the outlook for complete seizure control on a long-term basis is significantly improved if the seizures can be completely suppressed with anticonvulsant medication. The following factors are relevant to the probability of achieving complete seizure control.

1. The longer the illness lasts, the less likely control is to be complete.
2. The more seizures the patient experiences before initial treatment, the less likely control is to be complete.
3. The more different types of seizures a patient has, the less likely he is to be free of them.
4. The more abnormal the neurological and mental status examinations and the lower the IQ, the more difficult it is to control the seizures.
5. The younger the patient is at the time of onset of major seizures, the less likely control is to be complete.

Approximately 50 percent of those patients with major motor seizures *without* associated minor attacks will be free of seizures for at least 2 years. However, this figure drops to 20 to 30 percent if one deals with patients who have temporal lobe epilepsy.

The situation is appreciably different for children with petit mal absence or minor seizures. In children with absence seizures but no other type of seizures, 80 percent will be seizure free by adulthood. However, for those children with petit mal seizures who also develop grand mal seizures, only one-third will be seizure free. There is some evidence to indicate that, in the petit mal group, appropriate therapy will decrease the risk of developing grand mal.

FUNCTIONAL DISABILITIES

Physical Disabilities

Except for those persons whose epilepsy is secondary to stroke or cerebral trauma (see chaps. 9 and 10), no physical disabilities are present. Thus, persons with epilepsy are fully independent in all eating, dressing, transfer, ambulation, personal hygiene, and communication skills. While mechanical driving skills are also unimpaired, local laws dictate the seizure-free status required for issuance of driving licenses. Even immediately after a seizure, independence of action is preserved, although level of consciousness may be impaired.

Anticonvulsant medication may, however, influence physical function. Low-grade toxicity may produce some clumsiness of gait, hand coordination problems, and eye-focusing difficulty without loss of independence. Higher levels of toxicity (table 12-2, p. 163) can create dependency in physical functions. This dependency, however, is reversible with medical attention and alteration of drug regimens.

Psychosocial Disabilities

For many years, a number of psychologists discussed what they termed the "epileptoid personality," characterized by a flatness of affect, various distinctive physical characteristics, and other traits which they believed to be associated with a personality typology. Much of this thinking seems to have evolved in institutional settings where the psychologists were working with seizure patients who were often heavily medicated, had associated mental retardation, and were otherwise nonrepresentative. Today, this personality concept is refuted in psychological circles. It is generally agreed, however, that individuals with psychomotor, temporal lobe seizures can be prone to a number of characteristics which differentiate them from the normal population. These characteristics can include dependency, lack of humor, obsessionality, overconcern with religious and philosophic issues, and an emotional lability which often includes anger. Although the relationships are not clearly definable, the temporal lobe is involved with behavior and emotion. It is also agreed that there is a higher incidence of psychosocial problem areas among those with epilepsy when contrasted with a normal population. The relationships between neurological deficits and personality aberrations are difficult to establish.

The etiology of much psychosocial symptomatology seems to be related to the nature of an individual's seizures (type, severity, and age of onset) and the reaction of the person's environment (parents, siblings, teachers, employers, and peers) to the specific type of seizure disorder.

The major psychosocial disability of the grand mal seizure stems from the reaction of others in the vicinity at the time of occurrence. The observer is usually frightened, tends to overreact, and thereafter tends to treat the patient as someone very "different" from other human beings. In many cases, neither the individual nor society have adequate time to adapt, for unlike a paralysis problem, seizures are not present all the time. Other than the occasional seizure, many persons with epilepsy look and function like everyone else in society. The seizure problem, because of its occasional, unpredictable nature, creates a state of expectation and uncertainty. With most other disabilities, stability allows for the possibility of a fuller understanding of the nature of the disability. It is this lack of experience-based understanding and a tendency to categorize epilepsy as a psychiatric disturbance which has impaired rehabilitation efforts in this field.

The manner in which the family reacts to the child with epilepsy is a major determinant of later adjustment. Problems can arise from feelings of guilt and parental conflict regarding approach to childrearing (e.g., involvement in competitive sports, amount of independence to be fostered, whether or not to disclose the child's epilepsy, or the manner of discussing the disability with other siblings). Fear and concern based on ignorance may cause relatives, in a misplaced effort to be helpful and protective, to place restrictions on the activities of patients with seizures. The restrictions foster dependency and further isolate and alienate these individuals from the rest of society. The person with epilepsy who has been overly sheltered by the family is usually very naive regarding the world of work.

It is these social consequences of the seizures which form the significant disabling component of epilepsy. Adjusting to the change from the dependency status which was "licensed" by the seizures is often a problem for those who have become completely seizure free following surgery.

In the area of intellectual functioning, the randomly selected client with epilepsy will tend to function within the normal range, barring organic brain damage. Data suggests, however, that there tends to be a skew in functioning toward the lower end of the normal range. This tendency toward the lower end in both intellectual functioning and neuropsychological adaptive skills (e.g., problem solving) is due to the negative effect of a number of factors: the severity, duration, and type of seizures; early age of onset; and frequency of major seizures.

In addition to seizure activity, high (toxic) levels of anticonvulsants in the blood will impair motor functioning, attention, and memory, with subsequent decrements in intellectual and neuropsychological performance. Other factors, such as excessive fatigue or abnormal electrical brain discharging on the day of testing can also detract from performance on these measures.

Rehabilitation Potential

The rehabilitation potential for persons with epilepsy and no other chronic neurological impairment is governed by psychosocial factors. For those persons who do have chronic neurological impairment in addition to epilepsy, rehabilitation potential is governed by the nature of the neurological impairment.

Without question, most individuals with epilepsy are employable. Rehabilitation potential must be considered very good and not diminished from the perspective of the epilepsy itself, particularly if seizures are under good control. Hence, long-term planning and goals are appropriate.

STANDARDS OF EVALUATION

In considering the diagnosis and etiology of seizures in new patients, the age-related patterns of occurrence of different types of epilepsy are taken into account. The appearance during adolescence of seizures of focal origin, whether or not associated with major generalized seizures, generally implies a minor injury to the cerebral cortex at birth, without additional associated neurologic disease.

Seizures following major head trauma can occur at any age, but major head trauma is more common during adolescence and early adulthood. Again, there are no implications for major neurologic disease other than the obvious results of the trauma.

In middle to late adulthood, the possibility of a brain tumor assumes more importance when the history does not reveal obvious trauma. In the older age group, the possibility of tumor persists, but cerebral vascular disease assumes a progressively greater importance.

While all of the above statements are generally true for the population at large, any individual must receive a specific evaluation aimed at defining the background of his own seizure problem. Certain clinical manifestations of some kinds of seizures may be most difficult to distinguish from some ordinary nonepileptic behavior. Simple fainting episodes (syncope), for example, usually are due to vascular changes with a transient drop in blood pressure and are not epilepsy. Careful history-taking will usually indicate that such episodes are provoked by syncope and that the patient is not suffering from epilepsy. Certain cardiac problems or small strokes may also mimic epileptic phenomena.

Temporal lobe seizures may mimic psychiatric symptoms, such as anxiety attacks. However, unlike temporal lobe seizures, anxiety attacks are prolonged, are not associated with disturbances of consciousness, and are usually precipitated by environmental events. Similarly, outbursts of rage and violence associated with a seizure may be construed as a psychiatric disturbance. Such misinterpretations and inadequate diagnoses have repeatedly resulted in involuntary commitment of seizure patients to psychiatric hospitals. When episodic unusual behavior caused by temporal lobe epilepsy is thought to be due to mental illness, patients and their families may be subjected to untold anguish. The combination of a skilled history, neurological examination, and electroencephalogram (EEG) are essential and should differentiate between epilepsy and psychiatric conditions with similar manifestations.

Medical Evaluation

The clinical evaluation of seizure patients is appropriately carried out by a neurologist, although in some communities a neurosurgeon may also have an interest in epilepsy. In view of the potentially progressive nature of epilepsy, the new seizure patient should be seen promptly for an evaluation, appropriately scheduled as an outpatient visit rather than as an emergency.

There are two principal aims in the initial evaluation of the patient with epilepsy. The first aim is to define the etiology of the seizure disorder to separate those patients who are in need of therapy directed at an underlying disease (e.g., brain tumor) from those who have stable epilepsy amenable to drug suppression of seizure activity. The second aim is to classify the seizure type so that appropriate medical therapy can be chosen. Both etiology and classification are most readily determined by the neurologic examination, which consists of the neurologic history, the physical examination, and the EEG. The history and physical are generally carried out by the neurologist in his office and require approximately 1 hour. The EEG must be performed in a laboratory with the necessary equipment and also requires about an hour.

The major aim of the neurologic history is an accurate description of the seizure itself, since it is generally possible to determine the site of origin of the seizure discharge from the initial display of abnormal behavior. A description of the events following the active element of the seizure (the postictal phenomena) also has bearing on the location of the seizure focus. Another major objective of the neurologic history is a description of events which tend to precipitate seizures, either acutely or after a period of time.

The history also provides significant clues to the etiology of the seizure disorder. Seizures could represent a symptom of some other disease or a mechanical process within the brain requiring a surgical solution. The recent onset and progressive worsening of a focal neurologic deficit, such as a hemiparesis, tends to point to a localized intracranial mass, such as a tumor or subdural hematoma. The presence of additional symptoms related to other body systems might suggest a general medical disease requiring specific attention. In many patients, the history reveals an episode of brain injury which may be an adequate explanation for the subsequent appearance of seizures. Sometimes the history is obvious, such as the previous presence of encephalitis, meningitis, or a major head injury. Sometimes the history is inferential only, such as a story of a difficult labor at birth, coupled with slow development of motor skills and subsequent normal performance, all of which point to birth injuries as the cause of seizures.

The second element in the neurologic evaluation is a specialized physical examination directed at the nervous system. The activities of the motor system, the cranial nerves, the sensory system, the coordination system, the intactness of reflex arcs, and an overall estimate of mental status are reviewed in a physical examination requiring 20 to 30 minutes. The information gleaned from this examination is integrated with the patient's history to confirm or refute the initial diagnostic impression. The demonstration of localized neurological dysfunction of recent appearance without obvious recent trauma might suggest the presence of a progressive neurological disease, while a normal neurologic examination suggests the presence of an old or static process.

The electroencephalogram, a dynamic display of the brain's spontaneous electrical activity, has particular bearing on the evaluation of the patient with epilepsy. "Reading" the EEG consists of examining the recording of the brain's activity from several points on the skull simultaneously, in an effort to identify specific patterns. The information gleaned from the EEG has bearing on the location within the brain of the discharging focus. Less frequently, some inferences can be made concerning etiology and classification which might have bearing on the therapeutic agents chosen.

For the vast majority of patients, the above sequence of neurological history, examination, and EEG represents all the investigation that is necessary. In those instances, however, where there is a suggestion that generalized medical disease is present, certain laboratory blood tests might appropriately be chosen to evaluate the specific disease in question. If the tests suggest that further investigation is necessary, the patients are usually sent to an internist.

If the initial evaluation has suggested the possibility of a progressive neurological disease, further radiologic investigation may be undertaken. Skull films have only a small yield in this respect, but the new technique of computerized axial tomography (CAT scan) rapidly yields excellent information concerning structural abnormalities within the brain without danger, discomfort, or hospitalization. Depending on the findings, it may indeed be appropriate to hospitalize the patient for specific studies of the arteries leading to and supplying the brain (arteriogram) or the spaces within and over the brain as visualized by the injection of air into the spinal canal (pneumoencephalogram). These latter two studies are currently rarely done unless surgery is seriously contemplated for a given problem.

Psychosocial Evaluation

In a recent study of 369 outpatients, fewer than 25 percent were categorized as having "epilepsy only" without an associated problem, such as intellectual disturbance, neurological impairment, or behavior problems. Those in the "epilepsy only" category seemed to function very competently at work or in the school setting, while the other groups, especially those with brain damage, seemed to have difficulties in various aspects of living. It is those clients with epilepsy plus associated problems who will usually be seen in the rehabilitation setting. Therefore, a counselor having a client with epilepsy should procure as much information as possible from the person's family, the neurologist, and in many cases, a psychologist and social worker.

Neuropsychological evaluation, although not always readily available in all communities, can be invaluable. A rehabilitation agency's psychological consultant should be contacted regarding the appropriateness of this type of evaluation. The measures developed by Drs. Halstead and Reitan comprise the core neuropsychological battery. It is used to discriminate between normal performance and performance of brain-damaged populations. The neuropsychological assessment can provide the information regarding specific brain-behavior relationships (e.g., a determination of brain damage and the type of adaptive skills which the individual lacks, the efficiency of functioning of one side of the body versus the other, or particular patterns of ability). Decreased neuropsychological and intellectual functioning may result from seizure activity, fatigue, or toxic levels of anticonvulsants on the day of testing. The examiner should therefore check for these problems before administering the tests.

When the rehabilitation counselor is dealing with an epilepsy client, it becomes extremely important to identify the arena in which a behavioral problem occurs. For example, the problem may be related to the reactions of the client's family to his seizure disorder. Family difficulties in adjusting to the client's epilepsy can be a fertile area for counseling and involvement by the rehabilitation counselor. Adolescents with epilepsy can have their prospects for employment greatly improved through the active involvement of the rehabilitation counselor at a prevocational stage.

The behavior problem may be related to side effects of anticonvulsants, such as irritability, lethargy, and depression. Since these side effects may be subtle, the counselor should always be alert for their appearance and refer the client for evaluation of his anticonvulsant drug program if side effects are suspected.

In some cases, the behavioral characteristics are related to the focus of the seizure (e.g., with temporal lobe seizures). Abnormal behavior is sometimes actually part of a seizure or related to anticipation of a seizure. If the counselor is familiar with the client's seizure pattern, he will be able to recognize those behaviors which are clearly seizure related.

Finally, the maladaptive behavior may simply be related to a person's attempt to ''cloak'' the fact that he has epilepsy. In many cases, however, behavioral problems have no identifiable relationship to the disability, and one simply observes some of the personality aberrations noticeable in the general population. In any case, the more specific the information gathered, the better prepared the counselor is for a positive counseling intervention.

TOTAL TREATMENT

The absence seizure of childhood is so brief (a few seconds) that it may go unrecognized and, when identified, requires no attention. When a person has a generalized tonic-clonic seizure, there is little required of those around him. The goal is to let the seizure run its course without letting the individual hurt himself. For unknown reasons, the average onlooker often tries to insert some firm object between the teeth, presumably to prevent biting of the tongue. It is true that occasional biting of the tongue may occur, but this is a relatively minor problem and far less dangerous than the significant damage that has been produced by injudicious attempts to insert a spoon handle or other object between the jaws, which can easily result in broken teeth and other damage. If it is easily possible, insertion of a padded wooden tongue blade or its equivalent can be undertaken, but no attempt should be made to force the jaws open. The patient may be moved into a comfortable position, preferably on his side or semiprone, so that any excess salivation will drain to the outside. Something soft may be placed under the head. Beyond such simple measures, nothing else is necessary. The seizure will be over in a few minutes, and it is important not to overreact while reorienting the person.

Anticonvulsant Drugs

Repeated seizures are anatomically and physiologically bad for the brain, can produce irremedial neuropsychological deficits, and tend to facilitate the subsequent appearance of additional seizures. The therapeutic goal in the management of epilepsy, therefore, is suppression of all seizures before they can recur. This requires that appropriate anticonvulsant drugs be chosen for any given seizure type and administered on a steady basis. With an appropriately chosen and managed program and with cooperation on the part of the patient, it is possible for most patients to be entirely free of seizures on medication, with the remainder having only rare seizures under major precipitating circumstances.

Scientific drug therapy for epilepsy is only now developing, but certain guiding principles can be described. It must first be appreciated that not all anticonvulsant drugs operate equally well for all seizure types. It is therefore necessary to make an appropriate choice based on an accurate diagnosis.

The drugs appropriate to the several categories of seizures are listed in table 12-1. As the table indicates, most of the seizures of adulthood, all those of focal origin, and all the major convulsive seizures can be considered as one group for the purposes of therapy. Having chosen the proper drug, it is necessary to

TABLE 12-1
MOST COMMON ANTICONVULSANT DRUGS

Seizure Type	Primary Anticonvulsants	Secondary Anticonvulsants
Focal, Jacksonian, grand mal, and psychomotor	Phenytoin (Dilantin) Carbamazepine (Tegretol) Mephenytoin (Mesantoin)	Phenobarbital Primidone (Mysoline) Clorzepate (Tranxene) Methsuximide (Celontin)
Petit mal	Ethosuximide (Zarontin) Valproate (Depakene) Clonazepam (Clonipin)	Trimethadoine Tridione)

ensure that an adequate amount of the drug will be delivered to the circulation so that the blood level is sufficient to have the desired therapeutic effect. Dose alone is not a sufficient guide, since different patients have different body sizes, varied fluid-fat relationships within the body, and different capabilities of their livers (where most drugs are metabolized). Differences in rate of metabolic destruction of the drug can account for variation in serum levels between individuals. Furthermore, with the continued exposure of the patient to any drug, a progressive ability of that patient's liver to dispose of the drug will develop, resulting in slowly declining serum drug levels on stable doses. It is not uncommon that a dose initially providing adequate protection against seizures is subsequently no longer adequate. With various dose increase, and after some period of time, a long-term stable state is reachieved.

A problem which has immediate impact on the serum level and usually almost as rapid an impact on seizure control is the matter of compliance. Simply stated, if patients do not take their medicine, they are not protected, and the seizures will quite likely recur.

In order to assess whether lack of control of the seizure in a patient taking a specific drug is due to relative ineffectiveness of that drug for that patient or merely due to inadequate amounts of the drug being present, it is necessary to measure the level of the drug in the patient's serum. This gives an accurate guide to the amount of drug delivered to the brain, which is the effector site for anticonvulsant activity. The blood-level information must be interpreted with an understanding that the so-called therapeutic ranges are a rough guide only. The most effective way to deliver stable anticonvulsant protection is by the use of a single drug delivered in maximum tolerable doses. Those drugs

which are likely to control the appropriate types of seizures when given alone are *primary anticonvulsants* and are so indicated on table 12-1. The anticonvulsants which offer some measure of protection, but in most patients do not confer full protection when given alone, are called *secondary anticonvulsants*.

There are two problems associated with using more than one drug for the treatment of epilepsy, although it is necessary to do this on some ocassions. First, the use of more than one drug tends to promote more rapid destruction of both drugs than would tend to occur if either were given alone. Use of the second drug may, therefore, decrease the therapeutic effectiveness of a given program, rather than increase it. This can, to some extent, be overcome by increasing the doses of either or both of the drugs to the point at which the body's ability to dispose of the drugs is nearly saturated.

Secondly, drug side effects tend to be additive, presumably because all the drugs interfere with the coordination system and depress alertness. The therapeutic effects do not seem to add pharmacologically because they apparently operate via different mechanisms. It is therefore hard to achieve adequate therapeutic levels of any of the multiple drugs because of the addition of side effects.

It is now becoming more common practice to switch from one primary anticonvulsant to another, rather than merely to add more drugs to the first drug. When it is necessary to use secondary anticonvulsants, the trend has been away from more sedating ones, such as the barbiturates, and toward drugs with fewer side effects, which can then be added in sufficient quantity to achieve some degree of therapeutic effectiveness. Continued frequent followup and accurate controlling of prescribed drugs are critical for good control. It is

TABLE 12-2
CLASSIFICATION CRITERIA FOR SIDE EFFECTS AND INTOXICATION

Category Title	Findings
I None	I None
II Side effects	II Nystagmus without diplopia
	Minimal (barely perceptible) coordination disturbance
III Mild intoxication	III Symptomatic nystagmus
	Diplopia
	Mild to moderate coordination disturbances
IV Definite intoxication	IV Mental status change
	Severe/marked coordination disturbance
	Vomiting
V Encephalopathy	V Brain-stem and cerebellar signs
	Changes in level of consciousness
	Focal neurological signs
	Increase in seizure frequency

essential that every seizure patient have a knowledgeable physician who is seen regularly at least every 3 to 6 months.

The anticonvulsant side effects, which are listed in table 12-2, represent a major barrier to the easy control of seizures. All the drugs have essentially the same side effects which limit the progressive raising of drug doses and levels. Frequently, the side effects are represented by *impairment of coordination*, which can range from difficulty focusing the eyes, through mild clumsiness of the hands, to gait disturbances ranging from slight stumbling to a major difficulty in walking. These side effects are objectively apparent, and when drug dose is reduced, side effects diminish.

Much more subtle are the *mental and emotional side effects* related to many of the anticonvulsants. Some of the drugs are sedating, and it is only a complaint from the patient that will bring this to anyone's attention, since when the patient is sitting in the physician's office, he is sufficiently involved to remain alert. The same patient with the same drug level, however, might be incapable of remaining alert while performing a routine task. Additionally, noticeable deteriorations in intellectual performance are found on neuro-psychological evaluation which are related specifically to certain of the anticonvulsants. Although these are, as previously mentioned, to some degree dose-related as well, they may also occur even at small doses in some patients and not affect other patients at all. Sensi-

tivity to the complaints of the patient is again the best clue to the presence of such side effects.

Another rather common side effect is *depression*. This can be subtle in onset and may well be confused initially with depression related to the occupational and social limitations imposed on patients with seizures. Nevertheless, certain of the drugs, particularly the barbiturates, tend to promote emotional depression, which will disappear with the removal of those agents. Since many of these more subtle side effects will persist even at blood levels under those needed to achieve seizure control, it is now considered appropriate to shift drugs and attempt to achieve adequate therapeutic levels with an agent that does not produce side effects in the particular individual in question.

Another group of side effects are *idiosyncratic,* meaning that they are simply due to the mere presence of the drug. Most of these, such as rashes, are benign, but infrequently they may be dangerous, such as a failure of the bone marrow to produce blood cells (aplastic anemia). Idiosyncratic side effects require prompt termination of the offending drug and the substitution of another.

Problems of side effects tend to make seizure control in some patients difficult to achieve until a logical process of trial and error, aided by serum-level measurements, is pursued. Throughout, it must be recognized that unless the patient's report of side effects is taken into account, the patient himself may very well alter the dose of medicine and thereby interject an unknown and random factor into the attempt to control the seizures.

Surgery

Surgical treatment of epilepsy is now well established, the criteria for consideration are clear, and the results of treatment well documented.

The most important criterion for consideration of surgery is ineffective control of seizures by competent and aggressive treatment with anticonvulsant drugs. A trial on one or two of the common antiepileptic drugs does not satisfy this criterion. It is necessary that the patient receive a thorough trial on the best drugs effective for his type of seizure and that he receive adequate dosage as judged by quantitative tests of the amount of drug in his blood serum.

If the seizures cannot be controlled with medical treatment, the necessary diagnostic studies must be undertaken to determine the exact location of the seizure focus. This focus must be located on the surface of the brain, in an area of cortex which can be surgically removed without producing significant neurological deficit. Thus, a patient whose focus is located in the speech cortex is not a candidate for surgery because, while surgery might control the seizures, the patient would be left with an aphasia far more disabling than the seizures. The diagnostic studies to acquire the information to make these judgments require a short period of hospitalization. Of all patients with epilepsy, about 5 percent will qualify for surgery.

The surgery itself can almost be described as plastic surgery. Irritating scar is removed in a very delicate fashion so that the postoperative scar is as small as possible. The operation is lengthy and requires a complex team who have had special training and experience in the surgery of epilepsy. It also requires rather elaborate electronic instrumentation. For these reasons, there are relatively few centers in the United States that have the personnel and facilities to undertake surgery of this kind.

The success of the surgery depends to a large degree on the location of the focus and the type and degree of scarring causing the seizures. The overall results are that about 60 percent of all patients undergoing the surgery become seizure-free. Patients with temporal lobe epilepsy represent more than one-half of all adult epileptics and also represent the largest group receiving surgery. In this group, 71 percent become seizure free after surgery. The value is 77 percent for temporal lobe epilepsy due to birth trauma and 61 percent when the cause is unknown. In general, slightly more than 50 percent of patients are seizure free and taking no anticonvulsant medication more than 2 years after surgery. An additional group (about 20 percent) are seizure free, but still require medication. When one considers that the candidates for surgery are those with the most intractable seizures, such figures are impressive. Furthermore, surgery is the only treatment modality which can result in permanent eradication seizures.

If the surgery is to be undertaken, it is most effective if carried out fairly early in the course of the disease. Not only does early surgery improve the results in terms of seizure control, but it also inhibits the development of the social consequences of epilepsy, and hence a more optimal rehabilitation result becomes possible. On the other hand, patients who are seizure free following successful surgery may need psychological counseling to help them overcome their previous dependency.

VOCATIONAL IMPLICATIONS

A recent nationwide survey of persons with epilepsy, performed by the National Epilepsy League, indicated vocational counseling as the highest priority of direct services requested, substantially above the stated need even for medical services. Rehabilitation professionals must channel more energy and skill into providing the specific assessment and counseling services which these clients require.

The maturation of a person with epilepsy is often hindered, and he tends to enter the job market several years later than a normal peer. This delay must not be prolonged by waiting for the ideal situation of a seizure-free state before initiating rehabilitation planning efforts. Remaining seizure free is not certain, even if a client's seizures do cease for several months or even several years. In developing a rehabilitation plan, success is more likely if the counselor fully understands his client's seizure disorder, identifies the client's adaptive skills and job goals, coaches the client toward social competence, and, if necessary, assists in locating a "seizure tolerant" work environment. Enhancing the client's social skills is especially important, because the more socially acceptable he is, the less likely repeated seizures will result in a quickly contrived "lay-off" and social isolation from other employees.

The importance of seizure-related information cannot be overstressed. *Understanding how the seizure disorder may specifically affect functioning on a job is critical.* The counselor must be concerned with type and frequency of seizures; the existence, if any, of a warning on the day of a seizure; the time lapse between an aura and the onset of the seizure, and whether the client is conscious and capable of taking safety precautions during this period; any evidence of a relationship of seizure onset to other factors; and the amount of recovery time necessary following a seizure. Information regarding the possible precipitants of seizures (e.g., fatigue, flickering lights, alcohol intake, stress) should be carefully noted for discussion with a medical advisor and for analyzing the total work environment. Other factors, such as the direction an individual falls during a generalized grand mal seizure or whether this person has ever been injured during a seizure, should be considered when selecting a work station or job.

The more seizure-related information counselors have in regard to their clients, the better prepared they are to engage an employer for placement purposes. If a client has both grand mal and petit mal seizures, but it can be determined that the grand mal seizures occur late in the evening and the petit mal seizures are barely discernable (lasting only several seconds) during the day, client employability is significantly improved. The existence of a dependable aura and warning sensations is also important to an employer, as they provide time for the individual to withdraw from potentially unsafe work situations.

With regard to vocational evaluation techniques, traditional vocational interest inventories, various aptitude tests, and traditional education and training approaches can easily be utilized with this group. Further, a series of volunteer experiences in hospitals, nonprofit corporations, or workshops, for example, can provide both vocational exploration and work adjustment. Such experiences provide more precise seizure-related and social skills feedback through job supervisors. Job experiences can also serve to identify precise positive or negative information on performance which may be at variance with information provided by clients or their overly supportive families. While neuropsychological measures can identify organic deficits and provide the general directions with regard to adaptive strengths and weaknesses, they cannot predict performance on specific jobs. When using sheltered work settings for job experiences, care must be taken to avoid holding a client in a sheltered workshop longer than necessary due to workshop staff misconceptions about the disability.

Rehabilitation planning should have this solid assessment as a base, complemented by energetic counselor-client involvement. Since dependency is a significant problem of many clients with epilepsy, the assumption of personal responsibility for life and work planning by the client should be a consistent counseling focus.

There are a number of medical concerns to which the counselor should be especially attentive in the field of epilepsy rehabilitation. The counselor must understand the anticonvulsants used by his client. Deterioration in work performance may be due to side effects, especially those in category III on table 12-2. The counselor should not hesitate to refer the client promptly for medical re-evaluation if side effects are even in the least suspected.

Should seizure activity either recur or increase in frequency, it is attributable in many cases to self-medication by the client as opposed to the considered advice of a physician. Anticonvulsant side effects, costs of medication, and feelings of social discomfort may lead to the client's abandonment of his treatment regimen. These issues can often be addressed by the counselor. The counselor should also be aware of medically prescribed changes in primary or secondary anticonvulsants, for their influence on the client may affect vocational planning and performance.

Since neurological surgery for seizure reduction in some persons with severe and frequent seizures can radically improve their vocational potential, the counselor should ensure that this possibility is explored. The counselor should be aware, however, that although surgery often improves seizure control, the individual may undergo substantial psychological adjustment postoperatively that may require attention and time.

A decided majority of those with epilepsy prefer disclosure of their disability to an employer. If this is chosen, it is very helpful for clients to be able to explain the impact of seizures on their work performance clearly. Specificity of information is an extremely important tool for effective job placement. The employer often wants very complete information regarding a client's seizure disorder in relation to functioning on the job. The counselor and client may therefore wish to rehearse together the clear communication of this pertinent information.

In following up a client's job interview with an employer, seizure-related questions may often arise, and the counselor must be prepared to respond appropriately. In discussing seizure activity with an employer, it may be helpful to avoid some of the medical terminology and concentrate on a clear and specific description of the seizure, its aftermath, and what, if anything, those in the environment ought to do should it occur. Employers seem to appreciate this type of approach. If a client with active seizures never falls forward during a seizure (most persons with grand mal seizures fall to the side or backwards), has never injured himself while working, or has never used all available sick leave in previous jobs, this information should be carefully presented to the potential employer. A client's personal methods of coping with seizures in job settings should also be described to employers. Some will simply compensate for any "time out" due to a seizure by working overtime on the same day. The fact that approximately 50 percent of those with grand mal epilepsy consistently have a seizure warning aura greatly improves prospects for employment, if explained carefully to potential employers.

Many employers fear that their employee insurance rates will be raised if they hire an individual with epilepsy. This is not true, even if the company is privately insured, as opposed to having coverage through state Workers' Compensation. Insurance rate hikes are related chiefly to the frequency and severity of accidents which actually occur on a job site. Hiring an individual with epilepsy does not, in itself, increase insurance rates. A discussion of insurance coverage should always be preceded by statements affirming that employees with epilepsy have no more accidents on the job than their peers and that, in some instances, firms employing *only* individuals with epilepsy have actually been awarded reductions in insurance costs by private agents due to excellent safety records.

In general, although there is some variance among states, the Workers' Compensation Second Injury Fund will cover an employee with epilepsy who has an injury on the job resulting in total disability. This coverage is specifically for persons who already have a disability and are further disabled by an injury on the job. Therefore, if an employee is to be eligible to utilize this Second Injury Fund, an employer should have prior knowledge of the first disability (in this case, epilepsy), preferably documented in the firm's medical file.

Most persons with seizure disorders are especially attuned to potential dangers in a work environment and make extra efforts to avoid physically hazardous situations. The rehabilitation counselor, however, should be selective in job placement efforts with these clients, especially with those having more severe types of seizure activity or no seizure-related warnings. Working around heights, potentially dangerous machinery, or other situations in which these individuals can endanger themselves or others should be avoided. If an individual who is no longer having seizures desires to return to a potentially hazardous job, a medical consultant should review EEG results and the individual's natural propensity for seizures. Possible precipitants of seizures should also be taken into account in the placement process.

Although avoiding stress-inducing jobs is a concern for many clients, these same clients may also have frequent seizures when bored or tired sitting at home. It is often a better "trade off" for a person to have occasional seizures in a mildly stressful work environment than to sit alone at home with no appreciable lessening of seizure activity. Acclimation to the job and concentration on the work itself can result in a tapering off of seizure activity initially exacerbated by the stress of a new job.

There is no question that the counselor will be confronted with numerous additional problems in working in the field of epilepsy rehabilitation. Many individuals with epilepsy are not eligible to drive due to seizure activity. State laws vary regarding the length of time a person must be medically certified seizure free for license eligibility. If they are eligible to drive, epilepsy rehabilitants are often subject to more expensive assigned risk insurance rates. This group also has difficulty securing adequate health and life insurance. Local epilepsy associations can be helpful in the identification of insurance companies with more equitable rates.

Greater cohesiveness among those with epilepsy in lobbying for remediation of particular needs could definitely bring about improvement of services. There is a lack of consumer involvement, probably because of the "invisible" nature of the disability. The rehabilitation counselor should be aware that agencies serving the developmentally disabled (e.g., the cerebral palsied or mentally retarded) often are prepared or required by sponsors to make their services available to those with epilepsy as well.

Another problem area in employment is the existence of negative employer attitudes toward hiring those with epilepsy. A recent study suggests that employer education alone does not dispel this attitude. It appears that *less traditional* educational approaches are more effective and that the employer really has to be reached at an emotional level. Vocationally successful citizens with epilepsy, popular TV personalities, and established members of the business community might be used in more innovative programming focused on changing these negative employer attitudes.

The counselor has a number of tools which should help in placement of the client with epilepsy. New affirmative action legislation demands "accommodation" on the part of the employer. No longer can a seizure in a person with a physically hazardous job constitute sufficient grounds for dismissal, when altering the job or transferring the employee to other positions within a firm can result in safe and competent job performance.

Epilepsy rehabilitants who encounter negative attitudes from employers and others in the community and, additionally, must work through problem areas associated with their primary disability, can often profit from group involvement. Job-finding clubs allow clients to share job leads and confront or reinforce each other regarding vocational goals. Job-seeking-skills groups can also be useful to epilepsy rehabilitants, for they are often very naive regarding the world of work and can profit from coaching in job-seeking procedures. Finally, group social-skills training in areas such as assertiveness and conversational skills can have substantial impact on greater life satisfaction for the individual with epilepsy. Above all, the group setting fosters the development of emotional strength. When the person with epilepsy learns that he is not alone in encountering life and work barriers, his confidence improves.

BIBLIOGRAPHY

Barmore A (ed): *Epilepsy. . .Major Aspects: A Counseling Guide.* Wisconsin Epilepsy Association, 1954 E. Washington Avenue, Madison, WI 53704, 1977.

This counselor handbook offers a succinct overview of rehabilitation concerns for the client with epilepsy. Of particular interest are discussions of insurance, Workers' Compensation, Second Injury Fund, and driver's licensing.

Epilepsy Foundation of America: *Basic Statistics on the Epilepsies.* Philadelphia, Davis, 1975.

The Epilepsy Foundation of America has compiled an excellent overview of statistics related to this disability, framed within topical reviews of the literature. Chapters on psychological considerations, education, employment, and rehabilitation are particularly pertinent to the rehabilitation counselor. This text is an invaluable desk aid for grant writing or the development of project rationales.

Goldin GJ, Perry SL, Margolin RJ, Strotsky BA, Foster JC: *Rehabilitation of the Young Epileptic: Dimensions and Dynamics.* Lexington, MA, Lexington Books, 1971.

This book presents the results of an extensive survey study focused on identifying needs of the young person with epilepsy. Basic and psychosocial needs are reviewed within the context of educational, vocational, social, and family settings. The book concludes with specific recommendations for prevocational involvement by the rehabilitationist on behalf of the young person with epilepsy.

Laidlaw J, Richens A (eds): *Textbook on Epilepsy.* Edinburgh, Churchill Livingstone, 1976.

A comprehensive and current text on the medical treatment of epilepsy. The editors have succeeded in their purpose of making the present state of the art equally understandable to those in other than the medical profession.

Rodin EA: *The Prognosis of Patients with Epilepsy.* Springfield, IL, Thomas, 1968.

Dr. Rodin uses extensive data from the Michigan Epilepsy Center and thorough reviews of the literature to provide an excellent exposition of epilepsy and its associated problem areas. Chapters related to intelligence and prognosis for seizure control, behavior, and employment provide extremely useful and interesting information for the rehabilitation counselor.

Rodin EA, Shapiro HL, Lennox K: Epilepsy and life performance. Rehabil Lit **38**:34–39, 1977.

In this article, staff of the Michigan Epilepsy Center summarize data collected on 369 patients with a diagnosis of epilepsy during the years 1970–74. Patients were initially classified into an "epilepsy only" group or into another category, depending on an identified problem in addition to the primary disability. Statistical analysis of the data on various outcome measures compares the function of those with "epilepsy only" to the function of those with an additional problem (e.g., brain damage).

Schlesinger LE, Frank DS: *Epilepsy: On the Way to Work.* Washington, D.C., Artists and Writers Syndicate, 1976.

This book, sponsored by the Epilepsy Foundation of America, is written in a dramatic script format as a guide for the rehabilitation counselor. Dialogue is between experienced and inexperienced counselor or counselor and physician, and coverage includes: medical aspects of the disorder, epilepsy and the community, preparing the client for the job, reaching employers, and group vocational counseling. An "epilepsy quiz" with answers is included.

Schlesinger LE, Frank D: From demonstration to dissemination: Gateways to employment for epileptics. Rehabil Lit **35**:98–106 and 109, 1974.

This article describes the three-cities project, in which comprehensive vocational demonstration projects were established for those with epilepsy in Atlanta, Chicago, and San Antonio (1967-68). The article is particularly valuable because of the authors' description of the various vocational program components important in meeting the needs of this population.

Wright GN (ed): *Epilepsy Rehabilitation.* Boston, Little, Brown, 1975.

This is the most comprehensive reference text that currently exists in the field of epilepsy rehabilitation. Dr. Wright has judiciously utilized the talents of 16 well-known authorities in the medical and rehabilitation aspects of the disability. Within the chapters on vocational counseling and rehabilitation planning are various data protocols which can be valuable for use in intake, assessment, planning, or program-evaluation procedures.

13 AMPUTATION

Lawrence W. Friedmann, M.D.

INTRODUCTION

The term "amputation" means the complete loss of all limb elements below a certain point. In this chapter, however, the term also includes congenital limb deficiency. Congenital deficiencies may consist of an absence of all limb elements below a particular level, complete absence of only an intermediate section (e.g., upper arm), or the partial absence of a limb element (e.g., not all fingers present). The reader is referred to the section of chapter 3 on the musculoskeletal system for a review of the extremities.

The exact incidence and prevalence of limb amputation in the United States is difficult to ascertain. The National Center for Health Statistics of the U.S. Public Health Service estimated a prevalence of 311,000 amputees in 1970. An incidence of approximately 43,000 new amputations per year is estimated, of which 77 percent occur in males, and 90 percent involve the legs. In lower extremity amputations, 40 percent are above the knee, 50 percent are below the knee, and 10 percent are at the hip. Of particular interest is the fact that 58 percent of amputations occur in those between 21 and 65 years of age. If we include the late teenage population, two-thirds of all amputees are potential candidates for vocational rehabilitation.

Amputations may be traumatic or surgical. The traumatic amputations result from a sudden severe injury. Explosions, mangling in a machine, severance by a sharp object, or burns, for example, cause traumatic amputations. Surgical amputations are usually associated with cancer (see chap. 28) or peripheral arterial disease (see chap. 22). Surgical amputation for cancer is usually major, occurring at either the shoulder or hip and usually in young adults. Osteogenic sarcoma of bone is the most frequent cause. Vascular amputees comprise 89 percent of the amputee population over 50 years of age. Half of these patients have diabetes mellitus (see chap. 24). Progression of peripheral arterial disease is generally slow. Amputation becomes necessary when occlusion of the vessel either by progressive encroachment on its interior or by a sudden clotting (embolus) causes death (gangrene) of that part of the limb ordinarily nourished by the vessel.

Congenital limb deficiencies evolve largely from insults during pregnancy. Drugs (e.g., Thalidomide) and X-radiation have been implicated. Genetically induced limb deficiencies are not transmitted from generation to generation, as they are recessive traits or one-time changes in the genes.

In general, the disabilities, treatment, prosthetic prescription, and vocational implications of amputation are similar regardless of cause. Where special considerations for a specific cause exist, they are noted throughout the chapter. Otherwise, this chapter deals with amputations generally, regardless of cause. Psychosocial factors are considered first. Upper and lower extremity amputations, prosthetics, and vocational considerations are then discussed, followed by consideration of the complications of amputation and prosthesis use.

PSYCHOSOCIAL FACTORS

Amputation as punishment, common in ancient times, still occurs in isolated areas. The concept of amputation as punishment for sin persists, and a feeling of guilt and shame often accompanies an amputation. Further, the disfigurement and destruction of a previous self-image contribute to the possible development of introversion, self-pity, feelings of inferiority, and social isolation. Anger and frustration are also common responses. Not all of these psychological characteristics, of course, are seen in every patient.

A reactive depression, however, is natural after an amputation. Proper preoperative preparation and good guidance through the amputation, prosthesis fitting, and training phases helps prevent the depression from becoming chronic. The total treatment principles outlined in this chapter help avoid unnecessary delays in the development of skill in use of a prosthesis. This in turn also helps prevent chronic depression and social isolation due to lack of contact with family, friends, and employment opportunities.

The traumatic amputee has no psychological preparation for the loss of a limb and therefore experiences a sudden shock. Adjustment to the amputation may be more difficult for him than for those who have had some preparation. Additional concerns also exist for patients whose amputations were required by cancer or arterial disease. The counselor should be aware of the whole complex of psychological responses associated with cancer (see chap. 28) and the anxiety and fear of possible loss of a second limb from arterial disease.

Individuals with congenital limb deficiency have diverse problems quite different from those of individuals who lose limbs later in life. Sudden loss is not their concern. During their childhood, parental rejection or parental overprotectiveness may have been experienced if the parents were unable to successfully adjust to having a "deformed child." Both of these reactions inhibit social maturation of the child with congenital limb deficiency. Reduced mobility, if the lower extremities are involved, and reduced function, if the upper extremities are involved, limit the experiences of the growing child and contribute to relative immaturity as adulthood is reached.

Some methods of functioning which are acceptable in children with congenital limb deficiency are not acceptable in the adult. For example, the development of leg, foot, and toe dexterity to substitute for upper extremity deficiencies may be considered "cute and brave" in the child, but not in the adult. The adult may well be unprepared to handle the rejection by peers, parents, and friends of activities that were acceptable when he was younger. Withdrawal, depression, and feelings of inferiority may result.

In addition to restricted experiences, persons with congenital limb deficiency may also have missed a considerable amount of time in school due to hospitalization for surgery. They may therefore have educational deficiencies.

The counselor must be alert to the possible existence of the above psychosocial disability factors. If suspected, they require careful evaluation and treatment and incorporation into the vocational plan.

UPPER EXTREMITY AMPUTATION

Levels

An amputation in the upper limb may be at any level along its length. Figure 13-1 illustrates the varius amputation levels and the terminology used to describe them. The most severe level, the *forequarter* or *interscapular-thoracic* amputation (not shown in fig. 13-1), removes the entire arm, scapula, and clavicle, leaving the patient with only the rib cage. The shoulder is therefore eliminated. In the *shoulder disarticulation* (S/D) amputation, the arm is removed at the shoulder (glenohumeral) joint. The scapula and

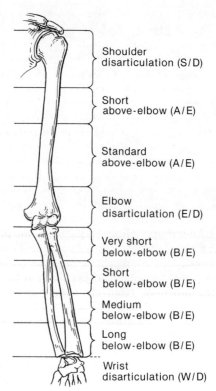

FIGURE 13-1. Classification of upper extremity amputation levels.

clavicle remain and the shoulder is preserved. The *above-elbow* (A/E) amputation refers to any level below the glenohumeral joint. The very short above-elbow amputation is functionally the same as the shoulder disarticulation because the short humerus is literally buried in the axilla. An above-elbow amputation below the anterior axillary fold leaves a bony and soft tissue stump which can be contained by an artificial limb socket.

The *elbow disarticulation* (E/D) amputation removes the arm through the elbow joint. This leaves an irregular bony end covered mainly by skin alone. The *below-elbow* (B/E) amputation passes through both bones of the forearm (radius and ulna). The more proximal the amputation, the greater the muscular covering of these two bones. The more distal the amputation, the more irregular the shape, for the radius and ulna are relatively more exposed. The *wrist disarticulation* (W/D) leaves an irregularly shaped distal forearm, with almost no soft tissue under the skin over the bone ends. Finally, the *partial hand* amputation may vary from loss of one or more digits to a loss of complete fingers or a loss of part of the palm and associated fingers.

Functional Disabilities

The functional disabilities associated with unilateral upper limb amputation at all levels are not as great as might be expected. Immediately after the amputation, impairments in eating, dressing, bathing, writing, and driving are apparent. Usually less than a week of training in new techniques with the use of adaptive devices is sufficient to restore independence in most functions, even without a prosthesis. Performance of these tasks is easier with a prosthesis, however. If the dominant hand has been amputated, redevelopment of writing skills takes longer. Activities that absolutely require bilateral skills cannot be performed until the prosthesis has been fitted, and if the dominant hand has been amputated, more extensive training is required for bilateral skills because dominance must be developed on the other side. The more proximal the amputation, the more difficult it is to restore bilateral skills.

With bilateral upper limb amputation, the problems multiply because the patient now has no hand to do fine manipulation. Nonetheless, the bilateral amputee can usually develop independence in all of the above-mentioned functions relatively easily. Even without prostheses, these skills can be achieved through more extensive use of modifications at home and adaptive clothing and equipment. Writing with a prosthesis is possible, but typing is not very practical, and a tape recorder is usually needed for notes at lectures or meetings. The bilateral amputee can be trained to drive, some even without prostheses.

The bilateral shoulder disarticulation amputee has the most serious problems with self-care and may never develop independence, even with prostheses. Special clothing adaptations are obviously required for this severe disability. Some can learn to independently dress, eat, bathe, write, take care of personal hygiene, and even drive by training their feet to act as hands. The hips, knees, and toes must be very limber, and such activities are therefore much more difficult for the adult who loses both arms at the shoulder level than for the child who is born with such a loss or had an early accident.

Principles of Management

Preoperative preparation. Before a surgical amputation, except in cases of acute emergency, the patient usually receives an outline of the immediate postoperative care, initial dependency to be expected, training required to achieve independence, a brief description of the prosthesis and of prosthesis training, and expected outcome. This presentation should incorporate knowledge of the patient's intellectual capacity, skills, current life and family responsibilities, and vocational and avocational requirements. When feasible, the patient is introduced to the treatment team to be involved in his recovery: physician, physical therapist, occupational therapist, psychologist, social worker, rehabilitation counselor, and prosthetist. Introducing him to another patient of similar age, level of amputation, and medical condition is also advisable,

if possible.

An amputation, even a therapeutic one, is often viewed as a treatment failure. This is stressful to both the patient and the physician. Total team treatment helps prevent severe reactions to this stress, and helps the patient achieve a positive but realistic attitude toward his future.

Maintenance of hope for the future is vital to the psychological well-being of the amputee. It enlists his cooperation and that of his family in therapeutic efforts on his behalf. Instilling an unrealistic concept of potential future function, however, creates a basis for later disillusionment that is sure to lead to depression, resentment, and even legal redress. Honest appraisal at all stages of the amputee's treatment is essential to retain respect and obtain cooperation.

The following items should be included in both preoperative and postoperative discussions with the patient and his family. This information cannot and should not be presented in too brief a form and perhaps not all at once. Patients cannot assimilate more than a few of the items at one time and the information must be repeated often after amputation.

1. The sensation that the amputated limb is still present ("phantom limb") is normal in all amputees and is not evidence of an emotional disturbance.

2. A functioning and happy life can be achieved and maintained after amputation.

3. Adjustments will have to be made in order to cope with the various problems engendered by amputation. These problems can be psychological, physical, social, vocational, and recreational.

4. Becoming accustomed to wearing the prosthesis takes several weeks, since it does not feel like a normal limb. It lacks sensation and, at the beginning, seems heavy.

5. There will be a training period to achieve skill with the prosthesis. Without training, the patient will be unable to use the prosthesis adequately.

6. The stump shrinks as a result of reduced use of residual muscles, bandaging, elastic "stump shrinkers," and pressure from the prosthesis. Prosthetic adjustments will therefore be required over an indefinite period in the future.

7. The prosthesis is basically cosmetic and partially functional. It will not wholly substitute for the amputated limb, and some frustration and disappointment with it should be expected.

8. Independence in most functions can be achieved in a few weeks with the help of the treatment team.

9. No cosmetic prosthesis is ever entirely natural looking, especially at close range.

The prosthesis must be viewed by the medical team and by the patient as a tool to perform certain tasks and not as a replacement for the human limb. Hope must be tempered with realism, so that this useful force is not converted into disappointment and resentment.

Surgery. Surgical amputations and stump revisions are usually performed by an orthopedic surgeon, but may also be performed by general or vascular surgeons. Wounds are bandaged with soft dressings either with or without elastic wraps to control postoperative edema. Some centers use plaster of Paris for final wrapping (rigid dressing). Others shape plaster of Paris into a socket of a temporary, detachable prosthesis. This temporary prosthesis, while different in nature from the later permanent prosthesis, allows the patient to begin rehabilitation efforts early.

Partial hand amputations are often revised to achieve pinch (prehension) or grasp without a prosthesis, thereby preserving sensation. Reconstruction after loss or congenital absence of a thumb is an example. In this procedure, the index finger and its metacarpal are rotated and displaced to perform as a thumb able to oppose the middle and other fingers (see fig. 32-7, p. 422).

Within a week or less after surgery, patients with uncomplicated unilateral upper limb amputations and revisions can be discharged from the hospital to continue their rehabilitation as outpatients.

Postoperative care. Within a day or two after surgery, the patient will begin physical therapy for posture training and an exercise program to maintain and improve the range of motion and muscle strength of the uninvolved joints of the limb. The patient will also receive retraining by an occupational therapist in activities such as personal hygiene, dressing, and eating, and in using the opposite limb if a shift in handedness is required. The daily training program is generally at least 2 hours in physical therapy and 2 hours in occupational therapy for perhaps 2 to 4 weeks.

A period of about a month after surgery may be necessary for the stump size to stabilize sufficiently to receive the final prosthetic socket. Elastic bandaging, elastic "stump shrinkers," and serial castings are often used to facilitate this maturation.

Prosthesis Description

The functions of the upper extremity which the prosthesis attempts to replace are very complex. The proximal portions of a normal upper extremity serve to position and stabilize the hand for action. The muscles, largely those at the shoulder and elbow but also those at the wrist, are used to move these joints so that the hand can be positioned for performance. Hooking, grasping, and pinching are the main modes by which objects are held. Manipulation is then performed by the many muscles controlling finger and wrist action.

In addition, adequate function requires sensory feedback not only from the skin of the hand, but also from the muscles themselves. Ordinarily, one of the upper extremities develops greater dexterity than the other. This is what is meant by "handedness." No prosthesis applied to the dominant extremity can achieve dexterity equivalent to prior function. Handedness must therefore shift after dominant extremity amputation.

The prosthesis, which attempts to duplicate lost function, has the following components: (a) suspension, a method to hold the prosthesis on the body; (b) a socket to interface with the stump skin; (c) mechanical joints to replace lost joints; (d) a terminal device to substitute for hand loss; and (e) a source of power both to pre-position the terminal device and to activate it. Feedback, although partially received from pressure of the socket, suspension apparatus, and power activation, is primarily received by the amputee through visual inspection.

Suspension. Methods of suspending the prosthesis to the body include straps, suction between the socket and the stump, or shaping of the socket over bony prominences to achieve a clamping effect. A common type of strap suspension is the so-called figure-8 harness, which anchors the prosthesis to the opposite shoulder via straps that cross over the back (fig. 13-2). Another variation is the "shoulder saddle chest strap harness." The latter may be less uncomfortable for carrying heavy loads.

Socket. The socket is always custom made of special plastic, and is shaped to the stump and underlying muscle and bone. Total contact is required, i.e., the socket must be in contact with the entire stump. This total contact may be hard, soft, or semisoft. Some sockets are made with a distal air chamber for special purposes. Total-contact sockets support the distal soft tissues, prevent edema, and provide additional sensory feedback. The socket usually has two walls, the inner wall or stump wall which is in intimate contact, and an outer cosmetic or structural wall designed to resemble the limb (fig. 13-3). To avoid additional weight, the space between the walls is not filled. Stump socks, of varying thicknesses, are often required. They absorb perspiration and protect the skin from friction.

Joint replacement. The joints of a prosthesis are relatively simple. They do not in any way approximate the complexity of the joints they replace and usually move in only one plane. A passive joint is one which is not provided with power that controls movement. Movement is achieved by gravity or positioning by the opposite arm. An active joint is provided with power. Joint stabilization is achieved, when desired, via mechanical locks or friction devices. Shoulder joints are usually passive but may be coupled with friction. Wrist joints are passive and contain friction devices for stabilization and positioning.

Terminal device. The most important part of the upper limb prosthesis is the terminal device, either a hook or a hand. Terminal devices mostly pinch, hold, or grasp.

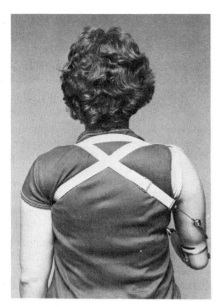

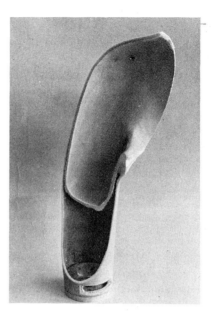

FIGURE 13-2. Figure-8 suspension harness on patient with right A/E prosthesis. Note cable attached to harness and passing into cable housing anchored to socket of prosthesis.

FIGURE 13-3. Above-elbow amputation socket cut open to show double-wall structure. Inner wall is in total contact with the stump and was custom made from a plaster cast of stump. Outer wall "fills out" the upper arm. The flat base serves as a place of attachment for prosthetic elbow joint.

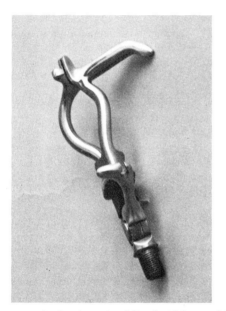

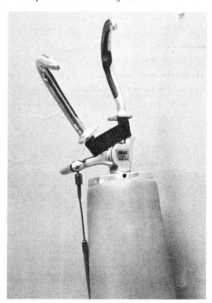

FIGURE 13-4. *(Left)* Aluminum hook lined with latex rubber (neoprene) in the open position. The cable is attached to the "thumb" of the hook which, when pulled, causes the "finger" on the left to move away from the "finger" on the right, which is always stationary. The patient's voluntary action creates the force in the cable to open the hook (V.O.). As the "fingers" separate, the wide rubber band at the base of the "fingers" stretches. When the cable force is relaxed, the rubber band causes the hook to close. The hook is screwed into the wrist unit and held in position by a rubber disc in the unit (friction wrist). *(Right)* Heavy-duty steel hook ("utility," "farmer's," or "carpenter's," hook) in the closed position. The surfaces of the "fingers" are serrated (not shown). The shape of the hook (compare with fig. at left) allows it to hold things such as nails, files, and hammers. The bolt at the base of hook screws into a wrist unit.

They cannot sense shape, texture, or temperature and they do not duplicate in any way the wide range of manipulation and dexterity of a normal hand.

Hooks are made of aluminum for lightness or steel for heavy use and come in a variety of sizes and shapes.

All are characterized by two opposing surfaces, one of which is movable. Steel hooks are used for heavy work, while the aluminum hooks are used for everyday life and sedentary, desk-type jobs. Aluminum hooks generally come with a latex rubber inner surface to add friction to enhance contact with such objects as doorknobs, paper, and pencils (fig. 13-4, *left*). Steel hooks may come with or without the rubber gripping surface. They may also be in different shapes for specific functions and have earned titles such as "utility hook" or "farmer's hook" (fig. 13-4, *right*).

A source of power is necessary for active terminal devices. Power may be used to open the device (voluntary opening, V.O.), with closure achieved passively via springs or rubber bands, or power can be used to close the device (voluntary closing, V.C.), with opening achieved passively. Some terminal devices can voluntarily open and close and also can be locked at various open positions.

The prosthetic hand resembles a normal hand only in appearance. It has a palm and five fingers but no real dexterity. The cosmetic hand is fully passive and does nothing. The functional hand has only one plane of motion, opposition of the thumb against the tips of index and middle fingers in a three-finger pinch (fig. 13-5). Encirclement of the three fingers around an object also adds grasp function.

Both cosmetic and functional hands are covered with cosmetic gloves designed to match a person's skin color. These gloves can be cut easily by sharp objects and are easily stained by newsprint, mustard, ink, and other dyes. They therefore can only be used in "clean" situations, as replacements are expensive.

The fine tips and carefully engineered flat opposing surfaces of hooks give them much greater utility than functional hands in a performance setting. Patients are usually fitted with hooks first and hands second. Many end up using both, hooks for "work" and hands for "play."

Power. Power to move active joints, activate locks, or open or close the terminal device may be obtained by harnessing movement produced by unamputated muscles. This is achieved by a cable running from the normal joint supplying the power to the part of the prosthesis to be moved. Power can also be supplied externally from compressed gas or from a battery source built into the prosthesis. Whether the power is wholly internal or external, control of its activation is achieved through movement of an uninvolved body part or from action potentials induced by muscle contraction (see p. 19).

Prosthesis Prescription

The specific prosthesis prescription will depend upon the patient's anticipated requirements for his activities of daily living, and his vocational, avocational, and cosmetic needs. The prosthesis will generally be prescribed by a physiatrist or orthopedic surgeon. Other physicians generally are not trained in prosthetics or knowledgeable on what is available. Input from the treatment team can help ensure that

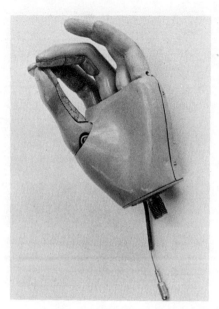

FIGURE 13-5. Northrup-Sierra voluntary opening functional hand without cosmetic cover. Thumb has two possible positions. The thumb position depicted allows for three-finger pinch. The second position, a more open one, allows for grasping of larger objects. Direct external pressure on the thumb controls the position. Using power harnessed from proximal normal joints and muscles, the amputee can voluntarily pull on the cable to move the index and middle fingers together away from the thumb. The ring and little fingers are passive and do not move.

prescriptions will be appropriate.

Fabrication of prostheses is usually performed by certified prosthetists or supervised technicians. Fabrication facilities may be found in most large cities and in some smaller ones. Artificial limbs can still be obtained in communities without such facilities if a certified prosthetist is available to send the prescription, measurements, and appropriate casts of the stump to a central fabricating facility. An adequate prosthesis may be obtained in this manner. Adjustments are then made locally for final fitting. Actual fabrication of a prosthesis takes no more than 1 to 2 weeks. Longer delays are generally due to administrative problems, lack of authorization for payment, or inefficiency in the prosthetic facility. This may include a lack of an adequate number of people to make the prosthesis more rapidly.

Fitting must be done carefully. A patient will abandon an upper limb prosthesis if it is not comfortable because he can manage so well with one arm. The longer the delay, the harder it is to replace inefficient one-handed techniques with bilateral techniques. This principle is incorporated in the care of congenital limb deficiency, where application of prostheses during infancy is advocated. While each prescription is specific to an individual patient, certain concepts apply to all prostheses for each of the

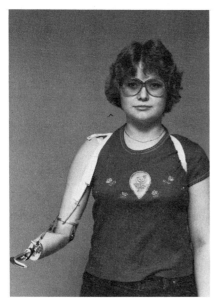 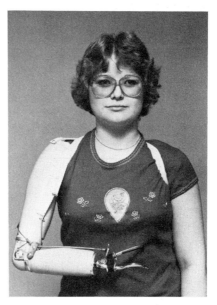

FIGURE 13-6. *(Left)* Front view of the same patient as in figure 13-2. Note how figure-8 harness anchors around normal shoulder. The cable extending to the hook is the same cable described in figure 13-2. The second cable, which enters the prosthesis at the elbow, controls the elbow lock. Forward movement of the stump (shoulder flexion) will bend the elbow into flexion. In this figure, the patient has flexed and locked the elbow. Shoulder flexion, if executed now, will open the hook. The turntable, shown just above the elbow lock cable, has been positioned in external rotation. *(Right)* The turntable is now in internal rotation, which places the hook in front of the body. The patient has now flexed the shoulder, causing the hook to open.

amputation levels with regard to suspension, socket, joint replacement, terminal devices, power, and control.

Shoulder disarticulation and interscapular-thoracic.

Both S/D and interscapular-thoracic amputations are extremely difficult to fit with a prosthesis for effective function. The prosthesis is often discarded unless it provides a clear advantage to the patient's work or avocation. The socket ("shoulder cap") covers a large area of what is left of the shoulder and trunk and is suspended via chest straps. At this level, harnessing of power from other joints is most difficult. To activate and move a cable attached to the limb, use of chest expansion or opposite arm movement is required. Use of a good normal arm to operate a prosthesis, however, is not particularly recommended. The shoulder joint replacement is passive and has limited motion in flexion and abduction. Positioning prior to use is usually done with the good arm, and friction to hold a specific position may be used for the shoulder joint. Use of the opposite hand for positioning elbow flexion or for operation of an elbow lock may be used. Power harnessed from other joints may only be used for the terminal device. External power may also be prescribed. The terminal devices that can be used are hands for cosmesis and lightweight aluminum hooks if an active device is required. The amount of body power that can be obtained is not sufficient to operate a functional hand. The prosthesis is heavy and difficult to put on. Cosmesis may be the only goal for most.

Above-elbow. Double-wall sockets are used for A/E

prostheses. Figure-8 suspension is used and stump socks are preferred. Elbow joint replacement is a prefabricated item. Its mechanism is internal, occupying the space distal to the stump. Since shoulder rotation cannot be transmitted to the terminal device because of the soft tissue in the stump, a turntable is added to the elbow mechanism. The turntable can be pre-positioned by the amputee to a desired position of rotation (fig. 13-6). A friction wrist or a mechanical wrist which can be locked into one of several positions of pronation and supination, using the opposite extremity, is preferred. The choice of a hook or a hand for the terminal device is governed by needs.

Power is required for three functions: elbow flexion, elbow locking, and terminal device operation. This power is obtained exclusively from harnessing shoulder motion via cable attachments to the forearm section, the elbow lock, and the terminal device. At least two motions (power sources) are required. The sequence of action is usually shoulder flexion to achieve elbow flexion, immediate shoulder depression and abduction to lock the elbow, and then shoulder flexion again to operate the terminal device. Cables are so attached that once the elbow is locked, the shoulder flexion action force can be transmitted to the terminal device. External power triggered by shoulder motion is increasingly being used for elbow flexion and automatic elbow locking. The devices are still experimental, expensive, and fragile.

Elbow disarticulation. Suspension of E/D prosthesis

is again achieved by a figure-8 type shoulder harness

and by socket shaping. The socket is shaped to the upper arm and is usually double-walled. The forearm section is usually prefabricated, and wrist units and terminal devices as described above are attached to it. Generally, voluntary opening terminal devices are preferred. An external elbow joint which can be locked in several positions connects the socket to the forearm section. Harnessing of power from proximal joints for operation of elbow flexion, elbow locking, and terminal device operation is the same as for A/E prostheses.

Below-elbow. Figure-8 suspension and a double-walled total-contact socket with a stump sock are usual for B/E prostheses. Unless the stump is quite long, a wrist unit as above is required for pronation and supination. A voluntary opening device can be prescribed. An elbow hinge connecting the forearm socket to an upper arm cuff anchors the cable. Rigid metal hinges are used if the stump is too short to achieve active pronation and supination. The hinge is made of flexible material when pronation and supination can still be actively achieved. Cable control is again by shoulder flexion.

A myoelectric prosthesis (fig. 13-7) should be carefully considered for B/E amputations. The prosthesis motor is activated by the myoelectric potentials produced by the muscles and picked up by electrodes situated over the skin covering the muscles to be used. It is suspended by shaping of the socket around bony prominences at the elbow. No shoulder straps are necessary. The electrical circuits, battery, and motor are contained within the prosthesis, making it heavy. Currently, hands are used which can be both V.O. and V.C., with locking at any position. The terminal device is activated by using the same muscles normally associated with opening and closing of the hand. Myoelectrically controlled hooks may also soon be available.

Wrist disarticulation. Suspension of W/D prostheses is mostly via socket shaping, although the figure-8 harness can assist. The socket is double walled, the inner wall shaped snugly over the forearm ends. A thin stump sock may also be used. The socket shape allows forearm pronation and supination motion to be actively achieved, and a friction wrist joint can be kept in any position. Interchangeable hooks and hands are used. Power is achieved by harnessing energy from proximal joints through a cable attached to the terminal device as above. A myoelectric prosthesis can also be considered for wrist disarticulation, but it is long and the functional gains are minimal.

Partial hand. Suspension of prostheses for partial hand amputations is achieved via straps and socket shaping about the wrist. The socket is usually applied without a stump sock. No joints are replaced. The terminal device may simply be a passive cosmetic completion of the hand or a passive, specifically designed post or surface against which parts of the

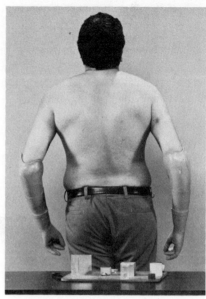

FIGURE 13-7. Bilateral below-elbow amputee, with two VA-Northwestern University Below-Elbow Myoelectric Prostheses. Harnesses are not necessary. No cables are required, and suspension is achieved by shaping the socket around the bony prominences at the elbow. The electrodes registering the electric signals from the muscles in the stump are buried in the socket walls and cannot be seen. The cosmetic cover extends to the mid-forearm level. The thumb and the index and middle fingers voluntarily open and close when the amputee contracts the muscles of the back and front sides of the stump, respectively. (Photograph courtesy of *Bulletin of Prosthetics Research,* Veterans Administration).

remaining hand are applied for grasp. No power is necessary.

Bilateral amputee prescription. In the bilateral amputee, all the above principles apply. In addition, it is rare that a bilateral amputee regularly uses two prosthetic hands because hands do not provide sufficient function. Hooks are therefore preferred. Further, at least one wrist flexion unit may be used. This is a passive device pre-positioned and locked in flexion before use to bring at least one terminal device in close to the body. Suspension of bilateral prostheses may be achieved by separately harnessing and suspending each prosthesis or by tying them together. The latter makes donning easier, but the former provides greater versatility and preserves at least one functioning arm should one of the prostheses be in need of repair.

Congenital limb deficiency. Prosthesis prescription for congenital limb deficiency becomes much more individualized to utilize all parts of the extremity, particualrly when the loss is of an intermediate part (e.g., elbow and wrist gone with hand residuals at the shoulder). Efforts are made to take advantage of even vestigial elements. Prosthesis prescription for such patients requires a center with professionals experienced with limb deficiency.

General. Each prosthesis must be custom made for the particular patient's needs. Many patients need multiple prostheses for different uses. Any prosthesis is a tool with which the patient performs one or more jobs, including not only work, but also play and personal care. Other things being equal, the prosthesis must be as good looking as possible and, in unilateral amputees, create a balanced appearance. However, the patient, his family, and his employers need to recognize that no prosthesis is truly cosmetic. There is always a balance between the appearance of a prosthesis and its function. Unfortunately, especially in upper limb prostheses, cosmesis decreases as function improves. The amount of attention that must be paid to appearance depends upon the individual patient, the society in which he lives, his ethnic group, and his job.

Each person's standards of what is appropriate will vary. Some are so disturbed by the fact of the amputation that they strive for perfection in appearance. This is not attainable since all pigments used for hand covers appear a different color under day, incandescent, and fluorescent light. Striving for less noticeability, rather than true cosmesis, is more appropriate.

The noticeability of an artificial hand may be decreased by the use of a wrist watch or a conservative ring to draw attention away from the abnormal appearance. The noticeability of the lack of dynamic movement of the hand may be diminished if the patient uses an adhesive bandage around one of the fingers. This creates the illusion of injury as a cause for lack of movement. Clothing is another way to draw attention elsewhere. While some patients may use such "tricks" initially to help them become accustomed to the prosthesis, they may soon find them pointless.

Prosthesis Checkout and Training

The prosthesis is best not given directly to the patient upon completion of fabrication, but should rather be delivered to the treatment facility. This avoids early failures and disappointment. The checkout and training for an upper limb prosthesis are usually done by an occupational therapist. Checkout proceeds according to a standard format, beginning with a check to see if all components are as prescribed. Systematic examination of suspension, socket fit, power operation and control, and joint and terminal device operation follows. Certain minimum standards have been established. The physician and treatment team then review for corrections. If the prosthesis is satisfactory, training can begin. As training proceeds, the occupational therapist may make suggestions for further improvements as the patient utilizes the device.

For a B/E prosthesis, the training program is a matter of about 2 weeks, when done on a daily basis. For the A/E amputee, up to 4 weeks may be necessary. Training of bilateral amputees and patients with more proximal amputations may take longer.

The training will include the care of the skin of the stump, maintenance of stump socks, an explanation of what the prosthetic components are and how they operate, and prosthesis maintenance. The patient first learns controls operation alone so that he understands how the power is transmitted from his own muscles or from external sources to the parts of the artificial limb. After achieving some skill in controls operation, the patient will be taught how to use the prosthesis for the activities of daily living, such as toileting, personal hygiene, eating, dressing, general housework, and driving. Subsequently, the patient is trained in more complex tasks related to actual vocational and recreational needs. The patient also spends progressively more time in public settings to establish confidence, with the knowledge that people will stare and may be inclined to turn away or ask questions. Guidance in these public forays, first with family members or with the occupational therapist and then alone, establishes confidence.

Followup Management

Physician followup will be required weekly at first and then at progressively longer intervals to ensure that there is no stump breakdown and that the prosthesis functions adequately for the patient's needs. In the first 1 to 2 years, followup visits will be required every 3 to 6 months to provide stump socks, to ensure the prosthesis still fits and is functioning properly, for routine professional cleaning and maintenance of the prosthetic components, and to guard against complications. The patient is also instructed to come in sooner if any problem or emergency arises.

A new socket may be needed twice in the first 2 years after provision of the prosthesis, depending upon use, due to a change in stump size caused by skin and muscle atrophy. The first new socket is usually required at 4 to 6 months, and the second at 24 months. Even without a need to change because of stump alteration, a prosthesis may last only 2 or more years, depending upon the severity of use and the care it is given. Whether the patient needs just a socket or a whole prosthesis, and whether any components can be salvaged, varies from patient to patient. Like any mechanical device, if the prosthesis is cared for and used judiciously, it lasts longer than if it is abused.

Vocational Implications

The majority of clients who were engaged in professional, managerial, or executive careers prior to a unilateral arm amputation return to their former employment, especially if they are under 50 years of age. Thus, those whose work is intellectual do well vocationally. The vocational disability of the loss of one or both upper limbs is much greater for those whose former occupation required manual labor.

The lower the educational level, the greater the problem. Careful vocational evaluation and guidance, job training, and education to prepare for white collar employment or more intellectual pursuits are usually required. The counselor must, however, first analyze the client's previous occupation to determine whether the amputation is a real, or only an apparent, vocational impediment. Frequently, modifications of the job task or of specific responsibilities can be made.

Clearly, the bilateral amputee will require an extensive review of his interests, aptitudes, educational level, and skills with prostheses, and perhaps also with his feet, if such dexterity has developed.

The client with congenital limb deficiency may need more extensive psychological review and educational assessment. Education may have been impaired because of multiple medical visits or prior hospitalizations for surgery. Social maturation may be inadequate due to a protective upbringing. These psychosocial factors, rather than physical inability to do a job, may well be the primary vocational problem. More extensive vocational preparation may therefore be required for these clients than for amputees in general.

No prosthesis provides real sensation, though some amputees do get some sense of what is happening at the terminal device from strap and harness pressure. All amputees, however, must use vision to get sensory feedback. Eye-hand coordination and finger-hand dexterity skills are impaired or absent. The client's interests in employment areas that require such skills cannot be developed, and exploration and development of other interests is necessary.

A client who works in an office will generally be advised to have an aluminum hook or a functional hand, while a person who works in a factory or who does heavy manual labor will generally be given a voluntary opening steel hook. A person in contact with the public will generally want a cosmetic hand, but it should be remembered that the cosmetic gloves cannot withstand heavy use. It is quite likely that the client will need different terminal devices for different vocational, recreational, and social activities. The concept of the prosthesis as a tool to perform a certain job is important in this context. Multiple terminal device prescription is therefore generally warranted.

The prosthesis is used for holding, while the normal hand is used for manipulation. If the client's dominant limb has been amputated, job performance will require training to shift dominance to the other side.

The climate in the client's place of residence and the nature of the work environment are very important. Hot, humid environments may induce skin maceration, due to excessive sweating and friction between stump and socket. Loss of heat by the body may be impaired, due both to the socket and to loss of surface area. The macerated skin is easily scraped by repetitive tasks. Working in wet locations may cause prosthesis deterioration. Dust or grit in the environment may be abrasive to the skin and grind the moving parts of the prosthesis. Provided wool stump socks are utilized, cold is less of a problem. The prosthesis must, however, be made of a material that does not transmit cold to the stump readily. The environment may determine the frequency of prosthetic repairs, especially if these factors were not taken into consideration in the initial prescription.

The physical demands of a job are particularly important for the amputee client. The general physical capabilities of clients with amputations at each level are discussed below.

Interscapular-thoracic and shoulder disarticulation. The prostheses for these high-level amputations are essentially cosmetic. The terminal device cannot be operated higher than desk level. Locks can be placed on the elbow to carry objects, but an object placed in the terminal device cannot be lifted by movement of the prosthetic joints (live lift). Lifting can only be accomplished by locking the elbow at an angle, bending down and securing an object in the terminal device, and then straightening up again. The maximum pinch force of the hook is usually only two pounds.

Above-elbow. The A/E amputee can position the terminal device somewhat below shoulder level. Lifting force actively increases to about two pounds greater than the weight of the forearm, but lifting is generally not done. Carrying capacity is considerable, however. Up to 50 or 60 pounds can be carried if the elbow is straight and locked. Pinch force can increase up to four pounds in exceptional cases.

Externally powered elbow joints now coming into use can add more live life at the elbow, up to about four to six pounds, but the rate of lift is slow.

Below-elbow and wrist disarticulation. The terminal device of a B/E prosthesis can be raised to shoulder height. If active motion above the shoulder is required, the shoulder saddle chest strap harness may be used. Lifting force approaches normal if the client has a long stump. The shorter the stump, the less the lifting force. With very short stumps, the lifting force may be no more than one or two pounds in addition to the weight of the prosthetic forearm and hand or hook. Maximum pinch force can be six pounds.

The myoelectric prostheses for B/E amputation with either hands or hooks are generally more suitable for office ("white collar") than for factory ("blue collar") activity. They are not suitable for heavy work.

Partial hand. The partial hand amputee treated with surgical revision or a custom prosthesis for pinch has the advantage of sensation. Special surgery may be needed to ensure that the part of the residual hand that is used for grasping has sensate skin. Lifting force and carrying force are normal.

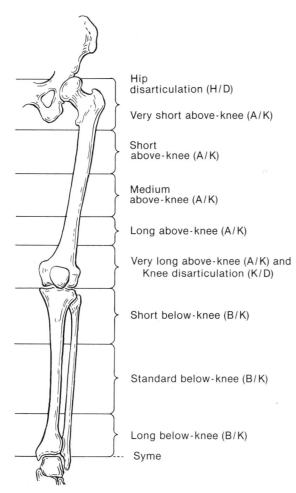

Hip
disarticulation (H/D)

Very short above-knee (A/K)

Short
above-knee (A/K)

Medium
above-knee (A/K)

Long above-knee (A/K)

Very long above-knee (A/K) and
Knee disarticulation (K/D)

Short below-knee (B/K)

Standard below-knee (B/K)

Long below-knee (B/K)

Syme

FIGURE 13-8. Classification of lower extremity amputation levels.

LOWER EXTREMITY AMPUTATION

Levels

The lower extremity amputation levels shown on figure 13-8 are analogous to the upper extremity levels. Congenital lower limb deficiencies, as in the upper limb, can include losses of intermediate segments or partial losses of the separate sections.

The most severe level of amputation is the *hemipelvectomy* (H/P), or *hindquarter* amputation, which removes the limb through half of the pelvis. The soft tissues of the buttock and sides of the trunk become the stump. The sitting bone (ischial tuberosity) is usually absent. The *hip disarticulation* (H/D) preserves the ischial tuberosity and pelvis. The stump remains mostly the soft tissue of the buttock. The *above-knee* (A/K) amputation is the first level to provide a movable stump. If the stump is long enough, the patient has good hip control. The *knee disarticulation* (K/D), a rare amputation, involves provision of healthy skin for weight bearing, and sometimes includes removal of the patella and shaping of the end

of the femur bone. The *below-knee* (B/K) amputation preserves the patella and leaves a functioning knee joint. The *Syme* amputation is a section through the ankle. The sharp projecting ends of the tibia and fibula are removed. Usually a firm soft tissue pad from the heel allows the amputee to walk indoors on the stump end without a prosthesis. *Transmetatarsal* or *partial foot* amputations are usually managed without a prosthesis. A firm shoe reinforced with a steel shank through the sole and simply filled with lamb's wool or other atraumatic material to take up the space is generally all that is required. Partial foot amputations, therefore, will not be further discussed.

The Syme amputation is done mainly for injury. Half of the Syme amputations done for vascular disease (see chap. 22) fail, and a reamputation below the knee, where blood supply is more adequate, is required.

The below-knee amputation is usually the procedure of choice for peripheral arterial disease and in most cases of foot injuries where salvage of the foot is not possible.

The knee disarticulation is generally done for trauma or malignancy in young individuals. If the patient is still growing, a K/D becomes equivalent to an A/K in adulthood due to reduced growth in bone length of the femur.

In the past, above-knee amputations were traditional for severe vascular disease. Improved surgical techniques for repair of clogged arteries and for the amputation itself have decreased the number of A/K procedures. Amputations for bone cancer are usually quite high. An H/D or at least a short A/K is usual.

Functional Disabilities

In lower extremity amputations, the basic function compromised is ambulation. In some patients, transfer skills are also impaired. Personal hygiene, dressing, and eating skills are unimpaired. Hemipelvectomy patients may have toileting problems due to a poor sitting surface. While unilateral amputees quickly achieve transfer skills, bilateral amputees need some time to learn transfers in and out of a wheelchair. Within a few days, unilateral amputees with healthy normal limbs can balance well on one leg and ambulate with underarm and forearm curtches. Bilateral amputees, of course, ambulate via wheelchairs prior to prostheses fitting.

Unilateral amputees, following prosthesis fitting and training, achieve full independence in level-ground ambulation, most stairs and ramps, and driving. The more proximal the amputation, the more difficult ambulation will be on rough, uneven terrain, and the greater the potential need for a cane. Unilateral hip disarticulation and hemipelvectomy patients frequently abandon their prostheses during work because crutch ambulation is faster. They may only use their prostheses for recreation and in social settings for better cosmesis.

Bilateral amputees do not all ambulate satisfactorily with prostheses. If ambulation is achieved, two canes are usually required, and uneven terrain can only rarely be handled. Fitness of the cardiovascular and pulmonary systems is necessary for ambulation because of high energy requirements to walk with two above-knee artificial limbs. All bilateral amputees will use a wheelchair some of the time, and those with limited ambulation will use wheelchairs a major part of the day.

Principles of Management

Preoperative preparation. Patient preparation for a lower extremity amputation is the same as for an upper extremity amputation. Since, however, practically all amputations for vascular disease occur in the lower extremities, the potential amputee with peripheral vascular disease is usually made aware of the following:

1. The physicians and surgeons did their best to save the leg, and at surgery every effort will be made to leave as long a stump as possible consistent with good healing and better function with a prosthesis.
2. The care of the other leg is vital, for while walking may be achieved with one leg amputated, it is difficult or impossible with two, particularly if amputated above the knee.
3. Continuous and indefinite medical supervision will be required, not only for care of the stump, but also for protection of the other leg and management of the arterial disease that necessitated the amputation.

Preoperative preparation includes information concerning the need to maintain range of motion and strength of the residual joints of the amputated as well as the normal leg after surgery. Instruction in necessary exercises can even start before amputation so that the patient understands what will be required.

Surgery. An orthopedic surgeon, a vascular surgeon, or a general surgeon will generally do the surgery. Dressings may include fashioning of a plaster of Paris "socket" over the stump with inclusion of a device to which a temporary prosthetic leg and foot can be attached (fig. 13-9). This early or immediate postoperative fitting technique allows for some standing, weight bearing, and crutch walking with minimal weight bearing within a week.

Postoperative care. The physical therapist works to improve walking function by concentrating not only on the amputated side, but also on general body conditioning. Exercises to strengthen and maintain range of motion of the leg are necessary. Less obvious, but just as important, are exercises to strengthen the abdominal and back muscles. Strengthening of the

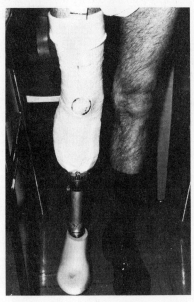

FIGURE 13-9. Below-knee amputation patient with an immediate postoperative prosthesis with plaster socket, leg pylon, and prosthetic foot. The hole in the plaster allows room for the knee cap (patella). By incorporating the knee joint, the plaster prevents knee motion during wound healing. The strap at the top of the plaster socket is tied to a waist belt for suspension. (Photograph courtesy of Prosthetics Research Study, Seattle, WA, Veterans Administration Contract No. V663P-937.)

arms is also required for successful use of the crutches, canes, or walker often required, at least on a temporary basis, after amputation. The physical therapist also works with the patient on transfer skills and crutch ambulation, and provides wheelchair training, if required. Occupational therapy assistance in dressing and personal hygiene skills may be necessary.

The patient is hospitalized at least 2 weeks, but usually longer, before outpatient care is possible. If the immediate-fit technique is used, usually two to three recastings are required. These are made every 1 to 2 weeks until stump shape matures and the patient is ready for a temporary or permanent prosthesis. If rigid plaster cast dressings are not used, a longer period of elastic wrappings is usually necessary, and a temporary prosthesis is used to condition the stump and train the patient.

Prosthesis Description

Walking, the basic lower extremity function, is much less complex than the multiple functions performed by the upper extremities. Prosthetic replacement is therefore easier. The components of the lower limb prosthesis fall into the same general categories as upper limb components and include suspension, socket, joint replacement, and, instead of a terminal device, an ankle-foot assembly.

Suspension. A lower limb prosthesis is heavier than

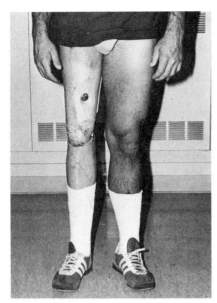

FIGURE 13-10. Patient in an above-knee prosthesis with suction socket suspension. The one-way valve shown at mid-thigh level is located close to the bottom of the total contact socket.

an upper limb prosthesis and therefore suspension is more difficult. Adequate suspension is critical to ensure that the prosthetic leg does not slip off during walking. The many types of suspension available are generally the same in principle as in upper limb prostheses, employing straps, suction, or socket shaping around bony prominences.

Socket. All sockets are made of special plastics. First, a plaster of Paris cast is made of the stump and then a mold of the stump is made from the cast. The socket is made over this mold, and is shaped to support the soft tissues and to transmit body weight to the floor. A special valve may be included in the socket for suction suspension (fig. 13-10).

For most prostheses, except those employing suction suspension, stump socks are required to protect the skin from friction and to absorb perspiration from the skin. They vary in thickness and are added as the stump shrinks. As a general rule, if more than two thick socks are necessary for total contact, a socket adjustment is required.

Joint replacement. Depending on the level of the amputation, the prosthesis replaces the ankle, knee, and hip joints. The ankle replacement may be immovable or movable in a single axis. More elaborate ankle joints are available, but are rarely useful. The many options for knee joint replacement will be discussed below. Hip joint replacements allows single-axis movement only.

Power. In lower extremity prostheses, external sources of power are not required. Energy for advance of the prosthesis during walking is obtained mainly from residual parts. Patients with H/D and H/P amputations advance the thigh portion of the prosthesis by thrusting the lower part of the body

forward. The lower portions of the prosthesis follow automatically. The A/K and B/K prostheses follow the movement of the stump.

Alignment. An additional factor essential in lower extremity prostheses is the vertical alignment of the different components. Balance and support of the body weight while standing on a prosthesis depends on proper alignment of the joints with relation to the patient's center of gravity. In particular, the knee joint axis must be at or behind a vertical line through the center of gravity. Most complaints of knee buckling and balance difficulties can be traced to a faulty alignment. This may be due to an error in fabrication or a reduction in range of motion of the joints remaining after amputation and even of the joints on the normal leg. Flexion contractures of the hip and knee, in particular, may thwart the achievement of a successful alignment. Alignment varies with heel heights of shoes. Therefore, once alignment is established, all shoes worn by the amputee must have identical heel heights. If both low heels and high heels are regularly worn by women, two removable prosthetic feet are required.

Prosthesis Prescription

The prescription of a lower extremity prosthesis takes into consideration the patient's vocational, avocational, and cosmetic needs, whether ambulation will include outdoors as well as indoors, the nature of the terrain expected, and whether canes will be required. Cosmetic factors relate more to how well the patient walks than to the appearance of the prosthesis. While the shape of the prosthesis attempts to reasonably match the normal limb, appearance is not an important issue except for women wearing dresses.

The options available in the various components are discussed below for each amputation level. Prosthesis prescription for congenital lower limb deficiency is consistent with the same principles, but the prostheses are further customized depending upon the character of the residual appendages.

Hemipelvectomy and hip disarticulation. Suspension of the H/P and H/D prosthesis is achieved by shaping the total-contact socket around bony prominences at the pelvis and above. The socket is also secured around the waist with a strap or an extension of the plastic socket. Rarely, straps over the shoulder are required for suspension.

In H/P amputation, the entire mass of soft tissue distributes weight to the prosthesis. In H/D amputation, weight is transmitted to the prosthesis predominantly at the ischial tuberosity. All H/P and H/D sockets include a stump sock.

Prostheses for these high-level amputations replace the hip, knee, and ankle joints. A special prosthesis called the "Canadian-type Hip Disarticulation Prosthesis" is used. It includes a single-axis hip and a knee joint. The stability of these joints in the upright posture is assisted by an elastic strap. The ankle-foot mechanism can be either the single-axis type or an immovable assembly called the Solid Ankle Cushion Heel, or SACH, foot.

A cane is required in most situations. Only one speed of ambulation (very slow) on level ground is possible. Many patients use the prosthesis only for special occasions, preferring to go without the prosthesis and use crutches or a wheelchair for work and more rapid ambulation.

Above-knee. Suction suspension is preferred for the above-knee prostheses (fig. 13-10). For suction suspension, the socket is shaped intimately to the stump in total contact to conform to underlying muscles, and a one-way valve is incorporated near the end of the socket. Air is expelled through the valve when the patient puts his body weight in the socket. When the leg is raised and swung, the force of gravity pulls the artificial leg down, but it does not fall off because the one-way valve does not permit air to rush back into the socket. Air also cannot enter through the top of the socket because of total contact. A relative negative pressure is thus created to hold the stump in the socket. No stump sock is worn with a suction socket. The donning of a prosthesis with suction suspension is difficult and requires good balance and arm strength. It is not advisable for elderly, infirm, or neurologically impaired patients.

Short A/K stumps and stumps that vary in volume do not handle suction suspension well. For these patients, a webbing Silesian band suspension may be added to the prosthesis. If more stability is needed, a metal or plastic joint (hip joint) that lines up with the patient's hip joint is tied to a belt that goes around the patient just below his waist (pelvic band, fig. 13-11). No valve is needed, a stump sock is worn, total contact is still preferred, and the prosthesis is put on more easily than when suction suspension is used. Sometimes a hip joint and pelvic band suspension is used together with suction and a valve.

The most common and preferred A/K socket is the total contact quadrilateral socket, so-called because of its four-sided shape. The older type socket, which was totally round, is rarely prescribed. A depression in the anterior wall of the quadrilateral socket supports the soft tissues and holds the stump so that the patient's ischial tuberosity can "sit" on the top of the posterior wall of the socket (ischial seat). The shape is modified depending upon the amount and nature of the soft tissue, the age of the patient, and the specific medical problem.

There are many possibilities for knee joint replacement to achieve a stable knee during standing and walking. Perhaps more critical than the type of joint selected is the alignment and the amputee's ability to extend his hip and drive the stump against the back

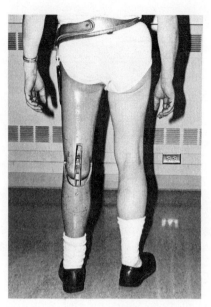

FIGURE 13-11. Patient in an above-knee prosthesis with pelvic band and hip joint suspension. The pelvic (waist) belt connects to the prosthesis via the hip joint on the side next to the patient's left hand. The top of the posterior wall of the socket is flat to provide a platform for the ischial tuberosity. The overhang of buttock skin blocks the view of this platform.

wall of the socket for knee stability. In addition to preventing the knee from buckling, knee joints control the amount of bend that occurs during leg swing.

The "conventional" joint has a single axis. The friction between the moving parts of the joint is set during training to control leg swing. Only one speed of walking is possible with such a constant-friction knee without adverse effects occurring.

Knee joints fitted with any of several types of hydraulic mechanisms have variable friction. The friction automatically increases as speed of walking increases, and decreases as the patient slows down. Walking is therefore more natural. A hydraulic mechanism which couples knee motion with ankle motion is also available and is sometimes preferred over the hydraulic knee alone with a SACH foot. Hydraulic mechanisms are best suited to active, healthy, usually younger A/K amputees who are quite able to maneuver without a cane and can handle suction suspension well. Occasionally, a knee joint will be prescribed with a lock that can be operated manually, not so much for walking, except for the infirm, but rather for standing activities associated with some hand and arm lifting requirements. A "safety knee" is like a constant-friction knee that has an additional component which inhibits buckling. It is sometimes also prescribed, especially for workers who must carry weights.

Ankle and foot replacement is usually with a SACH foot. A single-axis ankle joint may be prescribed for less agile amputees or for use where the terrain may

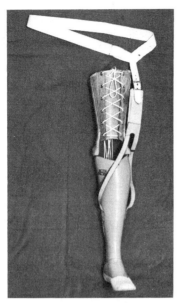

FIGURE 13-12. Below-knee prosthesis with thigh lacer, waist belt suspension, and single-axis ankle and foot.

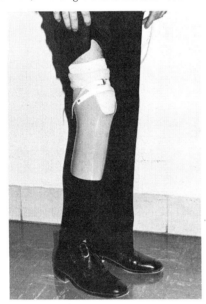

FIGURE 13-13. Below-knee prosthesis with cuff above the patella for suspension. Side-to-side (mediolateral) stability is achieved by extension of the sides of the socket across the knee joint rather than by the lacer and side joints as in figure 13-12.

not be quite flat. More complex ankle joints are available and should be carefully considered. They provide flexibility, but less stability.

Knee disarticulation. Suspension of the K/D prosthesis is achieved by waist belt and, in part, by socket shaping. The socket is shaped around the thigh if the end of the stump is bulbous, and may extend to include an ischial seat as in the A/K socket. More likely, weight transmits to the prosthesis from the end of the stump. The socket has a trap door or expandable walls to allow the femoral condyles to reach the bottom

of the socket.

The knee joint replacement is usually a hinge placed on the side of the socket above the end of the stump rather than at the end of the stump. This joint allows the knee to flex, but does not allow the prosthesis to extend beyond a straight position. Restraining straps are sometimes required to reduce the speed of the lower leg swing during ambulation. Polycentric hydraulic knee units are now available. Ankle-foot assemblies are usually SACH.

Below-knee. For suspension of the B/K prosthesis, the socket may be formed around the bony prominences about the knee joint. There are two types of such suspensions: the supracondylar, which shapes over the bony end of the femur, and the suprapatellar, which shapes over the patella. More commonly, suspension is achieved by a strap anchored above the patella. Waist belt suspension is also sometimes required, and when used, a leather thigh lacer may be added (fig. 13-12). The thigh lacer is tied to the prosthesis via metal joints that coincide with the knee joint.

The socket for B/K prostheses is designed so that the weight is borne almost entirely on the patellar tendon and the medial part of the tibia. Some weight is borne on the thigh if a thigh lacer is used. This is most important for obese patients and workers carrying heavy loads or walking a great deal. The socket must also be designed to relieve certain parts of the leg below the knee of pressure. The most common prosthetic socket design is the patellar tendon bearing, or PTB, socket (fig. 13-13). Variants of this design may assist slightly with weight bearing, but generally are variations in methods of suspension. The socket types, by name, include PTB with suprapetellar strap suspension, PTS (supracondylar-suprapatellar suspension), and PTB with thigh lacer and knee joints. Total contact, either soft, moderately firm, or hard, is used in most, but not all, below-knee sockets. An air cushion at the end of a socket is a variant of total contact.

In some B/K sockets, soft padding material is required. This may be cotton or wool prosthetic socks, a soft insert liner of sponge rubber and leather (Kemblo liner), or a sponge or foam plastic material. An insert liner also helps the prosthetist adjust the socket for stump changes. Its use to compensate for errors in fabrication is very undesirable.

A SACH foot is the ankle-foot mechanism of choice. A single-axis ankle is sometimes used for a short B/K or when a thigh lacer is used.

Syme amputation. Suspension of the prosthesis for Syme amputation is achieved by shaping the socket to the lower leg over the bulbous end of the stump (fig. 13-14). No straps are necessary.

Generally, the equivalent of a B/K prosthesis with a trap door or expandable walls to accommodate the bulbous distal end of the stump at the ankle is

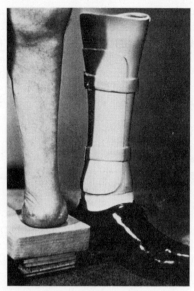

FIGURE 13-14. Syme amputation stump alongside the Syme prosthesis. Trap door allows the bulbous end of the stump to be inserted into the socket. The trap door is secured by Velcro straps after the stump is inserted.

required. The Syme socket widens the ankle and has a poor appearance. Body weight transmits to the prosthesis directly from the end of the stump, with some weight bearing at the patellar tendon. The SACH foot is used.

Prosthesis Checkout and Training

Prosthetic checkout is usually done by the physical therapist and reviewed by the physician, often with the prosthetist and the other treatment team members. Determining whether the prosthesis was made as prescribed is followed by review of socket fit, presence of total contact, adequacy of suspension, proper distribution of weight bearing to the prosthesis, and careful attention to the alignment. The prosthesis is best delivered to the patient at the center, so that initial wear proceeds under supervision of the physician and/or physical therapist. Often it is delivered unfinished to allow for changes in alignment based on what is seen during walking (dynamic alignment).

Ambulation training begins with simple standing balance training in the parallel bars. Training then progresses to walking, first in the bars with hand support, then out of the bars with cane support, and then without support. Training proceeds under supervision until good habits, stability, safety, and independence develop. Gradual increase in wear time helps in stump conditioning. Daily training for 3 to 6 weeks or longer may be required, particularly for A/K and higher amputations, before skills are sufficient for independent walking.

Techniques for climbing stairs and ramps are taught next. A/K and higher level amputees usually climb stairs one at a time, going up with the normal leg first and going down with the prosthetic leg first. Generalization of skills to outdoors, public transportation, automobiles, and work-related activities may then follow. The training period for bilateral amputees is longer than that required for unilateral amputees.

Throughout the training period, the stump is carefully examined for unusual pressure points requiring socket correction. Care of the prosthesis and the stump is taught simultaneously. The need to wash the stump daily, change and wash stump socks daily, and wash the inside of the socket every night is emphasized. The components of the prosthesis are explained to the patient, and danger signs that might appear on the stump or with the prosthesis are also explained.

Followup Management

Monthly followup visits are required intitially, and less often later, to monitor the patient's general condition, and for stump inspection, component checkout, and shoe wear. The physician will also examine the cancer patient for evidence of metastases and recommend any necessary additional treatment. For patients with peripheral arterial disease, followup must include inspection of the other limb. Further, underlying diabetes, if present, must be managed.

Stump shrinkage will require modifying the size of the socket. This can be accomplished initially by filling the socket in or by adding additional stump socks if they are worn. Eventually, a new socket will be required, usually after 6 months in the first year and every 1 to 2 years thereafter. A whole new prosthesis may be required in 3 to 5 years due to component breakdown.

Vocational Implications

Long-term planning can and should be considered for the amputee. However, clients whose amputations were associated with cancer and peripheral vascular disease may require short-term vocational training. Also, the eventual vocational evaluation and training of child amputees must not be neglected. For children over the age of 12, evaluation of interests and vocational potential by a vocational counselor, if one is available, is recommended. Such evaluation can help direct the child's education toward areas consistent with the amputation or limb deficiency. The earlier such planning begins, the less difficulty is encountered in the adult years.

The vocational plan for the amputee must take into consideration the environment in which the client will work. Unusually warm environments cause sweating of the stump and may cause skin problems. Stump volume may also change. Cold environments can be harmful, and excessively dusty or sandy areas may injure the prosthetic components.

The vocational implications of lower extremity amputation are primarily concerned with the physical demands of a job, particularly walking, climbing, standing, pushing, pulling, and balancing. These functions will be impaired to varying degrees, depending on the level of the amputation and whether the amputation is unilateral or bilateral.

Walking with a prosthesis is more difficult on uneven ground and on sand or mud. Climbing stairs, walking up and down ramps, and walking up hills usually present difficulties, and therefore jobs involving these activities to a considerable degree are best avoided.

Carrying objects is impossible if the client uses two canes, crutches, or a walker because his hands are occupied. Even with no cane, carrying capacity is limited because the weight of the carried object throws off the person's alignment.

Clients with unilateral amputations or bilateral below-knee amputations can drive a vehicle with automatic transmission with no difficulty. Clients with bilateral above-knee amputations will require a special vehicle with hand controls. Some jobs requiring driving may therefore be considered.

The following discussion deals with the more specific vocational implications of lower extremity amputations at the various levels.

Hemipelvectomy and hip disarticulation. With a prosthesis, clients with amputations at these high levels will expend 75 percent more energy than nonamputees to walk the same distance on level ground. Jobs in which the client will mainly be seated, with very little walking required, are appropriate. Such jobs will generally be indoors. Clients with bilateral amputations at these levels will require a wheelchair for work.

Above-knee. A client with bilateral above-knee amputations would expend so much energy to walk that he would frequently have no energy left for a job. A wheelchair is therefore required for employment, especially for clients middle aged or older. The unilateral above-knee amputee expends about 60 percent more energy walking with a prosthesis than a nonamputee walking the same distance. The higher the level of the unilateral amputation, the greater the need for a cane or a crutch, and consequently the greater the likelihood of carrying limitations. More sedentary occupations with slight walking or carrying requirements are therefore best.

Below-knee. With a prosthesis, the unilateral below-knee amputee will expend only 10 percent more energy than a nonamputee to walk on level ground. The only function definitely impaired is running, although walking on rough ground, especially if it is hilly, may also present some difficulties. Walking in sand may also cause some problems, but special prostheses can be

made for this activity. Stairs do not present a significant problem, and all-day standing and heavy work are possible.

Syme and partial foot. The vocational implications of these amputations are essentially the same as for the below-knee amputation.

COMPLICATIONS AND THEIR TREATMENT

The complications of amputation are the same for upper and lower extremity amputations. They include edema, skin ulceration, contractures, infections, pain, bone overgrowth, and scoliosis.

Edema

Stump edema in the immediate period after amputation needs to be controlled and resolved before a permanent prosthetic socket is fitted. Of greater concern is stump edema that develops in the course of prosthesis wear, which usually means that there is some constriction of the stump or greater pressures higher up on the stump than at the more terminal end. The higher pressures block the return of venous blood to the heart, causing a backup of blood in the veins of the stump and extrusion of fluid through the capillary walls into the tissues. Assuming the prosthesis socket was originally fitted correctly, the usual cause is shrinkage of the stump with time and wear. Constriction can occur when the shrinkage is uneven and the distal end of the stump has more room than the proximal end. In particular, proximal constriction can develop when the amputee increases the number of stump socks he wears to make up for shrinkage at the end.

Edema can occur with stump shrinkage as a direct result of trauma at the end of the stump, particularly in the lower extremity if the stump bears weight improperly.

Edema must be recognized early before it proceeds to ulceration. Chronic edema can be recognized by discoloration of the stump caused by rupture of the capillaries. Treatment requires re-establishment of a proper socket-stump fit and usually means a new socket, although sometimes modification of the old socket can suffice. Before the patient again wears the prosthesis with the new or modified socket, the edema must be resolved.

Ulceration

Ulceration in the skin of the stump occurring during prosthesis wear may be secondary either to excess pressure or to chronic edema. In the upper extremity, excess pressure may occur with chronic lifting or heavy use if stump shrinkage has destroyed total contact. Ulceration due to pressure also occurs in the lower extremity if socket fit is lost and parts of the stump take more pressure on weight bearing than they can withstand.

In both instances, the treatment required is usually a new socket. Some control of the ulceration may be necessary before the new socket can be fabricated, although in some cases the new socket can be fabricated and the prosthesis again worn even though the ulceration is still present. With a good fit, the ulceration can usually heal during prosthesis wear.

Contractures

Joint contractures are not a complication of prosthesis use, but rather a consequence of events prior to the amputation. In particular, contractures may occur as a result of efforts to save the limb over an extended perod of time during which the extremity is inactive and treatment needs prevent full joint range of motion. Failure to recognize that the uninvolved joints must have range-of-motion exercises to preserve their mobility can also result in contractures. In the upper extremity, contractures at the shoulder or elbow will interfere with operation of the prosthesis, and in the lower extremity, contractures at the hip or knee will reduce stability in standing and limit the patient's walking capability.

Physical therapeutic exercises can reverse contractures in most cases, and surgery to manipulate the joint or actually cut the tight structures may help. Contractures are always easier to prevent than to correct.

Limitations of joint motion may also occur secondary to scarring of the skin across the joint from healed burns or from major injury. Correction by plastic surgery (see chap. 32) may help improve the skin problem and subsequently the joint range of motion.

Infection

Stump infection may occur if an ulceration becomes contaminated, or simply through neglect of stump cleanliness leading to an infected hair follicle or sweat gland. Careful daily cleansing of the stump, stump socks, and the socket prevents such infections from developing. Treatment of stump infections may require surgical incision to drain the pus, and associated antibiotic treatment may be indicated.

Pain

The pain problems associated with amputation and prosthesis wear are many and varied. Relatively circumscribed local pain may be due to a neuroma. When an amputation is performed, the nerves, of course, are also cut. The ends of the cut nerves heal with the formation of a scar containing a bundle of nerve fibers called a neuroma. Under excess pressure,

these neuromas can produce pain, which the patient perceives as existing not only in the stump but also in the amputated limb (phantom limb) from which the cut nerve formerly carried impulses.

The first treatment approach to a painful neuroma is a correct socket fit. If this is not sufficient, efforts to desensitize the neuroma through injections and ultrasound therapy may help. Sometimes increasing the sensory stimulation coming from the limb by periodically rubbing, tapping, and massaging it can reduce the sensitivity of a neuroma. If these approaches are not successful, surgery may be necessary to excise the neuroma and place the residual nerve in a more protected location in the stump. Such a procedure may change the shape of the stump and therefore necessitate a new socket.

Pain localized in the stump but more diffuse than pain from a neuroma may also occur. In the absence of any underlying bone spur (see below), this type of pain is caused by improper socket fit.

Another type of pain associated with amputation is phantom pain. This must be distinguised from phantom sensation, which is the sensation that the amputated body part is still present and which is experienced by all adult amputees. Phantom sensation diminishes with time, but it may last a lifetime. Patients with congenital limb deficiency or who have had surgical or traumatic amputations before the age of 4 do not usually experience phantom sensation or phantom pain.

Unlike phantom sensation, phantom pain can be disabling. There are three types of phantom pain. The least serious type is a vaguely distributed discomfort in the phantom limb associated with muscle tenderness or spasm in the stump. This is commonly caused by improper socket fit, and correction of this problem usually eliminates the phantom pain. Exercise of the phantom is helpful.

The second type of phantom pain is an electric-shock-like discomfort in the phantom limb which lasts for a few moments and then disappears. It is generally associated with a neuroma under excess pressure and resolves with treatment of the neuroma itself. It may also be due to pressure on the nerve caused by an ill-fitting prosthesis.

The third and most severe type of phantom pain is a burning, agonizing discomfort throughout the stump and in the phantom limb. The stump may feel warm or cold or appear mottled, but it may appear quite normal. Clothing or a breath of air suddenly touching the stump can trigger the pain. The patient may find it necessary to wrap his stump in protective towels to avoid the sudden touch.

A gradual increase in the amount of sensation from the stump by more sustained prosthesis wear, or by rubbing, tapping, or heating the stump may block this agonizing discomfort. Surgical excision of the sympathetic nerves is sometimes helpful. Intractable phantom pain may require neurosurgical procedures on the spinal cord.

Back pain, particularly low back pain, can develop secondary to walking on a prosthesis for A/K amputation. This type of pain is caused by excessive motion of the pelvis and lower spine produced by hip flexion contractures or simply by improper prosthetic alignment. Careful examination by physicians skilled in both prosthesis use and back pain problems may be necessary to identify and correct the problem.

Finally, pain due to factors totally unrelated to the stump and the prosthesis may be perceived by the patient as coming from the stump or the phantom limb. When, for example, a herniated intervertebral disc (see chap. 15) impinges on a spinal nerve, referred pain is perceived in those areas where nerve fibers ordinarily contained in the spinal nerve originated. Again, a careful evaluation by a physician knowledgeable in prosthetics and vertebral column problems can help resolve and correct referred pain of this type.

Bone Overgrowth

There are two types of bone overgrowth, one associated with surgical amputation and one associated with congenital limb deficiency or amputation in the growing child. Surgical amputations require cutting of the bone and therefore cutting the periosteum, the covering of the bone which has the capacity of producing new bone elements. If shreds of periosteum are left in the stump at the time of surgery, they develop into bone spurs which change the effective shape of the stump and produce local pain. Correction requires surgery to remove the spur and the shreds of periosteum.

In the young amputee or the patient with congenital limb deficiency, bone overgrowth means that the stump bone increases in length faster than the skin of the stump grows. The bone end begins to push through the skin. When feasible, skin traction is the preferred treatment because, if successful, no stump shortening results. If stump shortening is necessary, surgery can be performed to put a bend in the bone and effectively reduce its length, or the end of the bone is cut off.

Scoliosis

In patients with high upper extremity amputations, spinal curvature (scoliosis) may occur secondary to imbalance of the trunk. In lower extremity amputees, scoliosis may occur secondary to unequal leg lengths or insufficient use and wear of the prosthesis. Trunk exercises as a regular routine for high upper extremity amputees and careful attention to length at the time of prosthesis prescription for lower extremity amputees helps prevent the development of scoliosis. Once scoliosis develops and becomes fixed, it is hard to reverse. If severe, particularly in the growing child,

surgical spinal fusion to prevent progression may be required if special bracing does not arrest or retard progression.

Other Complications

Some patients may have significant complications associated with their underlying diseases, which may in part have contributed to the amputation, rather than with the amputation or prosthesis wear itself. Patients with peripheral vascular disease, such as that associated with diabetes, may have visual problems, cardiac problems, or cerebral problems due to arterial disease elsewhere (see chaps. 22 and 24). Patients with heart and pulmonary disease in association with, or incidental to, amputation may become limited because of the extra energy requirements of walking with an artificial limb, particularly if the amputation is above the knee. The heart and lungs may not have sufficient reserve to handle the extra energy requirements and walking may therefore be more limited. Patients whose amputations are associated with arthritis (see chap. 14) may find themselves limited because the residual joints are not sufficiently normal to handle the extra demands placed on them. Patients with cancer (see chap. 28) may have additional difficulties.

CONCLUSION

The above review of amputations and prosthetics is simply the current picture. Perhaps more than with other disabilities, this picture is ever changing. Research by the Veterans Administration and in university and industrial laboratories has been productive in the past and promises to continue to be so in the future. Advances in the fields of prosthetics and in reconstructive surgical techniques is to be expected.

The counselor should be alert to new developments to ensure that his client receives those services likely to be of added benefit. The *Bulletin of Prosthetics Research*, a semiannual publication of the Veterans Administration which is available through the U.S. Government Printing Office, is currently the best source for keeping abreast of new developments.

BIBLIOGRAPHY

Barnett AJ, Twist E, Balfe A: Lower limb amputation in a general hospital: A comparative review. Med J Aust 2:14–18, 1976.
Report of a study of lower limb amputees from 1970-1973 compared with a similar 1964 study. Mobility, independence, use of prostheses, medical condition, and mortality are discussed.
Caine D: Psychological considerations affecting rehabilitation after amputation. Med J Aust 2:818–821, 1973.
Short article describing reactions to amputations in children, adolescents, adults, and the aged. Useful because it highlights the attitude and techniques most likely to aid

in the adjustment of amputee clients to their disability.

Friedmann LW: Rehabilitation of amputees. *In* Licht HM: *Rehabilitation and Medicine*, Licht, New Haven, 1968.

An extensive review of upper and lower extremity amputation and prosthetics. Useful for those needing greater elaboration of the material covered in this presentation. In particular, more training detail is given and a section on the juvenile amputee is included.

Friedmann LW: *The Psychological Rehabilitation of the Amputee*. Springfield, IL, Thomas, 1978.

Covers phantom limb sensation, phantom pain, and common emotional reactions to amputation and prosthesis wear.

Klopsteg PE, Wilson PD (eds): *Human Limbs and Their Substitutes*. New York, McGraw-Hill, 1954.

Presents results of engineering and medical studies of the human extremities and application of the data to the design and fitting of artificial limbs and to the care and training of amputees.

Miller LS, Naso F: Conditioning program for amputees with significant heart disease. Arch Phys Med Rehabil **57**:238–240, 1976.

Lower extremity amputees with heart disease were first stress tested and were then placed in a conditioning program. Reports the effect of the program on ambulation ability.

Murdoch G (ed): *Prosthetic and Orthotic Practice*. London, Arnold, 1970.

Detailed discussion of prosthetics and orthotics. Helpful for the counselor who requires additional information.

Parks CM: Psychosocial transitions: Comparison between reactions to loss of a limb and loss of a spouse. Brit J Psychiatry **127**:204–210, 1975.

A study of the similarities and differences between the experience of losing a limb and losing a spouse. Discusses the process of ''realizing the loss,'' which includes phases of numbness, pining, disorganization, and reorganization.

Parkes MC, Napier MM: Psychiatric sequelae of amputation. Br J Psychiatry Spec No **9**:440–446, 1975.

An excellent review of the psychological responses to amputations, psychosocial factors affecting employment, psychological factors associated with phantom limb pain, and methods of prevention and alleviation of these problems.

14 RHEUMATIC DISEASES

John J. Nicholas, M.D.

INTRODUCTION

The rheumatic diseases include all those diseases and syndromes that involve joints, chiefly the synovial joints, and/or the soft tissue structures around them (para-articular structures). In some of these conditions, the joint (rheumatic) complaints occur irregularly or constitute only a minor problem. In others, the joint disease may play an important or a dominant role in the patient's illness. The classification of the rheumatic diseases established by the American Rheumatism Association, the professional medical organization devoted to arthritis and rheumatism, actually lists 113 diseases and syndromes distributed over 13 general classes of disorders. With new knowledge, this classification undergoes periodic review.

The prevalence of the rheumatic diseases in the United States is quite large. A recent Arthritis Foundation survey indicated that 31.6 million persons in the United States suffer from rheumatic disease. The prevalence in persons under 45 years old was 48 per thousand, while in individuals over 45 and under 65 it was 333 per thousand. The prevalence rates for women were higher than those for men at every level, and two-thirds of those afflicted were women. The incidence of all forms of arthritis is now estimated at 900,000 new cases per year.

The three diseases discussed in this chapter, rheumatoid arthritis, ankylosing spondylitis, and degenerative joint disease (DJD), are particularly important because of their frequency, their disabling character, and their occurrence in the working age group. Rheumatoid arthritis and ankylosing spondylitis are both in the category "polyarthritis of unknown etiology," and degenerative joint disease occupies a category all its own. The latter appears both in primary and secondary forms (secondary meaning an occurrence as a result of some other problems).

The incidence of rheumatoid arthritis is estimated at 500 per 1 million population per year. It may be found in about 3.2 percent of the general population, with women having the disease three times as often as men. DJD is a ubiquitous condition which steadily increases in frequency with age and affects men and women equally.

The section on the musculoskeletal system in chapter 3 should be studied by the reader. An appreciation of the normal character of this system allows for a better understanding of the disturbances that occur in rheumatoid arthritis, ankylosing spondylitis, and degenerative joint disease.

RHEUMATOID ARTHRITIS

Disease Description

Rheumatoid arthritis is a total body (systemic) disease characterized chiefly by inflammation of the synovial joints. Since these joints are designed both to allow motion and to bear weight, motion restrictions and weight-bearing problems can be an early consequence of the disease. In particular, the shoulder, elbow, wrist, hip, knee, ankle, and the small joints of the hands and feet are affected by rheumatoid arthritis. In addition, many tendons and ligaments that are lined with synovial tissue are also inflamed in rheumatoid arthritis.

Rheumatoid arthritis may occur in persons of any age, but children aged 2 to 4, women in the fourth and fifth decade, and men and women over the age of 50 are the most susceptible.

Figure 3-17 and page 32 describe the anatomy of a synovial joint and the location of the thin synovial tissue layer. This tissue produces the fluid (synovial fluid) which lubricates the joints and provides cells that "eat up" the debris from normal wear. When a synovial joint develops rheumatoid arthritis, huge numbers of small round cells (lymphocytes) which manufacture antibodies invade the synovial tissue, accompanied by new blood vessels and often a collection of fibrin (a protein essential for blood clotting). As a result, the synovial tissue increases in size (hypertrophies) and bulges out under the skin covering the joint. Substances elaborated from the cells cause the joint cartilage to wear away and the joint capsule to stiffen and become thin. The cellular activity also causes the adjacent bone to thin and lose strength.

189

Further, the hypertrophied synovial tissue invades the bone and "eats it away," forming defects in the bone called *erosions*, which are noted on X-rays and are characteristic of rheumatoid arthritis. The synovial tissue around tendons and ligaments similarly thins and weakens these structures.

The disease may start suddenly with rapid onset of heat, swelling, pain, and tenderness in multiple joints. In other patients, a decrease in range of joint motion may be noted for many months or years before the heat, redness, tenderness, and swelling appear. Corresponding joints on both sides of the body are usually involved, and the inflammation is persistent.

The amount of synovial fluid increases in many of the involved joints and it is filled with white cells. Subcutaneous nodules characteristically develop at the elbow, but may also occur at other points where pressure is applied to the skin, e.g., over the bridge of the nose, on the sacrum or ischial tuberosities, or over the knuckles. The patient will usually report that use of the affected joint and weight bearing cause an increase in the inflammation and that he can predict a change in the weather by noting increased stiffness and pain.

The cause of rheumatoid arthritis is not known, but the bulk of the current evidence points to an immune or allergic reaction by the body to an unknown invader (antigen). Currently, it is thought that this antigen is probably a virus that persists in the body, causing an immunity to develop which is transferred to some of the body's own structures. In other words, the body's usual defenders against allergy attack the joints, tendons, and bones as if they were the invaders. This theory is supported by the existence of an antibody called "the rheumatoid factor," which is found in the blood of about 80 percent of patients who have had arthritis for several months. This antibody is usually a large protein molecule that interacts with the patient's normal gamma globulins (antibodies). The rheumatoid factor is manufactured by inflammatory cells in the synovial tissue. Experimental animals develop a persistent arthritis similar to rheumatoid arthritis after being inoculated with various protein substances similar to these antibodies, verifying this hypothesis in part.

Muscle weakness and reduction in muscle size (atrophy) appears in many patients soon after the onset of arthritis. The muscles within the hand, for instance, weaken early and can rarely be strengthened. When the shoulder joint becomes inflamed, the shoulder muscles weaken and also remain weak. The exact cause of the muscle wasting and weakness in patients with rheumatoid arthritis is not clear. The avoidance of motion to prevent pain, the invasion of lymphocytes into the muscle, and perhaps a lack of nerve impulses all contribute to muscle weakness.

Loss of joint movement is the impairment in rheumatoid arthritis. Some patients report they are "paralyzed," but they are not. There is simply so much pain on motion that they cannot make themselves move and the lack of movement allows their muscles to become weak and atrophic. The combination of unwillingness to move and muscle weakness diminishes the patient's ability to perform activities requiring both strength and dexterity. The functional and vocational skills of the patient may be impaired early by the inflammation, pain, lack of movement, and weakness.

If the inflammation clears after several weeks, there may be no residual impairment. If, however, the inflammation persists, the patient will find he has developed a permanent loss of joint motion. If the inflammation in a particular joint cannot be satisfactorily treated, the early loss of joint motion will persist and lead to the gross and readily observable deformities which are characteristic of patients with rheumatoid arthritis. These permanent deformities change the mechanics of the joint so that it cannot function well, even though pain and inflammation may have subsided.

The early and late deformities have been well described for many years and should be recognized by those involved in the care of patients with rheumatoid arthritis. In the hand, a common initial deformity is the inability to bend (flex) the knuckles fully. Subsequently, an exaggerated flexion of the middle knuckle (the boutonniere deformity) may appear (fig. 14-1). In other patients, the "swan's neck" deformity, with exaggerated straightening of the middle knuckle, develops (fig. 14-2). The knuckle (metacarpophalangeal) joint of the hand may fail and the finger bones slip underneath it (metacarpophalangeal subluxation, fig. 14-3). Also at this same joint, the fingers may bend over toward the little finger side of the hand (ulnar deviation, fig. 14-4). Surprisingly, many patients with these deformities are able to continue performing their various activities of daily living as well as nondexterous vocational tasks.

At the wrist, the deformity is an inability to bend (flex) or straighten (extend). With severe disease, an exaggerated flexion occurs and the joint may be nearly dislocated (subluxed).

Deformities also occur at other joints. At the neck, they may limit rotation, and at the hip, they may limit rotation or extension. Other deformities cause the knee to become permanently flexed, the ankle to bend outward, and the foot to become flat.

These deformities occur singly or at many joints. While it is impossible to predict which patient will get which deformity, it is possible to predict which deformities will occur at which joint. The efforts of physicians and allied health professionals are required to perhaps prevent, but more likely to delay and possibly correct, these deformities. Their efforts should be supported throughout by the counselor.

Patients frequently act on two misconceptions with which the counselor should be thoroughly familiar.

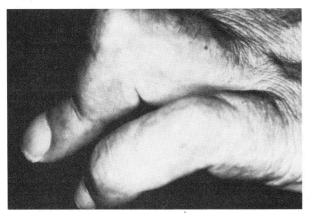

FIGURE 14-1. Ring and little fingers of left hand of a patient with rheumatoid arthritis. So-called "boutonniere" deformity is present in the ring finger (top). Proximal interphalangeal joint (see p. 35) is fixed in flexion, and distal interphalangeal joint is fixed in extension. This hand, therefore, does not fully open.

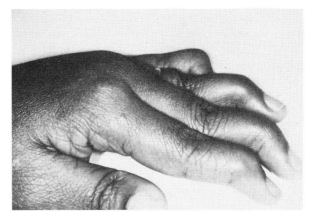

FIGURE 14-2. Left hand of a patient with rheumatoid arthritis. So-called "swan's neck" deformity is present in all four fingers. The proximal interphalangeal joint is fixed in extension. The distal interphalangeal joint is fixed in flexion. This hand, therefore, does not fully close.

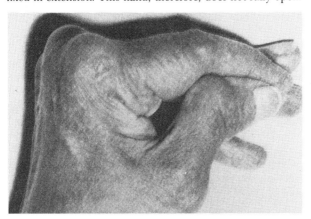

FIGURE 14-3. Left hand of a patient with rheumatoid arthritis showing near dislocation (subluxation) of knuckle (metacarpophalangeal) joints and distal joint of the thumb. This hand will not fully open and will have weak pinch force.

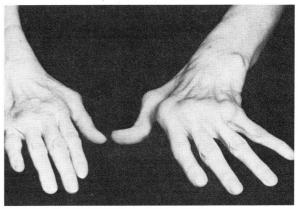

FIGURE 14-4. Hands of a patient with rheumatoid arthritis. Left hand demonstrates subluxation of knuckle (metacarpophalangeal) joints with deviation of fingers away from the thumb (ulnar deviation). This hand will have weak pinch and grasp and will open incompletely.

The first is that it is mandatory for them to "keep going" or they will stiffen up and become deformed. At the heart of this misconception is the subjective feeling of stiffness that rheumatoid patients notice on arising in the morning. However, there is no evidence that this morning stiffness leads to permanent deformity, especially if the patient performs his prescribed exercises conscientiously. The patient may be motivated by morning stiffness to pace up and down or perform activities that may lessen his feeling of stiffness, but may actually increase the inflammation and joint destruction.

The second misconception patients frequently have is that their ordinary work and play activities are as beneficial as any special therapeutic exercise. This is not true. Therapeutic exercise allows the patient to move a joint in a direction that he has neglected because of pain. During work or play, this motion is usually ignored or avoided because of pain. A therapeutic exercise may be directed at strengthening a muscle by graded maximum contractions that fall short of exhaustion and are designed to cause minimum joint motion. During work or play, the patient must follow whatever motions are required by the activity and may contract his muscles to the point of fatigue. A therapeutic exercise is not designed to force the patient to move his joint so frequently that the inflammation is increased, whereas a particular activity may require that the patient repeat the same maneuver over and over until his joint "cries out" in pain. This "work equals exercise" misconception is as common among housewives as among laborers. The counselor may reinforce the suggestions of the therapist by recommending that his client avoid work which leaves him inflamed and fatigued and perhaps unable to perform the exercises that could strengthen and correct deformities and weakness of his joints.

Complications. There are a number of complications

of rheumatoid arthritis. These include the carpal tunnel syndrome, Sjögren's syndrome, peripheral neuropathy, pleural effusion, Baker's cyst, and anemia.

The *carpal tunnel syndrome* is characterized by numbness and tingling and eventual loss of feeling in the thumb, index finger, and middle finger. The small muscles of the thumb may fail to function. This syndrome occurs when the hypertrophied synovial tissue fills the narrow tunnel at the wrist through which the median nerve (see p. 104) travels from the forearm to the hand. Failure of the function of the compressed median nerve causes the tingling and loss of strength.

In *Sjögren's (show-grens) syndrome,* multitudes of lymphocytes invade the glands of the mouth, nose, eyes, throat, and lungs and cause the patient to suffer dry eyes (keratoconjuntivitis sicca) and dry mouth (xerostomia). The loss of the glandular function may cause ulcers of the eye tissue, serious dental caries, and an inability to chew food normally. When dry eyes and dry mouth occur alone, the "sicca syndrome" is said to be present. When the sicca syndrome is accompanied by rheumatoid arthritis, the condition is termed Sjögrens syndrome. The lymphocytes also invade the kidney, liver, and lungs, causing these organs to function poorly.

Many rheumatoid arthritis patients with *peripheral neuropathy* complain of mild numbness and tingling in their fingers and toes (see chap. 7). Rarely, however, do they lose complete function of a major nerve. This loss of nerve function is due to inflammation of the blood vessels that supply these nerves. When one nerve is involved, it is termed a *mononeuritis,* and when more than one are involved, it is termed a *mononeuritis multiplex.* This condition may remit spontaneously or require drastic medical treatment. *Vasculitis,* the blood vessel inflammation, it also thought to be the cause of both the subcutaneous nodules and the shallow, painful ulcers which may occur on the patient's ankles. These ulcers probably occur following minor trauma. They then may become infected and fail to heal. Many days of disability may result, and prolonged hospitalization may be required.

Pleural effusion may occur in rheumatoid arthritis patients. Commonly, patients will have X-rays showing some mild accumulations of scars in the lungs, but these findings are rarely of significance. However, on occasion the patient may develop a collection of fluid (pleural effusion) in the pleural space (see p. 44). This accumulation causes little harm but must be carefully distinguished from cancer, tuberculosis, bacterial infection, and heart failure. In addition, nodules may also develop in the lungs and these must be distinguished from the more serious but similar-looking nodules of cancer, tuberculosis, fungus infection, and pneumonia.

Baker's cyst occurs when inflamed synovial fluid escapes from the knee and collects in the space behind the knee, with extension into the calf. Patients who have only recently developed rheumatoid arthritis may complain of sudden pain and swelling in the calf of the leg caused by this escape of fluid. Baker's cyst must be distinguished from thrombophlebitis of the calf veins (see chap. 22). Patients who have had rheumatoid arthritis for a longer period of time may develop a chronic escape of fluid in the calf. This may respond to treatment of the knee disease. Surgical removal of the cyst is occasionally required.

The *anemia* of rheumatoid arthritis has two sources. Chronic inflammation can affect the production of the red cell elements of the bone marrow. Further, the various medications used in the treatment of this disease may contribute to chronic, very low-grade blood leakage from the stomach walls. In some patients, actual ulceration of the stomach walls can occur. Anemia may contribute to the fatigue experienced by the patient with rheumatoid arthritis. If anemia is severe, it can weaken the patient sufficiently to cause him to become more susceptible to other diseases.

Prognosis. The general course of rheumatoid arthritis is characterized by gradual diminution of inflammation and progression of deformity and crippling. The speed with which the deformities occur varies from patient to patient, but their progression can be anticipated, observed, and measured. On occasion, patients with rheumatoid arthritis appear to lose all signs of inflammation and are said to have undergone a remission. The usual course, however, is for the deformities to progress and persist.

A physician who has observed a patient with active rheumatoid arthritis for several months is in a position to evaluate the prognosis and to discuss this cautiously, yet realistically, with the patient and the rehabilitation counselor. Factors associated with a poor prognosis include persistent disease of more than 1 year's duration and an age below 30, coupled with the presence of subcutaneous nodules and high titers of rheumatoid factor. On the whole, however, about 50 percent of the patients are in the so-called stationary or unimproved category after 10 years of the disease. If there is no improvement by that time, there is little likelihood that it will occur. The counselor can assume that the course of the client's disease will be no better and that deformities probably will be worse in subsequent years.

Functional Disabilities

Physical Disabilities. The interference in motion induced by pain, the loss of proper mechanical joint motion due to deformities, and the loss of strength all may markedly limit the patient's activities. The particular activity impaired depends upon which joints are involved. If the shoulders and hands are involved, activities such as dressing, combing hair, using wrenches, and peeling vegetables may be limited or impossible. If the knees, hips, or feet are involved, walking may be limited, as will bending, stooping, and lifting. While the patient may have no difficulty getting around within limited enclosures, for example, walking longer distances may be impossible. In severe cases, even transferring from bed to chair, chair to toilet, and chair to car will become impaired, and daily bathing, feeding, and grooming activities will be limited. Certainly persistent joint pain or deformity of the hips, feet, or knees will limit the patient's ability to use public transportation.

These disabilities are usually caused by inability to continue the customary way of doing things. As new techniques are learned, many of these disabilities can be overcome.

Psychosocial disabilities. Psychologists frequently characterize patients with rheumatoid arthritis as hostile, repressed, angry, and frustrated. Generally, it is believed that these characteristics are caused by constant pain with movement, rather than that a particular person with a propensity for hostile or repressed feelings gets rheumatoid arthritis. Patients who are chronically limited by pain have difficulties with their personal feelings and social interactions. Marital, parent-child, and other relationships may be seriously affected.

Some patients adapt to their disease and disability and function well with limited abilities, while other patients seem incapacitated by fairly minimal involvement. Adaptation to rheumatoid arthritis requires the patient to give up a former self-image and life style, without giving up those efforts required to achieve and sustain maximum independence. Maintenance of effort requires a tolerance for pain. This adaptation is difficult, and may be thwarted by denial, depression, or dependence.

Many patients who are in almost constant pain may never entirely give up the hope that one morning the pain will all vanish. This type of denial may lead to unrealistic expectations and resistance to altering behavior patterns. The patients may presume that once their "pain goes away" and their strength returns, their vocational problems will disappear.

Another reaction to the limitations imposed on the patient by his disease is increased dependency. Faced with the prospect of progressive deformities and pain on movement, the patient may decide to avoid pain and give up trying to remain active by increasingly depending on others for care.

However, for some patients, increased dependency may conflict with their previous active, independent self-image. When such a patient resists a desire to become excessively dependent and is willing to tolerate pain in order to continue with activities, he may become frustrated and depressed. The frustration occurs because, despite the effort, it becomes increasingly difficult or impossible to maintain previous activities, due to the accumulation of deformities. Patients become particularly frustrated when they discover that certain physical outlets and exercise activities are no longer feasible. The patient's inability to accept diminished activity *and* continued pain often leads to depression.

Rehabilitation potential. Longevity of rheumatoid arthritis patients is somewhat less than that of the normal population because of an apparent increased susceptibility to bacterial infection. Longevity is sufficient, however, so that the counselor can plan in terms of 2 or 4 years, rather than 6 or fewer months, for possible education and/or retraining.

After the counselor is assured that appropriate consultation and evaluation have been obtained from physicians and allied health personnel and is satisfied that the standards of evaluation have been met, he must consider several factors. The problem is not how long the patient will live but how he will function. Many patients seem to function well with severe deformities, while others with lesser deformities are more impaired in their functioning.

The prognosis for work is of course better for patients who possess highly trained skills which do not depend upon manual dexterity or strength. Those who possess more intellectual skills before the onset of their disease will likely have more skills afterwards.

Standards of Evaluation

A patient with rheumatoid arthritis should have certain evaluations performed to aid in diagnosis and treatment and to assess the extent of disease. An internist specializing in rheumatology (rheumatologist) is likely to be best equipped to do this. The patient requires a complete medical history and a physical examination, and descriptions of inflamed joints, of any joints which have less than normal range of motion, and of any weakness present. Deformities in the most seriously involved joints should be noted so that excessive use can be avoided. Complications should be sought.

A history should include all drug treatment, past and present. The duration of morning stiffness should be recorded. A complete blood count will disclose anemia, if present. A hematocrit of less than 30 percent suggests that at least part of the anemia is due to blood loss, and the source of the loss must therefore be sought. Also, this degree of anemia should be further investigated by study of the bone marrow and life span of red blood cells.

The urinalysis is usually normal. If blood is present in the urine (hematuria), it may mean that the patient is having an adverse reaction to a drug or perhaps is ingesting too much of a drug. For example, ingestion of compounds containing both salicylate (aspirin) and acetaminophen (e.g., Tylenol) may cause destruction of the renal collecting system (see p. 329). Also, if protein is present in the urine, the cause must be sought.

The erythrocyte sedimentation rate (ESR) is a very useful measure regularly obtained to help assess the degree of inflammation and the effect of any particular medication regime. This test is a nonspecific general measure of inflammation and is quite simple. A blood sample is mixed with an anticoagulant to prevent clotting and a column of blood is then set in a rack to keep it perfectly vertical. The red blood cells (erythrocytes) gradually settle to the bottom of the container. The sedimentation rate is expressed in millimeters of plasma remaining (i.e., the clear area above the settling blood cells) per unit of time, usually 1 hour. In normal persons, sedimentation occurs slowly. The normal sedimentation rate for males is less than 10 mm per hour and for females, less than 20 mm per hour. The ESR will be elevated proportionately to the degree of inflammation in rheumatoid arthritis and may decrease with effective treatment. The sedimentation rate for rheumatoid arthritis patients can be as high as 150 mm per hour.

Other tests assist in analysis of the extent and severity of the disease. The rheumatoid factor test (latex fixation) becomes positive during the first year in approximately 80 percent of patients with rheumatoid arthritis. The sheep cell agglutination titer (SCAT), while positive less frequently, is thought to be more specific for rheumatoid arthritis.

The lupus erythematosus preparation (LE prep) and antinuclear antibody tests are also performed in all patients thought to have rheumatoid arthritis. The connective tissue disease, systemic lupus erythematosus, frequently begins with an arthritis identical to rheumatoid arthritis, but the presence of a positive LE prep or antinuclear antibody test and the absence of the bony erosions characteristic of rheumatoid arthritis serve to separate these two diseases. Because the course, treatment, and prognosis of systemic lupus erythematosus and rheumatoid arthritis are quite different, diagnosis must be accurate.

A uric acid test should be obtained. Results are usually normal in patients with rheumatoid arthritis (or low in those taking large doses of aspirin). The test is elevated in patients with gout, renal disease, and other problems that are themselves associated with joint disease.

X-rays should be taken of all involved joints to determine if erosions or cartilage destruction are present. Subsequent X-rays should be obtained at yearly intervals to assess the degree of joint destruction and to be used as a guide to treatment.

The patient should be referred by his physician to a physical therapist to assist in evaluation of the joint range-of-motion limitations and muscle strength. A physical therapist should continue to periodically assess the patient's progress or lack of it under prescribed treatment for range-of-motion and strength limitations.

Rheumatoid arthritis patients should also be referred to an occupational therapist, who can evaluate activities of daily living, such as dressing, eating, personal hygiene, and housekeeping, and recommend training and techniques to achieve improved independence and to minimize joint damage. The therapist will be able to provide information regarding the likelihood that the patient will benefit from assistive devices, whether splints can be fitted, and what changes in the home or work place may be useful.

A clinical psychologist can assess the patient's adjustment to his disease, and search for the existence of the psychosocial disabilities discussed above. In most cases, patients and their families will benefit from referral to a social worker who can identify problems in family relationships and/or financial difficulties due to the patient's disabilities.

When a patient has multiple problems, a thorough evaluation may be best carried out in a comprehensive rehabilitation setting under the direction of a physiatrist. In such a setting, all professionals, physicians and the allied health group, simultaneously and in concert evolve a comprehensive treatment plan that incorporates an attack on all the problems that the evaluations uncover.

Total Treatment

Drugs. Drugs used in rheumatoid arthritis primarily function to control the inflammation. Many drugs are available because no single drug is completely effective for all patients. The patient very likely will be given several drugs simulataneously, as the effect of several seems additive.

Aspirin or another form of salicylate is most commonly prescribed first. Many preparations are available: plain aspirin, buffered aspirin, liquid preparations, and rectally administered aspirin. Each relieves pain, lowers the body temperature, and may reduce inflammation. All may cause side-effects in sufficiently high doses. Buffered, liquid, and rectally administered preparations cause less stomach upset and gastrointestinal bleeding. Excessive doses which may have been taken with suicidal intent cause marked derangements of the body's mineral and salt metabolism and require hospital treatment.

The appropriate dose of a salicylate preparation is that which almost causes ringing in the ears (tinnitus). At the level of tinnitus, the amount of aspirin has exceeded the liver's ability to metabolize and eliminate it and hence more is available to exert a therapeutic affect. Up to 15 or more aspirin tablets a day may be prescribed. Concentration levels of aspirin in the blood are periodically measured to determine whether they are high enough for anti-inflammatory effects.

Recently, several new anti-inflammatory drugs (Motrin, Nalfon, Indocin, Clinoril, Tolectin, and Naprosyn) have become available. As a group, they are called the *nonsteroidal anti-inflammatory drugs*. They relieve pain and decrease inflammation as well as salicylates, but no better. Their side effects are similar but perphaps less common. They are, however, considerably more expensive. Butazolidine, an older nonsteroidal anti-inflammatory drug, has been available for many years. It is usually used for only a few days, as it has caused skin rashes and bone marrow depression, a serious complication that can result in death.

Adrenocorticosteroid preparations (cortisone, prednisone, methylprednisone, triamcinolone, dexamethasone) are the most effective anti-inflammatory drugs available. In high doses, they may practically eliminate the clinical symptoms of rheumatoid arthritis. They do not, unfortunately, stop the formation of erosions, the loss of cartilage, or the weakening of ligaments or joint capsules. In spite of their good anti-inflammatory action, their use is avoided if possible because of their major side-effects. These side-effects include cataracts (see chap. 29), thinning of the bones (osteoporosis), peptic ulcers with bleeding, augmentation or initiation of high blood pressure and diabetes, thinning of the skin and delayed wound healing, muscle weakness, unsightly weight gain of the face and the trunk, and poor resistance to bacterial and tuberculous infection. Doses higher than that equivalent to roughly 7.5 mg of prednisone consistently result in undesirable side-effects and require cessation of the drug whenever possible. In an attempt to avoid these side-effects, steroids may be given in a double dose every second day. When inflammation is brought under control, the physician usually attempts to taper steroids and substitute the nonsteroidal medications for maintenance.

Special steroid preparations may also be injected locally into particularly involved joints. The injections may be repeated three or four times a year without fear of damaging the joint.

Chloroquine, an antimalarial drug, may also be prescribed. Its beneficial effect occurs only after several months of use. Because of the frequent occurrence of permanent retinal damage when used regularly, ophthalmological examination is necessary.

A more commonly used drug whose effect is noticed only after several months is *gold*. The two most commonly used compounds are Myochrysine and Solganol. They are given intramuscularly, usually 50 mg weekly for about 20 weeks. If there is no response, it is stopped. If the patient has improved, the drug is continued, although often in smaller doses and at wider intervals.

Side-effects of gold are serious, and weekly examination of the urine for protein, and of the blood hematocrit, white blood count, and platelet count are required to avoid serious complications. If the urine contains abnormal amounts of protein, gold must be stopped before severe kidney damage occurs. If the red or white blood cell or platelet count falls, the drug must be stopped. The most common side-effect is skin rash. Since it is difficult to tell whether or not a rash is due to gold, the gold is stopped and then readministered. If the rash recurs upon the readministration of gold and is extensive, gold must no longer be given.

Penicillamine is a new antirheumatic drug whose long-term benefit has not been fully established. *Anticancer drugs* (Cytoxin, Immuran, see chap. 28) are also given to patients with rheumatoid arthritis. These drugs seem to decrease the signs and symptoms of rheumatoid arthritis but have many distressing side-effects, which include liver poisoning, hair loss, bloody urine, and bone-marrow poisoning. These drugs may increase the risk of infection, predispose to malignancy, and increase mutations in offspring.

While aspirin is the mainstay of drug treatment, patients during the course of their disease usually are exposed to one or more of the others. Frequent followup visits for drug management are necessary, since the disease has a variable course for each patient and drug prescription needs to be revised. At each visit (anywhere from weekly to three or four times per year), the physician assesses the degree of inflammation present by examining the patient's joints and obtaining blood samples. The sedimentation rate (ESR) is a useful measure to assess degree of inflammation and to assist in adjusting medications.

Surgery. Surgical treatment in rheumatoid arthritis is of two types, one to control or remove inflammation and the other to correct deformity.

To control inflammation, removal of the synovial tissue to as great a degree as possible (synovectomy) prior to the occurrence of joint destruction and the formation of major erosions is indicated when conservative measures fail. The two most common joints for which synovectomies are done by orthopedic surgeons are the knee joint and the knuckle (metacarpophalangeal) joints of the hand. While results are often rewarding, synovial tissue regenerates and therefore the procedure is not a curative.

When surgery is performed to correct deformities, the goals are decreased pain and greater functional use. Some of these surgical procedures include:

1. Resection and removal of the distal ends of the metatarsal heads ("balls") of the feet to reduce foot pain and improve comfort and walking. This is a consistently successful procedure.
2. Fusion of the metacarpophalangeal and/or interphalangeal joint of the thumb to convert an unstable thumb into one quite able to sustain fingertip pressure from the other fingers as objects are grasped.

3. Replacement of the metacarpophalangeal joints with plastic "joints" to allow realignment and a better ability to grasp larger objects.
4. Fusion of the proximal interphalangeal joints of the fingers to relieve pain and increase the angle of flexion so the patient can function securely.
5. Sophisticated surgery to correct boutonniere and swan's neck deformities of the proximal interphalangeal joints which, if performed early, have given quite good results.
6. Surgical fusion of the wrist to provide a stable, painless wrist improves function in many cases.
7. Shoulder and elbow surgery are also performed, although less frequently.

Prostheses. The recent development of the *total hip prosthesis* (hip arthroplasty) holds great advantages for patients with rheumatoid arthritis. The procedure has few postoperative complications and causes improvement in motion and diminution in pain. The total hip prosthesis has been implanted bilaterally in many patients. The long-term durability of this prosthesis has not yet been determined, but the results are so good to date that the counselor should support the patient for hip arthroplasty, as it likely will add 5 to 15 more years of useful hip function.

The *total knee prosthesis* (knee arthroplasty) is constantly improving, and several successful models have been devised. These knee operations result in joints with less than optimum stability in many cases and have more complications than the total hip operations. Nonetheless, in a patient with a largely destroyed knee who cannot ambulate, surgery is clearly indicated. A failure will result only in knee fusion, which in itself is not a catastrophe and will also allow ambulation to a greater extent than is possible with a painful, destroyed, inflamed rheumatoid knee.

Total wrist prostheses have been recently devised but are still in an experimental state. In time, other joint replacements are likely to become successful, such as those for the elbow, shoulder, ankle, and hand.

Rehabilitation treatment. Rehabilitation medicine treatment may be classified into five categories: (a) measures to reduce pain and inflammation; (b) measures to prevent deformities; (c) measures to correct deformities; (d) measures to increase strength; and (e) measures to improve functional skills.

Measures to reduce pain and inflammation, such as moist heat, paraffin baths, contrast baths, and cold packs, decrease the heat and swelling around a joint and allow motion and exercise to be performed more extensively with less discomfort. The choice of which treatment to use depends upon patient preference, as there is no substantial body of data upon which to base the choice. The pain relief from these treatments is temporary and may last only 2 to 4 hours. The patient should be taught to perform these treatments in his home so he will not be limited to visiting the office of a physician or therapist unless, of course, the inflammation is too severe.

Placing a joint in plastic, fiberglass, or plaster splints or casts will also diminish the inflammation. The devices may need to be worn for several weeks to achieve maximum benefit, however, and therefore are cumbersome and unacceptable to many patients. For some, night use only may be sufficient. Splints or casts are most conveniently placed on the wrists, hands, and knees. Such splints also can control the severity of deformity progression. Design is critical, as is repeated checking of splint fit. If splints interfere with function to the degree that greater disability results, the patient is likely to discard them. Close followup can allow for a balance between function and joint protection.

Hydrotherapy in Hubbard tanks, walking tanks, pools, and spas has given relief to patients for centuries. While beneficial effect has been attributed to the mineral content or radioactivity of the spring, probably it is only the hot water which causes the soothing effect. Hydrotherapy can be expensive and inconvenient and is usually reserved for hospitalized patients.

Measures to prevent deformities can be taken, since an observer can predict which kind of deformities are going to occur. The patient who does not balance rest and activity well may actually increase inflammation and joint destruction. Exercises taught by the physical therapist will prevent loss of motion at the joints and help maintain strength. Various joint protection techniques are also taught. For example, the patient will be advised not to sleep with his knees bent or with a pillow beneath them, but rather to sleep on his abdomen. He will then be less likely to develop hip and knee flexion deformities.

The effect of exercises and splints or casts is dependent upon their use and repetition. The counselor may therefore wish to review his client's treatment program and urge him to comply with it.

Measures to correct deformities include the use of serial casts or splints which place the joints in more and more extension to correct flexion deformities at the wrist and knee. Casts and splints are awkward at the shoulder, and if this joint has lost motion and has become deformed, stretching exercises by the physical therapist are the only available treatment. The application of heat or cold prior to corrective exercises increases the motion which may be gained and decreases the pain. Shoe inserts may be used to correct flat feet.

Measures to increase strength in some muscles can be performed by the physical therapist. Although weakness in the hand muscles and shoulder muscles is difficult to improve, exercise can decrease the weakness that occurs in the knee muscles and in the muscles which extend the hip. Efforts should be concentrated upon increasing strength in these muscles. Exercise while moving the joints as little as possible (isometric exercises) will allow for an increase in strength without joint inflammation. This type of exercise requires diligence on the part of the patient and skilled coaching on the part of the therapist. The therapist can also advise the patient on which sorts of work or other activity increase his inflammation and should therefore be avoided or minimized, as well as those specific therapeutic exercises to strengthen muscles without joint stress.

The counselor can reinforce the suggestions of the therapist by recommending his client avoid work that leaves him inflamed and fatigued and perhaps unable to perform the exercises that could strengthen his joints. Further, if the client reports to the counselor that he is pacing or performing other activities in the morning to alleviate his feeling of stiffness, the counselor should advise the client to consult his physician. Such morning activities may be harmful.

Measures to improve function can be recommended by both the physical and occupational therapists, the former dealing with ambulation and transfer techniques and the latter concentrating on activities of daily living. When the problems are carefully outlined, devices such as reachers, hooks, and built-up utensil handles can be provided.

The occupational therapist may also visit the homemaker in the home to determine in what ways labor-saving and energy-saving reorganization may be accomplished. Recommendations such as the raising or lowering of table tops, the lowering of storage cabinets, and provisions of more easily activated faucet handles may be appropriate. Similarly, a visit by an experienced occupational therapist to a client's place of employment may yield recommendations for the worker's station that will yield increased productivity with less joint strain.

Followup treatment. Good total care of the patient with rheumatoid arthritis unfortunately rarely results in a complete absence of pain and inflammation. This fact, coupled with the unpredictable nature of the course of the disease, requires regular followup for increases in pain, inflammation, deformity, and reduced functional skills. Monthly visits to the physician are quite usual for evaluation of results of prior treatment and recommendations for additions and changes. The sedimentation rate is usually repeated frequently to assess degree of inflammation. Low values mean good control. The hematocrit or hemoglobin test adequately checks for anemia. If there is a drop in either of these, bleeding from the gastrointestinal tract secondary to medication or bone marrow depression should be sought and treated. The occurrence of proteins in the urine (proteinuria) suggests the complication of gold or penicillamine

therapy. Review of joint range of motion status, strength and functional skills, and of splints the patient may be using are also performed at regular followup visits.

Psychosocial treatment. The rheumatoid arthritis client needs understanding while he is grieving for his previous self-image and life style, and he needs help and support during the transition to a more limited range of activities. It is not sufficient for the counselor simply to tell the client to go out and do things differently. The counselor needs to be understanding and listen to the exact nature of the particular problems the client may have. He must also attempt to help the client achieve a resolution of the problems and an alteration in the type and degree of physical activity that realistically conforms to the client's limitations. He should encourage the client to avoid those activities believed to increase his deformities and disability and help him find activities that allow him to continue as active a life as his arthritis will allow. If a client has unrealistic expectations due to denial, the counselor may need to be forthright in a supportive way in explaining to the client that it is unlikely his arthritis will vanish to such an extent that he will not have to alter his life style.

Clients who are obsessed with performing their daily jobs, tasks, or housework, and by so doing ignore all advice about protecting their joints, may be helped by psychotherapy with a clinical psychologist or psychiatrist. Also, psychotherapy may be useful in helping clients adjust to their disability. A skilled social worker experienced in counseling clients with rheumatoid arthritis will let the client ventilate his feelings and advise him and his significant "others" of ways to attempt to work out the marital, parent-child, and/or other family problems associated with the client's disability.

Vocational Implications

The signs and symptoms of rheumatoid arthritis are not static. Unlike the client with an amputation, paraplegia, or a stroke, the client with rheumatoid arthritis has a condition that varies. The counselor must therefore observe and understand his client's changing condition and provide vocational goals and support appropriate to the more difficult periods so that employment can be sustained.

Not all clients with rheumatoid arthritis progress unremittingly to disability. The counselor should be alert for the client with only a few involved joints who seems to undergo a remission. Such a client is more easily provided with vocational goals and supports. This discussion of specific vocational implications will assume, however, that the client has a persistent, generalized involvement with a slow, steady, but inexorably progressive course.

Education. Advanced or additional educational goals should be a strong consideration both for clients with recent-onset rheumatoid arthritis and those with long-standing disease. The longevity of the client with rheumatoid arthritis is diminished, but not sufficiently to make long-term educational goals unreasonable. Vocational training and/or college courses of 2 to 4 years should clearly be considered. If the client is in the third or fourth decade of life, the common age of onset of rheumatoid arthritis, educational goals should be guided by his past intellectual skills and experience, rather than limited by the fear of death or total disability.

A further consideration is that manual labor and many vocations requiring chiefly physical skills may cause exacerbations of rheumatoid arthritis. A client who has this experience would appear to be a likely candidate for rehabilitation to a vocation where mental rather than manual skills are paramount.

Aptitudes. There is nothing inherent in rheumatoid arthritis that affects the client's intellect, learning ability, verbal skills, numerical skills, color discrimination, or form and space perception, except the constant frustration of pain with nearly every movement.

Motor coordination, finger and hand dexterity, and eye-hand-foot coordination are adversely affected by rheumatoid arthritis. Loss of motion and pain on motion certainly slow the client's movements and diminish coordination.

Later in the course of the disease, ligament, tendon, and muscle weakness will affect coordination. Deformities subsequent to destruction decrease mechanical advantages (e.g., weakening of the grip when the wrist is subluxed in a palmar direction and when the fingers are distorted or stiff). Clients lose the ability to raise the arms and hands above the shoulder level due to contractures of the shoulder joint. The loss of stability of the thumb decreases the force of pinch. Vocational goals dependent upon fine, dexterous, or coordinated movement of the hand are therefore not good choices for clients with rheumatoid arthritis. The operation of machines requiring dexterous, rapid, repeated movements probably also is a bad choice. Nevertheless, if the force required is quite low, dexterous tasks, including the use of an electric typewriter, may be accomplished.

Interests. The counselor must remember that the client with rheumatoid arthritis is likely to be in his third or fourth decade. By the fifth or sixth decade, the client will have progressed from the inflammatory phase to the stage of persistent deformity where movement will be limited by mechanical failures of the joints to support weight and allow motion. The counselor thus will have to guide the interests of his younger clients into areas where frequent use of joints will not aggravate the disease and increase the clients'

rage and frustration. Some younger clients more inclined to anger may succeed best when dealing with objects or with scientific or technical activities rather than with people.

It is likely that the client with rheumatoid arthritis would fare better with activities of an abstract, creative nature, rather than with routine organzied activity, if such interests and aptitudes are present. Routine activities are frequently associated with repetitive mechanical motions, which may induce overuse of an inflamed joint. Certainly, the client with rheumatoid arthritis will have difficulty succeeding when productivity is the chief criterion for success. In all likelihood, he will be frustrated even if his interests and personality traits suit him to high performance, piece work, or production-oriented tasks. The counselor may well try to seek situations where prestige and esteem are the rewards. Clients with rheumatoid arthritis may have diminished self-images, which would be enhanced by rewards of esteem.

Jobs with continuous stresses, both to the joints and to the person, are not recommended. They may cause exacerbations of both disease and frustration. The management of rheumatoid arthritis usually requires rest periods, and a combination of rest and exercise often must be available on the job as well as at home. Some clients may even require a nap at noon or in the afternoon. In addition, they also benefit from frequent changes of position.

The solo or group nature of a job minimally affects the client with rheumatoid arthritis. Some clients will be buoyed up by companions and others plunged into despair, self-pity, and hostile antagonism. If the client responds to a fellow sufferer or a well person with increased self-pity, he should likely work alone. The client who obtains support and inspiration from others should be placed with a group.

Physical demands. Most clients with rheumatoid arthritis will be better employed in vocations with sedentary or, at most, light work. While most of the clients who respond to treatment will be able to perform medium or heavy work, the counselor must keep in mind that the progressive nature of this disease is toward further crippling and disability. Thus a client who initially may do medium work (i.e., lift 25 to 50 lb, or 11.3 to 22.5 kg) or even heavy work (i.e., lift 100 lb, or 45 kg) will not be able to do so throughout his working career. Many clients may be able to continue sedentary or light work until retirement, and should not be encouraged to continue medium or heavy work which will perhaps further inflame their joints and result in total disability before the usual age of retirement.

Climbing skills, balancing skills, stooping, and kneeling are all hampered by pain on weight bearing or with motion. All these activities may be accomplished by most clients with rheumatoid arthritis, but activities that repeatedly overuse joints without periods of rest and recovery should be avoided. Reaching, handling, and fingering will be clumsy, painful, weak, and awkward in clients whose hand joints are inflamed.

A further consideration concerns which joints are the most seriously involved. Unfortunately, at onset this is somewhat difficult to predict or determine. However, if the arthritis seems to attack particular joints and spare others, the counselor may consider recommending vocations that utilize the less affected joints. Thus, if the fingers are spared but the hips and knees are seriously involved, a sedentary clerical job might be appropriate.

Unless the rare occurrence of peripheral neuropathy, mononeuritis, or the carpal tunnel syndrome decreases finger sensation, no loss of sensation should interfere with the rheumatoid arthritis client's ability to work. Speech and hearing are also not impaired. Vision is unaffected unless steroid-induced cataracts occur, or if a toxic response to chloroquine appears.

Environment. It is usual for clients with rheumatoid arthritis to detect changes in humidity, temperature, or barometric pressure. An indoor climate where the environment is relatively controlled is therefore well advised. Extremes of weather or temperature with abrupt variation probably should be avoided. Whether the climate is wet, humid, dry, warm, or cold is apparently less important to a client's comfort than the frequency of abrupt changes. The occurrence of excessive noise, vibration, fumes, gases, dust, and poor ventilation have no specific effects on clients with rheumatoid arthritis.

Many clients with rheumatoid arthritis may not be industrially competitive but are able to work in a sheltered workshop. This experience may enable them to work in an environment consistent with their level of productivity and may also support them until they acquire the skills that will enable them to gain access to the competitive commercial world.

Above all, the counselor must realize that the client with rheumatoid arthritis does not have a permanent disability with clearly defined limits, but rather a changing disability with frequent pain, varying from day to day, but generally resulting in an unfavorable, disabled outcome. Such clients require a combination of analysis, sympathy, encouragement, and adequate evaluation and treatment. The vocational counselor who skillfully coordinates these issues will be amply rewarded.

ANKYLOSING SPONDYLITIS

Disease Description

Ankylosing spondylitis is a form of inflammatory joint disease which most affects the joints and ligaments of the spine. Ankylosis refers to bony or fibrous union, and spondylitis means inflammation of the joints of the spine. The disease usually occurs in young men in the first through third decades and frequently affects members of the same family.

The cause of ankylosing spondylitis is unknown, but it is thought that an allergic reaction occurs, causing the body's immune cells (lymphocytes) to invade joints and tendons. The presence of immune cells in the joints and tendons is accompanied by the elaboration of various substances which start an inflammatory reaction. The inflammatory reaction is followed by repair and healing with new bone formation. The disease is thus characterized by erosion and destruction of tendons and joints, particularly in the spine, with the formation of bony bridges and reduced motion.

The sacroiliac joints, or posterior pelvic joints, are the most frequently involved at first, manifested by low back pain. Since these joints have little motion normally, there is little motion impairment when they become fused. Subsequently, the lumbar spine, thoracic spine, and eventually the cervical spine are involved in ascending order, although the process may skip over parts. At first the spine is painful and tender, but later, when it is completely fused and the patient has lost his ability to rotate or bend it, pain may disappear. As the patient develops a stiff or "poker" spine, the joints where the ribs attach to the vertebrae also are inflamed and subsequently heal with bone formation and loss of motion. The patient therefore cannot expand his chest well and takes in less air with each breath.

Less frequently, other joints, including the hips, shoulders, and, more rarely, the peripheral joints, such as elbows, hands, feet, and ankles, are involved. This inflammation is usually not as destructive as in rheumatoid arthritis, but on occasion hip joints are solidly fused and other joints are damaged and lose motion.

Some patients complain little of pain, and physical examination and X-rays are necessary to diagnose ankylosing spondylitis. Some of these patients progress to relatively marked loss of motion quite insidiously.

Two features of this disease as it affects the vertebral column contribute to the degree of disability produced: (a) pain is less when the vertebral column is flexed, and (b) the disease progresses continuously to fusion of the vertebral column. Since fusion will occur in the usual position of the back, a severe flexion deformity of the trunk may result. A patient might progress to the point where fusion occurs with his head in so much flexion that he cannot look around and can focus only on the floor.

Ankylosing spondylitis is not only the name of a particular inflammation of the spine which occurs in young men, but is also a descriptive term which is applied to other diseases in which inflammatory stiffening of the spine occurs. Among these are regional enteritis, ulcerative colitis, Reiter's syndrome, and psoriasis. They are briefly discussed here, since spondylitis may be the predominant finding for which the patient is referred to the vocational counselor.

Regional enteritis and *ulcerative colitis* are both inflammatory diseases of the bowel. They are distinguished by X-ray evidence of bowel inflammation, persistent bloody diarrhea, and characteristic findings on direct visual examination of the sigmoid colon. *Reiter's syndrome*, like anklyosing spondylitis, is a disease mostly of young men. It is characterized by inflammation of the eye (uveitis), inflammation of the lower urinary passage (urethritis), and inflammation of peripheral joints (arthritis). Skin eruptions on the sole of the foot or the penis are often found. *Psoriasis* is a very common skin disease. The spondylitis of Reiter's syndrome and psoriasis differs from that of inflammatory bowel disease and primary ankylosing spondylitis in having less complete involvement of the spine with more ''skip'' areas. Motion is therefore less restricted.

All forms of ankylosing spondylitis demonstrate a gradually worsening course in which the pain lessens but the stiffness and lack of motion increase. Currently, no form of treatment protects the patient from ultimately developing a stiff spine.

Patients with ankylosing spondylitis may also have inflammation of the aortic semilunar valves (see chap. 3). If this is sufficiently extensive, blood will leak from the aorta back into the heart through the damaged valve (aortic insufficiency), and the patient may develop heart failure. The electrical conduction system for activating the heart may also become partially blocked, causing various forms of irregular heartbeat which will require medical treatment. On occasion, patients will have inflammation of the tissues of the eye and develop pain on viewing and, if untreated, may develop blindness. Pain in the heel may occur from inflammation of the attachment of the tough tissues of the sole of the foot to the heel bone (calcaneous), and painful bone spurs may develop.

Functional Disabilities

Loss of motion of the spine or pain in the spine with motion may greatly affect a patient's mobility. Walking, however, will be unimpaired unless the hips and knees become inflamed and stiffen. A stiff spine may make certain chores difficult, and certainly frequent stooping and bending will be impossible. Toilet activities and dressing may be difficult, but rarely does the patient become less than self-sufficient. In fact, a characteristic of patients with ankylosing spondylitis is that, in spite of progressive stiffness, they are able to continue their chosen vocational activity unless it requires significant back mobility.

There are no specific psychological or social impairments ascribed to patients with ankylosing spondylitis except those that may develop in any disability where there are major functional losses. As the spine stiffens, the patient's posture may become unsightly. Patients with ankylosing spondylitis and psoriasis may become socially isolated or resentful.

The rehabilitation potential of the patient with ankylosing spondylitis is relatively good. Patients may have to change their vocations if their jobs require flexed postures or much back movement. The prognosis for life approaches that of normal individuals, so that if the patient can no longer perform his duties because of back pain or stiffness, he may be supported in training programs of any length. No goal which is appropriate to the patient's resources, skills, and aspirations should be denied because of the time required for its attainment.

Standards of Evaluation

The patient with ankylosing spondylitis must have X-rays of the sacroiliac joints, the entire spine, and any other joints that demonstrate pain and swelling. Besides a complete history and physical examination, it is imperative that the patient with suspected ankylosing spondylitis have precise measurements made and recorded of his ability to expand his chest and of the distance between the back of his skull (occiput) and a wall against which he is standing as erect as possible. His ability to flex his spine should be measured at frequent intervals. These three measurements characterize the degree of physical impairment and measure its progress. In addition, respiratory function and involvement of other joints need to be evaluated. An internist with special interest in rheumatology is usually best able to assess the disease.

A recently described association between patients with ankylosing spondylitis and the tissue typing antigens has revealed that the antigen HLA-B27 occurs in 95 percent of patients with ankylosing spondylitis, 90 percent of patients with Reiter's syndrome, and about 50 percent of patients with bowel inflammation and psoriasis who develop anklyosing spondylitis. It is not essential for the HLA-B27 test to be ordered on all patients with obvious ankylosing spondylitis. However, for the young patient with early arthritis in whom the diagnosis is unclear, the test may provide evidence that the arthritis will eventually turn out to be ankylosing spondylitis.

Cardiac and eye examinations should be performed routinely. All patients should be referred to a physical therapist for posture evaluation. Patients with psoriasis must be referred to a dermatologist for care of the skin problem, and patients with an inflammatory bowel disease should have gastroenterological consultation.

Total Treatment

The patient is usually treated with the appropriate medicines to control pain. Aspirin is still the first choice and is used in the highest tolerable doses to achieve the best effect. If aspirin is inadequate, the addition or substitution of the nonsteroidal anti-inflammatory drugs should be tried (see above). Indocin and phenylbutazone appear to work especially well in patients with spondylitis. Phenylbutazone (Butazolidine), however, has considerably more dangerous side-effects and its choice is therefore less frequent. Adrenocorticosteroids (e.g., prednisone) are also quite effective, but because of the more frequent and more serious side-effects, they are considered less desirable than Indocin, but preferable to phenylbutazone. The side-effects of these drugs, their doses, and the responses are discussed in greater detail on page 195.

If the spine pain of ankylosing spondylitis does not respond to anti-inflammatory medication, radiation treatment may be considered. Radiating the spine certainly eliminates pain and inflammation in many resistant cases, but an increased incidence of leukemia at a later date in these patients has been reported.

Physical therapy treatment includes instruction in exercises which will enable the patient to maintain as erect a posture as possible, to expand his chest and fill his lungs to as great a degree and for as long as possible, and also to vigorously and deeply exhale in order to expand the thorax. It is felt by rheumatologists that if the exercises are performed diligently and daily, the patient will have better posture and lung expansion than a patient who does not exercise. Braces have been found ineffective in passively keeping the spine extended.

When a marked flexion posture has developed (a forward slump), surgical correction may be considered. On occasion, removal of a piece of the bony spine has allowed a bent spine to be straightened, but this operation must be performed only by the most experienced surgeon. In addition, it must be determined if the patient is properly educated, motivated, and has had adequate conservative treatment in order to benefit from this operation.

The treatment of Reiter's syndrome is similar to that of ankylosing spondylitis, but more attention to peripheral joint arthritis is required because these joints are more frequently inflamed. Treatment of psoriasis includes many skin medications, ultraviolet light, and anticancer drugs.

Inflammatory bowel disease requires more vigorous treatment than the accompanying spondylitis. On occasion, surgical removal of the inflamed and bleeding bowel is required. Since there is an increased incidence of cancer in inflammatory bowel diseases, repeated X-ray observations must be performed.

Rarely, patients with ankylosing spondylitis develop limited motion in the hip and shoulder joints secondary to synovial inflammation similar to that of rheumatoid arthritis, with bony bridging across the joint. When this occurs at the hip, surgical implantation of a total hip prosthesis has been used successfully. Sometimes the bone re-forms, undoing the surgeon's work.

Vocational Implications

The client with spondylitis may be considered for vocational, college, or professional training as his resources indicate. Spondylitis will not affect the client's mental aptitudes, learning ability, verbal skills, numerical skills, or form and space perception. However, although motor coordination, eye-hand coordination, and eye-hand-foot coordination will not be impaired, a stiff back will limit the client's twisting, turning, and perhaps reaching in such a way that dexterity may be limited. The client will be quite dexterous with tasks placed directly in front of him but may have difficulty with tasks requiring reaching or bending. Color discrimination should be unimpaired, although the complication of inflammation of the eye (uveitis) may diminish vision.

Severe deformity may cause embarrassment in interpersonal relations, but this is hard to predict. The client's preference for technical versus personal work would depend on his particular personality characteristics. In addition personal characteristics will determine whether or not the client will do better with tasks of a routine or a more creative nature. Tasks which require piecework or are production oriented often require a person to maintain a fixed position while working rapidly with the hands. The client with spondylitis may not do well with such tasks because he often requires frequent changes of position.

A client with a persistently painful back probably will do less well in a situation of chronic emotional stress. Associated muscle tension, for example, can increase pain and further reduce motion. In such a situation, the client may become too preoccupied to attend to the need to pull himself erect and practice his exercises during the course of the day.

Clients with spondylitis should not be offered tasks requiring lifting over 10 to 15 pounds (4.5 to 6.8 kg). Even lifting 20 pounds (9 kg) with significant walking or standing (light work) may cause intolerable back pain. Some clients, however, have little pain. Although their spines become quite stiff, they must pay careful attention to posture. Lifting and bending will not be well tolerated and may even enhance the spine flexion. Clients with arthritis of the hips and knees certainly should not be required to perform consistent or prolonged walking.

Climbing skills, balancing skills, stooping, and kneeling may be tolerated by some clients but not by others. The counselor should avoid suggesting vocational opportunities which require these activities. Reaching, handling, fingering, and feeling will not be impaired, but as spinal motion is often an integral part of these maneuvers, they may be well tolerated. Tasks requiring dexterous activity without reaching, standing, stooping, or bending are certainly within the vocational reach of clients with ankylosing spondylitis. However, even with sedentary tasks, the client must be allowed the opportunity to stretch his spine frequently.

While many arthritic clients describe joint pain in relation to weather changes, clients with spondylitis should not necessarily require an indoor environment. Some noise, vibration, fumes, gas, dust, and poor ventilation should be no more troublesome than they would be to an ordinary worker.

A sheltered workshop will be required only by the clients with severe spinal deformity who cannot perform at industrial levels. Clients with advanced education or clerical skills will frequently be able to continue employment, while those with only manual skills will become disabled.

DEGENERATIVE JOINT DISEASE

Disease Description

Degenerative joint disease (DJD; osteoarthritis) is usually a disease of patients in their sixth or seventh decade. It affects joints singly or in pairs, but rarely involves more than one to three joints in an individual. Commonly, the patient notes the gradual onset of pain on use or weight bearing in a hip, knee, carpometacarpal joint at the base of the thumb, or distal or proximal interphalangeal joints of the fingers. The shoulder is rarely involved. In the spine, the term degenerative disc disease is preferred, and this disease is discussed in chapter 15.

When swelling occurs around the joint, it is usually due to bony overgrowth rather than to increased synovial tissue or joint fluid accumulation as in rheumatoid arthritis. DJD begins as a roughening of the surface cartilage of the joint. There follows an increase in water content of the cartilage, a proliferation of cartilage cells, and an increase in cellular metabolism. Subsequently, the bone under the cartilage proliferates, with the development of "spurs" of bone growing out from the margin of the joints, an apparent attempt of the body to repair or replace the damaged joint. The cartilage does not regenerate or repair itself and does not become stronger, despite the increased number of cells and increased metabolism. It progressively frays, thins, weakens, and becomes disarrayed until the cartilaginous cushion which normally protects the bones of the body from shock becomes ineffective. The bony surfaces then rest and rub painfully on each other. There often is a little fluid in the joint and a few inflammatory cells, and hence anti-inflammatory arthritis medication is often beneficial.

The cause of DJD is entirely unclear. It is thought to occur as a consequence of some earlier, perhaps unnoticed, damage to the joint, which then fails to withstand wear and use with time. Overweight is often associated with DJD of the hip and knee, and DJD of the proximal interphalangeal and distal interphalangeal joints seems to be hereditary.

Some diseases predispose an individual to DJD. Ochronosis, a hereditary defect in the metabolism of the amino acids phenylalanine and tyrosine, results in a deposition of a dark pigment in connective tissue and joint cartilage, leading to cartilage breakdown and the development of DJD. In addition, diabetes, syphilis, syringomyelia, and other neurological conditions which affect the nerve supply and sensation of a joint lead to rapid and extreme DJD. This appears to be due to lack of protective nerve impulses from the joint. Thus use, loss of innervation, hereditary cartilage defects, joint trauma, and probably other as yet unknown factors lead to this condition.

The occurrence of DJD in multiple finger joints is common and should not be alarming. Rarely are these joints a site of intense inflammation. When it does occur, the condition is known as erosive osteoarthritis (EOA). This condition should not be confused with rheumatoid arthritis because the treatment, prognosis, and vocational implications are radically different. Even inflammatory DJD of the fingers with bony proliferation is an isolated condition for which local treatment is indicated, and unless marked finger dexterity is required by the patient, he should not otherwise be limited in his vocational capabilities.

The course of DJD is generally progressive and unremitting. The patient will have good days and bad days. Weather, overuse, and unknown factors will cause exacerbations from time to time, and rest and proper treatment will diminish symptoms. DJD does not shorten life expectancy.

Functional Disabilities

DJD affects the patient's performance by impeding use of the involved joint. Since the hips and knees are common sites of DJD, walking and transfer activities may be impaired. At first the patient will be able to function well in a limited area, but as joint damage increases, he will be less and less able to walk to the parking lot, the bus, or the shopping center. Dressing, eating, and other activities of daily living, however, will be little impaired. Although DJD of the jaw joint (temporomandibular joint) may occur, talking and even eating are rarely impaired. DJD of the hip may interfere with perineal hygiene due to limited motion of the hip, and sexual activities may be difficult due to hip pain.

Decreased ability to walk or perform related activities and the associated pain can certainly lead to despair, frustration, anger, and depression. Treatment of the primary condition can considerably alter both function and these psychological responses. Unlike rheumatoid arthritis, acute attacks do not occur. The course of the disease is slow, with gradually increasing impairment as pain increases and joint motion decreases.

The rehabilitation potential of a patient with DJD is generally limited by his age and the results of medical and surgical treatment. Since walking is the function most commonly impaired in patients with DJD, treatment that improves ambulation may allow continued employment. If treatment cannot eliminate the pain, the long- and short-term goals and vocational aspirations should be guided by the patient's age and interest. The presence of DJD will not decrease the number of a patient's working years.

Standards of Evaluation

The evaluation of the patient with DJD includes X-rays of each involved joint and its mate on the opposite side for comparison. Repeat films at annual intervals help assess the progress of the disease. A medical history should elicit any history of trauma, diabetes, syphilis, or sensory abnormalities. The history will point out which joints are involved, the duration of pain, and factors, such as use or increased weight, which influence symptoms. Laboratory data obtained for evaluation should include tests for syphilis and diabetes. No tests other than X-rays are needed to confirm the presence and extent of DJD in a joint. The physical examination includes a detailed examination of joint range of motion and strength and an assessment of walking limitations.

While an internist or family practitioner usually can easily make the diagnosis, evaluation by physicians with special interest in the musculoskeletal system, such as orthopedic surgeons and physiatrists, should be obtained prior to vocational rehabilitation planning.

The patient might also be referred to the physical therapist for evaluation and instruction in hip and knee exercises, and for gait training if gait is impaired. The occupational therapist may be useful for evaluation of self-care skills and provision of splints, such as a thumb splint for those with carpometacarpal DJD of the thumb. Dieticians may be helpful if the patient is overweight. If functional losses are severe, psychological and social evaluations may be appropriate.

Total Treatment

Total treatment begins with the administration of antiarthritic drugs to decrease the pain. The same drugs described for rheumatoid arthritis are utilized,

and aspirin again is the mainstay. The injection of steroids directly into the involved joint is also an effective treatment, but should be limited to about four times annually so as not to advance joint destruction. Weight reduction and some curtailment of weight bearing is essential. Judicious use of canes and crutches, for example, protects against progression. The patient should be taught by the physical therapist to exercise the muscles around the knee and hip to maintain strength and range of motion.

When nonsurgical treatment fails to decrease the pain sufficiently, referral to an orthopedic surgeon for consideration of joint replacement arthroplasty is appropriate (see p. 196). Complications of surgery include dislocation, infection, or failure to achieve the pain relief, motion, or function hoped for.

Vocational Implications

Since DJD is not a systemic disease, successful treatment of a single involved joint may result in continued employment in the client's current job or a resumption of the same or related activity. The client is therefore likely to be able to perform those tasks which fit his education, aptitudes, and interests unless they require dexterous or heavy use of an involved joint. Even if surgical or medical treatment of the affected joint results in an increased range of motion, diminished pain, and ability to walk further, the use of that joint should be limited. Heavy lifting, which repeatedly places unusual stresses on the hips and knees, is best avoided. Light to medium work, however, should be possible.

Return of the client to work after undergoing successful surgery requires careful consideration. The pain and the need to limit activity will be less and his ability to walk will probably be increased. Nonetheless, the client's activity should be limited, as the durability of the prosthetic implants has not yet been measured. While further surgery might be attempted, it is not yet clear that a second, replacement prosthesis will be as successful as the initial prosthesis.

Climbing, balancing skills, stooping, and kneeling will be impaired in many patients with DJD unless treatment removes the pain and consequent unsteadiness of hip and knee. Stooping and kneeling may be accomplished without pain following surgery but should be limited. Certain motions involved with stooping and kneeling may cause an implanted hip prosthesis to become dislocated. Climbing and balancing can be accomplished, but are hazardous and should not be allowed to make up the bulk of the client's vocational activity.

Dexterity will be impaired or limited so slightly by surgical fusion of the carpometacarpal joint of the thumb that only occupations requiring unusual finger dexterity need be eliminated from consideration.

The environment has no significant effect on

patients with DJD. Changes in relative humidity, barometric pressure, and temperature may cause joint discomfort as they do in other form of arthritis, but these are not influential enough to lead to a change of residence in most cases.

If the client cannot have surgical replacement of the hip and knee joint and medication does not suppress the pain sufficiently, sedentary or sheltered workshop activity may be advisable. Unless there is severe involvement, however, the client should be able to pursue competitive industrial tasks.

BIBLIOGRAPHY

Harris R: Rehabilitation. *In* Licht S (ed): *Arthritis and Physical Medicine*. Baltimore, Waverly Press, 1969, pp. 458–481.
A general review of rehabilitation medicine techniques applied to the patient with rheumatoid arthritis. The section describing vocational modifications and restrictions is brief.

Hill AGS: General management of rheumatoid arthritis. *In* Scott JT (ed): *Copeman's Textbook of the Rheumatic Diseases*. Ed 5, Edinburgh, London, New York, Livingstone, 1978, pp. 391–403.
A discussion of the identification of problems and questions of communication. It introduces methods of treatment and a general guide to overall management.

Nichols PJR: Rehabilitation. *In* Scott JT (ed): *Copeman's Textbook of the Rheumatic Diseases*. Ed 5, Edinburgh, London, New York, Livingstone, 1978, pp. 491–508.
A detailed description of many aids and devices and a brief statement about feasibility of particular jobs.

Robinson HS: Prognosis: Return to work—arthritis. *In* Erlich, GE (ed): *Total Management of the Arthritic Patient*, Philadelphia, Lippincott, 1973, pp. 183–192.
This brief chapter gives citations of available employment statistics for arthritic patients.

Vignos PJ Jr, Thompson HM, Katz S, Moskowitz RW, Fink S, Svec KH: Comprehensive care and psychosocial factors in rehabilitation in chronic rheumatoid arthritis: A controlled study. J Chronic Dis **25**:457–467, 1972.
Forty rheumatoid arthritis patients were divided into two groups. One group received additional intensive treatment, including visiting nurse services, and the control group did not. For both groups, the interrelationships among social adjustment, personal adjustment, intelligence, and motivation were studied. The influence of these factors and intensive treatment on medical condition and maintenance or improvement of function in activities of daily living was also studied.

15 ORGANIC MUSCULOSKELETAL BACK DISORDERS

Rene Cailliet, M.D.
Loren A. Helberg, Ph.D.

INTRODUCTION

Pain in the low back, with or without radiation into the lower extremity, is a frequent symptom that affects approximately 80 percent of all persons sometime during their lifetime. Back problems constitute a large percentage of all disabilities. They are perhaps the most nebulous of all musculoskeletal disorders, and affect persons of both sexes at any age.

The location of the discomfort is usually in the lumbosacral area. It may be at the midline, on either or both sides of the midline, or across the entire low back. Radiation (spread) of the discomfort, if present, may extend into the buttocks or the groin, down the posterior or posterolateral thigh, or into the calf, ankle, and foot. In many cases, there are not objective findings on physical examination and the various specific tests of the neurological, musculoskeletal, and other related systems are normal. Diagnosis in such situations is usually based on the details of the patient's description of his discomfort and its history. The absence of positive pathology on examinations or tests is, however, not entirely without value, for it assists in eliminating some potential causes of back pain.

Many of the labels applied to problems of low back pain are not always accurate or meaningful from the point of view of management. Patients and even physicians might interpret the condition as a slipped disc, bulging disc, ruptured disc, disintegrating or degenerated disc, lumbago, and/or sciatica, often without true documentation. Others might more rightfully simply apply the symptom itself as the diagnosis. Hence, "chronic low back pain" may appear on the records as the diagnosis.

In this chapter, the normal spine will be discussed first to provide a basis for understanding the pathology of the major specific back disorders described later. The sections of chapter 3 on the musculoskeletal and nervous systems and pages 65 to 68 in chapter 5 also provide additional helpful background information.

THE NORMAL SPINE

The vertebral column has 7 cervical vertebrae, 12 thoracic vertebrae, 5 lumbar vertebrae, the sacrum, and the coccyx. It is useful to consider as a functional unit any two neighboring vertebrae and their connections (fig. 15-1). Each of these two vertebrae consists of a body, two pedicles, two laminae, two transverse processes, one spinous process, and two articular processes with their facets. The two vertebrae are connected by the anterior longitudinal ligament, the intervertebral disc interposed between the two bodies, the ligaments attached to the transverse and spinous processes, and the posterior, or neural arch, joints. These posterior joints are formed by the articulation of the facets of one vertebra on the facets of its neighbor. The facets are covered by articular cartilage and are surrounded by a joint capsule much like any synovial joint (see p. 32).

The intervertebral discs are remarkable structures. They are 88 percent water retained in a matrix of protein and complex sugar compounds. This matrix is reinforced by concentric layers of tough collagen fibers (*annulus fibrosus*). The central portion of the disc, the *nucleus pulposus*, is well contained within the annulus. The nucleus is an amorphous gel under pressure and it keeps the bodies of the vertebrae apart and the connecting ligaments taut.

The spinal cord lies within the vertebral canal formed by the vertebral bodies, pedicles, and laminae. As discussed on page 65 and as illustrated in figure 15-2, each spinal nerve leaves the vertebral canal through an opening (intervertebral foramen) between the pedicles of the two vertebrae of a functional unit.

A number of tissues in and around each functional unit can cause localized or radiating pain if they are irritated, injured, or inflamed. These tissues are the posterior longitudinal ligament, the outer layers of the annulus fibrosis, the spinal nerve passing through the intervertebral foramen, the posterior synovial joints and capsules, the interspinous ligaments, and the back muscles themselves. The skin and subcutaneous fat overlying the back muscles can also be a source of discomfort. Figure 15-2 illustrates how these tissues receive their nerve supply and hence how they are able to "communicate" discomfort perceived as coming

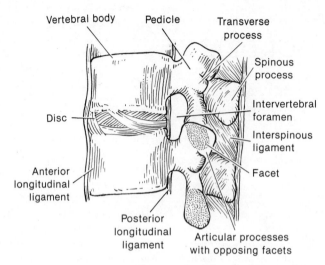

FIGURE 15-1. Lateral (side) view of the functional unit of the vertebral column. Two vertebrae and one disc make up the unit. The spinal cord (not shown) is located behind the posterior longitudinal ligament. The spinal nerve (also not shown) exits through the intervertebral foramen.

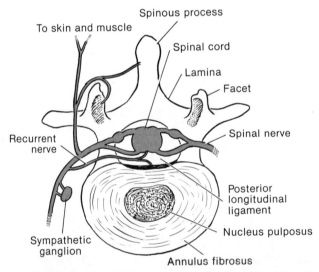

FIGURE 15-2. Top view of functional unit showing nerve connections to the soft tissues of the functional unit. The spinal nerve leaving the vertebral canal branches into an anterior and a posterior division. The posterior division serves the facet joints, the interspinous ligaments, and the skin and muscle of the back. The anterior division sends a nerve branch back into the vertebral canal to serve the posterior longitudinal ligament, annulus fibrosis, and meninges (coverings) of spinal cord. The anterior division goes on to connect to the sympathetic nervous system (see fig. 3-12, p. 29) and to innervate muscle function and sensation in the limbs.

from the local area of damage or as radiating pain. Radiating pain seemingly comes from areas away from the local damage which receive their nerve supply from the same spinal nerve associated with the damaged tissues.

The Erect Spine

The erect vertebral column is composed of four curves. The curves created by the cervical and lumbar vertebrae are convex toward the front of the body and

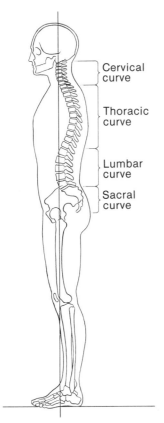

FIGURE 15-3. Lateral view of the erect normal spine, pelvis, and lower extremity. The normal curves (cervical lordosis, thoracic kyphosis, lumbar lordosis, and sacral kyphosis) are seen in relation to a gravity force line.

concave toward the back and are termed *lordotic curves*. The curves created by the thoracic vertebrae and the sacrum are in the opposite direction and are termed *kyphotic curves*. Figure 15-3 shows the relationship of these curves to a vertical line passing through the center of gravity of the body. This vertical line passes from the ear down through the entire spine behind the hip joint and in front of the knee joint. Any excessive

curvature in any one of the four curves must produce a compensatory increase in the curvature of the neighboring curve in order for the head to remain oriented over the feet.

The cervical, thoracic, and lumbar vertebrae are supported at their base by the sacrum. The basic angle or orientation of the sacrum (*lumbrosacral angle*) is one factor that determines the degree of curvature of the lumbar lordotic curve, the thoracic kyphotic curve, and the cervical lordotic curve. The lumbosacral angle is formed by a horizontal line and a line parallel to the top surface of the sacrum (fig. 15-4). Since the sacrum, for all practical purposes, is rigidly attached to the pelvis, all muscles and ligaments attached from the thigh to the pelvis can influence the degree and the size of the lumbosacral angle. These muscles are the hip extensors, namely, the muscles of the buttock (glutei) and the posterior thigh (hamstrings), and the hip flexors (iliopsoas). The dominant ligament influencing this angle is the *iliofemoral ligament* in front of the hip joint extending from the pelvis to the femur.

The influence of the size of the lumbosacral angle and the orientation of the sacrum to the curvature of the lumbar spine in the low back is illustrated in figure 15-4. An increased lumbosacral angle results in an exaggeration of the lumbar lordosis (''swayback''), and a smaller lumbosacral angle reduces the curvature of the lumbar lordosis. As already mentioned, exaggerations or reductions of this type will also influence the magnitude of the curves in the thoracic and cervical areas.

The body weight above any particular functional unit is supported by the vertebral body and the surfaces (facets) of the posterior synovial joints. The vertebral body, with its large surface area, is better designed to support the superincumbent body weight than is the smaller surface area of the posterior joint. As figure 15-5 shows, the greater the lordosis, the greater the amount of the body weight supported by the joints, and the smaller the amount supported by the

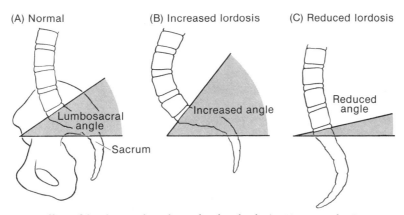

FIGURE 15-4. Effect of lumbosacral angle on lumbar lordosis. *(A)* Normal, *(B)* Increased, *(C)* Decreased.

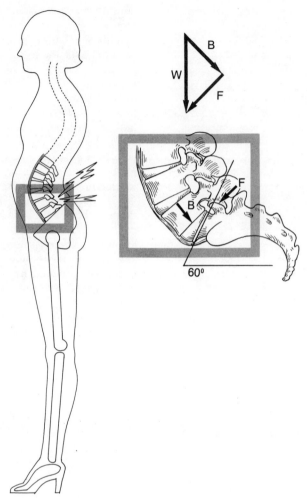

FIGURE 15-5. Effect of an increased lumbar lordosis on the forces acting on the posterior neural arch joints. The super-incumbent body weight, *W,* can be viewed as made up of two components: *B,* the force perpendicular to the vertebral body, and *F,* the force parallel to the surface of the vertebral body which is absorbed at the facets. The greater the lordosis, the greater the force *F.*

vertebral body. An excessive lumbar lordosis, in addition to putting greater weight-bearing demands upon the facets, also induces more pressure on the posterior portions of the disc and tends to narrow the intervertebral foramen through which the spinal nerve emerges. For all these reasons, an excessively lordotic posture can induce back pain.

Low back pain noted in the erect nonmoving spine is termed "static" or postural pain. Occupations that require relatively erect nonmoving postures would therefore be less than desirable for persons with static pain.

The Moving Spine

The lumbar spine allows movement in three directions; sideways, forward, and backward. The forward movement, such as occurs during bending and lifting, and the backward movement, such as occurs on the resumption of the erect posture, are the most important. Figure 15-6 indicates what happens to the lumbar spine when forward bending occurs. Normally, the lordosis of the erect posture fully reverses and becomes kyphotic at the end of a full forward movement. For this curvature change to be achieved, the discs must be flexible and the posterior longitudinal ligament, interspinous ligaments, and back muscles must be able to lengthen sufficiently.

Full forward flexion is also associated with rotation of the pelvis about the hip joint axes and hence also requires the full length of the hamstrings. Resumption of the erect posture from a forward flexed position is ordinarily a smooth action as the pelvis rotates and the lumbar spine simultaneously resumes its lordosis.

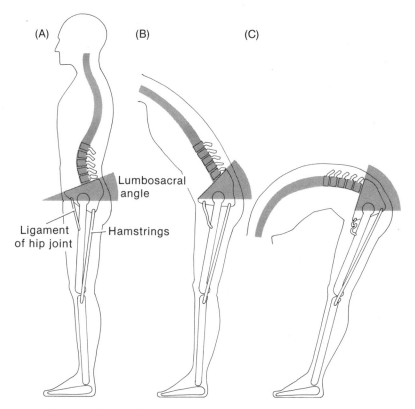

FIGURE 15-6. Schematic display of lumbar spine, pelvis, and lower extremities during forward flexion. *(A)* Erect spine showing normal lumbar lordosis and lumbosacral angle. The iliofemoral ligament is fully stretched and the hamstrings are relatively slack. *(B)* As flexion begins, the lumbar lordosis disappears. The lumbosacral angle increases as the pelvis begins to rotate around the hips. The iliofemoral ligament becomes redundant and the hamstring muscles increase in length. *(C)* In full forward flexion, the lumbar curve is kyphotic, the lumbosacral angle is maximum, and the hamstring muscles are at maximum length.

Low back pain that occurs during movement, either during forward bending or during resumption of the erect posture, is termed "kinetic" or functional back pain. Occupations associated with such movement therefore would be considered less desirable for clients with kinetic pain.

SPECIFIC SYNDROMES

Introduction

A normal individual will be free of static and/or kinetic pain under the following conditions:

1. No abnormality in the structures of the functional unit
2. Adequate but not excessive length in the ligaments
3. Proper strength and endurance of the musculature
4. Body weight consistent with the individual's size
5. Posture that, over the years, has developed without excessive curvatures
6. Acute and chronic stresses and demands well within the capacity of the various tissues to respond.

Clearly, then back pain may result: (a) from stresses exceeding the capacity of the tissues to respond, even if the individual's action was properly performed; (b) from less severe stresses on tissues with prior degeneration or injury; or (c) from improper performance of an activity, such as a bend or a lift, even with fully normal structures and stresses otherwise well tolerated.

Fatigue, anxiety, anger, depression, and other distractions may induce improper performance and cause an injury. The likelihood of back pain is greater with even small stresses if individual muscles and ligaments are in poor condition due to a prior history of insufficient exercise and activity, or if the tissues were previously damaged. Injury may produce actual ligament tears (sprains), overuse without actual tears (strains), intervertebral disc rupture, and joint inflammation.

It must always be kept in mind that back pain may be secondary to other conditions, such as cancers or infections originating in bone or seeding into bone from other areas; kidney disease; bowel and gall bladder conditions; and diseases of the bladder and uterus. Ankylosing spondylitis (see chap. 14) should also be considered when back pain complaints appear.

Osteoporosis is another condition that may cause low back pain. In osteoporosis, the amount of calcium in the bone is reduced and the bone is weakened. The manner in which osteoporotic vertebrae might cause back pain is not always clear. It is felt by some that osteoporosis may produce pain through tiny microfractures not apparent on X-ray examination. Frank obvious fractures can also occur if the bone is sufficiently weakened through loss of calcium to be unable to withstand the stress to which it is subject. Such stresses need not be great. In relatively severe osteoporosis, the simple action of getting out of bed or bending forward, even in a normal controlled manner, may be sufficient to produce fractures visible on X-ray. Osteoporosis is likely to produce both static and kinetic back pain. If a client has this condition, the counselor must deal directly with the physician involved with regard to any vocational planning. More often than not, osteoporosis requires relatively sedentary activities until treatment restores bone strength, if possible.

To understand a major dimension of chronic low back pain from a behavioral point of view, chapter 16 should be read. The following sections are limited to several specific syndromes that can cause low back pain with or without radiation into the buttock and the lower extremities. The salient features of acute sprains without disc rupture, chronic strains, herniated nucleus pulposus, degenerative disc disease, and spondylolisthesis are discussed.

Acute Sprain Without Disc Rupture

The counselor will find that the concepts of strain and sprain are not always explained or defined in the same way. For purposes of this discussion, a sprain, usually the result of an acute or sudden stress, invariably means that tissue has torn. A strain on the other hand, is a discomfort originating out of a chronic, repeating stress not excessive but occurring over a sufficiently long period of time to exceed the endurance capacity of the tissues involved. A strain, therefore, is not viewed as a frank tear or rupture. The following relatively common statements can help clarify these definitions.

"I tripped and fell and *sprained* my ankle."

"I jogged for six miles, and the doctor said I *strained* my ankle."

"I lifted the motor out of my car and *sprained* my back."

"I stood in line for 6 hours waiting to buy football tickets, and the doctor said it *strained* my back."

The terms "acute sprain" and "chronic strain" are redundant, given these definitions for strain and sprain. It is useful, however, to use these terms to help avoid confusion.

Acute low back sprain without disc rupture therefore implies the occurrence of an excessive stress on a normal well-conditioned back, a minor stress on a normal but unprepared back, or a relatively minor stress on an unconditioned or diseased back. The tears referred to in this condition are localized to the muscles, the ligaments, and the capsules of the neural arch joints.

The pain associated with such tears is usually appreciated at the instant of the stress, although the initial pain may not be severe and might abate, only to become more intense within about 2 hours. Hemorrhage, edema, and inflammation following the tear cause increased pressure in the tissue and intense pain shortly thereafter. The muscles around the site will usually go into a spasm as a reflex response to splint the area and reduce movement. Chronic contractions of even the relatively healthy muscles may add additional secondary pain. The discomfort usually causes activity to cease and will cause any but the most stoic individual to seek medical attention, if not the same day, then certainly a day later. The pain, while initially located at the site of the tear, may also be experienced as radiating. Both static and kinetic pain are present.

The key issue with acute sprains is adequate treatment and reduced use to allow healing to occur and hopefully to ultimately restore the tissue to a normal state. Lack of adequate treatment can result in unhealed tissue and predispose the back to further injury from less severe stresses and to chronic strain problems.

A counselor's client is not likely still to be in the acute phase. However, he may well have an initial history of an acute sprain which did not fully heal, resulting in a chronic pain problem.

Chronic Strain

With static pain. A chronic strain problem exists when the onset and persistence of static low back pain is associated with a history of prolonged standing and sitting, superimposed on tissues no longer able to sustain such stresses. Prior sprains, poor posture, or general deconditioning may be the cause. The discomfort is described as aching or throbbing, possibly even sharp or excruciating. It is aggravated by prolonged activity and is eased by frequent changes in position. The pain may be referred into the buttock area, but rarely into the legs.

Patients with this condition often have an increased lumbar lordosis, and the pain is aggravated by further arching or extension of the back, high heels, or a protuberant abdomen (fig. 15-5). Persistence of the swayback posture without a program of exercises to reverse it may cause the back to lose flexibility on forward bending and introduce kinetic pain as well.

With kinetic pain. Chronic kinetic low back strain is

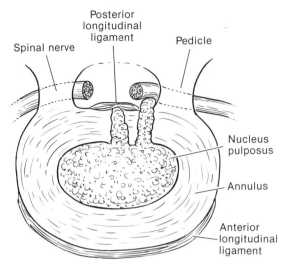

Spinal nerve

Posterior longitudinal ligament

Pedicle

Nucleus pulposus

Annulus

Anterior longitudinal ligament

FIGURE 15-7. Top view of an intervertebral disc whose annulus fibrosis has ruptured in two places. On the left, extruding nucleus pulposus material abuts against the posterior longitudinal ligament. On the right, the extruding material bulges against the spinal nerve.

associated with, and develops as a result of, repeated activities requiring forward bending. The pain may centralize in the low back, but may also refer into the buttocks and the legs. The variation depends upon which structures involved with the chronic activity are less able to handle the continued stresses. The pain, once it develops, is aggravated by forward flexion and resumption of the erect posture, and may also be present in the static sitting and standing postures.

Patients with chronic kinetic low back pain usually demonstrate limited low back flexibility. The normal lumbar lordosis does not reverse on forward bending (fig. 15-6). If the hamstring muscles behind the thigh are tight, an added burden is placed on the lumbar spine during forward bending, which aggravates the flexibility limitation.

The condition may develop after acute sprains or in deconditioned persons subjected to continuing stresses which, for them, are excessive. Poor techniques when executing forward bending and extension can aggravate the condition. Patients with increasing kinetic low back pain may develop secondary muscle spasm to inhibit further forward bending, creating back rigidity. If rigidity occurs only on one side, it will induce a scoliosis.

Herniated Nucleus Pulposus (HNP)

Herniation of the nucleus pulposus of the intervertebral disc refers to its extrusion through a tear in the annulus fibrosis (fig. 15-7). The tear may be secondary to an acute high-level stress (acute sprain) or to a long-standing chronic strain problem. Trunk rotation stresses are more likely to induce a tear or rupture in the annulus fibrosis than forward and

backward forces. As the nucleus pulposus herniates through the tear, it may bulge against the posterior longitudinal ligament in the midline or rupture somewhat laterally to cause pressure on the spinal nerve exiting through the intervertebral foramen.

The pain of a herniated nucleus pulposus (ruptured disc) is usually more severe than that of the other conditions discussed above. Spasm of the back muscles may be particularly marked and the patient may stand with a tilt and be unable to flex forward. The location of the pain in herniated or bulging discs depends upon which tissues are being pressed upon. Most commonly, herniated discs occur between the L4 and L5 vertebrae and between the L5 vertebra and the sacrum.

In addition to the signs of kinetic low back pain, particularly if nerve pressure exists, pain will radiate down the extremity along the usual course of the particular nerve involved. Pain may be aggravated by straight leg raising, coughing, sneezing, and straining. In addition, weakness of the leg muscles served by the involved nerve, and numbness, tingling, and loss of sensation over the skin of the area ordinarily served by the nerve may also be present. Reflexes can also be affected and, in extreme situations, problems with bowel and bladder function may result.

Degenerative Disc Disease

Degenerative disc disease (DDD) is a condition of aging, and occurs in all individuals. A history of acute sprains and chronic strains can aggravate the progression of the degeneration. With aging, the intervertebral disc gradually dehydrates and the collagen fibers of the annulus fibrosis may gradually fray. Pressure within the nucleus pulposus causes it to gradually encroach outward into the annulus. This dissipates the pressure in the nucleus, the disc therefore begins to collapse, and the vertebrae begin to approximate each other (fig. 15-8). The anterior and posterior longitudinal ligaments become slack and the facets of the neural arch joint compress together, inducing degenerative joint disease (see chap. 14). Bone overgrowth occurs at the facet joints and at the vertebral bodies on either side of the degenerating disc. These bony overgrowths (osteophytes) appear on the anterior and posterior surfaces of the intervertebral foramen and may trap the emerging spinal nerve roots. The collapse of the vertebrae on each other restricts their mobility, resulting in somewhat more rigidity in the back and development of both static and kinetic pain.

Movement of the lumbar spine is limited, particularly in extension. In the majority of situations, the degenerative process is greater on one side, and scoliosis may therefore occur. If the nerve roots are trapped, pain will radiate into the involved extremity, with numbness, tingling, loss of sensation, and muscle weakness, as in HNP.

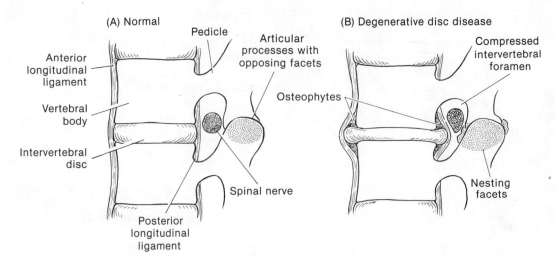

FIGURE 15-8. Effect of degenerative disc disease. *(A)* Normal lateral view of functional unit showing spinal nerve exiting through intervertebral foramen. *(B)* Degenerative disc disease showing narrowed disc, bulging anterior and posterior longitudinal ligaments, nesting of facets, osteophyte production, narrowing of intervertebral foramen, and distorted spinal nerve.

Unlike acute sprains, chronic strains, and HNP, which are exclusively diseases of the soft tissues, degenerative disc disease represents actual changes in the bone and joint structure. Hence, the condition is always there and is neither reversible nor correctable. Fortunately, degenerative disc disease, although present in practically everyone as a function of aging, is not necessarily symptomatic and painful for everyone. While it is not always completely clear why some patients with degenerative disc disease have pain and others do not, one of the factors is the degree of static or kinetic stress on the more rigid back. Hopefully, proper conditioning and proper control of the static and kinetic stresses can allow the patient to function without pain.

Spondylolisthesis

Spondylolisthesis is a condition that may have its onset in the late teens and be present at the beginning of the working years. It is a unique mechanical abnormality of the lower lumbar spine.

If the lumbosacral angle were zero, the lumbar spine would be perfectly vertical and all the superincumbent body weight would be directed straight through the center of the vertebral bodies. Since the lumbosacral angel is rarely ever zero and a lumbar lordotic curve almost invariably exists, the superincumbent body weight creates a stress that is chronically attempting to cause the L4 vertebra to slide forward on the L5 vertebra, or the L5 vertebra to slide forward on the sacrum. Forward slipping is prevented by the locking of the articular facets (fig. 15-9A). The inferior facet of the uppermost vertebra of the functional unit locks behind the superior facet of the lower vertebra of the functional unit, preventing the forward slippage.

If forward slippage does occur, spondylolisthesis is said to be present. Forward slippage can occur if there are defects (spondylolysis) in the locking mechanism. Figure 15-9B demonstrates one of these sypondolysis defects which can lead to spondylolisthesis. In this defect, the facet and the articular processes are separated from the bodies. Thus, while the facets may remain locked, the bodies still can slide forward.

The sliding forward of one body on the other stretches the anterior and posterior longitudinal ligaments and the annulus fibrosis, producing pain. The interspinous ligaments can also be stretched and cause pain. Further, if the spinal nerve roots are trapped by the forward sliding, the same symptoms that occur in HNP or in DDD can be present, namely, pain referred into the leg, thigh, and hip, numbness, tingling, loss of sensation, and weakness. An increased lumbar lordosis, reduced lumbar spine mobility, and a depression in the back above the sacrum where the slip is occurring may be palpable.

The various conditions associated with spondylolysis and the presence of forward slippage can be seen by X-ray. Spondylolisthesis, like degenerative disc disease, is a bony abnormality and cannot be reversed. The pain of spondylolisthesis, however, can often be corrected.

Chronic Low Back Pain

The presence of chronic low back pain after surgery may mean an earlier incorrect preoperative diagnosis, a failure to completely remove an extruded disc, or a failure to explore both sides of an offending disc or more than one level, all of which require proper diagnosis and correction. Persistent chronic low back pain which is not associated with any of the specific

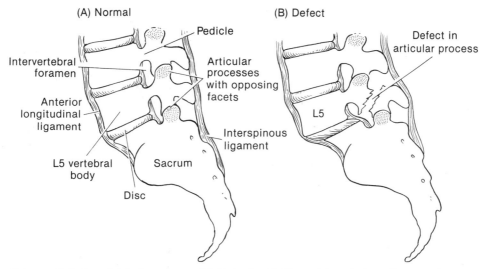

FIGURE 15-9. Spondylolysis and spondylolisthesis. *(A)* Normal lateral view of L5 vertebra and sacrum. *(B)* Defect in articular process of L5 (spondylolysis) with forward slippage of body of L5 on the sacrum (spondylolisthesis).

syndromes discussed in this chapter can also occur. Such chronic pain may well be considered a disease in itself, and one that is particularly disabling, even though objective signs do not seem to "justify" the degree of disability. Chapter 16 deals with the nature of this condition, its causal factors, and the techniques available for treatment and rehabilitation.

FUNCTIONAL DISABILITIES

Physical Disabilities

All of the specific syndromes listed above produce, to a varying degree, reduced levels of function in standing and walking, and possibly also in dressing, bathing, and other tasks that require general trunk mobility. Negotiation on uneven ground, slopes, and stairs may also be impaired. In the majority of cases, the ordinary requirements of dressing, walking, and standing can be met. Those activities associated with the patient's particular employment activity are likely to be impaired, since they are often the activity requirements contributing to the back problem initially.

Pyschosocial Disabilities

Back pain, psychological disturbances, and social upheaval frequently go together. Anxiety, depression, anger, and fear influence how a person uses his musculoskeletal system. All these emotional factors may increase the person's estimation of his disability and may in themselves aggravate the discomfort. Legal factors, compensation factors, and fear of supervisors all contribute to the psychological response and may interfere with an effective rehabilitation. Attitudes of spouse and family, co-workers, and others may influence how a patient responds to his discomfort. In the male, it is not unusual to find psychological impotency as part of the picture.

STANDARDS OF EVALUATION

Medical Evaluation

Orthopedic surgeons and physiatrists are usually the physicians most able to evaluate the back and lower extremities. Since there are other than mechanical causes of back pain, a complete physical examination also needs to be included in addition to the localized examination of the back and the legs. When other causes might be suspected, an internist, urologist, or gynecologist might well be asked to see the patient if the diagnosis is unclear.

The evaluation includes a careful history which characterizes the back pain, indicates factors that make it better or worse, analyzes the relationship of the pain to activities at work, play, or in the home, and a review of the details of an accident, if one has occurred. Examinations of posture, leg length, back mobility, hip range of motion, knee range of motion, and strength of the back, abdomen, and legs are generally included. A neurological examination of the lower extremities is mandatory for the presence or absence of spinal nerve disease. The search for causes might also include a number of blood and urine tests.

X-ray examination of the back and sometimes the hips is standard. Part of the X-ray examination searches for congenital defects, such as: spina bifida occulta, a failure of the posterior elements of the vertebrae to fuse; sacralization, a condition in which the L5 vertebra is fused to the sacrum rather than existing alone; lumbarization, a condition in which the

S1 vertebra, rather than being part of the sacrum, is separated out as a vertebra on its own; degenerative disc disease; spondylolysis; and spondylolisthesis.

Additional special tests may include electromyography, an examination of electrical activity in the muscles of the lower extremity which can be altered due to spinal nerve involvement. A special X-ray examination, during which dye is injected into the vertebral canal (myelography), may be considered and is usually done after the decision to operate has already been made. The outline of the column of dye after injection is viewed by X-rays and can suggest injury to spinal nerves by herniated discs, narrow intervertebral foramina, spondylolisthesis, and degenerative disc disease.

If posture abnormalities or significant obesity problems are superimposed on the back pain problem, the primary physician might ask for assessment by a physical therapist to review posture and lifting techniques, and by a dietician to recommend modification of eating habits.

Psychosocial Evaluation

There is a clear interrelationship between emotional and social factors and back pain and disability. Therefore, all back pain patients with discomfort of a chronic nature and all who respond poorly to management and are still uncomfortable within 2 to 4 months of an initial episode should have psychological or psychiatric consultation for review of contributing factors. It has been suggested by many that no patient should be operated upon who has not yet had careful psychological and personality review. Too often, psychological and psychiatric consultation is considered too late.

Review by a medical social worker of social adjustment, the health of spouse and family, financial status, and any litigation factors can be valuable in understanding the entire milieu in which the back problem is occurring. Careful review of vocational history and performance also contributes to the understanding of the overall adjustment of the patient prior to the back discomfort.

TOTAL TREATMENT

Acute Sprain Without Disc Rupture

Acute sprains require 6 to 8 weeks of immobilization for proper healing. The first 2 weeks might well include total bed rest, and hospitalization may be required for some patients. The remaining period of immobilization may not require full bed rest, but will require reduced activity and the support of a corset. Medications to ensure relaxation and to control inflammation and pain are usually included during the acute phase. Judicious medication prescriptions are

required and are best limited in duration to guard against drug abuse. Mild superficial heat and light massage are also useful.

As the initial acute phase subsides, exercises are introduced to restore appropriate length to the muscles and ligaments involved in the area of the sprain or to restore mobility to the back and hips, and to restore strength and endurance to the back, abdominal, and leg muscles. For many patients, the remobilization and strength restoration activities may not begin until after 8 weeks of relative immobilization.

The physician may instruct the patient in a home exercise program, ask a physical therapist to do so, or suggest that the patient regularly receive such treatment by a physical therapist until full range of motion and strength are restored. Instructions must also include proper posture, lifting techniques, and stooping techniques. Lifting techniques for back pain patients involve holding the object close in front of the body, with the pelvis tucked under the trunk and the lifting done largely with the legs rather than with the back. The amount of lifting allowed is often difficult to determine and is best assessed by starting with smaller weights and building up gradually to larger ones. The lifting of excessively bulky objects and those weighing over 25 pounds (11.3 kg) is usually discouraged.

During the remobilization and strengthening program, the patient is gradually weaned off his corset. Depending upon the severity of the acute sprain, full resumption of all activities might not be achieved until 4 months after the initial episode. Static and kinetic stresses associated with work, play, or home activities need to be carefully reviewed for modification, if suggested by the severity of the patient's sprain. Patients who have experienced acute sprains may well be advised to maintain a regular exercise program indefinitely to ensure future protection of their backs.

Chronic Strain

The back pain associated with chronic strain requires a shorter immobilization period than acute sprains, and rarely requires hospitalization. Cessation of the repetitive activity is important initially. Medication for pain relief might consist simply of aspirin or other mild analgesics. More important in the treatment of the chronic strain is usually a 2-month period of full reconditioning. This includes a physical exercise program to increase flexibility and strength, posture training, and training in lifting and bending techniques. A careful review of the activity productive of the strain can suggest alternative approaches to reduce the likelihood of a repetition.

Herniated Nucleus Pulposus

Herniated discs with nerve root irritation require

complete bed rest with the hips and knees slightly flexed. At least a 2-week period should be considered to determine whether rest will prevent damage. While complete bed rest may be possible at home for some patients, others may require hospitalization to ensure complete rest. Pain medications and relaxants assist control of discomfort and anxiety during this period. If relief results, the patient might be allowed up with a corset and be managed subsequently as in acute sprain. A successful nonsurgical treatment program may require a term of 3 months for healing and restoration of back health. During this period, various anti-inflammatory medications of the type discussed in chapter 14 might be considered.

If nonsurgical treatment is failing, surgery is considered. A lamintomy (laminectomy), an opening in the lamina (see fig. 15-2), exposes the vertebral canal to the surgeon. This exposes the disc and the region of the compressed nerve. The herniated fragment of the disc is removed.

Convalescence after successful surgery is usually a 1- to 3-month period, depending upon the severity of the findings and the extent of nerve damage. After the first month, the convalescence reconditioning exercises may begin. These exercises are prescribed by the surgeon and outlined and performed with the assistance of the physical therapist. As in the prior conditions, these exercises are aimed at regaining low back flexibility and muscle strength. Proper bending and lifting techniques are also taught.

Degenerative Disc Disease

If degenerative disc disease is associated with spinal nerve root irritation, the treatment program outlined for herniated nucleus pulposus is followed. If nonsurgical conservative management does not succeed, surgical intervention is required to relieve the nerve of the pressure. Postoperative recovery may take longer. The various anti-inflammatory agents discussed in chapter 14 may also be regularly prescribed. Indefinite corset wear might be prescribed, and the reduced mobility produced by the corset must be considered in later activity and work planning.

Spondylolisthesis

When mild, spondylolisthesis may be manged with a period of bed rest followed by exercises to promote reduced lumbar lordosis and to prevent further slippage. However, it may be necessary to fuse the involved vertebrae surgically. If nerve root pressure is present and causing pain, surgery to relieve the pressure by widening the intervertebral foramen (foraminotomy) may also be required. When fusion is performed, as much as a 6-month period may be required for healing. Conditioning exercises for the back are also required after surgical fusion.

General

In addition to the specifics for each of the above conditions, some techniques may be applied to all of them. Local injections into painful back areas are sometimes useful. More recently, relatively less major surgical techniques have been introduced. In chemonucleolysis, a chemical is injected directly into the disc and is a potentially useful substitute for open surgery for a relatively minor herniated nucleus pulposus. An anesthetic agent, steriod medication, or a destructive chemical can be directly injected into the neural arch joint. Other techniques that destroy the nerve to the facet and reduce pain are also sometimes used. The procedures may be helpful simultaneously as a diagnosis and as a treatment.

Special medication regimes for chronic pain have recently been found to be helpful where a source of pain is reasonably clearly documented but cannot be removed surgically. These medications include Dilantin, Tegretol, Elavil, and Prolixin, all of which require careful monitoring by a physician familiar with their use. Treatment techniques based on behavior modification are discussed in chapter 16.

Psychosocial Treatment

Depending upon psychological, psychiatric, and medical social work evaluations, simultaneous psychotherapy and family and marital counseling may assist patient recovery.

VOCATIONAL IMPLICATIONS

Evaluation of the suitability of potential employment for a client with current or prior back pain requires a particularly careful analysis of the sitting, standing, moving, lifting, pulling, pushing, and climbing requirements of the job. These specific requirements should be reviewed with the client's physician to determine whether they are compatible with the client's condition. If not, the counselor must then determine whether job environment modifications or work simplification can make a particular employment suitable. The counselor may also wish to consult the physician about prognosis, for any known anticipated change in the client's condition over time should be incorporated into the vocational plan.

During the recovery phase of any one of the back syndromes, it may be possible to return the client to work either part time, or full time with temporary modifications in his job. This may ensure the continuation of the work habit and make it easier to resume full activities later. Some employers may prefer this approach to a longer layoff period.

An industrial engineer or perhaps the counselor himself, equipped with knowledge of the client's limits and the job requirements, can suggest modifications in the work environment. Such things as proper elevation of tables, desks, and chairs, and adequate space for the client to utilize the movement techniques he has learned, can be considered. It may also be possible to modify the frequency and duration of any bending, lifting, carrying, pulling, shoving, or other weight-bearing activities and the size of objects to be handled by the worker. The amount of weight to be lifted is often not as important as the bulk of the object, the lifting technique, the height and direction of the lift, and the frequency and rapidity of the lifting process. For example, lifting an object measuring 2 feet by 4 feet by 2 feet weighing only 12 pounds may be more detrimental than lifting a small 25-pound object. The heavier object can be held close in to the body to minimize back stress. Experience has suggested that lifting weights greater than 25 pounds requires caution and careful assessment of whether this is within the client's limits.

If psychosocial assessment suggests that psychological stress is an aggravating factor in the client's back problem, it is important to identify potential sources of stress in the client's job, and to reduce or eliminate them. Productivity requirements, personality clashes, and less esthetic physical environments are examples of stress-provoking issues to consider. For some clients, it may well be that these stress factors, rather than the physical requirements of the job, may govern the choice amongst various employment possibilities.

The following additional guidelines should help the counselor in vocational planning with back pain clients:

1. For clients with back disorders, the physical demands of employment will usually have to be reduced, and more sedentary employment sought.

2. The counselor should assume that the client will be less able to handle acute and chronic physical stresses as well as he did prior to the onset of his back problem, even after optimal treatment.

3. Educational or vocational retraining into less physically strenuous occupations is indicated, particularly for clients in the younger age groups, if such retraining is consistent with the client's interests, aptitudes, intellect, and personality.

4. After a prolonged period of unemployment, a gradual reintroduction of employment through successive experiences in job stations, sheltered workshops, and on-the-job training is more likely to lead to successful job placement. Through this process, the client is able to build up his confidence and his physical endurance before re-entering the competitive job market.

5. The client will attain his maximum strength, endurance, flexibility, and skill in body mechanic techniques from a regular physical therapy program within 3 months. The counselor should recognize that additional physical therapy is not likely to increase the client's function after the completion of such a remobilization program. Improvement in functional level can, however, be anticipated if a physical therapy program is established with a client who has not had adequate physical therapy previously. Further, the counselor should ascertain whether the client requires a continued home exercise program to maintain his functional level and whether the exercises are being performed. Clients who are not regularly performing their prescribed home program can also be expected to improve with the resumption of exercises.

6. Any medical treatment plan which includes surgery and is expected to improve the client's work potential should be delayed until psychological, psychiatric, and social work evaluations have been performed. Surgery is not likely to produce the expected improvement if psychosocial issues contributing significantly to the client's disability are not first resolved or concurrently managed.

7. The counselor should pay particular attention to whether the client's back pain is primarily related to static or kinetic activity, and consider employment possibilities accordingly. Further, jobs requiring frequent changes of position are generally beneficial, while those requiring maintenance of the same position for long time periods are generally detrimental.

CONCLUSION

The client with chronic back pain poses a unique and difficult challenge to the counselor. The disease component is often nebulous, the visibility of the handicap is relatively small when compared to such conditions as spinal cord injury and amputation, and yet the disability is quite profound. The counselor able to successfully return his back pain client to work and sustain such employment has indeed achieved a success.

BIBLIOGRAPHY

Beals RR, Hickman NW: Industrial injuries of the back and extremities. J Bone Joint Surg **54A**:1593–1611, 1972.
This study of 180 industrially injured men compares those with extremity injuries to those with back injuries. All received comprehensive evaluation. The relation to return to work of such factors as duration of unemployment, number of operations, and psychosocial problems, and the predictive value of the MMPI are discussed. Documents the importance of psychological evaluation for optimum results.

Cailliet R: *Low Back Pain Syndrome*. Ed 2, Philadelphia, Davis, 1968.
Covers causes, evaluation, and treatment of low back pain in greater detail than this chapter. Includes an illustrated chapter on therapeutic exercises which the counselor may find helpful.

Kokan PJ, Wing PC, Thompson WJ: Factors associated with failure of lumbar spine fusion. Can J Surg **17**:294-298, 1974.

Reviews medical, vocational, psychological, and economic factors associated with success and failure of spinal fusion. Success is defined relative to postoperative disability, rather than to stability of the fusion.

McNab I: *Backache*. Baltimore, Williams & Wilkins, 1977.

Although written for physicians, this book is not too technical for the counselor. Clearly presents some of the causes of low back pain and discusses the management of several syndromes. Useful for counselors desiring more detail than this chapter.

Rosenthal AM: Rehabilitation of the patient with chronic low back pain. Ill Med J **146**:189-190 and 223, 1974.

Short, concise article describing a treatment program for chronic low back pain. Emphasizes the need for evaluation and treatment of psychological, social, and vocational problems in addition to the medical problem.

Westrin CG, Hirsch C, Lindegard B: The personality of the back patient. Clin Orthop **87**:209-216, 1972.

Description of a study of patients who were absent from work for at least 8 days during the year 1964 due to low back pain. Using matched controls, factors which might be causes of absenteeism were identified.

Wilfling FJ, Klonoff H, Kokan P: Psychological, demographic and orthopaedic factors associated with prediction of outcome of spinal fusion. Clin Orthop **90**:153-160, 1973.

A study of 26 male chronic back pain patients. One group had a single previous spinal fusion and a second group had multiple previous fusions. Identifies factors differentiating patients with good, fair, and poor surgical outcome. Supports previous research indicating the value of the MMPI in predicting surgical outcome.

16 CHRONIC PAIN

Wilbert E. Fordyce, Ph.D.

DISEASE DESCRIPTION

Chronic pain cannot be approached in quite the same way as other disabilities described in this text because it does not respect the usual body boundaries evolved by medical practitioners to support specialization. The site of the pain and the circumstances which first caused it are often of secondary importance and have diminishing relevance after the problem has persisted for months or years (i.e., has become chronic).

The distinction between acute and chronic pain must be made clear. Acute pain, also called time-limited or recent-onset pain, represents the pain prototype most often written about and studied, in which a known or approximately known noxious stimulus is applied for a time-limited period. In experimental pain studies, the stimulus can be measured precisely and is applied for limited and clearly defined time intervals. Pain from a wound, a bruise, a fracture, or an infected tooth are examples of typical acute pain.

One of the differences between chronic pain and acute pain is that, in the case of chronic pain, the noxious stimulus is typically not observed or precisely known, but may only be inferred from previous medical examinations, without direct confirmation that those findings are currently valid. Also, the individual has little basis for estimating when, or even whether, the pain problem and associated disruption of his life will end. Finally, chronicity ensures that learning or conditioning effects will have had an opportunity to become established and to complicate an understanding of the problem. In this chapter, the term "chronic pain" represents a set of problems involving a complex interaction of organic or physical factors, environmental influences, and psychological factors, principally learning or conditioning.

Another way of describing pain problems is to make a functional distinction between respondent pain and operant pain. *Respondents* are actions of an organism which are reflexive in nature. If an adequate stimulus occurs, the response will automatically follow. Respondents are controlled by antecedent stimuli, and usually involve glandular or smooth muscle functions of the body. *Operants*, on the other hand, are responses that are under voluntary control. Operants may also be elicited by antecedent stimuli, but they are influenced by the consequences of the response. Therefore, operants can come under the control of those consequences. Operants mainly involve striated or voluntary muscles (e.g., speech, body movements, and facial expressions).

Neurophysiologically, the distinction between operants and respondents is becoming less important. Work in recent years on automatic or glandular conditioning has demonstrated that many actions that were previously classified as respondent can be conditioned, and therefore have the functional characteristics of operants. However, making a distinction between problems of respondent pain and operant pain is useful in determining the appropriate approach to the problem. When the expression of pain is found to be influenced or controlled to a significant degree by environmental consequences, the problem is one of *operant pain* and the solution to the problem must necessarily consider the role of these environmental consequences. In contrast, expressions of pain found to be influenced or controlled by antecedent environmental stimuli reflect *respondent pain.*

Through careful evaluation and analysis, a patient's pain can generally be classified as either predominantly respondent or predominantly operant in nature. The distinction can only be made after carefully assessing information relating to both body damage factors and the environmental consequences of the patient's expressions of pain. Using the terms "respondent" and "operant" pain avoids the issue of whether a patient's pain is "real" or "imaginary." Pain is what is felt and reported by the patient. The proper question is not whether the pain is real, but rather what factors influence it.

Respondent Pain Model

Traditionally, chronic pain has been viewed from the perspective of a disease or medical model. During the diagnostic process, it is usually assumed that the indicators of the pain problem, the symptoms, occur because of some underlying body damage process. In other words, it is assumed that the problem is one of respondent pain. Further, it is assumed that if the body damage factors were eliminated, the pain would cease. This conceptual model works well with most problems of acute pain, but its effectiveness diminishes as time passes and the pain becomes chronic.

There are, however, some chronic pain problems that may respond to medical treatment and a traditional approach to pain problems. These include headaches, limb or extremity pain, phantom limb pain, and pain associated with spinal cord injury.

Headaches. When headaches are sufficiently severe to immobilize a person and occur frequently enough to make a major difference in routine activities, such as employment, a significant functional impairment results. Headaches tend to fall into four subgroups. The first is associated with the growth of tumors in the cranial cavity. Individuals with this type of headache are rarely candidates for rehabilitation, either because the tumors are untreatable and have a dire prognosis or because they have been successfully treated and leave no residual pain problems.

The second subgroup is called cluster headaches because the headaches occur episodically but in groups (e.g., several over consecutive days, followed by weeks with no occurrence). If medication can alleviate the problem, there is no functional impairment. Patients with cluster headaches rarely appear as candidates for vocational rehabilitation.

Migraine or vascular headaches make up the third subgroup. They may occur at any time, often awakening the person from a sound sleep, but they are more likely to occur following an emotional crisis. These headaches are often preceded by a signal, or "aura," such as visual blurring or spots before the eyes. They tend to be asymmetrical in pain distribution, and the individual's hands are usually cold. The present treatment for migraine headaches is generally medication, biofeedback, or a combination of the two. The combination has a better than 50 percent chance of reducing the problem to manageable levels. In many cases, migraine headaches are so infrequent that they do not cause a vocational problem. There may, however, be a momentary problem if an individual with infrequent headaches does have one while at work.

The final and most common subgroup is tension headaches. They tend to be symmetrical, involving both sides of the head and/or neck. Tension headaches tend to occur during the day, particularly in the later afternoon after tensions have accumulated for a number of hours. Muscle relaxants are often helpful. In recent years, with the advent of biofeedback and other forms of relaxation training, the symptoms often can be brought under effective control. When they cannot, the person usually is highly vulnerable to emotional upset, with very limited capability for coping with stress. Often when these treatment methods fail to resolve or control the problem, the person is also found to have a psychiatric problem.

A brief mention should be made of facial pain. Aside from dental problems, facial pain tends to take the form of either tic douloureux or so-called atypical facial pain. Neurosurgical treatment methods for tic douloureux are effective in about 80 percent of cases. For the remaining 20 percent of patients, there is little likelihood of their being able to work at all. The atypical facial pain problems can be considered with chronic pain in general.

Limb pain. Chronic pain problems which stem from injuries to the upper and lower extremities are usually found to be respondent in nature. Even late in the problem's history, the pain is substantially more influenced by body damage factors than conditioning or environmental factors. Elbow, wrist, hand, knee, ankle, or foot pain problems which interfere significantly with activity "cost" the individual a great deal, for nearly every self-care act can be hindered. Most persons push to restore function and activity once the injured limb begins to heal. Therefore, those who come to vocational rehabilitation programs or pain evaluation centers are likely to have impairments that are respondent, rather than operant, in nature.

The major exceptions to this are (a) cases in which careful evaluation of the functional impairment reported by the patient reveals inconsistencies (e.g., the patient cannot grasp a pair of pliers but can hold a full stein of beer); and (b) cases in which the "impairment" is primarily a visual display of pain other than inactivity (e.g., the patient walks with a pronounced limp, signaling to his environment that he has pain, but nonetheless moves around and does things). In either of these instances, an operant component is likely and a detailed behavioral analysis will be necessary.

It is more difficult to generalize about shoulder pain. Many shoulder pain problems originate with body trauma and persist because of associated muscle tension. The individual's tendency to guard against movement by tensing the involved shoulder may make the problem worse. In such cases, biofeedback relaxation training may significantly reduce or resolve the problem.

Phantom pain. Following amputation of a limb or part of a limb, phantom sensations of the missing part are very common. These sensations may persist indefinitely to some degree, although intensity is likely to diminish with time. Not all phantom sensations are painful; phantom sensations and phantom limb pain should not be confused (see chap. 13, p. 186).

Fitting an amputee with a prosthetic limb very soon after surgery markedly reduces the frequency, intensity, and duration of phantom pain. If persistent and interfering phantom limb pain does occur, the treatment of choice is chemotherapy, such as Dilantin or Tegretol. Phantom limb pain is rarely a problem of lasting significance in vocational rehabilitation.

Pain associated with spinal cord injury. Two different forms of pain are often reported by spinal cord injured persons. The first is a sharp, burning pain which occurs episodically and often lasts only a few seconds. These episodes usually occur several times a day, although several days may pass without any occurrence. This form of post-injury pain seems similar to an epileptic seizure. Again Dilantin or Tegretol is the medication of choice and often adequately controls the problem.

The second type of pain is a deep, dull aching pain which tends to persist for hours, days, weeks, or even months, and generally increases with activity. This type appears to function more like operant pain and should be treated in the same way as other operant pain problems (see below).

It should be emphasized here that these respondent pain problems should not be confused with those associated with chronic systemic illness, such as rheumatoid arthritis or degenerative joint disease. However, the extent to which the functional impairment displayed seems warranted by the current state of the disease should be considered.

Treatment of chronic pain based on an analysis of the patient's problem by the medical/disease model often fails. When this happens, the physician committed to that model is in a dilemma, for he has few options. In most situations, he will simply refer the patient to another physician. However, the second physician is likely to apply the same conceptual model, and unless the first physician made an error or the second has some special skill or method unknown to the first, it is unlikely that the referral will lead to a successful "cure."

The physician's second option is to repeat the therapy which originally failed. Often a second surgery or a second course of such conservative management techniques as heat, massage, traction, or an alternation of these treatment modalities is attempted. Although sometimes successful, these techniques will likely have been tried repeatedly on most chronic pain patients without major changes in either self-reports of pain or functional ability.

A third option, not generally used until other therapies have been tried and found unsuccessful, is to infer that the pain problem is not real. This is often communicated to the patient by telling him the problem is "all in his head." This option may lead to one or more responses.

One response is to label the pain problem "psychogenic," which implies that the pain symptoms are influenced by some personality problem. The patient may then be referred for psychotherapy. Patients often reject this recommendation. If they accept, it is generally with reluctance and their participation in the therapy process is unenthusiastic.

Even if psychotherapy is accepted and followed diligently, it is indeed unusual to find a chronic pain patient whose problem is resolved by this treatment.

The most common response of physicians who have inferred that the patient's pain is imaginary when traditional treatment methods have failed to solve the problem is to tell the patient there is nothing more he can do. The patient is then given a medication regimen of renewable prescriptions, some recommendations regarding rest and exercise, and told he is going to have to go home and learn to live with the pain. The intent is to reduce fruitless pursuit of new diagnostic and treatment interventions, but it tends to have the opposite effect. Challenging the authenticity of the patient's pain in this way often serves to increase, rather than decrease, his use of health care providers because he is placed in the position of having to prove that he really hurts.

Persisting with traditional approaches to chronic pain occurs, therefore, primarily because physicians find themselves with few alternatives. There is, however, another way of considering a chronic pain problem, which is to deal with those behaviors of the patient which indicate to others that he is in pain. This approach to the problem of chronic pain may be called an operant pain model, in contrast to the respondent pain model traditionally used.

Operant Pain Model

There are persistent and repeated signals from the chronic pain patient to the environment that he has a pain problem. Such signals include grimacing, moaning, gasping, limping, giving verbal descriptions of pain, moving in a guarded manner, or spending much of the day reclining. Such signals, or *pain behaviors,* are operants and subject to the same influences as any other behavior.

Pain behaviors rarely are controlled exclusively by body damage factors (respondent pain), with no influence from environmental consequences (operant pain). There is now considerable evidence to indicate that pain behaviors which began as a response to a body damage stimulus often persist because of the influence of environmental consequences.

A positive consequence which systematically follows a particular behavior and which is contingent on that behavior is a *reinforcer.* Behaviors tend to recur more frequently or consistently if there is some prospect of again achieving a reinforcer. Conversely, a behavior which has been occurring but is no longer reinforced will begin to fade and ultimately will disappear. This process is known as *extinction.*

This is not to suggest that simple, or even complex, changes in environmental consequences automatically have immediate and unlimited impact on behavior. The relationships between the human organism, the learning process, and the residual effects of prior learning are too complex for this to be the case. However, persons are sensitive to consequences and their behavior does show change under the impact of systematic and persisting modification of environmental consequences.

Conditioning plays a role in the establishment of pain behaviors in three basic ways. First, pain behaviors may be *directly reinforced.* For example, a pain patient displaying distress may receive special attention which would not occur otherwise. The special attention is contingent upon display of pain behaviors.

A second and probably more important source of conditioning involves *avoidance conditioning.* When an individual is faced with an aversive or noxious event, he takes action to avoid it, if possible. Consider what may happen to a pain patient with a sore back. He reclines to rest it, thereby avoiding the pain which would occur if he went to work. Suppose that this person had a poor job or had recently been promoted beyond his competence and was anxious about keeping his new job. Staying home from work is reinforced not only by avoiding pain but also by avoiding the stress or anxiety caused by being at work. Either source of reinforcement is capable of effectively strengthening the pain behaviors.

For the majority of chronic pain patients, their pain behaviors not only guard against or reduce pain but also avoid other noxious events. When the body damage factor which originally triggered the pain heals or is effectively treated, the avoidance behaviors are no longer being reinforced by avoiding pain. Most pain behaviors are awkward and cumbersome and thus are themselves somewhat aversive to the patient. However, if the alternatives to being sick are *more* aversive, the pain behaviors would continue to be effectively reinforced by the avoidance of these aversive alternatives. If being sick or impaired with pain does not result in other hardships for the person, the risk of the avoidance pattern persisting is even higher. For example, if disability compensation benefits maintain an adequate level of income, the pain problem will probably be less aversive. If, in addition, the patient avoids returning to an aversive job by continuing to demonstrate evidence of persisting pain, these behaviors would be further strengthened.

There is a third and less important way in which conditioning may play a role. Some patients find that being more active is *directly punished.* Family members may insist that the patient take it easy to avoid making the pain worse, and physicians may prescribe rest for longer than is actually necessary.

Two additional observations may substantiate the importance of conditioning and learning factors in chronic pain. One almost never finds young persons under age 22 with chronic pain, except those affected by a disease process such as juvenile arthritis. They are too active, energetic, and involved in things requiring action and mobility to be immobilized by pain for more than a few days. Unless complications set in, a sprained back or ankle usually heals quickly in this age group, after which normal activity levels are resumed. The probability of rapid recovery and resumption of normal activity begins to diminish as age advances.

One might also consider the professional football player's response to pain. During the course of a game, there are stimuli far exceeding those sufficient to produce severe pain under other circumstances. But the player gets up, shakes it off, and continues to play. There appear to be three reasons why this occurs. Neurological and biochemical mechanisms undoubtedly play a short-term role. An ingenious neurological theory, the Gate Control Theory, contends that the nervous system is capable of generating nerve impulses from the brain "downstream" on the spinal cord. These impulses have the effect of partially or completely closing the "gate" of the brain, so that pain impulses arising from the site of body damage cannot get through to the brain or get through only in a reduced amount. More recent biochemical research indicates that the brain is capable of releasing substances which act much like morphine to reduce the pain experience. These mechanisms, however, are unlikely to persist through a full game, much less over a season. A second factor is that the player has had years of experience and prior conditioning against the display of pain behaviors. Third, pain behaviors would "cost" too much—he would not be able to play if he repeatedly signalled that he was experiencing severe pain.

Examination of some of the failures of the traditional medical (respondent pain) model for approaching problems of chronic pain will further highlight the principles of conditioning underlying the behavioral approach to this problem. One such failure involves medication. Medical students learn that pain medications carry the hazard of addiction or habituation. The traditional safeguard is to require patients to limit their use of pain medications to only those times when they are needed; that is, the patient must hurt before getting the medication. This is written on a prescription as *p.r.n.,* "take only as needed." The *p.r.n.* regimen seems sensible, but it often fails. Experience in clinics specializing in chronic pain problems suggests that nearly 50 percent of clinic patients give evidence of addiction or habituation to pain medications. Nearly all of them have been on *p.r.n.* regimens.

Examining the *p.r.n.* plan from a behavioral or conditioning viewpoint suggests a possible explanation for the high addiction/habituation rate. The *p.r.n.* plan makes medication *pain contingent.* The patient does something, hurts, and then requests medication. The activity-hurting sequence is systematically followed by a particular consequence: medication. If the medication makes the patient feel better, it could be considered a reinforcement for pain. This is likely to make the pain behaviors, which signal the presence of pain and the need for medication, to become conditioned. Clinical experience indicates that this is often the case.

Traditional methods for handling rest and exercise also present problems. Whether by formal prescription or their own devices, pain patients for whom a specific exercise or physical activity makes the pain worse tend to fall into a "work-to-tolerance" pattern. They will engage in an activity or exercise until pain begins or reaches an intensity they no longer wish to tolerate, then stop to rest. Activity or exercise is systematically followed by expressions of pain, which are in turn systematically *and contingently* followed by rest, avoidance of further work, and the associated beneficial results. As with pain-contingent medications, pain-contingent rest is likely to strengthen or increase (i.e., condition) the pain behavior which leads to the reinforcer.

FUNCTIONAL DISABILITIES

The functional disabilities associated with chronic pain vary considerably from patient to patient. They may be physical and/or psychosocial, and are caused by the pain behaviors which limit activity or lead others to encourage activity restriction.

Physical Disabilities

Many pain behaviors interfere with physical movement, vigor, and speed. For example, ambulation may be impaired by a limp, or the distance a patient can walk may be limited by the need to rest frequently. Pain behaviors may limit both the extent and duration of body motions, such as lifting, bending, twisting, and reaching. In addition, actions guarding against pain or the residual effects of surgeries to alleviate the problem may result in selective limitations. A person with a back fusion, for example, may not be impaired by pain but may be mechanically restricted in twisting or bending.

Pain medications significantly interfere with alertness or body control, and may cause dizziness, changes in intellectual and cognitive function, or lethargy. Judgment and memory may also be affected. These in turn may affect ambulation and coordination, and may impair reading, writing, driving, and fine motor skills.

Psychosocial Disabilities

The communication of pain, either verbally or nonverbally by movements or facial expression, is likely to elicit oversolicitous responses from family members, co-workers, and others. This reaction may reinforce the pain behavior and cause activity to be limited more than necessary. The patient's spouse or other family members may provide much pain-contingent support or attention for pain behaviors, encourage the use of medication, or discourage the patient's attempts to become more active. Spouses may also be strongly supportive of efforts to maintain compensation income in lieu of wages.

Chronic pain patients may be unnecessarily inactive because of fear of incurring additional body damage or pain. If continued activity increased the patient's pain early in the history of his pain problem, he may continue to fear activity as a source of pain even when this is no longer necessarily true.

Chronic pain patients are often depressed. Sometimes the patient's problem is really depression rather than pain, but it is often difficult for the patient or those who observe and examine him to differentiate between the two. For example, one often finds a chronic pain patient with markedly lowered activity level, allegedly because physical movement results in increased pain, who displays greatly increased activity level and tolerance when the only treatment has been antidepressant medications. Thus, sometimes a problem is mislabeled pain when it actually is depression.

Many chronic pain patients have other problems which would give them much distress if they were not limited by pain. The first-ranking functional disabilities are the pain behaviors and the immediate impairments associated with them, but the functional impairments characterized by limited ability to be effectively well are not less important. This relates to avoidance learning and corresponds to what is often termed "secondary gain." For example, some workers disabled by pain and receiving wage-replacement compensation find those funds sufficient reinforcement to maintain their pain behaviors, particularly when return to work might be aversive because of poor job skills, conflict with their employers, or aversive change in job responsibilities. In effect, being sick does not "cost" enough to offset the reinforcement from avoiding the aversive consequences of work.

Another source of aversive stimuli which may reinforce pain behaviors is the existence of another disability more aversive to the patient than pain. For example, some older pain patients are found to have memory deficits associated with minor strokes or arteriosclerosis. Were they not disabled by "pain," they would risk revealing intellectual deterioration. Similarly, patients with multiple sclerosis or spinal cord injury often will attribute their limited performance ability to pain when the real problem is that they find being seen in public in a wheelchair aversive. "Pain" rationalizes their immobilization.

Rehabilitation Potential

The presence of pain or a pain problem by itself often has little direct influence on rehabilitation potential, which is determined primarily by what each person does about the pain. The kind of action taken when pain arises varies among individuals and affects the level of physical disability. Some persons get up, move around, and change body position when they feel pain. They tend to have high activity levels and are therefore called "pacers." Usually they have either tension headaches or pain problems in the high back, neck, shoulder, and arms. Most pacers maintain their usual activity patterns, and do not have functional disabilities. These patients are not likely to require vocational rehabilitation services.

Persons who rest when pain arises are called "recliners." They tend to have low activity levels and more functional impairments. Their pain is more likely to be located in the low back or abdomen. There is usually a marked difference in the kinds and amounts of physical work recliners can and will do compared with pacers. Recliners will require treatment to increase their activity level. They are also more likely to require vocational rehabilitation services.

Assuming that treatment has restored an optimal level and range of activity, or that evaluation indicates that such a restoration is feasible, the potential for rehabilitation is likely to be influenced mainly by avoidance learning factors. Restoration of activity level with treatment and reduction of the various pain behaviors will not suffice if personality functioning is not also brought to a level compatible with job demands. One must ask what the person would be required to do if he were not limited by pain and then assess the extent to which he could cope with the situation.

Not all pain patients, even though effectively treated, can return to their previous level of employment. This is generally due to inconsistencies between the basic characteristics and strengths of the individual and the specific demands and requirements of the job. Once pain behaviors have been minimized, care should be taken not to reinstate the individual into the environment which may partially have been responsible for the initial maintenance of those behaviors.

STANDARDS OF EVALUATION

The proper evaluation of chronic pain can rarely be adequately accomplished solely by a physician's examination. By the time a pain problem has become chronic, it is rarely merely a disease or respondent pain problem which requires only the identification of the body-damage factor stimulating the pain behaviors. Both medical and nonmedical factors need to be evaluated. Therefore, evaluation of long-standing pain problems usually is best accomplished in a facility using a multidisciplinary approach. Further, it is essential that an evaluation unit be organized to ensure there is adequate communication among those contributing to the evaluation process. If they do not communicate with each other, the evaluation is likely to reflect only the potentially narrow perspective of the dominant figure in the evaluation team.

Some chronic pain patients are essentially intoxicated from pain medications. Effective evaluation of the pain problem cannot be carried out under these conditions. The pain evaluation unit should implement a rapid detoxifying regimen for such patients so that communications are clear and evaluation can proceed. Methods for accomplishing this can be found in the professional literature. Pain evaluation units which do not have access to inpatient facilities will be unable to deal adequately with evaluation of the toxic patient.

Medical evaluation will require a specialist trained to assess the body system or parts involved. For example, an orthopedic surgeon or physiatrist should evaluate back or limb pain and an internist should evaluate abdominal pain.

The frequency with which tension plays a role in pain indicates that a comprehensive evaluation unit should also have a biofeedback component to assess this factor. Tension headaches and the muscle tension pain problems often associated with neck, shoulder, and high back pain should be examined via biofeedback trials, using the EMG mode.

Some pain evaluation programs attempt to evaluate nonmedical factors solely by use of the Minnesota Multiphasic Personality Inventory (MMPI). Studies have been published alleging that the MMPI adequately identifies who will or will not profit from surgery for pain, but other studies fail to support this. Extensive clinical experience with hundreds of chronic pain patients makes it apparent that there are too many contributing factors for any single device to be considered as an adequate appraisal tool. The MMPI should be used, as it is very helpful in gaining an understanding of the personality factors which influence the individual and will also identify the severity of a patient's depression. However, the MMPI needs to be analyzed by persons expert in its use. There are computer-based memory banks from which MMPI interpretations can be obtained, although most of these systems are based upon, and address themselves to, psychiatric problems. Unfortunately these are only sometimes relevant in evaluation of chronic pain. Therefore, availability of staff experienced in using the MMPI with chronic pain patients is helpful.

Adequate evaluation of nonmedical aspects requires careful consideration of the patient's total situation. This can be broken down into two parts: (a) What good things happen if there is pain behavior? This refers to the direct positive reinforcement of pain behaviors. (b) What bad things do not happen if there is pain behavior? This refers to the avoidance learning issue.

Examination of the direct reinforcers for pain behavior requires assessment of previously prescribed medication and rest/exercise regimens to determine whether they have been producing physician-induced problems. Further, the family's response to the patient's pain behaviors and the compensation/litigation issues should be assessed. This evaluation should be performed by a person skilled in interviewing and sensitive to the special problems of chronic pain, such as a social worker, psychiatrist, or psychologist.

Examination of avoidance learning factors is more complex and usually will require the expertise of an experienced psychiatrist or psychologist. The examiner needs to be aware that when a pain problem (i.e., the expression of pain behaviors) cannot be adequately accounted for on the basis of clearly identified and currently active physical findings, the alternative is *not* simply some form of mental illness, personality problem, or motivation problem. Each of those *may* be playing a role, perhaps even a dominant one, but they also may not.

Evaluation of chronic pain should include gathering information about *actual* activity levels: what activities are engaged in, how often, for how long, and at what rate or speed. Although it is generally not practical to obtain direct observations, careful interviewing of the patient and spouse can often help to pinpoint how much activity is possible and how much impairment exists. A pain evaluation which uses only a brief statement by the patient regarding what he can and cannot do is not likely to be accurate or effective because there is often a discrepancy between what the patient says and what he does. A "diary" to record when the person sits, stands, walks, or reclines, completed by patients prior to evaluation, is much more useful.

TOTAL TREATMENT

In keeping with the conceptual model used thus far, the approach to describing treatment of chronic pain will consider the behaviors that need to be changed. Although not all of the treatment methods are necessarily behavioral in nature, treatment objectives can only be discussed in terms of the effects on behavior they are intended to produce.

If the pain problem is largely respondent in nature, with the pain behaviors predominantly under the control of currently active body damage factors, traditional therapies will presumably have been tried and found inadequate. It is possible, but not likely, that the problem may still be responsive to medical intervention and that the medical system failed to properly diagnose the problem. If, after compre-

hensive evaluation, a physician is prepared to assert confidently that there is a definitive treatment available with a high likelihood of a positive outcome, then that course should receive serious consideration and be followed if it has not been tried previously with the patient and found inadequate.

In most cases, however, additional traditional medical intervention is not likely to be fruitful. Furthermore, pain behaviors which were originally elicited by chronic systemic disease, such as rheumatoid arthritis or degenerative joint disease, are still pain behaviors and, as such, may be influenced by partial or substantial control of the environmental consequences of the behaviors. Thus, even when the problem is largely respondent in nature, treatment should address itself to the same set of issues discussed below that must be faced when the pain problem has significant operant elements.

Activity Restriction

Restriction in body movement, position, or range of motion of a limb should be treated with physical therapy and/or occupational therapy. Guided, selectively prescribed exercise has several objectives. First, it is generally important that reduced activity levels be increased to a point where re-employment is feasible. Reduced strength and stamina due to disuse of a limb or body parts will need to be restored. Secondly, as discussed before, many pain patients continue to regard the pain they experience upon moving a limb or body part as a warning signal which should be responded to with rest to prevent increased pain and further body damage. The patient now needs to be taught that it is safe to move about and increase activity without incurring future pain and body damage. Graduated exercise, starting at low levels and systematically increasing, will accomplish this. A third function of exercise is to help the patient's family realize that activity will not prove harmful so that they can provide support and additional encouragement for increased activity.

Procedures for programming exercise plans for chronic pain patients are now well established. First, current exercise tolerance is established through a series of observed exercise trials (baseline tolerance). This information is then used by the patient and therapist together to set goals or quotas. The patient initially does less work than that observed in the baseline tolerance sessions and is rewarded by rest, therapist attention, and effective avoidance of pain. The quotas are then gradually and systematically raised by, for example, an increment of one repetition of each exercise for each treatment session. By working to quota, rest, attention, and the avoidance of pain become work contingent rather than pain contingent. The patient learns to stop when a certain amount of activity is completed, independently of how he feels.

Medication Toxicity

Toxicity or intoxication from narcotics and other pain medications must be eliminated in order to proceed with evaluation and/or treatment. This is most easily accomplished by the so-called "pain-cocktail" method, in which all medications are shifted to oral form. Narcotics, if used, are changed from rapid- to slow-acting types. Methadone is usually the preferred substitute. All other analgesics are shifted to phenobarbiturate equivalents and tranquilizers are eliminated. The ensuing mix is incorporated into a color- and taste-masking vehicle and taken every six hours. Active ingredients may then be systematically reduced at a rate of approximately 10 percent each day until medication is low enough to allow precise patient evaluation or treatment.

This detoxifying method is usually too rapid to permit a lasting deconditioning of long-established drug habits. If there is evidence of addiction or habituation, a more gradual form of withdrawal, continuing with the pain cocktail format, is indicated. When the patient enters treatment following the evaluation phase, the active ingredients are restored to a level providing comfortable coverage for the pain. Still delivered in the color- and taste-masking vehicle (usually cherry syrup), the active ingredients are now reduced approximately 10 percent every 7 to 10 days. The slower rate provides sufficient time for activity level to build up and for the patient to learn he can indeed handle movement without dire consequences. The process should always be carefully explained to patients at the outset of the program.

Overt Pain Behaviors

Patients need to be helped to eliminate endless complaints of pain by word, gesture, or facial expression. This usually can be best handled by (a) ensuring that treatment staff are nonresponsive to signals of pain by avoiding reassuring or comforting comments; and (b) by being responsive to effective effort and activity. This part of the treatment is explained to the patient and family. It is usually simple for treatment personnel to adopt a posture of nonresponsiveness to pain behavior while providing positive attention to activity accomplishments.

Family members of some pain patients are militantly protective and supportive of pain behaviors and ready to discourage or limit activity for fear more pain and body damage will be produced. It is usually essential to the success of treatment that they be helped to learn new ways of responding to the patient's pain behaviors.

In addition, where there is a severe limp or a history of "knee buckling" which has been established as operant in character, it is important to help the patient eliminate such behaviors by systematic gait retraining. If these behaviors are not minimized, the display of such pain behaviors on a job is likely to elicit excessive concern or overprotection from fellow workers, thereby reinstituting social reinforcement of pain behaviors and making the pain problem again worsen.

Depression

In the context of operant pain, depression should not be seen as a form of mental illness for which psychotherapy is indicated, but simply as the natural result of a deprivation of reinforcers resulting from reduced activity level. Therefore, treatment of depression is fairly simple. If the depression is mild, re-establishing activity levels, resulting in increased access to work and play, may well alleviate it. If the depression is more severe, chemotherapy is also used. Antidepressants (usually Elavil and Sinequan) are added to the pain cocktail at levels sufficient to help "energize" the patient, and are reduced at a much slower rate than other elements. If there is real concern about the depression, reduction of the antidepressants should not start until the patient is actually re-engaged in the vocational and avocational activities which are the aim of treatment.

"Avoidance" Problems

Where it has been established that pain behaviors were being significantly supported by the "time out" they yielded from aversive events or activities, it is essential to reduce either those events or activities or their aversiveness to the patient. For example, a worker may be promoted or shifted to new job responsibilities he cannot handle or which produce much anxiety. The emergence of a pain problem has the side effect of helping to avoid the now-aversive job. Treatment for pain which restores activity level and reduces medication intake must also help the person find work he can handle effectively. The treatment plan is more likely to be successful and probably more cost-effective if the vocational counselor focuses on elements of the job (i.e., either altering the job demands or finding the client a more suitable job), rather than trying to alter the worker to fit the aversive job.

Some chronic pain patients are found to be highly vulnerable to confusion and emotional upset, functioning in ways often termed "inadequate personality" or "borderline schizophrenic." Both terms are used to describe persons who are functioning marginally in their environments. Their pre-onset work histories are likely to be marked by marginal performance and frequent job failures. Restoration of activity level and reduction of pain behaviors and medication intake will not likely yield enduring gains unless these marginally functioning persons are helped to find work with limited demands.

''Avoidance'' problems need to be identified, coordinated, and integrated with the overall pain treatment. If it is to be accomplished by referral to another facility or individual, planning for this and obtaining the client's approval must be done in the earliest stages of pain treatment, rather than at the end. The transfer must also be closely monitored to ensure that the new therapist is well aware of the main features of the just-completed pain treatment program.

Muscle Tension

Muscle tension components of pain problems require specialized treatment. There are a number of techniques for training persons to relax, such as direct relaxation instruction, hypnosis, training in self-hypnosis, yoga, or transcendental meditation. The easiest and most effective technique for a wide variety of patients is EMG-mode biofeedback. Surface electrodes are placed on the skin above the hyperactive muscles. The amount of electrical activity in those muscles is then communicated back to the patient by a tone which varies in pitch with the intensity of muscle activity, by a needle moving on a dial, or by both. Using the feedback information, the patient then experiments with ways of reducing the tension or level of muscle activity until one is found that works for him.

Biofeedback treatment for muscle tension is fairly effective with high back, neck, and shoulder pain, tension headaches, and the jaw pain associated with teeth clenching. For tension headaches, electrodes are usually attached to the trapezius muscles supporting the head or on the frontalis muscle on the forehead. For jaw pain, the electrodes are attached to the masseter muscle of the jaw, and for other muscle tension pain sites that can be clearly identified, the electrodes are positioned as appropriate. Biofeedback is rarely effective with low back pain.

Generalization of Performance

The objective of pain treatment is the restoration of performance. Although reduction of pain is usually one step along the way, it does not always lead to restored and maintained performance or activity. Reliance solely on physical therapy and occupational therapy exercise programs often is not sufficient. The increased activity level generated in an exercise program needs to be generalized from the treatment center to the world of work.

Effective treatment of chronic pain usually requires linking increasing exercise level and tolerance in treatment with opportunities to practice the new activity level in work-related activities while still within the treatment program. This may occur in specially arranged situations in the hospital; in community facilities, such as sheltered workshops, where work-related activity levels can be practiced and strengthened; or by arrangement with the employer to provide graduated return to full work demands under the guidance of the treatment team.

Effective pain treatment programs also work at generalization of activity gains through programmed weekend passes and recreational activities. These are important, but are not likely to be adequate substitutes for work-related rehearsal.

Other Treatment Modalities

While chronic pain problems are only occasionally alleviated by additional surgery or nerve blocks, there are three other treatment approaches which have gained a fair amount of attention and should be mentioned here.

Transcutaneous stimulation (TCS). The basic concept of TCS is to provide electrical stimulation to nerve fibers. Although this is usually accomplished through the use of surface electrodes, the transmitter can be introduced into a nerve trunk by surgical means. Numerous studies have been carried out in what appears to be a fruitless effort to identify which pain problems and which patients will benefit. As many as 25 percent may report significant benefit from TCS or some variation, but the findings of various review studies are scattered and variable. Certain generalizations about this approach can be made:

1. TCS, a noninvasive technique as distinguished from surgical implantation of transmitters, is not likely to be harmful.
2. TCS is relatively inexpensive and therefore warrants at least an exploratory trial.
3. Many patients report an initial benefit which subsequently declines, often to no benefit at all, after 2 to 6 weeks. A TCS device, therefore, probably should not be purchased until at least 6 weeks of tryout have elapsed and there is some indication that it produces a discernible effect on a previously limited activity or on medication consumption. Verbal reports of significant relief of pain, if unaccompanied by alleviation of activity constraints, are of questionable merit.
4. Significant benefits from TCS do not necessarily preclude proceeding with further treatment aimed at producing additional gains.

Acupuncture. There are not as yet reliable and scientifically sound data which indicate lasting and significant benefit on functional performance and/or medication consumption from acupuncture treatment applied to problems of chronic pain. Some patients report subjective benefit from periodic acupuncture treatments but those few have not yet been shown to perform significantly differently in work or daily living activities.

Hypnosis. Hypnosis is a potentially powerful, but as yet not well-understood, tool. Only a handful of clinicians have been able to demonstrate lasting benefits from the use of hypnosis for persisting problems of chronic pain. Most hypnosis achievements in relation to pain have been with such time-limited problems as toothaches or childbirth. The major contribution of hypnosis to a spectrum of chronic pain patients has been in assisting reduction of muscle tension. As knowledge expands and skill progresses, perhaps more success will be achieved with this method.

VOCATIONAL IMPLICATIONS

Education

The chronic pain patient will likely have been unemployed for several years. Taking additional "time out" for further education is risky, particularly immediately following a treatment program which has restored activity level. Unless that increased activity level is related to such positive environmental consequences as wages, and the desirable things those wages make accessible, treatment gains can quickly fade. Further education is indicated only where acceptable vocational alternatives are not found and there is compelling evidence to indicate that the newly restored activity level will be sustained during the educational program. If brief training (e.g., 3 months) is undertaken, efforts should be made to continue exercise treatment during this period in order to keep the activity level up.

Aptitudes

Chronic pain, per se, is unlikely to influence aptitudes. The exception would be permanent loss of some body movement or skill due to the effect of surgery. For example, a fused neck will limit head turning.

Interests

The basic question to address here concerns the client for whom pre-onset work proved to be aversive. The counselor must determine the characteristics of that type of work which made it aversive and also identify transferable skills and other interests which would lead to a more satisfactory vocational placement. The methods the counselor will use in dealing with these problems are not different than those used with any other type of client.

Physical Demands

Body changes resulting from surgery or medically prescribed limitation of motion or activity must be considered. A comprehensive treatment program will have addressed itself to restoring physical function to some practical maximum, which can then be translated to specific job demands. There may be some constraints on physical activity even with successful treatment, such as those imposed by surgery. If the chronic pain patient continues to have some visible residual of the pain problem (e.g., the consistently rigidly postured fused back or the limited head turning associated with neck fusion), co-workers may have a tendency to overprotect. Once the work limits have been defined, all involved should be made aware of them and no special accommodation should be made beyond those prescribed.

Chronic pain patients are likely to be more vulnerable to recurrence of pain problems than other persons, and some prudence in regard to physical activity should be prescribed. The translation of those prescriptions into categories ranging from "sedentary" to "very heavy work" will vary according to the specific circumstances of each client.

Employment Opportunities

The vocational counselor working with a client with chronic pain may meet an additional obstacle that he must overcome. Many employers may take the position either officially or unofficially that chronic pain patients are too high a risk with regard to future medical liability. The employers may therefore choose not to employ them, however effectively they may be functioning. Such policies are often influenced by the insurance carrier providing medical coverage for the company's employees. Insurance policies themselves frequently have a clause stating that chronic pain patients may not be hired or, if hired, they will not receive medical coverage. While these policies present further constraints on potential success of the vocational rehabilitation program, the counselor ought not simply to avoid working with chronic pain clients and necessarily assume that he will not be able to place them. Careful documentation of the client's performance ability and his job experiences in workshops or job station, coupled with an appropriate probationary period, may well overcome this obstacle and lead to successful placement.

BIBLIOGRAPHY

A symposium of the chronic pain syndrome in problem low back cases. J Occup Med 17:654–663, 1975.
Four articles by different authors dealing with the eval-

uation, treatment, and prevention of chronic low back pain. The descriptions of typical chronic pain patients and their life situations are especially helpful for understanding the many facets of chronic pain problems.

Bonica JJ (ed): International symposium on pain. *Advances in Neurology,* Vol. 4, New York, Raven Press, 1974. A series of papers by the world leaders in the study and treatment of pain, based on an international symposium held in 1973.

Chapman CR: Psychological aspects of pain patient treatment. Arch Surg **112**:767–772, 1977. Review of the psychological aspects of both acute and chronic pain. In problems of chronic pain, the author emphasizes an interrelation among four dimensions: noxious sensory input, motivational-emotional, conceptual-judgmental, and social-cultural. Pain caused by psychosocial stress and pain maintained by the social environment (operant pain) are also discussed.

Clark WC, Hunt HF: Pain. *In* Downey JA, Darling RC (eds): *Physiological Basis of Rehabilitation Medicine.* Philadelphia, Saunders, 1971, pp. 373–401.

A short, intensive, scholarly review of the subject of pain.

Fordyce WE: *Behavioral Methods for Chronic Pain and Illness.* St Louis, Mosby, 1976.

An analysis of conceptual background and rudiments of behavioral methods, followed by details of their application to the evaluation and treatment of chronic pain problems.

Gottlieb H, Strite LC, Kollar R, Madorsky A, Hockersmith V, Kleeman M, Wagner J: Comprehensive rehabilitation of patients having chronic low back pain. Arch Phys Med Rehabil **58**:101–108, 1977.

This article describes a program in which 72 chronic low back pain patients participated. Biofeedback, counseling, medication reduction, case conferences, physical reconditioning, vocational counseling, educational lectures, and therapeutic milieu were included in the self-regulation program. Treatment was considered successful for 50 of the 72 patients at the end of the program.

Management of pain: Postgrad Med **53** (6), 1973. This entire issue is devoted to a select series of papers by experts in the evaluation and treatment of pain. It is short but comprehensive.

Sternbach RA: *Pain Patients: Traits and Treatments.* New York, Academic Press, 1974.

An innovative view of chronic pain and the special problems of chronic pain patients.

Swanson DW, Floreen AC, Swenson WM: Program for managing chronic pain. Part I: Program description and characteristics of patients; Part II: Short-term results. Mayo Clin Proc **51**:401–411, 1976.

Description of an inpatient operant pain treatment program and short-term followup results. The level of functional improvement at discharge is compared with the level 3 to 6 months later to determine the success of the program.

Swanson DW: Less obvious aspects of chronic pain. Postgrad Med **60** (5): 130–134, 1976.

This article presents the hypothesis that the suffering of chronic pain patients is the product of both (a) some input signal from the periphery, and (b) the attention the patient focuses on the pain site. Economic, sociocultural, and legal considerations relevant to pain and the patient's attention to it are discussed. Treatment measures are considered.

17 ALCOHOLISM

Vernelle Fox, M.D.
James P. Conway, M.S.
Jeri Schweigler, M.S.

DISEASE DESCRIPTION

Alcoholism, with or without a simultaneous drug abuse problem, is one of the most prevalent disabilities in the United States. More often than not, the alcoholic client's stated reason for seeking vocational rehabilitation services will *not* be a candid declaration of alcoholism, but this disease will be the major disability after the client has been adequately evaluated. If the alcoholism is not diagnosed and realistically dealt with, as opposed to simply treating the complications or presenting symptoms, there is virtually no chance of the individual being rehabilitated.

Alcoholism occurs in all ethnic, socioeconomic, and age groups. However, the incidence of the disease is higher in some groups (for example, Irish and native Americans) and lower in others (for example, Jews and Chinese), and is reported three times more often in men than in women. It has been estimated that one-quarter to one-third of the persons who have alcoholism also abuse other drugs, usually sedatives or tranquilizers prescribed for them in an attempt to control their alcoholism. The disease is seen in persons of all occupations, but tends to be higher in some occupational groups, such as physicians, career and service personnel, painters, and short-order cooks. Although speculations have been made, the reason for higher incidence in persons in these vocational areas is not known.

The total number of alcoholics in the United States is estimated to be nine million. About 5 percent of all employed persons are thought to have the disease, while the "skid row" or homeless male with frequent arrests, often thought of as "the alcoholic," constitutes only 3–5 percent of the alcoholic population. During recent years, there has been an increased prevalence of alcoholism among women and youth.

Definition

Alcoholism can be the person's only disability, or it can occur with one or more other physical or psychiatric disabilities. The label "alcoholism" is frequently loosely applied to several groups of disabilities and does not always refer to the disease "alcohol addiction." Much of the confusion and pessimism surrounding this illness is due to the fact that we label abusive drinking as alcoholism without trying to differentially diagnose the mechanism by which the individual developed the alcohol addiction or the specific manifestations and prognosis for that individual. Prior to the mid-1950's, alcoholism was only regarded as willful misconduct rather than as a disease, and alcoholics were handled punitively by the legal system. The individual was blamed for his lack of will power, and medical treatment was only available for the advanced complications of alcoholism.

In this chapter, the terms "alcoholism," "alcohol abuse" and "alcohol addiction," and the terms "alcoholic" and "alcohol addict" are synonymous. The National Council on Alcoholism (NCA) and the American Medical Society on Alcoholism (AMSA) have defined alcoholism as "a chronic, progressive and potentially fatal disease . . . characterized by: tolerance, physical dependency and/or pathological organ changes, all of which are the direct or indirect consequences of the alcohol ingested."

Tolerance is that phenomenon whereby a much greater and more toxic amount of alcohol (or any drug) is required to produce the same subjective effects that a smaller amount originally produced. The exact mechanism for tolerance is not proven, but it is known that certain changes occur in the liver and that persons develop central nervous system adaptation to the sedative effects of alcohol. How much tolerance is due to altered liver metabolism and how much to central nervous system adaptation is not yet known.

Alcohol addicts usually develop *cross tolerance* to other sedative drugs and sometimes to narcotics. The individual who develops a high tolerance for one sedative drug will subsequently nearly always have a higher tolerance, from the beginning, for related drugs. For example, an individual whose metabolism is so changed that it takes a fifth of whiskey to make him drunk will also probably require two or three sleeping pills to put him to sleep, more morphine to kill pain, and more anesthetic to induce unconsciousness than a person with normal metabolism. Also, a person

231

addicted to one drug obviously has a much higher risk of becoming addicted to other drugs.

Withdrawal symptoms begin to occur 6 to 12 hours after the long-term heavy intake of alcohol has ceased. The symptoms reach their peak in 1 to 2 days and gradually subside after 3 to 6 days. The symptoms of withdrawal can be quite mild, such as lack of appetite, sweating, and nervousness, or they can be very severe and potentially fatal, such as severe tremors, hallucinations, convulsions, cardiac irregularity, and shock.

Physical dependency on alcohol is defined by the appearance of some withdrawal symptoms when the individual decreases or ceases alcohol consumption. In addition, an *alcoholic* is generally a person whose drinking repeatedly and seriously interferes with one or more major spheres of his life, such as work, health, or interpersonal relationships.

The NCA has developed groupings of signs, symptoms, and criteria for the diagnosis of this disease. During the early stages of the disease, the individual often drinks increasing amounts to feel a "glow," gulps and sneaks drinks, looks for more occasions to drink, lies about the amount consumed, misses more work and shows decreased performance when at work, has morning shakes, and shows a loss of appetite. In the later stages, the alcoholic typically stays drunk for weeks at a time, is unable to go a day without drinking, displays severe withdrawal symptoms lasting for days (sometimes including convulsions and hallucinations), and shows physical damage to the liver, nerves, heart, gastrointestinal tract, and other major organs.

Etiology

There are three distinct ways a person can develop alcoholism. Most commonly, however, a combination of these mechanisms is present.

Physiological susceptibility. A certain portion of the alcoholic population appears to be biologically abnormal in their physiologic response to alcohol. They appear to have a potential at birth for developing abnormal metabolism and tolerance to alcohol if they are exposed to it. Persons with high susceptibility may develop gross tolerance and withdrawal symptoms after only brief exposure, while those with only slight susceptibility would take longer exposure to develop the same set of clinical symptoms that we call alcoholism. There is substantial evidence that this physiological susceptibility to alcoholism is familial.

Peer group pressure. The drinking culture in which the individual lives has a substantial influence on the development of and recovery from alcoholism. In some subcultures in the United States, drinking is so much a way of life that the abstinent individual is viewed as a social deviant and regarded with suspicion by his peers.

A great deal of sociological research has been done regarding drinking habits and other behavioral patterns of subcultures. Drinking patterns are so influenced by peer pressure and cultural value systems that it is impossible to answer such pertinent questions as whether children who are taught responsible drinking, such as wine with meals or an occasional cocktail, are less likely to develop alcoholism than those who are taught total abstinence. Although it is known that the incidence of alcoholism is very high in environments where drunkenness is "normal" and sobriety "abnormal," not all individuals who live in these environments become alcoholics. There is obviously a great deal yet to be learned about the influence of the environment in the development of alcoholism.

Reality avoidance. Some persons develop their high exposure to alcohol by learning to use the drug as a tranquilizer, a means to avoid reality. They control their anxiety or depression by drinking, and alcohol increasingly becomes their most effective coping skill. Gradually, as their tolerance develops, they stay in a state of low-grade chronic withdrawal, with a resultant craving for the drug. They drink in order to avoid withdrawal symptoms and to be able to maintain routine functions. Eventually, alcohol may become the most important thing in their lives and they frequently become preoccupied with getting a drink, stopping drinking, or staying sober.

Complications

Alcohol is a relatively short-acting drug that is rapidly absorbed and circulates unchanged in the blood stream and cerebrospinal fluid. The most common acute complications of alcoholism are falling and driving accidents causing bruises, broken bones, and other injuries.

Every organ system in the body is affected to some degree by alcohol, and prolonged heavy usage often causes pathological changes in the brain, liver, stomach, pancreas, peripheral nerves, and heart. Anemia, gastritis, pancreatitis, neuritis, and fatty changes of the liver can occur. There can also be impaired brain function, resulting in confusion and memory loss. Cirrhosis of the liver, a devastating, destructive disease, is not as common as it was once thought to be.

Individuals have great variance in their organ susceptibility to alcohol damage. It is not known why two alcoholics drinking approximately the same amount over the same number of years will develop different complications. For example, one individual may have severe gastritis or ulcers, while another develops some level of brain damage and associated symptoms, such as impaired judgment, loss of recent memory, irritability, or emotional instability. Organs are not affected in any specific pattern, nor is there a specific relationship between the amount or duration of drinking and the development of organ damage. Undoubtedly, the degree of malnutrition and vitamin deficiency that the person suffers to some extent governs the severity of organic pathology that will develop.

Since the complications of alcoholism can mimic almost any disease, it would require several textbooks of medicine to completely describe all the organ damage that can be caused. If a client reports high levels of alcohol ingestion and has multiple other diagnoses, the counselor should suspect alcoholism and request a thorough medical evaluation.

Although major complications and organ changes usually develop in the later stages of alcohol addiction, work problems can be diagnosed much earlier. With earlier recognition and appropriate treatment leading to abstinence, these complications are usually preventable or easily reversible. The majority of physical complications are reversible with long abstinence and good nutrition, even in the more advanced stages.

In addition to these medical complications, the social and economic costs of alcoholism are awesome. The NCA estimates that 50 percent of all fatal accidents involve the use of alcohol, with two-thirds related directly to the actions of alcoholics. In addition, a conservative estimate of the cost of alcoholism to industry is 25 percent of each employed alcoholic's salary when such factors as absenteeism, tardiness, spoiled materials, decreased efficiency, on-the-job accidents, and medical benefits are taken into account.

Prognosis

Alcoholism is a slowly progressive disease. The typical male alcoholic has been drinking abusively for 8 to 12 years before he develops complications or otherwise deteriorates sufficiently to seek help. For women, the time period is usually somewhat shorter. Individuals with serious psychiatric disorders who become more disturbed when they drink and individuals who have previously been, or currently are, addicted to other sedative or narcotic drugs also require a shorter exposure time to develop alcoholism. For example, the former heroin abuser or the methadone maintenance patient is virtually an instant alcoholic if he begins to drink any appreciable amount. This is due, at least in part, to cross tolerance, but there may also be specific biochemical alterations that result in this difference.

The natural course of addiction is quite variable across individuals. Although it is commonly believed that, once developed, addiction is steadily progressive and the individual's condition worsens in an uninterrupted fashion, this is not necessarily true.

Some persons "mature out" and virtually stop drinking unassisted, while others have variable periods of spontaneous remissions. Since there are no reliable indicators or characteristics to predict the natural course of the disease, remission should never be relied upon for the individual's recovery. However, the majority of alcoholics can show improvement or completely recover with abstinence and appropriate treatment over a sufficient period of time.

FUNCTIONAL DISABILITIES

Physical Disabilities

The degree of physical disability may be severe for the alcoholic even in the early stages of the disease. During drinking episodes, motor functions, such as memory and judgment, will obviously be affected. As organ involvement becomes more pronounced, the magnitude of symptoms and resultant impairment of functional abilities increases.

Impairment of fine or even gross forms of motor coordination generally do not interfere with activities of daily living. In the first 6 to 12 months of recovery, clients may have tremors which interfere with their ability to write, or they may experience lapses in short-term memory and the ability to concentrate.

Physical restoration will be gradual and is predicated on the client's ability to remain abstinent. Milder forms of dysfunction will reverse within a few months after abstinence, while more pronounced dysfunction may require 6 to 12 months. Although uninterrupted alcoholism over a long period of time can result in irreversible organ damage and physical disability, in most cases are fairly temporary in nature if the individual can achieve and maintain abstinence. If the client has impairment in self-care, ambulation, and gross motor performance after several weeks of proven abstinence, advanced complications or another disability must be suspected. In these cases, the counselor should refer the client for complete medical evaluation.

Psychosocial Disabilities

Long-term combined alcohol/sedative addiction can produce manifestations of severe psychopathology during the addiction and for as much as 6 months afterwards. When these manifestations occur, they may be suggestive of severe debilitating mental illness and may possibly even require acute temporary intervention. The severity of the symptoms, sometimes accompanied by a self-destructive component, may lead the counselor to assume that an underlying chronic psychiatric disability is surfacing. This determination cannot accurately be made until all the organic brain syndrome secondary to alcohol and drug abuse has reversed. The vast majority of alcoholics who come for services have the potential for becoming emotionally adjusted and functioning adequately in their environments.

Other psychosocial disabilities are often observed in the untreated alcoholic and often also extend into the early stages of recovery (0–12 months). These include pathological dependency, marked anxiety, pathological isolation, denial, and decreased ability to establish long-term goals, proceed in a step-wise manner, and handle responsibility.

Dependency. Alcoholism reduces the person's ability to act effectively in his own behalf. As a result, alcoholics become increasingly dependent on others for both economic and physical support. They may expect to have their dependency needs met in all their relationships and may attempt to develop new relationships for this purpose. Accompanying the dependency is often a feeling of resentment toward those who are viewed as having power or authority over them. Even after abstinence begins, many alcoholics will continue to seek the same sort of dependent relationships with people or institutions, often including the counselor and rehabilitation agency. The client may want the counselor to do things that he could do for himself, such as make contacts with agencies and communicate with family members. Since reduction of dependency is nearly always desirable, the counselor should avoid doing things for the client that he honestly believes the client could do himself.

In many instances, the client's family may contribute to his alcoholism. Often in their effort to help, family members perpetuate the alcoholic's dependency and lack of responsibility by rescuing him from the consequences of his drinking behavior. Examples of rescuing behavior include making excuses to employers, bailing the alcoholic out of jail, providing money, and covering bad checks.

Anxiety. The tension-reducing properties of alcohol also deplete the alcoholic's natural coping abilities and leave the recovering person vulnerable and prone to crisis. Anxiety states may render the person temporarily dysfunctional and interrupt his ability to perform in a job or training setting. Often the anxiety will be cyclic and related to trying to remain sober. At other times the anxiety will be related to new situations and responsibilities resulting from sobriety. Whenever the client is undergoing some type of change, stress and anxiety are likely to increase.

Isolation. Alcohol is widely regarded as a social "lubricant" that facilitates communication and personal contact. Often the alcoholic has learned to depend on alcohol as an aid either in making social contacts or tolerating a dearth of social contacts. Alcohol consumption is frequently the alcoholic's most effective way of communicating with persons around him and of relieving the pain caused, in part, by lack of meaningful communication. He may have established his entire social life around alcohol consumption and find that, in recovery, his ability to maintain old contacts or develop new relationships and communicate meaningfully with others is impaired or lost.

The recovering alcoholic has often been given ponderous amounts of unsolicited critical advice which he has generally learned to ignore effectively. Typically, he doesn't trust people and seemingly is more concerned with getting something from them than in genuinely relating to them. This is often misinterpreted by the counselor or consultants to be indicative of surfacing psychopathology. Both the client and the counselor should recognize that it takes time to develop new avenues for social contact and meaningful interpersonal relationships.

Denial. The alcoholic can be particularly adept at denying reality. Misperceptions of reality can be an effective tool in defending himself against pain and avoiding some of the unpleasant aspects of the alcoholic life style. For example, he may have convinced himself that if he stops drinking, everything will be rectified, the pain he has inflicted and suffered will be healed, and his life will automatically readjust to normal. This type of oversimplification can often hamper his commitment to a total treatment plan.

Inaccurate self-appraisal. The alcoholic is often unrealistic in assessing his own aptitudes and skills and in setting suitable goals for himself. He may overestimate his abilities and have unrealistically high achievement expectations. Further, his level of functioning is often not congruent with his potential as measured by psychometric instruments. It is not uncommon for trained and experienced professionals to be misled by the apparent abilities of an alcoholic. It is important for the professionals evaluating the client to guard against overestimating the alcoholic's functional abilities.

Impatience. In addition to his unrealistic expectations, the alcoholic is impatient and seeks immediate rewards for his efforts. He is not only likely to have a firm concept of what he wants but also will demand immediate action. Although the recovering alcoholic has begun to live without alcohol, he usually does not simultaneously give up his need for quick solutions. In fact, in giving up alcohol, his attention may be drawn even more acutely to other needs which he may honestly feel must be satisfied without delay if he is to remain sober. He may have great difficulty understanding why others do not respond immediately to his needs. The amount of pressure that such a client can exert on the counselor can be appreciated only by those who have encountered this force. All too often, these pressures can result in the counselor either giving what is being requested without proper evaluation or rejecting the request, and possibly the client, entirely. Both these extremes should obviously be avoided.

To complicate matters, drinking is not always the worst possible course of action for the alcoholic to follow. He may have reached a point of crisis in his life when his alternatives are reduced to three perceived courses: (a) become openly psychotic and require hospitalization; (b) kill himself and/or someone else; or (c) drink. In such a context, the client may view drinking as the only choice by which he can retain some degree of control over himself and his environment. It is easy for the professional to see treatment as a preferred course and to encourage the client to seek help. But while this seems an acceptable alternative to someone else, it may be completely impossible for the client. Many reach a point in their recovery when their feelings toward the treatment person or group are so intense that contact with these "helpers" is the least tolerable thing they can imagine. From the alcoholic's perception, then, drinking becomes not just a "good" choice, but the only choice available.

Any of these psychosocial disabilities can contribute to the occurrence of a relapse in which the recovering alcoholic returns to the use of alcohol. As such, they should not be regarded as isolated from the disease itself. The counselor should anticipate the possibility of their occurrence, develop the rehabilitation plan accordingly, and integrate his planning with other treatment resources in the community.

Rehabilitation Potential

The stage of the client's alcoholism or treatment must be taken into account to accurately appraise an individual's feasibility for rehabilitation services. For the vast majority of clients, the ability to achieve and maintain abstinence is the critical difference between success and failure. Major clues in determining the probability of success are to be found in the client's response to general interview questions and specific treatment elements. Among questions the counselor should ask are:

1. Does the client accept the fact that he has a serious drinking problem?
2. Is the client able to accept the need for a long-term recovery plan which includes a new peer group identity?
3. Is the client willing to take deterrent medication?
4. Can significant others be involved in the client's recovery process?

If most of the above are answered positively, the client has a relatively good prognosis for success. However, the counselor should be wary of too rapid acceptance of the total treatment plan and anticipate a certain amount of limit testing and acting out.

The initial struggle for the alcoholic is maintaining sobriety, which is a prerequisite of any realistic and meaningful evaluation and planning. No one has yet learned how to *make* an alcoholic stay sober. In fact, it seems that the harder people try to keep him away from alcohol, the more intent he becomes on asserting his independence by drinking.

Drinking can occasionally serve a kind of therapeutic purpose for the client. An occasional "slip" can help to convince an addicted person who has been sober for a relatively long time that he still has a problem with alcohol, and that there is no "cure" that will allow him to drink with impunity or without destructive consequences. The counselor has the task of deciphering the reasons for any drinking episode and relating the episode to the other observations by which he is determining the feasibility or prognosis.

The rehabilitation potential of an alcoholic is affected more by his psychosocial disabilities than by his physical disabilities. This is particularly true of the impatience, lack of realistic self-appraisal, and limited ability to handle stress so often characteristic of alcoholics. Prior to recovery, the practicing alcoholic lived a life marked by increasing irresponsibility and impulsive behavior, and a decreased ability to set long-term goals. In early sobriety, he may wish to "make up for lost time" by resuming a job or career at a previously achieved level. Also, as a rehabilitation client, he may wish to establish vocational goals with quite unrealistic time frames.

The counselor should be prepared to deal with such expectations and to regard them as natural for a recovering person in the first year. He should guard against either (a) considering the client as unfeasible, or (b) being manipulated into poor planning and potential crises. Agencies with short-term rehabilitation production goals are especially vulnerable. The alcoholic may be able to exert heroic efforts for short periods of time while pressures are simultaneously building up toward a relapse. It is extremely important that counselors and agencies not encourage the recovering alcoholic to achieve too rapid a "success."

The recovering alcoholic needs both long- and short-term goals, a sense of the long-range process of his rehabilitation, and a continued source of ongoing reinforcement. The longer the alcoholic continues his involvement in a total treatment process, the more stability he gains in all areas of functioning. This stability is accompanied by increasing capacity to make long-range plans and to handle emotional stress. During the course of treatment, the counselor should regularly reassess the client's changing ability to assume more responsibility and independence and plan the next phase of vocational rehabilitation accordingly.

STANDARDS OF EVALUATION

Behavioral impairment and the development of physical organ damage are usually viewed as the major criteria for diagnosis of alcoholism. Evaluation should consist of a complete general medical examination including standard blood tests, urinalysis, and liver function studies. In addition, an electrocardiogram should be included if the client is over 40 years of age.

Although nearly all physicians can be expected to perform an accurate appraisal of physical status, most will not be equipped to provide long-range treatment for the client with alcoholism. The counselor should identify specifically trained and interested physicians in the community and encourage them to become involved in the treatment plan. Unfortunately, there is not yet a board or certified specialty in the area of addictions. Although this may evolve, at present the counselor must personally inquire about the physician's training and interest in this field. Reliable indicators are membership in the American Medical Society on Alcoholism and recent attendance at any alcohol and drug abuse conferences. These conferences are often sponsored by organizations such as the Alcohol and Drug Abuse Problems Association of North America, the National Council on Alcoholism, and the National Drug Abuse Conference.

Each state has a special agency dealing with alcoholism information and treatment referral. These agencies are partially funded through the National Institute for Alcohol Abuse and Alcoholism (NIAAA). The State agencies, in turn, support organized community alcoholism treatment programs, and can provide the counselor with a directory of State and local resources. Research directed toward the development of improved alcoholism treatment techniques is also supported by NIAAA. The counselor should be aware of all these resources and establish a working relationship with the staff of these programs.

If gross psychiatric and behavioral symptoms are manifested, a psychiatric evaluation, with or without psychological testing, can provide valuable treatment and prognostic information. However, it is essential that the client be recovered from the organic brain syndrome associated with alcohol and drug abuse before interpreting tests or psychiatric evaluations. Experience has shown that routine or extensive psychological testing frequently offers little useful information. For example, intelligence tests or aptitude batteries can be so responsive to the temporary intellectual impairment associated with an acute or intermediate brain syndrome that they give an inaccurate and misleading indication of the real aptitudes of the recovering alcoholic. Similarly, personality inventories such as the Minnestoa Multiphasic Personality Inventory (MMPI) can often give an erroneous prediction of the recovering alcoholic's stability.

A trained counselor's clinical evaluation of the client's attitudes and intellectual functioning obtained through routine interviews is usually sufficiently accurate to serve his practical needs in developing a preliminary rehabilitation plan. In fact, the client's ability to function in the environment, especially the vocational environment, is usually a more significant indicator of impairment than either the physical or psychiatric pathologies. This environment may be the client's job, if he has remained employed, or a variety of work evaluation/adjustment settings, depending on the individual needs of the client and the community resources available.

If an individual is referred for evaluation and services immediately after entering alcoholism treatment for the first time, it is virtually impossible to make an accurate evaluation in a brief period. In most instances, a period of several months to observe the client's response to alcoholism treatment is the preferred course of action. Data obtained during this period should include feedback from clinical staff regarding his attendance and level of active participation in the treatment program. If the client has a sponsor for Alcoholics Anonymous, or if contact can be made with close family members, these lines of information should also be established. In addition, the counselor should make direct observations by attending open Alcoholics Anonymous and treatment staff meetings with the client. Taken together, these behavioral factors can provide meaningful evaluative material for timing of rehabilitation efforts and establishment of vocational goals.

TOTAL TREATMENT

Alcoholism treatment is an ongoing process rather than a single act. The alcoholic has many obstacles to overcome and a total process is the key to gaining stability in all areas of functioning. It is important that the rehabilitation counselor have a full understanding of this concept and of his role in the multistaged process. Without this base, he is likely to respond to the client's instant solutions, fantasies, and overinvestments. If this happens, the counselor may subsequently become disillusioned and reject the client he is trying hardest to help. The counselor can be instrumental in the client's rehabilitation by recognizing the many facets of the problem and being willing to help the client organize and integrate a recovery process.

A continuum of services is essential, and each client needs a different combination of services at the various stages of recovery. The rehabilitation counselor can play a critical role in the delivery of services at any stage by serving as the client's advocate and/or case manager. Almost never is it desirable for the counselor to assume a solitary or prime therapist relationship with the recovering alcoholic client. This may be difficult since it is not uncommon for the alcoholic to seek out one thing or one person to solve all his problems. When the counselor avoids solving all the client's problems, it decreases the client's dependency and supports his efforts to solve problems and take responsibility for his own behavior.

The critical first step of treatment is early diagnosis and motivation by the client to seek help to change. For a great many years, alcoholism was only acknowledged in its terminal stages, as manifested by repeated legal problems or advanced medical complications. In the past two decades, however, industrial, drunk driving, and armed services alcoholism programs have sprung up across the country. These programs have made a great deal of progress in the development of effective techniques of early diagnosis based on performance factors, such as tardiness, absenteeism, and decreased productivity on the job, rather than on complications. In these programs, emphasis is placed upon identifying the troubled employee and providing early intervention and treatment.

The rehabilitation counselor has a great deal to contribute in this area by helping to establish such detection programs, by working closely with the industrial counselor, and by being a source of counseling for the disabled employee. It is desirable that counselors become familiar with industrial "troubled employee" programs and the activities and materials of local branches of the National Council on Alcoholism and local Alcohol Safety Action Programs. When diagnosed early, a great many persons with uncomplicated alcoholism may recover with the help of their industrial counselor and a self-help group.

For clients who have been drinking recently, the first stage of any treatment program is *acute detoxification*. This refers to the treatment of the withdrawal syndrome. Mild withdrawal symptoms are sometimes treated on an outpatient basis in a medical facility or in a nonmedical detoxification facility. More severe withdrawal symptoms, however, do require medical supervision and usually hospitalization. Tranquilizers are commonly administered to reduce the symptoms and prevent the development of delirium tremens. Medical management usually also includes the administration of fluids, electrolytes, and vitamins.

Individuals with more severe withdrawal symptoms and greater organic damage will require *chronic detoxification* for 3 to 6 months. Medical monitoring will be needed intermittently to counter the adverse effects of alcohol on the digestive, nervous, and endocrine systems. The physician may prescribe vitamins, special diets, and specific drugs.

In addition, alcoholics may have associated illnesses, such as psychiatric disorders or emphysema, which require appropriate treatment. Because the needs of clients will vary so widely, it is important that the counselor identify at least one physician he can rely upon for this aspect of the total treatment plan.

After detoxification, the client is best served by a thorough evaluation of his individual needs and selection of the appropriate services to meet those needs. There are many approaches to the treatment of alcoholism; for example, medical, psychological, and social. Most alcoholics will benefit from a combination of these services, which will be available in different forms in different communities. In general, the following are the major components of alcoholism treatment which can be combined, as appropriate, for an individual client.

Environmental manipulation in varying degrees may be needed, depending upon the individual circumstances of the client. When the alcoholic comes for rehabilitation services, he is often immersed in a variety of life crises, such as divorce, dental problems, legal actions, overdue bills, and revoked driver's license. The client can be helped to solve these problems and thereby create an environment more conducive to abstinence.

Internal change therapy may be provided through a wide range of psychotherapeutic techniques aimed at the development of insight and the modification of behavior. These treatment modalities are not required by the majority of clients and are inappropriate for a large number at the beginning of recovery. An exception is those programs designed to prepare the alcoholic to enter a regular treatment program.

Involvement in the treatment plan of significant other persons, such as spouse, children, probation officer, sexual partner, or anyone else in a position to contribute positively or negatively to the client's recovery, is essential. Often these persons also need treatment in order to increase the prospects of the client's success. If the client has a family, alcoholism and its treatment is a family matter.

Antabuse (disulfiram) is a drug that interferes with the normal metabolism of alcohol, thereby causing acute gastrointestinal distress. When taken daily, it acts as a deterrent to alcoholism because ingestion of alcohol will produce the unpleasant reaction. It can be extremely helpful in support of other program elements. The courts may require individuals to take Antabuse regularly in order to retain or get back their driver's licenses. In some cases, it may be appropriate for the counselor to require Antabuse maintenance to help alcoholic clients keep their jobs, stay in school, and the like.

Modification of peer group identity may be achieved through membership in a self-help group which, for many alcoholics, will be the mainstay of treatment. In this country, the established, effective, and available self-help group is Alcoholics Anonymous (AA). This group is based on the philosophy that alcoholics can gather together and provide each other with support for sobriety and recovery. The principles and methods for recovery are incorporated in a 12-step program. Alcoholics Anonymous and its companion organizations, Alanon for adult family members and Alateen and Alatot for their offspring, are highly available, virtually free, and indisputedly effective for a great many alcoholics and their families. Especially when family members are inadvertently contributing to the client's alcoholism and dependency, they should be strongly encouraged to become involved in the Alanon and Alateen programs to help them understand their role in the total treatment program to the greatest degree possible.

Any counselor who is going to accept even one client a year with alcoholism is grossly negligent if he does not develop a working knowledge of, and relationship with, Alcoholics Anonymous. This can be simply and pleasantly accomplished. Local chapters usually have at least one open meeting a week to which most members would be delighted to invite a counselor. AA literature is easily available, inexpensive, and quite readable, and every community has many stable members who would be most willing to sponsor an appropriate new member. Groups have their own traditions and procedures which they adhere to quite rigidly. If the counselor becomes familiar with these traditions and procedures and respects them, the AA group will be an excellent ally for his client's recovery.

Some clients, for physical, psychological, or other reasons, are not able to use Alcoholics Anonymous as their recovery mainstay. This is especially likely to be true early in the recovery process. These individuals may need various levels of professional treatment directed toward preparing them for entry into a regular alcoholism treatment program. This preparation usually takes 1 to 4 months, and can be provided by some combination of medical, psychological, spiritual, and social service. Usually a combination of hospital, day care, outpatient, and residential settings is needed for this type of preparatory treatment.

VOCATIONAL IMPLICATIONS

Progressive loss of work skills or inability to develop new skills is often the best early indication of alcohol addiction. Industry leaders have estimated that 60–80 percent of persistent job performance problems are a direct result of alcoholism. Although the disease is more prevalent in certain occupations, virtually no group is immune. Actual or impending job loss is quite frequently the reason individuals seek treatment for their alcoholism. The counselor can often intervene at this point to help the client retain his job while he participates in a treatment program.

During the early phases of recovery, the alcoholic is unrealistic in assessing his readiness and capability to re-establish vocational, social, and emotional involvement. A great many alcoholics bring only one or two commonly heard requests to a rehabilitation counselor: (a) help me get a job, or (b) help me get vocational training. The applicant makes these requests quite firmly and expects the counselor to make a decision immediately. Any attempt on the counselor's part to evaluate such requests against the applicant's vocational, social, educational, and medical background is apt to be met with bewilderment or anger.

Vocational planning is dependent upon first, a reasonable amount of sobriety, and second, the assessment of individual strengths and problem areas. It is essential that the counselor help the client recognize that entering and maintaining a program designed to help him remain abstinent must be accomplished before any job seeking or retraining is undertaken. The counselor must then determine what the individual client's past job difficulties were. Common problems include inability to tolerate stress, lack of job skills, or attempting to achieve beyond ability level. With this information, the counselor and client should develop rehabilitation plans.

There is great variance in individual client's responses to different situations. Some are more successful working with people, and others are more successful working with data and things. Careful work history, vocational assessment, and individual evaluation are critical. Consultation with other members of the client's treatment team is most important in making these determinations.

In general, alcoholics must be helped to avoid three common pitfalls: (a) believing that an appropriate job will "cure" their alcoholism; (b) overcommitting themselves by working too many hours or too many days; and (c) taking on more responsibility than they are stable enough to handle. Usually the alcoholic should not be encouraged to undertake retraining or a new type of job until he has achieved sobriety for 6 to 12 months. Planning must be directed toward helping the individual establish an environment of low pressure. Continued observation and supervision by the counselor while the client participates in treatment and retains an easily managed job can be a most useful technique.

The client's potential skills frequently exceed his ability to tolerate stress. It is important to remember that stress tolerance is usually lowest early in treatment but can be expected to improve slowly over the next 3 years. Often the client does not adequately perceive his low stress tolerance and the counselor must continuously monitor the client's tendency to overextend. The stressfulness of the client's environment can be increased gradually as his tolerance increases. A series of short-term, easily attainable goals is the best way to achieve this.

The counselor should be aware that stress and anxiety are likely to increase whenever the client is undergoing some type of change and he should be prepared to offer greater structure and support during these periods. Repeated crisis counseling regarding work relationships and job stresses can be a mainstay of the client's recovery. Practicing and recovering alcoholics are excellent in short-term employment or training situations. Many have excellent job-finding skills, and it is not atypical to encounter an alcoholic who is able to get one or more jobs per month. However, poor long-term job performance patterns can be expected.

The vocational counselor is an essential component of the comprehensive alcoholic treatment team. In the preventive maintenance period of recovery, the counselor-client relationship will be most critical. The vocational counselor is most able to relate to the recovering person during the early period of re-employment and is therefore in a key position to positively influence the final rehabilitation outcome.

BIBLIOGRAPHY

Alcoholics Anonymous World Services, Inc. Alcoholics Anonymous, Box 459, Grand Central Station, New York, NY 10017
Commonly referred to as "The Big Book," this is the basic text and description of the AA program. As AA is the most widely available and inexpensive resource for the recovering person, it is incumbent upon the counselor to be familiar with it.

Catanzaro RJ: General aspects of treatment. *In* Cantanzaro RJ (ed): *Alcoholism: The Total Treatment Approach,* Thomas, Springfield, IL, 1968.
An overview of the multidisciplinary, multiphased approach to alcoholism treatment. The counselor can find important information on the acute phase, family involvement, and AA in the total treatment approach.

Estes NJ, Hanson KJ: Sobriety: Problems, challenges and solutions. Am J Psychother **30**(2):256–66, 1976.
Ten wives of alcoholics participated in group therapy for 2 years. The new problems they encountered as a result of their husbands' sobriety are described in this article.

Hough GS: A behavioral approach to alcoholism. Nurs Clin North Am **11**: 507–516, 1976.
This article describes a behavioral approach used in the treatment of alcoholism. The goals of the program include either abstinence or controlled drinking for problem drinkers who do not have any medical reason for abstinence.

Lowe WC, Thomas SD: Assessing alcoholism treatment effectiveness. A comparison of three evaluative measures. J Stud Alcohol **37**:883–889, 1976.
This article describes three criteria which were used to evaluate the success rate of an alcoholism treatment program: vocational rehabilitation, abstinence, and behavior (such as number of drinking episodes, family and marital adjustment, and participation in outpatient program).

Mullan H: Vocational counseling with the alcoholic. *In* Mullan H, Sanguiliano I: *Alcoholism: Group Psychotherapy and Rehabilitation,* Springfield, IL, 175–204. Thomas, 1966.
This chapter offers a comparative analysis of the vocational counselor's role and approach and that of the psychotherapist.

National Clearinghouse for Alcohol Information (NCALI), PO Box 2345 Rockville, MD 20850.
The clearinghouse is a major source of current information in all areas of alcoholism. The annotated bibliographies (Grouped Interest Guides) are periodically updated, and the one entitled Rehabilitation Strategies for Alcohol Abusers is particularly valuable. In addition, the clearinghouse provides an ongoing awareness service to its subscribers. This resource is free.

National Council on Alcoholism Criteria Committee: Criteria for the diagnosing of alcoholism. AM J Psychiatry **192**:127–135, 1972.
This effort by the council expands the basis for the diagnosis of alcoholism, which commonly has been delayed until the late stages when body organs are damaged. The criteria include behavioral, social, and physical trends in the patient which can aid in the early recognition of the illness.

Rowntree GR, Brand J: The employee with alcohol, drug, and emotional problems. A Kentucky occupational program. J Occup Med **17**:329–332, 1975.
This article describes a program designed to identify "troubled employees," 50 percent of whom will have alcoholism, on the basis of deteriorating job performance. Early intervention and referral are discussed.

Seixas FA Cadoret R, Eggleston S (eds): *The Person with Alcoholism.* Ann NY Acad Sci **233,** 15 Apr. 1974.
The issue is devoted to the psychiatric aspects of alcoholism. There are articles on various psychological characteristics and problems of alcoholics and on various psychotherapeutic approaches to alcoholism treatment.

Wiseman JP: *Stations of the Lost: The Treatment of Skid Row Alcoholics.* Prentice-Hall, Englewood Cliffs, NJ, 1970.
Dr. Wiseman offers two views, often contradictory, of rehabilitation; namely, the view of the providers and the view of the consumers of services in the Skid Row subpopulation. Chapters 1 and 9 provide descriptions of these separate perspectives, which can be generalized to other alcoholic populations seeking services.

18 DRUG ABUSE

R. Raymond Knowles, M.B.

DISEASE DESCRIPTION

A drug is any substance that, when taken into the living organism, may modify one or more of its functions. A dependence-producing drug is one having the capacity to interact with a living organism to produce a state of psychological and/or physical dependence. Such a drug may be used medically or nonmedically without necessarily producing such a state. *Psychological dependence* is a condition in which a drug produces a feeling of satisfaction and a psychic drive that requires periodic or continuous administration of the drug to produce pleasure or to avoid discomfort. *Physical dependence* is an adaptive state that manifests itself by intense physical disturbances when the administration of the drug is suspended. These effects constitute the *withdrawal syndrome*, and the form it takes varies with the class of drug causing the dependence. *Tolerance* may or may not be present. When present, the drug-dependent person requires increasing amounts of the drug to obtain drug effects previously experienced with smaller doses.

The term "drug addict" is obsolete because it implies physical dependence solely. We now know that dependence is rarely, if ever, free of a psychological component. "Drug dependent" has not found common acceptance as an updated term for drug addict, but "drug abuser" appears to have gained acceptance as its current equivalent.

The use of drugs of dependence may be (a) *experimental,* in which case use is terminated before dependence occurs; (b) *casual,* when use is discontinuous; or (c) *dependent,* when use is continuous. Not all drug dependence is necessarily harmful. For example, tea and coffee do not produce the individual, public, health, and social problems associated with alcohol, barbiturates, or heroin.

The World Health Organization classifies drugs of dependency as follows:

1. Alcohol and barbiturate-type drugs (e.g., Nembutal, Seconal)
2. Amphetamine-type drugs (Benzedrine, Desoxyn, Dexedrine)
3. Cannabis-type drugs (marihuana, hashish)
4. Cocaine
5. Hallucinogen-type drugs (LSD, mescaline, PCP)
6. Khat
7. Opiate-type drugs (heroin, morphine, Dilaudid)
8. Volatile-solvent-type drugs (toluene, acetone, freon)

Defining drug abuse as a disease exempts it from the assignment of moral transgression and the inseparable guilt. It ensures the abuser identity as a patient, hopefully ensures humane treatment, and gives him access to health and social service agencies. Some authors have defined drug abuse as learned deviant behavior resulting primarily from environmental influences. Finally, drug abuse has been appropriately defined as a social problem. However defined, drug abuse has multiple determinants and gives rise to medical, legal, educational, economic, and social consequences.

Incidence and Prevalence

Incidence and prevalence are terms customarily used in the field of public health to measure the rate at which new cases of a disease are occurring, and the number of cases in a study population at a given point in time, respectively. Studies of narcotic (opiate-type) dependency showed that the incidence was highest for those in the 14–15, 19–20, and 21–24 year age groups (15.5, 15.3, and 15.2 percent, respectively). For 1.7 percent of the study population, the age of onset was 11 or less, and for 5.9 percent, age 30 or more. It is estimated that in excess of 100,000 narcotics abusers reside in New York City alone.

Heroin use occurred in epidemic proportions from 1965 to 1970. It had its begininngs in the inner cities of major metropolitan areas and quickly spread to adjacent suburban areas and smaller communities. A decline in heroin use occurred in 1972 and 1973, primarily on the East Coast, associated with a sharp reduction in availability.

There is evidence that the rates of abuse of barbiturates and amphetamines are growing steadily in the young adult population. Overall rates of marihuana use have been increasing steadily but there may be signs of leveling off in the school-age

241

population. It is estimated that more than 15 percent of the general population in the United States have had experience with this drug. Although users of hallucinogens tend to discontinue after a few years, the available surveys indicate there has not been any decline in the extent of overall use.

Etiology

Professionals dealing with drug abuse attribute the onset in youth to the risk-taking behavior and rebelliousness characteristics of adolescence. As noted above, this experimental use may lead to casual use, frequent use, regular (dependent) use, or, hopefully, termination of use.

The pattern of dependent drug use is generally considered to be due to one or more of the following factors:

1. A manifestation of an underlying character disorder in which immediate satisfaction is sought, regardless of the long-term consequences
2. A manifestation of delinquency, when personal pleasure is obtained without regard to social norms and expectations
3. An attempt at self-treatment of a condition which is causing the abuser physical or emotional distress
4. The price of winning social acceptance in a peer group subculture
5. The consequence of a disturbance of the body's metabolism
6. An expression of rebellion against society's values of success and status
7. A reaction to socioeconomic pressures, in the absence of underlying psychopathology
8. Learned deviant behavior

Drug abuse is a persisting behavioral pattern because of the variety of rewards provided. A number of social and pharmacologic sources of reinforcement have been proposed. Participation in the drug-abusing subculture satisfies a "need to belong" in the neophyte abuser and thereby constitutes a significant source of reinforcement. One pharmacologic reinforcer is the feeling state ("high") that follows use of the drug. A more common pharmacologic reinforcer is the termination of withdrawal symptoms in the physically dependent individual. Finally, there is pharmacologic reinforcement because use of the drug facilitates emergence of behavior desired by the abuser. For example, he may become indifferent to a situation which would otherwise be threatening or frightening to him. This allows the individual to escape aversive aspects of the environment and enter instead into a state of pleasure.

A recent research development finds evidence for the existence of pain-killing substances (endorphins) which are manufactured by the body. Their actions may underlie the phenomena of compulsive use and withdrawal distress associated with narcotic dependence.

In the remainder of this chapter, the pathology, complications, functional disabilities, and rehabilitation potential associated with abuse of narcotics, stimulants, depressants, hallucinogens, cannabis, and volatile solvents will be discussed individually. A discussion of standards of evaluation, total treatment, and vocational implications of drug abuse in general then follows.

NARCOTICS

Pathology

Drugs such as morphine, heroin, methadone, and Demerol are central nervous system depressants. They are very useful drugs in medicine because they reduce awareness of pain and calm the emotional responses that generally accompany severe pain. Less desirable is their depression of the depth and frequency of respiration. Other side-effects produced include vomiting, itching, sweating, constipation, and pupil contraction.

The withdrawal syndrome associated with narcotic dependence begins within hours of the last administration of the drug (heroin 4 hours, morphine 6 hours, methadone 12 hours). A typical symptom array includes yawning, eye-tearing, runny nose, perspiration, muscle twitching, gooseflesh, loss of appetite, restlessness, irritability, diarrhea, rapid breathing, and large pupils. Not surprisingly, these symptoms are nearly always accompanied by overt behaviors directed toward obtaining drugs.

Complications

Narcotic drug dependency can be a fatal disease and has a definite mortality rate. Death may result from intentional or unintentional overdose, and is due to gradual slowing of respiration and finally complete failure of breathing. This condition is a medical emergency which can be successfully treated with narcotic antagonist drugs. A related and also fatal condition is pulmonary edema, in which the lungs fill with fluid, asphyxiating the narcotic abuser.

Many of the complications associated with narcotic dependence result from the manner of administration rather than the direct effects of the drug. Nonsterile injections may result in infection at the site (abscess) or at a distance (septicemia, infected clots, pulmonary embolism, endocarditis). The virus of infectious hepatitis is commonly transmitted from an abuser who is infected to fellow abusers who share needles and syringes. When insoluble materials are injected, they may cause blockage of the small blood vessels supplying vital organs or even compromise the blood supply of a limb with resultant gangrene. Sniffing ("snorting") heroin may cause perforation of the nasal septum.

After hepatitis, pneumonia is the most common diagnosis made on narcotic abusers admitted to the hospital. It has also been observed that tuberculosis afflicts narcotic abusers at a rate markedly greater than that expected for the general population. Because of the effects of narcotics on the body's immune mechanisms, abusers show a high rate of false positive tests for syphilis.

Neglect of personal health and hygiene, typical of narcotic abusers, aided by the pain-killing aspects of the drug, often lead to dental sepsis and decay. Physical signs of dependency characteristically include track marks along the superficial veins, residual scars of abscesses, and cigarette burns on the fingers, hands, and arms. By contrast, stabilized narcotic users under medical supervision who are paying attention to their diet and personal hygiene do not appear to suffer any of these obvious physical injuries.

Functional Disabilities

The physical consequences of narcotic dependency may result in significant disability. Fortunately, the majority of the abuser population are youthful and much of the disability inseparable from the associated pathology is largely reversible, given appropriate treatment. Where a serious physical illness (e.g., endocarditis, glomerulonephritis, or septicemia) has supervened, the physical impairment will obviously depend on the course of the complicating condition.

For the narcotic drug abuser, the psychological aspects present the most critical area of impairment. The abuser had membership in an antisocial subculture which, at best, did not share the value system of the larger society and, at worst, preyed on it. While some may have had sociopathic traits preceding their drug careers, the majority manifest such traits secondary to their drug dependence. The cost of supporting a narcotic habit is much higher than the cost of other drug habits, and it is unlikely that regular employment could provide enough money to sustain it. Inevitably, the male narcotic abuser is drawn into illegal activities, and the female abuser commonly supports her habit through prostitution. Associated with this criminality may be such character traits as unreliability and untruthfulness. The consequence of the abusers' amorality is the inevitable rejection and stereotyping by the society to which they no longer belong.

Rehabilitation Potential

Recent studies indicate that previous estimates of the rehabilitation potential of narcotic abusers were overly pessimistic. The improved results are attributed to a better understanding of the disabled population, the cooperation of professionals in meeting clients' needs, and a strengthening of the rehabilitation model for service, together with improved client management and the increased availability of facilities and resources. It is not uncommon for treatment programs to report that, while only a third of their clients were employed at onset of treatment, more than two-thirds were working or in training programs within a year.

A contributing factor to this improved outlook is the recent concern industry has shown with the problem of drug abusing employees. When confronted with their drug abuse problem, the individuals often terminate employment and enter a treatment program. In these instances, the rehabilitation counselor finds he is dealing with a different type of abuser client, one with a recent work record and skills that qualify him for further employment. Rehabilitation potential is much greater for these clients than for the more typical clients who have dropped out of school and, having supported themselves and their habit through illegal activities, have no history of regular employment.

The counselor may find himself under pressure for immediate placement, despite his awareness that the client is neither psychosocially nor vocationally prepared. Placement, in fact, should be viewed as a long-term goal after the more realistic intermediate goals of evaluation, work adjustment preparation, and skills training are established. The counselor will also identify special health, family casework, education, and counseling needs. Fulfillment of these needs also constitutes a series of appropriate intermediate goals. These guidelines are also relevant to abusers of depressants, hallucinogens, and cannabis.

STIMULANTS

Pathology

Drugs such as cocaine, amphetamines, methylphenidate (Ritalin), and caffeine (tea, coffee) are central nervous system stimulants. They increase the state of arousal so that the brain is exposed to a much larger input of information from the environment, and mental processes are speeded up. Their effects are often experienced as unpleasant. Feelings of nervousness and restlessness and an inability to sleep are common. The abuser, unless in a state of withdrawal, is alert, overactive, and talkative. He may also be anxious, irritable, hostile, or aggressive. Physical signs include dry mouth, dilated pupils, rapid heart rate, increased blood pressure, and weight loss. There may be lip and tongue ulcers or signs of needle marks and tracks.

Withdrawal from chronic use of stimulants is associated with excessive sleeping, due to a sleep debt which has accumulated during the extended insomnia associated with "speeding." There is profound mood depression ("crashing") with apathy, lack of energy, and lack of initiative. These symptoms may persist for 2 to 4 months after cessation of drug use.

Abuse of stimulants may result in the development of paranoid psychosis with delusions of persecution, false beliefs that objects and events in the abuser's environments have been contrived and have special meanings applicable to him (ideas of reference), auditory and visual hallucinations, hyperactivity, and excitement. In addition, there may be inappropriate cheerfulness, overactivity, and talkativeness (hypomania), depression, obsessive-compulsive reactions, or catatonic schizophrenia. Unlike other drug-induced toxic psychoses, there is no clouding of memory nor is there decreased ability to locate oneself in time and place (i.e., orientation is intact). This maintenance of orientation, a highly developed and fixed delusional system, and occurrence of repetitive behaviors (compulsive cleaning, for example) distinguish the amphetamine psychosis.

Complications

While stimulant drugs may be taken by mouth, there is often a change to injection as the preferred route of administration. Thus, the general medical complications of nonsterile intravenous injections of drugs of unknown quality are encountered: hepatitis, pneumonia, lung abscess, endocarditis, tetanus, syphilis, and septicemia. The intravenous administration of amphetamines (in particular methamphetamine "crystal") appears to cause spasm of blood vessels, leading to their blockage and hemorrhage. As with heroin, sniffing cocaine may cause nasal septum perforation. Deaths generally result from stroke, acute heart failure, high fever, and the complications of intravenous injection.

Toxic doses may cause dizziness, tremulousness, confusion, hostility, hallucinations, panic states, skin flushing, chest pain, palpitations, high blood pressure, vomiting, and abdominal cramps. There may also be high fever, convulsions, collapse, and ultimately death.

Functional Disabilities

The physical disabilities associated with stimulant drug abuse are generally the same as those mentioned above for narcotic drug abuse.

The psychosocial disabilities of stimulant abuse may be profound during both the phases of abuse and withdrawal. The marked deterioration of the personality and blunted moral sense was first observed with cocaine. While the development of physical dependence does not occur, the great psychological dependence makes relapse probable. It should be noted that seemingly motiveless crimes of violence may be committed by stimulant abusers in the grip of drug-induced paranoid delusions. Indeed, the behavior of

the stimulant subculture has been viewed as violently antisocial with respect to the larger society from which it is derived. For example, some motorcycle gangs are known for their amphetamine abuse. Studies show that there may be residual bizarre thinking associated with emotional apathy in the abstaining chronic stimulant abuser.

Rehabilitation Potential

Individuals who abuse stimulants become severely drug dependent, with the duration of the dependence persisting as long as with heroin. Generally the abuser either "burns out" within 2 to 3 years or develops a drug-induced psychosis which effectively terminates drug-seeking behavior. Any rehabilitation program must necessarily include regular urine testing as a method of monitoring the client's success in abstaining from further drug use. Rehabilitation potential increases as the severity and duration of abuse decreases.

The counselor should carefully assess the readiness of his client to renounce the life style he followed during his abuse career and his willingness to accept, to some extent, the values of the society he seeks to reenter. Verbal assurances are less encouraging than actual evidence of changes toward more preferable behavior patterns. The termination of associations with friends in the drug subculture and acceptance of a schedule of daily activities more appropriate to the working world than to the nightlife of the abuser should be strongly supported.

DEPRESSANTS

Pathology

Drugs such as alcohol, barbiturates, nonbarbiturate sedatives (Doriden, Equanil, Quaalude, Placidyl, chloral hydrate, paraldehyde), and large doses of minor tranquilizers (Librium, Valium) are central nervous system depressants. (Although narcotics also have depressant effects, it is customary to classify them separately because they have pain-diminishing properties and the depressants lack this analgesic aspect.) The barbiturates are classified as (a) long-acting (e.g., phenobarbital); (b) intermediate (e.g., Amytal, Butisol); (c) short-acting (e.g., Nembutal, Seconal); and (d) ultra-short-acting (e.g, Pentothal).

Regular use of high doses of barbiturates produces dependency in 5 weeks, Valium in 6 weeks, and Equanil in 38 weeks. If the drugs are abruptly terminated after dependency has been established, a life-threatening withdrawal syndrome occurs. This syndrome is virtually indistinguishable from the delirium tremens of alcohol withdrawal seen in chronic alcoholism, and is characterized by delusions, hallucinations, excitement, restlessness, incoherence, anxiety, mental distress, sweating, and gastrointestinal symptoms. Withdrawal from sedatives therefore requires a gradual reduction in dosage, which is best achieved in a hospital setting.

Chronic use results in a series of symptoms resembling the picture of acute intoxication with alcohol (disorientation, unsteady gait, and pathologic cheerfulness, or euphoria). When the eyes are looking to either side, there is a characteristic rapid to-and-fro movement (nystagmus). Signs of nervous system abnormality mimicking parkinsonism, multiple sclerosis, and brain tumor may be seen, such as confusion, poor memory, signs of intellectual impairment, and incoherent speech.

Psychopathology may be manifested by such behavioral and personality defects as (a) *egocentricity*: the individual is self-centered and narcissistic; (b) *inconsistency*: the individual is undependable and impulsive; (c) *ambivalence of feelings*: the individual may, for example, both seek and reject help, or he may show alternating love and hate toward significant others; (d) *lack of insight or awareness of abnormalities*: the individual rationalizes excessively and is unable to distinguish between the fantasy of promises and the reality of behavior. In extreme cases, the individual manifests arrogance and deviance, being grandiose and acting out hostility with physical violence. He may have paranoid thoughts and perhaps misinterpret what has been said to him or, worse, harbor delusions (for example, of his spouse's infidelity).

Complications

When depressants are medically prescribed and administered, side effects such as skin rashes, nausea and vomiting, restlessness, and excitement are occasionally encountered. Overdosage can cause coma and death due to depression of the main centers controlling vital life functions, such as breathing.

Barbiturates and, to a lesser degree, nonbarbiturate sedatives are notorious for their frequent use in attempted and successful suicides. When two depressants (one commonly being alcohol) are taken together, the effect is greater than would be expected from simple summation of their individual effects.

Functional Disabilities

As discussed above, the physical disabilities accompanying depressant drug abuse may be substantial. A continuum of effects may be encountered in depressant abusers, ranging from mild sedation not incompatible with normal functioning to profound central nervous system depression of life-threatening proportion.

Psychosocial deficits parallel such physical effects.

The development of drug tolerance may well obscure the nature of the individual's disability, but dependence is invariably accompanied by compromising of attention and concentration, memory impairment, blunting of sensitivity to environmental stimuli, indifference, loss of adaptive behavior patterns, loss of mechanical dexterity, and disregard for potential dangers.

Rehabilitation Potential

The prognosis for depressant abusers is usually regarded as more favorable than for narcotic abusers. Alcohol is a typical member of this class of drugs of abuse and those criteria which apply in evaluating rehabilitation potential in an individual with dependence on alcohol are equally applicable to dependence on other drugs in this class. Such criteria would include: age; duration of dependence; socioenvironmental resources, such as family, home, and finances; job skills; and concomitant pathology (see chap. 17).

The existence of psychopathology preceding or secondary to established depressant drug dependence constitutes a limiting factor which diminishes the individual's prospects for a favorable outcome. This does not, however, contraindicate rehabilitation attempts and improvement. With appropriate therapy, even recovery may be anticipated if compensatory rehabilitative assets are present.

The rehabilitation counselor must approach his client with the understanding that depressant drug dependence is a chronic illness characterized by relapses and remissions. When the traditional criterion of treatment success, abstinence from all drug use, is not achieved, the counselor can measure success in terms of drug-free days. In practice, the duration of the periods of remission become more extended and an occasional return to drug use should be accepted as part of the natural history of the disease. The relationship between counselor and client should not be jeopardized during these periods. In fact, the confidence of the client in his counselor will lead him to seek the counselor's help in terminating the episode rather than concealing the transgression from him.

HALLUCINOGENS

Pathology

Hallucinogens are sometimes also referred to as psychedelics or psychotomimetics. Some are found in plants (psilocybin is found in some mushrooms, mescaline in the peyote cactus, and lysergic acid diethylamide in the seeds of the morning glory), and others are synthesized in the laboratory (STP, PCP, and LSD). Lysergic acid diethylamide (LSD) was first synthesized in 1938, and its hallucinogenic properties were discovered in 1943.

These drugs are usually taken by mouth. Within 30 minutes, stimulant-type effects such as increased heart rate, enlarged pupils, dry mouth, nervousness, and overactive reflexes are observed. Next a phase of altered perception occurs: colors are brighter, sounds are more distinct, and there is increased awareness of all bodily feelings and sensations. A period of visual distortion then follows, during which perceptions of size, shape, and colors of objects may constantly change. Also, objects may seem to undulate and change their relation to each other (e.g., parts of the body may seem enormous and close up or minute and far away). Distortion of thought processes generally follows. This phase is often accompanied by hallucinations of the illusion of separation of mind and body.

Despite the severe disturbance of logical thought, individuals frequently report insights into the mysteries of nature or the universe. The mood of the subject varies. He may be overcome with awe at this experience and be ecstatic, or he may be horrified and fearful. There may be such terror that a panic state supervenes (the "bad trip") or the individual may pass into a true psychotic reaction. Minute doses of these potent drugs may induce disturbances as described which last 24 hours, but the duration is usually shorter.

Phencyclidine (PCP, "angel dust") may induce a state of motor inhibition so that the individual is inert and stares blankly. Physiologic responses to this drug may include elevated blood pressure, vomiting, increased salivary secretion, seizures, and respiratory rhythm disturbances.

Notwithstanding these powerful effects, the hallucinogens have developed a reputation they probably do not deserve. Although LSD use has been credited with high rates of suicide, such deaths have generally been the consequences of the bizarre behavior caused by the drug rather than a toxic effect of the drug itself. The occurrence of the LSD psychosis may also have been misrepresented. One researcher found an incidence of LSD-induced psychoses lasting more than 48 hours in only 0.8 per 1,000 persons. The danger of chromosome damage causing genetic defects has been misrepresented, and the contention that LSD causes brain damage also remains dubious. LSD may have gained its sinister reputation because of the presence of impurities or even because it was actually another drug whose effects were more toxic. It is nearly impossible to predict the composition of drugs purchased on the street. PCP is substituted for almost any of the others.

There may, however, be support for the fear that adolescents suffer personality changes as a result of LSD abuse. These changes may include increased susceptibility to irrational beliefs and behavior, regressive magical thinking, indifference to the demands of reality, and indifference to the consequences of their behavior.

Complications

The life style frequently associated with hallucinogen abuse may lead to neglect of physical health, poor hygiene, and poor nutrition. Poor nutrition often results from a tendency to food faddism, leading to an unbalanced or deficient diet.

Flashbacks develop in a small percentage of hallucinogen users. These are brief periods, usually a few seconds or minutes, during which delusions or hallucinations resembling the hallucinogen experience occur without drug ingestion. They may occur when the subject is fatigued and may continue intermittently for some time. Usually they are self-limiting and cease after a few months.

Mortality has been reported in a few cases following ingestion of very high doses of LSD and PCP. There is usually onset of a very high fever, convulsions, and ultimately coma and death.

Functional Disabilities

As noted earlier, the physical consequences of persistent hallucinogen abuse are not significant. The psychosocial consequences of continued hallucinogen use have also been alluded to. Examination of users shows several common characteristics, some no doubt representing aspects of the pre-drug-use personality which contributed to the onset of drug taking, and others representing direct effects of the drug. Users are less conventional in attitudes and behavior than nonusers. They are less likely to live at home, and they show an unstable life style with respect to stability of address, school career, and work record. They relate less well to their parents, belong to fewer organizations, and are more promiscuous sexually. They are more liberal in their political beliefs, have less respect for authority, and believe more strongly in supernatural phenomena. When tested psychologically, they show proneness to being impulsive, pleasure seeking, and rebellious. Frequent hallucinogen users consistently show high unemployment and general underachievement. It is to be noted that these same traits are shared by heavy marihuana users.

Rehabilitation Potential

It is uncommon for a drug abuser to limit his use solely to hallucinogens. Were he to attempt to do so, use of the drug would be self-limiting because of its properties. No physical dependence results and there is a rapid build-up of tolerance, so that the drug becomes ineffective if used daily. Effects are less on the second successive day of use and almost absent on the third administration. A period of 4 to 6 days must elapse before effects are experienced again. Unlike other drugs of abuse, the effects of hallucinogens are unpredictable, so that they cannot be taken to achieve a predictable pleasure experience. Finally, the hallucinogen "trip," if repeated many times, becomes commonplace and loses its appeal. For these reasons, it appears that the majority of hallucinogen users tend to terminate this abuse within a few years. It naturally follows that a favorable rehabilitation potential should be anticipated. However, in those instances where the individual is a polydrug user or manifests the personality traits common to hallucinogen abusers, the outlook will be less favorable.

CANNABIS

Pathology

Hashish and marihuana are derived from the hemp plant (*Cannabis sativa*). The plant produces a sticky resin rich in the active compound tetra-hydrocannabinol (THC), which is harvested as hashish. The flowering tops and leaves of the plant are dried to produce marihuana. When marihuana is smoked as cigarettes or in a pipe, THC in the smoke is inhaled. Hashish has five or six times the potency of marihuana. While smoking is the most effective means of administration, the drug can be taken by mouth. Attempts to administer the drug intravenously are ineffective and dangerous because it is insoluable in water.

The effect of small doses of marihuana resembles mild alcohol intoxication. As with alcohol, the user feels relaxed and less inhibited. There is a loosening of conventions, frequently accompanied by euphoria and laughter. There may be heightened sensation, particularly of sight and hearing. With higher doses there are perceptual effects resembling those of LSD. It should be noted that marihuana itself is a mild hallucinogen. The passing of time seems slowed, distance seems stretched out, shapes and colors are distorted, and hallucinations of an organized kind (in contrast to the colors and shapes associated with LSD use) are experienced. The next stage, fatigue and sleepiness, signals the end of drug action. The user will report enjoyment of music, cinema cartoons, and heightened appreciation of food tastes and texture.

A majority of users will report occasionally experiencing anxiety symptoms, strange feelings of detachment from reality (derealization), and memory impairment. Occasionally, acute panic states will develop. The more potent form of the drug, hashish, is sometimes associated with psychotic behavior.

Complications

Rapid heart rate, tremor, and conjunctivitis are regularly observed in marihuana users. Less often, dryness of the mouth and urinary frequency occur. Observations of heavy users of cannabis in India found a high incidence of lung disorders, anemias, malnutrition, and behavior problems. Very few deaths directly attributable to cannabis toxicity are recorded.

Functional Disabilities

With the dosage forms available in the U.S., cannabis abuse does not appear to result in serious physical disability. The psychosocial consequences are generally proportional to the extent of use. Infrequent use, even if regular, appears not to be associated with untoward consequences. With daily use, it is probable that symptoms of apathy and indolence (amotivational syndrome) will supervene. The abuser's age is significant. The adolescent jeopardizes his psychosocial maturation and may suffer underdevelopment or impairment of his coping skills. He is unlikely to maintain his grades and probably will fall behind his nonabusing peers scholastically.

Rehabilitation Potential

The pure marihuana abuser is a rarity. Since marihuana is a mild hallucinogen, the comments on rehabilitation potential for hallucinogen abuse are also applicable here. Where a true psychological dependence develops, the abuser will tend to deal with any stress by turning to marihuana, thus insulating himself against painful reality. The amotivational syndrome constitutes a late stage of heavy use in which the abuser lacks the motivation to undertake activities to change his own condition or that of the society he needs to rejoin.

There is little data to show how effective rehabilitation programs are when dealing with heavy marihuana abusers because this form of drug dependence is seldom encountered in isolation from use of other types of drugs. Since tolerance develops slowly, if at all, use is not self-limiting, as is true with the hallucinogen drugs.

VOLATILE SOLVENTS

Pathology

Volatile solvents appear to be used principally by young males aged 11 to 18. They include gasoline, varnish, paint thinner, cleaning fluids, aerosol sprays, glue, chloroform, ether, amyl nitrite, nitrous oxide, and toluene. Usually some of the volatile solvent is placed in the bottom of a plastic bag from which the fumes are inhaled. Following intake, there is a brief period of intoxication characterized by stupor or "drunk" behavior (staggering gait, incoordination of extremities, falls, slurred speech, and memory disturbance).

Complications

Reported complications of inhalation of volatile substances include a variety of blood disturbances, such as anemia, overproduction or underproduction of white blood cells, and abnormalities of white cell counts. There are also reports of brain damage, liver and kidney damage, pancreatitis, and lesions of the upper respiratory tract. A chemical pneumonia may occur. There may be disturbances of the heart rhythm, which probably account for occasional deaths. A more common cause of death is from asphyxiation resulting from inhaling fumes from a plastic bag; the individual loses consciousness while inhaling from the bag and is usually found with it still covering his face. It has been reported that inhalation of freon may freeze the vocal cords and block passage to the trachea with fatal consequences.

Functional Disabilities

Due to the youth of the group involved in this form of drug abuse, severe disturbance of the abuser's education and psychosocial maturation often results. Further, this type of abuse often appears to be a concomitant of quite serious degrees of personality disturbance.

Rehabilitation Potential

The abuse of volatile solvents has been less well studied than other forms of drug abuse but the outlook for abusers, because of the coexisting psychopathology, appears grave. Treatment of the underlying emotional disturbance is urgent, and the prognosis may be determined by that of the primary condition. Generally, the extent of use in these cases will be significant. Occasional use of these drugs probably represents a form of adolescent risk-taking and has a favorable prognosis. When the abuse is symptomatic of an underlying sociopathic illness, the outlook is less hopeful.

STANDARDS OF EVALUATION

It will not be unusual for the drug abuser client to have symptoms of physical illness, psychological maladjustment, educational underachievement, limited or absent job skills, legal entanglements, and a family receiving welfare support. Any one of this catalog of disasters might deter a counselor's

optimism. Collectively, they constitute a year or more of work for the professional team with whom the counselor will be associated.

Commonly, the counselor's assistance will be sought by the facility referring the client. This facility may be a community mental health center; a free-standing drug abuse clinic; the emergency room of a general hospital or its medical, surgical, or psychiatric inpatient service. The probation and parole service of a correctional facility or the officers of a court in which the abuser has been tried may also serve as sources of referral. The abuser's family may have called a "hot line" or sought the assistance of the community's welfare agency or a voluntary organization such as the local mental health association.

The counselor should review the social, medical, and psychiatric history provided by the referring facility. He will obtain data on past and present physical and mental health as determined by the physician from his review of body systems, physical and mental status examinations, radiologic findings, and clinical pathology testing. Where such evaluations are lacking, appropriate examinations should be scheduled. The services of an internist, psychiatrist, clinical psychologist, vocational psychologist, social worker, probation officer, attorney, welfare worker, and drug abuse counselor may all be needed.

When assembling the information and developing a rehabilitation plan, the counselor should ask a number of related questions. What medical and psychiatric diagnoses have been made? Is there an active disease and is it being treated? What medications is the client receiving and do side effects place constraints on potential skills, training, or work placement? Are evaluations of hospital, occupational, and recreational therapists available? Are psychological evaluations present in the psychiatric history and examination or should intelligence and personality testing be obtained?

The social history will identify the major milestones in the abuser's early development, the family structure and dynamics, and the client's vocational and marital history. Care should be taken to assess family support and available resources. A report of individual or group therapy and counseling may be available if the client has had inpatient or outpatient treatment. The abuser may have a history of penal incarceration during which he obtained further education or skills training. Is he on parole or probation? Does he have trials or pre-sentence investigations pending?

The answers to all these questions and the information received from the various consultants will enable the counselor to highlight the client's strengths and weaknesses and establish priorities so that a systematic program of rehabilitation can be undertaken. In most cases, the client will continue in a drug abuse treatment program after referral to the vocational counselor. Close cooperation between the counselor and the treatment program is essential for the client's successful rehabilitation.

TOTAL TREATMENT

The terms primary, secondary, and tertiary prevention have been derived from public health and are often used in developing programs for the prevention of contagious diseases. These terms are sometimes employed in considering the treatment of drug dependency.

Primary prevention seeks to eliminate a disease by preventing its occurrence (e.g., preventing poliomyelitis by immunization). It is outside the scope of this chapter to discuss methods of primary prevention in drug abuse.

Secondary prevention refers to the identification and treatment of all individuals in a population suffering from the disease. With respect to drug dependency, this has been the major public health advance of the last decade. Drug abuse was previously regarded as a crime rather than as a disease and was handled through correctional institutions rather than specialized treatment facilities.

Tertiary prevention refers to the process of reducing the residual disability caused by a disease and returning the affected individual to his optimal functioning level. With respect to drug dependency, it refers to that range of rehabilitation measures undertaken to restore the individual to society as a contributing rather than a dependent member.

There are essentially two types of drug-abuse treatment programs: methadone maintenance and therapeutic communities. These programs are philosophically opposed, since one works by substituting the narcotic methadone for the narcotic heroin, and the other by withdrawing the addict from narcotics to the drug-free state. Because of this, the former program is limited to the treatment of narcotic dependence, while the therapeutic community approach is also applicable to other types of drug dependency.

Methadone Maintenance

Currently, there are more than 100,000 patients enrolled in methadone programs. These programs are operated in accordance with strict guidelines established by the Federal Government and supervised by State governmental agencies. The drug is simply part of a spectrum of treatment services offered by the methadone clinic, which usually is a program of a city-wide drug treatment agency, a university, a community mental health center, or a hospital. Treatment often includes group and individual psychotherapy, family therapy, vocational counseling, and legal and medical services. The clinic usually has access to inpatient services to provide hospital care to narcotic-dependent patients who have drug-related medical needs, such as withdrawal from either heroin or methadone maintenance to the drug-free state (detoxification) or treatment of overdose. However, methadone maintenance is essentially an outpatient program, and hospitalization is generally not necessary for initiating and maintaining treatment. The primary advantages of methadone programs are the low cost per patient, minimal disruption of the patient's schedule, and increased likelihood of employment during the treatment process.

The goal of methadone maintenance is primarily to effect social rehabilitation and secondarily to ultimately achieve the drug-free state. Studies to date show that this latter goal is difficult to achieve, since less than a third of the patients successfully withdraw at their first attempt. That methadone is a successful treatment method is supported by statistics showing a substantial increase in the number of persons engaged in socially useful occupations after treatment. However, methadone, particularly in conjunction with alcohol, has become a major drug of abuse.

After some years of use, the most commonly occurring side-effects of methadone maintenance are: increased sweating (48 percent); constipation (17 percent); decreased libido (22 percent); and orgasmic difficulty (14 percent).

More recently, a second pharmacologic approach to narcotic dependency has been tested. Antagonist drugs, such as naloxone, which block the action of narcotics, have been synthesized. By taking such drugs daily, the narcotic abuser is rendered immune to the effects of heroin and other narcotics.

Therapeutic Communities

Therapeutic communities are residential facilities for the rehabilitation of drug abusers. The basic goal of these communities is to provide a 24-hour-a-day influence on its residents to help them completely change their life style. Changes include drug abstinence, elimination of criminal behavior, development of vocational skills, and acquisition of positive attitudes and values, such as honesty, responsibility, nonviolence, and self-reliance. Initially, the therapeutic communities were staffed solely by rehabilitated drug abusers, but recently they have undergone some professionalization of personnel.

The title "therapeutic communities" was originally used in psychiatry to refer to egalitatian treatment environments. In fact, the traditional drug therapeutic communities are highly structured social organizations which mirror the outside world in their use of titles, privileges of rank, and authoritarianism. The treatment method is confrontation, in which the drug abuser is forced to surrender his "sick" identity and reconstitute his personality in a more "healthy" fashion.

Synanon, established in the late 1950's, was one of the earliest of the traditional therapeutic communities. It developed a residential rehabilitation and resocialization program which was substantially adopted by numerous other treatment facilities. The essential elements of this type of community are: (a) individual entry and indoctrination (the newcomer enters because of acceptance by the peer group rather than by agency directive); (b) caste and stratification (one's position in the community is a correlate of social maturity): (c) intensive group psychotherapy; and (d) participation in real work. Inappropriate behavior may be dealt with by administering a "haircut" (i.e., a method of "attack therapy" using verbal hyperbole, ridicule, or direct verbal onslaught). An important goal of this method is to alter the abuser's "criminal-tough-guy pose" toward a more socially acceptable posture.

Generally, there are three stages in the treatment program in traditional therapeutic communities. During the first stage, the newcomer's relationships are closely watched and regulated for his own benefit and personal protection. In the second stage, he has learned how to conduct such relationships on his own, and as he assumes more responsibility for his behavior, he is given elevated social status and privileges. The third stage, or graduation, applies to individuals who live and work in the community and have complete freedom to come and go as they please. The duration of the treatment program varies greatly, but most persons who have been in the community more than 6 months are free to do their own work either in or out of the community.

Most contemporary therapeutic communities have not fully accepted the traditional model and differ from it in a number of ways. One difference is that many current communities provide family counseling and involvement, whereas the families were not involved in the traditional therapeutic communities. Involvement of the families is based on the awareness that, particularly for the younger residents, family problems have often been a cause of the drug abuse problem. Young persons have usually come to the community from their families and will return to them. If the family problems have not been alleviated, a young person is more likely to relapse into drug abuse after returning home.

In the contemporary therapeutic communities, individual therapy is considered more appropriate than encounter group therapy for some residents and/or for some areas of concern. The emphasis is more on the causes of drug abuse than strictly on altering drug-abusing behavior. Discipline is less rigid, and there is more flexibility, more effort to create an atmosphere of caring, love, and physical closeness.

The more recent therapeutic communities are more oriented to the outside world and re-entry into it, whereas the orientation of the more traditional communities was inward, toward the community itself. Treatment and training are directed toward the expectations of the "real world," and there is a strong emphasis on education and vocational training.

Traditional therapeutic communities are, for the most part, autonomous and independent, operating outside the medical model. More contemporary communities are often more integrated with larger health care facilities.

Both methadone maintenance programs and therapeutic communities have high drop-out rates, but the rate is higher for the communities. Some commonly cited disadvantages of therapeutic communities are the high cost per client, accountability problems, and unsuitability for many types of clients. They also have been attacked as high-cost services aimed at the needs of the middle class. Therapeutic communities therefore constitute a valuable but controversial part of the therapy spectrum.

Hospitalization

Treatment of dependence on drugs of the depressant group is best undertaken in a hospital setting, due to the risk of serious complications of the withdrawal process. Abrupt termination of such drugs may precipitate withdrawal seizures, so a progressive reduction (tapering) of the dose is called for. In the case of alcohol, another central nervous system depressant (usually a minor tranquilizer) is substituted. Detoxification of amphetamine abusers does not require hospitalization unless they show serious disturbance of mood (depression) or of thought (delusions and hallucinations). Abusers of hallucinogens and marihuana should not require hospitalization for detoxification unless complications are present.

In addition to the management of detoxification and complications of drug abuse, hospitalization provides for optimal overall care, since the consequences of drug abuse often include neglect of personal hygiene, poor diet, and loss of sleep. It offers opportunities to broaden the range of interests and to involve the drug-dependent person in supervised recreational activities, group and individual psychotherapy, and occupational therapy. By providing an opportunity to abruptly discontinue participation in a drug-oriented milieu, the abuser's own environment, his best intentions to change his life style are reinforced.

Followup

Upon discharge from a hospital or following outpatient detoxification, provision must be made for followup care, including establishment of a supportive relationship with a counselor, social worker, psychologist, nurse, or physician on the treatment staff. During the difficult transition from drug dependency to the drug-free state, visits may need to be weekly or more frequently. When problems of daily living create stresses that formerly would have resulted in drug use, counseling within the supportive relationship is available as a preferable alternative.

Since drug abuse is a notoriously relapsing condition, therapeutic approaches aimed at extinguishing drug-seeking behavior and reinforcing maintenance of the drug-free state have been devised. These techniques have been derived from the field of behavior modification and include covert sensitization and contingency contracting. The reader is referred to the literature of behavior modification for additional information.

VOCATIONAL IMPLICATIONS

The rehabilitation counselor plays a critical role in aiding the recovering drug abuser to make the transition from the treatment milieu to the work environment successfully. To do this, the client must give up the role of patient for the role of employee. As previously indicated, the client may show a fluctuating level of motivation with respect to rehabilitation. This quality, when coupled with a long history of discrimination and rejection, may result in attempts to manipulate the counselor into also rejecting him. The counselor may have to deal with immature and regressive behavior at a primitive level (i.e., acting out, shouting, and threatening).

A favorable trend in the field of drug abuse rehabilitation has been the increasing number of abusers in treatment who are either currently employed or have marketable job skills and/or a recent history of employment. This latter group will obviously present less of a challenge to the expertise of the counselor than those with no past history of employment. The difficulty is compounded if such individuals have supported themselves and their drug habits with lucrative "hustles" so that they are accustomed to a large, although illegal, income. Their first vocational placements will most often be at wages they find demeaning to their self-image. Such clients may well have been narcotic abusers who trafficked in drugs, an activity incompatible with the life style they now seek to adopt.

By contrast, some young adult polydrug users will have come from a counter culture that challenged the materialistic values of the larger society and therefore have been accustomed to the subsistence wages that their unskilled labor provided. It is not unusual for this group to have a record of casual labor consequent upon their indifference to the value orientation of their nonabusing peer group. They have not been motivated by goals of achievement and success and, for them, the work ethic exemplifies a socioeconomic system to which they do not subscribe.

Personnel involved in vocational rehabilitation of drug abusers caution against complying with insistent demands of these clients for early job placement. It is clear that a psychological transition must be made from the attitudes inseparable from the abuser life style to attitudes appropriate to an employee. The evaluation of the client's job readiness is based upon both general and specific employability factors. The former refer to such qualities as social development, grooming and hygiene, relation to supervisors and fellow workers, frustration tolerance, reaction to instructions and criticism, physical tolerance, performance rate, and general work habits. The specific factors refer to the skills, aptitudes, achievements, and interests which are directly related to a particular job class or area.

The counselor should encourage his client to complete the high school equivalence (GED) if he is not a high school graduate. He may, from time to time, recommend higher education, but this calls for a high degree of self-motivation and might reasonably be postponed until it is apparent that the client's recovery is established and sustained.

A job-seeking client may ask the counselor whether he should volunteer information about his abuse history, fearing that to reveal it is to court rejection because of prejudice. Hopefully, the counselor will have developed outreach services to educate the business community and may have encouraged the development of programs within industry so that an identified drug abuser might remain on the job while he is receiving help. The final decision regarding disclosure will necessarily be an individual decision made by client and counselor. Care should be taken, however, not to counsel the client to be evasive or defensive and, by all means, not to falsify the information provided the prospective employer.

Since both methadone maintenance and therapeutic community treatments are of extended duration, the question of the feasibility of combining employment with treatment arises. If a satisfactory degree of job readiness is present, there is no contraindication. The therapeutic community resident, however, must have reached the late second or third stage of recovery. Employers may express some concern about the effect of methadone on a client's manual dexterity, reaction time, and reasoning ability. Narcotic drug abusers learn to take their methadone at a time which permits them to experience the highest blood level when it will least affect them on the job.

When the drug abuser is abstinent, his counselor should seek confirmation that he is maintaining his affiliation with the treatment program and that, therefore, any recurrence of drug abusing behavior will be identified through urine drug screenings. The counselor should schedule regular followup interviews with his client, weekly initially and subsequently at less frequent intervals. The abstinent drug abuser who has been successfully returned to work remains very much in need of the services of the rehabilitation counselor as he attempts to deal with day-to-day on-the-job stresses. The counselor should remember that the drug abuser is less likely than other clients to tolerate ambiguity in the job situation, and problems with authority figures in the past may create difficulty in current supervision. It is also desirable that the client's work schedule be clearly defined, since his ability to deal with a relatively unstructured situation is limited.

It has been the practice for many narcotic drug abusers to seek employment in the drug abuse field. Although this has not been an unqualified success, some clients have succeeded very well. In most cases this was because they furthered their education and rose to positions of responsibility and trust. In another program, the successful placement of rehabilitated abusers in New York's off-track betting facility demonstrated that they can be trusted to work with money.

We might conclude that while some rehabilitated abusers have the same potential to achieve as their nonabusing peers, others will have great difficulty in entering the world of work. For the majority, their level of motivation, the vocational opportunities available, and the nature of professional support and assistance will determine the outcome.

BIBLIOGRAPHY

Arkin S: Drug patients vs employers: The confidentiality dilemma. Natl Conf Methadone Treat Proc 2:865–74, 1973.
This article discusses the employer's right to obtain drug treatment information as compared to the client's right to have his privacy maintained. Some guidelines are given for the kind of information employers should be given and under what circumstances they should be given the information.

Boudin HM, Valentine VE, Inghram RD, Brantley JM, Ruiz MR, Smith GG, Catlin RP, Regan EJ: Contingency contracting with drug abusers in the natural environment. Int J Addict 12:1–16, 1977.
Describes contingency contracting with drug abusers in the community. Clients must look for employment or continue their present employment to remain in the program.

Davidson S, Robinson J, Stegbauer V: Behavioral contracting workshop. Natl Conf Methadone Treat Proc 1:1203–1206, 1973.
This short article outlines the components of a behavioral contract and briefly explains some of the benefits of using this technique.

Dole VP, Wolkstein EC: Vocational rehabilitation of patients on the Beth Israel Methadone Maintenance Program. Mt. Sinai J Med NY 41:267–271, 1974.
Examines the role of job readiness, marketable skills, and job opportunities in the Beth Israel abuser rehabilitation program.

Hardy RE, Cull JG (eds): *Drug Dependence and Rehabilitation Approaches*. Springfield, IL, Thomas, 1973.
This book contains valuable material on rehabilitation needs of abusers, in particular, chapters by Jacks (The Public Vocational Rehabilitation Program and the Drug Abuser), Bowden (Clinical Counseling Problems in Drug Abuse), Murray and Trotter (Treatment in Drug Abuse, Counseling Approaches and Special Programs).

Josephson E, Carroll EE (eds): *Drug Use: Epidemiological and Sociological Approaches*. Washington, D.C., Hemisphere, 1974.
A standard work which is the "state of the art" in the epidemiology of drug abuse.

Kalant H, Kalant O: *Drugs, Society and Personal Choices*. Toronto, Addiction Research Foundation, 1971.
An excellent introductory text for understanding the pharmacological, social, and psychological aspects of drug abuse.

Morton FL: Employing ex-addicts: Determinants of support and opposition. Int J Addict 11:681–694, 1976.
A valuable contribution to a poorly researched area. The author reports on a symposium held to improve the employment opportunities and to examine the attitudes of the symposium attendees.

Scher JM, Crown B, Lee J. McAuley P: "Over-employment," mobility, and rehabilitation in methadone maintenance. Natl Conf Methadone Treat Proc 2:836–857, 1973.
Describes the program requirements, amount of methadone used, and dosage requirements in a private methadone maintenance clinic. Acceptance into this program requires employment. Federal regulations are also discussed briefly.

Wilmarth SS, Goldstein A: *Therapeutic Effectiveness of Methadone Maintenance Programs in the Management of Drug Dependence of Morphine Type in the U.S.A.* Geneva, W.H.O., 1974.
An objective evaluation of methadone in the rehabilitation of narcotic drug abusers.

19 MENTAL ILLNESS

H. Richard Lamb, M.D.
Cecile Mackota

INTRODUCTION

This chapter will provide a brief survey of some of the main categories of mental illness, the characteristics of psychiatric clients most important to the rehabilitation process, and some general principles for effectively helping severely disabled psychiatric clients deal with life in community settings. With some knowledge of the major mental disorders and the behaviors accompanying them, rehabilitation counselors will find work with the psychiatrically disabled less difficult and more meaningful and rewarding.

Mental illnesses are grouped into diagnostic categories. The four main categories—the *psychoses,* the *neuroses,* the *organic brain syndromes,* and the *personality disorders*—are discussed here.

Patients are diagnosed as neurotic or psychotic to distinguish between those who are in touch with reality and those who are not. The difference between neuroses and psychoses can be described in many ways. We will limit ourselves here to just a few major points. The psychoses usually involve a loss of a person's ability to distinguish what is actually taking place in his external environment from his own internal fantasies and impulses. For instance, a psychotic person may have an auditory hallucination. He may "hear" a voice which he thinks is a real voice, but which in reality comes from his own inner psyche. Other frequent, though not invariable, manifestations of psychoses are: marked disorganization of the personality; marked loss of impulse control; extreme and often total withdrawal from other people; and preoccupation with one's own thoughts and fantasies. There is generally a fairly marked distortion of reality. For example, a patient riding on a bus may be convinced that all the people on the bus are thinking about how fat and ugly he is.

On the other hand, the neurotic, while in touch with reality and his environment, suffers from many conflicts in fulfilling his needs. He has difficulty dealing with his emotions, may have specific neurotic symptoms, such as phobias and compulsions, often has poor impulse control, and is tense and anxious. Neuroses are generally less incapacitating than psychoses and the personality remains fairly intact.

Both psychotic and nonpsychotic disorders caused by damage to brain tissue are categorized as organic brain syndromes. Deeply ingrained maladaptive behavior patterns characterize the personality disorder category.

FUNCTIONAL PSYCHOSES

At this point in the state of our knowledge, functional psychoses are not associated with any physiological or structural change in the brain that can be demonstrated, as opposed to the organic brain syndromes which are usually accompanied by demonstrable changes in the brain. (Research in the biochemistry of brain functioning is fast revealing differences between mentally ill and "normal" persons, but this is beyond the scope of this chapter.) There has long been a controversy over the role of hereditary or genetic factors vs. environmental factors in the etiology of the functional psychoses. Research has now clearly established the existence of the genetic component. Most convincing have been carefully controlled studies of children of schizophrenic parents adopted away compared to children of nonschizophrenic parents adopted away; the incidence of schizophrenia in the adopted-away children of schizophrenic parents is significantly higher. We also know, however, that the course of these illnesses can be influenced by environmental factors throughout life. The consensus of opinion of most psychiatrists is that both genetic and environmental factors play a role in varying degrees in each case.

Schizophrenia

Schizophrenia has been defined as an upheaval from within the personality, a fragmenting of the mental functions, an overwhelming experience that separates thought, mood, and behavior from reality. There is some question whether schizophrenia is one illness or a group of related illnesses. For this reason, it is often referred to as the group of schizophrenias. Etiologic factors are thought to include heredity, deficiencies in the mother-infant relationship, the nature of later family interactions, and stresses outside the family in the various periods of development. The most frequent age of onset of overt schizophrenia is adolescence and early adult life, though the age of onset can be from late childhood to late middle age.

The schizophrenic usually has very low self-esteem and strong feelings of being rejected by those around him. Characteristically, he protects himself by withdrawal from emotional involvement or even communication with others. He may become isolated, sometimes not able to leave home, and may no longer trust or confide in anyone. He often shows an increasing indifference to members of his family, accustomed interests, and the demands and opportunities of his environment. There may be a deterioration in his ability to work. Friends and family often mistakenly attribute the patient's listlessness and loss of spontaneity, ambition, and sustained effort in pursuit of former goals to laziness.

Disturbances of affect (feelings and emotional expression) are characteristic of schizophrenia. There is usually a paucity of emotional responsiveness and a decrease in the variety of emotional expression. The patient becomes unable to feel and show emotions. A flatness of affect is often described, in which the patient displays no feeling whatsoever, regardless of what is happening around him. Inappropriate affect is also frequently described; e.g., the patient may giggle when told of the death of a loved one.

Problems of attention are usually evident. The patient may be oblivious to the world around him and instead be preoccupied with his inner fantasies. Thinking becomes primarily self-centered, with day dreams taking over for reality. Disorders of thinking are also typical. Normally, ideas follow one another with a definite logical connection, progressing to an ultimate completeness of thought. In schizophrenia, both thinking and speech may be in the form of "free association," or a loosening of thought processes. Ideas no longer follow one another with a definite logical connection and there is no apparent relationship among ideas presented. This may progress to the point where the patient's utterances become fragmentary, disconnected, or even unintelligible.

Other symptoms often seen in schizophrenia are false beliefs (delusions) and hallucinations. Still another important symptom of schizophrenia may be the loss of self-control resulting in unpredictable and highly bizarre behavior. There is often evidence that the patient is purposely concealing his feelings from a "hostile world."

Types. The schizophrenias are usually divided into types. The *simple type* is characterized by a slow and insidious reduction of external attachments and interests and by apathy and indifference leading to impoverishment of interpersonal relations, mental deterioration, and adjustment at a lower level of functioning. In general, this type is less dramatically psychotic than the other types of schizophrenia, but tends to become more exaggerated with aging.

The *hebephrenic type* is characterized by disorganized thinking, shallow and inappropriate affect, unpredictable giggling, silly and regressive behavior and mannerisms, and frequent hypochondriacal complaints. Delusions and hallucinations, if present, are transient and not well organized.

The *catatonic type* is usually divided into two subtypes. One is marked by excessive and sometimes violent motor activity and excitement. The other subtype, which is more common, is characterized by generalized inhibition of movement, stupor, mutism, and negativism. The patient of the latter type will probably stay in bed if allowed to. If he is forced to get up, he will stand or sit in one position, sometimes without any movement of any kind for hours. Delusions and hallucinations are usually present.

The *paranoid type* is characterized primarily by the presence of delusions of persecution or grandeur. Hallucinations are often present. Excessive religiosity is sometimes seen. The patient's attitude is frequently hostile and aggressive, and his behavior tends to be influenced by his delusions. In general, the disorder does manifest the gross personality disorganization of the hebephrenic and catatonic types.

The *chronic undifferentiated type* is characterized by symptoms associated with one or more of the other types mentioned. The symptoms may vary, with some symptoms most prominent at one time and others most prominent at other times.

When seen by the vocational counselor at the point of referral, the patient is often in partial or total remission; the syndromes and symptoms described above may remain only in subtle forms or may not be in evidence at all. Sometimes the patient will be rational and seem completely "normal" until a particular subject arises. Generally, the patient is abnormally ambivalent about almost everything and thus has great difficulty making decisions.

There is usually an element of depression present in persons suffering from schizophrenia, and a great deal of ruminating and agonizing over various problems. Sometimes the depression is the most prominent feature, along with such psychotic symptoms as delusions and hallucinations. This is referred to as a *psychotic depression* and is especially common in the middle years, or involutional period, in which case it may be related to the patient's reactions to middle age and its problems. It is usually precipitated by a loss of some sort. Strong and sometimes inappropriate feelings of guilt are present, together with feelings of inadequacy and unworthiness. Frequently, hypochondriasis is prominent and severe. There is further discussion of the classical signs and symptoms of depression below under Affective Disorders.

Prognosis. The prognosis of schizophrenia depends in large part on the severity of the illness in relation to the strengths of the personality. If treatment is started early, chances of remission are much greater. Also, it is generally believed that if the onset is very rapid, chances of recovery are greater. A trauma as a precipitating cause, rather than a slow, unfocused deterioration, heralds a more positive result. The patient's personality before illness and the relative strength of his ego have a very real significance in regard to what progress can be expected. The more successful the life before illness, the more likely the recovery. Many therapists believe that the greater the prominence of symptoms such as anxiety or depression, the more likely remission will occur.

Treatment. Just a few decades ago, a diagnosis of schizophrenia would more often than not have meant a lifetime in a state hospital. Today this is no longer true. Treatment of schizophrenia has been revolutionized by the modern psychoactive drugs and by an emphasis in recent years on social forms of treatment.

The psychoactive drugs in most widespread use for the treatment of schizophrenia include the phenothiazines, the thioxanthenes, and the butyrophenones. These are the antischizophrenic tranquilizers, often referred to as the major tranquilizers. The most commonly used phenothiazines are chlorpromazine (Trilafon), trifluoperazine (Stelazine), and thioridazine (Mellaril); the most commonly used thioxanthenes are chlorprothixene (Taractan) and thiothixene (Navane); and the most widely used butyrophenone is Haldol. All these drugs correct thought disorders and prevent full-blown schizophrenic episodes. Some act on all levels of the CNS, and others act on a specific part of the CNS, but the precise mechanism is unknown.

The most frequently encountered side effects of these drugs are: dryness of the mouth; dizziness and sometimes fainting caused by sudden drop in blood pressure when the patient sits up or stands up (postural hypotension); blurring of vision, especially in regard to near objects, and consequent interference with reading; constipation; impotence and decreased libido; symptoms similar to those found in Parkinson's disease (tremor and rigidity of the muscles, including the facial muscles, with decreased facial expression); increased sun sensitivity; and akathisia. Akathisia is a disorder in which the patient is not able to sit still. He suffers from "restless legs" and is forced to stand up and move around. The patient often describes his condition as "wanting to get outside his skin." Some of the medications may also interact unfavorably with alcohol. Parkinsonian symptoms and akathisia can be controlled by drugs such as trihexyphenidyl (Artane) and benztropine (Cogentin).

Tardive dyskinesia is a complication that can occur in connection with the long-term use of the major tranquilizers. It consists of slow, sometimes stereotyped, involuntary movements of the nose, tongue, mouth, or face, and sometimes other parts of the body. The movements are writhing, purposeless, and may or may not be continuous. Sucking, licking, lip pursing, blowing, and chewing are commonly seen. Tardive dyskinesia may subside a few months after discontinuation of the drug or it may be permanent.

Despite this impressive list of side effects, it should be emphasized that the major tranquilizers, properly used, can make the difference between an actively psychotic individual and one who can function in the community. For this reason, counselors should be continually alert to the possibility that their clients may have arbitrarily discontinued their medication. Should this occur, the counselor should make every effort to encourage his client to take his medication as prescribed.

Social forms of treatment include psychiatric day treatment centers, social and vocational rehabilitation, and therapeutic living arrangements. Also, it has been recognized that schizophrenics can and should be involved in individual and group psychotherapy. The vocational counselor works with other members of the psychiatric treatment team: the therapist, who may be a psychiatrist, psychologist, social worker, or, in some instances, a paraprofessional; and other persons involved with the patient, such as the halfway house director and welfare department worker.

The stresses in the patient's environment, the attitude of persons around him, and the supports given him also have important implications for treatment and rehabilitation. Schizophrenics appear to have much less capacity than others to deal with the ordinary stresses of life. This results in what has come to be known as the "revolving door syndrome"—frequent relapses, with patients being shuttled in and out of hospitals.

After a careful assessment of the patient and his environment, measures can be taken to reduce the stresses (e.g., resolution of family conflicts, reduction of social demands, helping the patient to find and accept a less stressful work situation) and to increase supports (e.g., medication, therapy, and supportive work and living situations, such as sheltered workshops and halfway houses). When schizophrenics are helped to find an equilibrium with increased supports and decreased stress, they can stabilize in the community and establish a base from which they can begin to work on social and vocational goals.

Affective Disorders

The group of affective disorders is characterized by a primary disturbance of mood, either elation or depression, and a resulting increase or decrease in activity and thought processes. These disturbances are clearly differentiated from the patient's prior functioning. When extreme and, especially in the case of depression, when accompanied by hallucinations or delusions, these disorders are classified as psychoses.

Types. There are three types of affective disorders. A *bipolar affective disorder* is characterized by the occurrence of both manic and depressive episodes at different times. In *manic disorders,* only manic episodes occur, and in *depressive disorders,* only depressive episodes occur (these are sometimes called unipolar affective disorders).

Prior to an acute manic episode, the patient usually has been a self-satisfied, confident, aggressive, effervescing extrovert, at ease with other people. He has been inclined to scatter his energy over a wide field of interests. His affective attitude has been one of emotional expression and responsiveness.

In a full-blown episode of mania, the affective picture is one of eagerness, exaltation, and extreme joyous excitement. The whole tempo of the personality is quickened. The patient sings, dances about, and whistles, and may be exhilarated and elated. The stream of thought is characterized by an extremely rapid association of ideas which is referred to as "flight of ideas" and there can be extreme pressure of speech. There is also a marked increase in motor activity and thought processes, extreme distractibility, and decreased need for sleep. Inflated self-esteem is typical. Hallucinations and delusions may occur, but they are not the most prominent part of this clinical picture.

Depressive episodes can vary in severity, and include the classical signs and symptoms of depression: the subjective feeling of depression; loss of interest or pleasure; decreased energy; sleep disturbance (early morning awakening, initial insomnia, fitful sleep, or excessive sleep); loss of appetite; tired, expressionless appearance; decreased

self-esteem (including feelings of worthlessness or guilt); and thoughts of death or suicide.

Manic-depressive psychoses usually begin in the twenties and early thirties. A manic or depressive attack may last from a few weeks to a year. Usually the condition does not become chronic; rather it is recurring. In fairly rare instances there is only one attack. Manic-depressive patients may need brief and recurring hospitalizations throughout their lives.

There have been problems in psychiatry in the differential diagnosis of schizophrenia and the affective disorders. For instance, in England the affective disorders have been diagnosed much more frequently and schizophrenia much less frequently than in the United States because of different diagnostic criteria. With the advent of specific drugs for the treatment of the affective disorders, in particular lithium, there appears to be an increasing interest in the United States in identifying affective disorders, with the result that diagnostic practice here is becoming more like that in England.

Treatment. Lithium has proven effective in both the treatment and prevention of the affective disorders, more so in the bipolar than in the unipolar type. Its use is monitored by taking blood samples to determine if the patient has a therapeutic blood lithium level. Diarrhea, vomiting, muscular weakness, tremor, lack of coordination, and excessive urination are symptoms of a blood lithium level that has risen too high.

Persons with affective disorders appear to share with schizophrenics a diminished capacity to cope with the routine stresses of life. While the drugs for the affective disorders are different, other treatment and rehabilitation considerations are similar to those for schizophrenics.

ORGANIC BRAIN SYNDROMES

Organic brain syndromes result from demonstrable physiological or structural changes in the brain. They are caused by a wide variety of conditions, including stroke, arteriosclerosis, head injury, senility, syphilis of the brain, and encephalitis. In many cases, the damage is irreversible. Symptoms of organic brain syndrome may appear as well with infections; alcohol, drug, or poison intoxication; epilepsy; metabolic changes; or brain tumors.

Unlike the functional psychoses, organic brain syndromes are manifested by impairment of orientation to time, place, and person (the patient may not know who he is, where he is, or what year it is); impairment of memory; impairment of all intellectual functions, such as comprehension, ability to calculate, general knowledge, and ability to learn; and gross impairment of judgment.

Organic brain syndromes are classified as nonpsychotic and psychotic. Some examples of the latter are senile dementia; the alcoholic psychoses, including delirium tremens and alcoholic deterioration; and psychoses caused by encephalitis and syphilis of the CNS.

Organic brain syndromes (for instance, many of those resulting from stroke, head injury, and alcoholism), are often at least partly reversible. Reversal of those caused by alcoholism, of course, assume cessation of drinking.

Treatment.

A most important aspect of treatment is eliminating causative factors, such as hypertension and alcoholism. Otherwise, supportive medical management and time are indicated. Techniques have been developed to help persons with brain damage ''relearn'' areas of mental functioning lost to them and to learn alternative ways of accomplishing the everyday routines of living to compensate for lost intellectual functioning. Counselors need to be aware that assessment must take premorbid functioning into account in measuring the degree of impairment and making judgments about the use of residual aptitudes. As an example, a patient whose functioning was at a professional level may, even with impairment, now function at an average level and be able to use many of his skills. On the other hand, a patient who was functioning at a low level and suffers brain trauma may have much more severe disabilities.

NEUROSES

Generally, the neuroses are recognized by the patient as symptoms. He realizes there is something wrong, experiences subjective distress, and desires relief. As mentioned earlier, the neuroses, as contrasted with the psychoses, do not manifest gross distortion or misinterpretation of external reality (reality testing is not impaired), nor is there gross personality disorganization. They are generally characterized as being less severe. Although uncomfortable, most patients remain employable. However, the patient is preoccupied with anxiety, which is the chief characteristic of the neuroses, and is therefore not functioning at his best. In some patients, the neurosis is severely incapacitating.

Types.

Anxiety neurosis. The anxiety may be felt and expressed directly as an anxiety neurosis with accompanying dread and apprehension, sometimes panic.

Usually there are symptoms like palpitations, tremulousness, pounding of the heart, rapid breathing, restlessness, increased perspiration, and muscle tension.

Phobic neurosis. Often anxiety may underlie the other neuroses and express itself in pathological defense mechanisms. One of these is phobic neurosis, characterized by an intense fear of an object or a situation which constitutes no real danger to the patient. A phobia is thus an irrational fear, a symptom that is a transformation of free-floating anxiety which could not be handled in a healthy way. A considerable portion of the person's energy may be devoted to avoiding the phobic object or situation. The fear is usually displaced onto the phobic object from some person or situation which the patient unconsciously fears. For example, a phobia of spiders is thought to stem from a fear of the mother. The patient is not, as a rule, aware of the psychological source or significance of his fear, and while he may acknowledge that his fear is irrational, he is quite unable to regulate his life except as dictated by the phobia.

Obsessive-compulsive neurosis. The obsessive-compulsive neurosis is characterized by the persistent intrusion of unwanted thoughts (obsessions) or actions (compulsions) that the patient is unable to stop. The thoughts may consist of single words or ideas, ruminations, or trains of thoughts that intrude into consciousness. The patient cannot stop them even though he often perceives them as nonsensical or even horrifying (as, for instance, a recurring thought about a loved one having cancer). A compulsion is an irresistible urge to perform an apparently unreasonable act repetitiously. It may be of a simple nature, such as touching a particular piece of furniture three times or going back again and again to check a locked door, or it may take the form of a complex ritual. Anxiety and distress are often present either if the patient is prevented from completing his compulsive ritual or if he is concerned about being unable to control it. The compulsion is the psyche's way of controlling and defending against the underlying anxiety.

Hysterical neurosis. In the hysterical neurosis, or conversion reaction, anxiety is ''converted'' into functional symptoms of the special senses or voluntary nervous system rather than being consciously experienced or displaced. This conversion of anxiety causes symptoms such as blindness, deafness, or paralysis. The conversion symptoms serve to prevent or lessen any conscious, felt anxiety, and usually symbolize the underlying mental conflict that is productive of anxiety. The hysterical symptoms may be regarded as expressing a conflict or an idea in symbolic form. A mental concept may be converted into a significant body symptom. For example, hysterical paralysis of an arm may express a wish to do a forbidden act—for instance, masturbation or striking a loved one—yet ambivalently prevent accomplishing the act. The conversion reaction does not merely serve as a defense against anxiety but usually provides some more or less obvious "secondary gain" (see p. 223).

In dealing with severe illness of any kind, the counselor must be alert to the possibility of secondary gain. This means that a person finds it socially and psychologically advantageous to remain in the regressed, disabled role, especially if his dependency needs are gratified and he is relieved of his normal work and family responsibilities. Anyone who has lain helpless in a hospital bed because of surgery or a physical illness has experienced difficulty in giving up the dependent role in which all his needs were met by the hospital staff, even though there may have been physical pain and emotional discomfort and conflict about being in the dependent role. When the time comes to resume normal responsibilities, it can be a wrenching experience, even for the most conscientious and adequate personality.

Consider, for example, the case of a patient with a hysterical paralysis of both legs. The origin of this symptom lay in an intrapsychic conflict of this man. From the point of view of rehabilitation, however, the secondary gain was crucial, for the patient was a mailman who felt trapped in a job he detested and in which he was becoming increasingly depressed. The paralysis prevented him from returning to work. It also resulted in his receiving a great deal of attention and care and being relieved of his family responsibilities.

Depressive neurosis. An excessive reaction of depression due to an internal psychic conflict or to an identifiable event such as the loss of a loved one or cherished possession is manifested in depressive neurosis. It is not as severe as psychotic depression, and is to be distinguished from manic-depressive psychoses.

Treatment

Generally, the neuroses are treated with psychotherapy, sometimes in conjunction with antianxiety tranquilizers (often referred to as minor tranquilizers) such as chlordiazepoxide (Librium) and diazepam (Valium).

Depressive neurosis is treated with psychotherapy, often in conjunction with the antidepressant drugs such as imipramine (Tofranil), amitriptyline (Elavil), desipramine (Norpramin or Pertofrane), protriptyline (Vivactil), and nortriptyline (Aventyl).

PERSONALITY DISORDERS

There is a wide range of personality disorders, including the *antisocial personality*, the *passive-dependent personality*, the *passive-aggressive personality*, the *paranoid personality*, and a number of others. These are nonpsychotic disorders which manifest themselves in disturbances of *behavior* rather than in *symptoms*. For example, as the names imply, the passive-dependent personality is manifested by passivity and dependency, and the passive-aggressive personality by aggressiveness expressed passively by such means as obstructionism, stubbornness, and intentional inefficiency.

The antisocial personality, formerly called the psychopathic or sociopathic personality, presents an especially difficult problem. The life style of such patients is characterized by antisocial behavior. They are callous, given to immediate pleasures, appear devoid of a sense of responsibility, and in spite of repeated humiliations and punishments, fail to learn to modify their behavior. They frequently possess a great deal of personal charm and persuasive ability. The essential defect in their character structure is a failure to develop an adequate conscience.

Persons with personality disorders may or may not be aware of their problems, may or may not have subjective anxiety, and may or may not be motivated for treatment and rehabilitation. They often rationalize their actions in order not to have to recognize the nature of their behavior, and thus may not seek help unless prodded to do so. They project their failures onto circumstances or other people. In some cases, these individuals can benefit by honest feedback from counselors and other helping professionals, but their maladjustment is usually lifelong and their rehabilitation difficult. When they do seek treatment and rehabilitation, however, the results can be gratifying indeed.

NATURE OF SEVERE DISABILITY

Having briefly described some of the major mental illnesses, let us look at the seriously disabled psychiatric patient in more depth. By seriously disabled we mean the psychotic, the borderline psychotic, and sometimes the severe neurotic and person with a severe personality disorder. Seriously disabled persons are often described as marginal, socially isolated, vocationally inadequate, and possessing exaggerated dependency needs. They lack self-confidence and the social skills necessary to communicate with others. They lack ego strength in terms of the ability to withstand pressure and to cope with the usual crises of life. Thus, they have a limited repertoire of problem-solving techniques and develop severe psychiatric symptoms when confronted with only a moderate amount of life stress. Most have a need for structure, and many require direction and control. In many cases, the seriously disabled person's illness may be a way of communicating his needs to other people and getting society to take care of him.

The problems of the seriously disabled person may be further compounded by the effects of prolonged hospitalization. The symptoms of what is referred to as *institutionalism* include lack of initiative, apathy, withdrawal, oversubmissiveness to authority, excessive dependence upon the institution, feelings of worthlessness and dehumanization, and the acceptance of limitations which are not really necessary. Many of the disabilities often attributed to institutionalism can actually be a product of the illness itself and the person's earlier life experiences, but the current environment in which the person lives also has a profound impact. The counselor should not lose sight of the fact that the same changes described as a result of prolonged hospitalization can occur when a person is institutionalized in a facility "in the community," such as a poor-quality board and care home, or is allowed to become overly dependent on a day treatment center.

Recognizing that a person has limited capabilities should not mean that nothing is expected of him. Central to the successful treatment of seriously disabled persons is the guiding principle that high, but realistic, expectations should be maintained so that they strive to reach their full social and vocational potential even though this potential may be limited. There is a tendency for patients to rise to the expectations of the environment in which they find themselves. This principle maximizes their participation in the mainstream of the community, enhances their self-esteem, and generally improves the quality of their lives.

A graphic example is provided by patients who are in transition from a day treatment center to a vocational workshop and who spend half a day in each facility. The contrast in behavior is remarkable. Since behaving like a patient is not acceptable in the workshop, given the expected role of worker, the person behaves like a worker. But at the day treatment center in the morning, the same person is fulfilling the role of patient and acts like a patient, exhibiting symptoms and bizarre behavior never seen in the workshop later the same day. In many settings, treated like "a poor thing" who needs constant care, watching, and attention, the person does not act independently and loses what confidence he had. To the layman, letting the patient know how far he can go (limit-setting) and requiring him to meet standards may seem cold and without feeling. But in fact, asking a person to live up to his potential may give him the strongest possible evidence that he has some ability.

Although it is important to expect a person to realize his potential, it is equally important not to expect more than he can realistically achieve because this may set him up for another failure. High expectations are frequently confused with unrealistic expectations. For instance, many therapeutic housing programs require a full daytime activity outside the facility. But what if it is a struggle for the person just to live outside the hospital? Even then, he may be able to tolerate only limited interaction which allows him to maintain social distance from other participants. All too often, what is lacking is an accurate assessment of the person's current capabilities and sufficient flexibility in the program to take account of his limitations. As a result, the person is often asked to do more than is realistically possible for him at that time. His failure to meet these expectations is a painful experience and a further blow to his already low self-esteem. To avoid a repetition, he may flee from the program. Still another possibility is that the pressure of these unrealistic expectations may cause the person to again become symptomatic.

The mentally ill person and the professionals entrusted with his care therefore need to avoid the problems attendant on unrealistically high expectations on the one hand, and a lack of expectations and stimulation on the other. The latter leads to the problems of institutionalism as described above and exaggerates any tendency already present toward social withdrawal, underactivity, and an apparent lack of motivation. Under these circumstances, unnecessary social withdrawal may result as the person loses incentive to be active and interact with other people. It must be remembered, however, that social withdrawal is not always to be discouraged; it can also be an adaptive mechanism used by seriously disabled persons to find relief and sanctuary from pressures and interpersonal relationships which they cannot handle.

The wise counselor assesses a client carefully to gauge how much and in which areas vocational planning can proceed. Timing is also important, and the counselor should confer with other members of the treatment team on these issues. Equally important is an analysis of the kinds of competence needed in work activity and the kinds of competence possessed by the client. Counselor and client can then formulate realistic goals with which the client can feel reasonably comfortable. For example, a draftsman does not necessarily need to develop social skills and get along well with his co-workers to do his job. Pressing this type of competence may make success impossible. Becoming part of the coffee or lunch group may be far too much for the client to handle, and a clear message that this is not expected can do much to give him confidence to try.

The concept of ego strength is crucial. For instance, evaluating a client's vocational and intellectual capacity, apart from his emotional strengths and weaknesses, provides an incomplete picture of what the client can do vocationally. This seems almost self-evident, and yet failure to take into account a client's emotional capacity is a leading cause of unsuccessful vocational plans. An example would be a schizophrenic graduate engineer with an excellent intellectual grasp of his field but an inability to handle the pressure and responsibility of actually working as an engineer. As used here, ego strength means the ability to adjust to a variety of environment situations, to control one's impulses, to seek satisfaction in healthy nondestructive ways, and the ability to make both large and small decisions reasonably well. A lack of ego strength must be a major consideration in vocational rehabilitation.

Involved in this concept of ego strength is the person's ability to withstand pressure and cope with the usual crises of life without cracking under the strain and fleeing from the situation through an overt mental illness, either psychotic or neurotic; through a psychosomatic condition, such as a peptic ulcer; by having a serious "accident" that removes him from the situation; or by getting drunk and forcing the employer to fire him. Additionally, ego strength involves the ability to be independent. Most of us take for granted our ability to be in competitive employment, to live independently in the community, and to take on the responsibilities of a family. For a person with limited ego strength, however, any one or all of these activities may produce overwhelming pressures.

The symptoms of severe mental illness, such as delusions, hallucinations, and disorganization of thought patterns, may seem unintelligible. Frequently, mental health professionals spend a considerable time trying to understand the unconscious and symbolic meanings of these symptoms. While such meanings can be found and, if analyzed carefully, are probably correct or close to being correct, there is another approach which has much more practical value for both the mentally ill person and those responsible for his rehabilitation and treatment. The symptoms can make sense when their appearance is considered a signal that the person is under more stress than he can handle and that some intervention is necessary. It can come as a great relief to a person to understand that his symptoms are his way of reacting to stress. He is no longer overwhelmed by mysterious, frightening, all-powerful forces beyond his control. The symptoms become a signal to him, too, that he is under too much pressure or does not have enough supports, or both, and that, in any case, he needs and should seek help.

REHABILITATION PROGRAM

It is the firm belief of the authors that even severely disabled psychiatric patients can be helped to alter and improve their lives through work. Rehabilitation counselors dealing with this population find that the same theories and techniques used with other clients are equally valid with the mentally ill. Once they have some familiarity with the major mental disorders and the behaviors to be expected, counselors often find it easier to work with the psychiatrically disabled than with other clients. There is a freedom to discuss the illness and its symptoms openly with clients, and the counselor can thus more quickly come to grips with realities. In most cases, psychiatric clients have been in treatment before referral to counselors and have become accustomed to discussing their illness individually and in groups. They are therefore less inclined to deny or rationalize their problems than the client who, for instance, is physically disabled but also has serious emotional problems.

Referral

Any psychiatric patient who expresses any interest in vocational rehabilitation and who has access to a facility should at least have the opportunity to be considered for these services. Assessment by a professional vocational rehabilitation counselor may bring different results than the referring therapist might have expected. Sometimes, the patient who appeared to the therapist to be a questionable referral seems highly appropriate in the judgment of the counselor, and vice versa. Counselor and therapist see the patient from different perspectives. Moreover, the patient may present himself very differently to the counselor. When the patient sees a therapist in a psychiatric setting, he usually will conform to the role expectations of his environment and behave like a patient, so his employment potential may not be evident. On the other hand, he may be expressing to the therapist a desire to work because he wants the therapist to perceive him as a person who wants to work, although he actually may be extremely fearful of work and not ready to consider it. In their discussion about work, these realities may become plain to both the counselor and the patient.

Although referral of the chronic patient should be made as early as possible, it should not be made at an unpropitious time. The patient can derive little benefit from vocational rehabilitation if his energies are totally involved with a divorce, a separation, the loss of a loved one, or a major change in his life style. The therapist, however, should be sensitive to the very beginnings of recovery from crisis and help the patient become involved in work activity before he settles into a life pattern of apathy and inactivity.

At the time of referral and shortly thereafter, mental health clients will respond to how clearly they perceive what will be expected of them. If they see the referral as a short step removed from the full responsibility of a job, a step they do not feel ready to take, their response may well be negative. However, if they have specific knowledge of what their activities will be, some assurance that they can proceed at a pace they can handle, and some knowledge of what structure will be available to guide them in their behavior, they will be far less fearful.

In the intake interview, as counselor and client are exploring what training programs might be considered, it would be well to provide details about daily activities of the programs contemplated. It is crucial for the client to feel that he will have the support of a clear delineation of tasks, so that he is not left with a feeling of having to map his own course in a vague undefined territory. The referral will much more likely "take" if handled in this way.

Evaluation and Planning

Many rehabilitation counselors have commented on the relative lack of physical disability in the mental health clients referred to them. Usually only an extremely small percentage will have any physical disabilities at all. Some psychiatrists believe this is because they meet their psychological needs in the manifestations of mental illness rather than in psychosomatic illness, "accidents," hypertension, or "whiplash" injuries.

Restrictions placed on mental health clients will generally relate to degree of job pressure, working alone or with others, or working with and being supervised by males or females, rather than to physical disabilities. With the mental health population, the two most important judgments the counselor will make are, first, determining the pace at which the client can proceed; and second, gauging his emotional strength, as well as his intellect and aptitude, to determine what level of occupation is appropriate.

Pace. With regard to pace, much will depend on the counselor and client assessing each other and working together to formulate plans. Work evaluations can be obtained in many rehabilitation and mental health facilities. For the seriously disabled person, an evaluation in a workshop is often a good beginning. At this point, the counselor's concern will be that the client is clear about what he hopes to accomplish in the workshop and what is being looked for in an evaluation. The counselor will have reviewed the client's employment history and made judgments about employment potential, as well as which behaviors need to be adjusted before successful and satisfying employment can be reached or skill training started. With these judgments in mind, the counselor can help the client identify problems to be dealt with in the workshop. The counselor needs to be cautious in this determination and plan for simple goals that are within the client's reach. For example, a first goal might be to determine how many hours of work a client can tolerate.

During the time the client is in the workshop, regular meetings with the counselor should be scheduled so that progress, or lack of it, can be assessed and new goals can be set, if necessary. It will be advantageous for the counselor to be very open with the client, because the client is then likely to respond with a similar openness and to deal with the real issues.

To illustrate, a workshop client on medication producing side effects of tremulousness consistently came to the workshop without taking the special medications prescribed to counteract the side effects. He would say he had forgotten and would have to go home to take it, thus losing several hours of work time. The counselor felt free to say, "Several times in the past 2 weeks you have missed hours of work because you had to return home for your medication. I think you are trying to tell us you do not want to be here." With the situation clearly articulated and in the open, the client could then talk about his real concerns: not really wanting to work, feeling resentment because he felt his wife and therapist were forcing him to come, and the fear that eventually he would have to face a job that was beyond his capabilities.

Emotional strength. Whether the counselor can or should rely on the therapist to determine the client's emotional strengths and weaknesses in the context of his work potential is questionable. Certainly, if the counselor probes, he can elicit information revealing the client's ability to withstand pressure, his anticipated reaction to authority, or other information which sheds light on specific work issues. In the authors' opinion, the actual determination must come from the collaborative effort of the client and the counselor. When a relationship of trust has been established, allowing for exploration of reality, and when the client's need for defensiveness is diminished, the client and the counselor are in the best position to examine or discover the client's emotional strengths and weaknesses as they relate to a job or an occupation.

This does not imply that the therapist should not be involved. It is essential that the counselor keep the therapist informed and that communication be continuous, so that each professional's work with the client does not conflict with the other's. Furthermore, the therapist can prevent unpropitious planning. He can advise the counselor to slow down or give the go-ahead, depending upon what may be occurring in therapy or in the individual's life which might affect the timing of an important vocational step.

VOCATIONAL PLANNING

Evaluation

The counselor's judgment in career choice, based on specific knowledge and training in the vocational field, is far more reliable than that of other professionals. In making decisions with the client, however, it is extremely important that the counselor take information supplied by the therapist into account. For example, to encourage cosmetology as an occupation for a young man prone to recurring homosexual panic is highly inadvisable, regardless of how great his natural aptitudes for that kind of work appear to be. As another example, exquisite skill and knowledge in the field of music will not make teaching music an appropriate choice for the individual who has difficulty with interpersonal relationships.

The counselor's in-depth knowledge of the competencies required for success in occupational fields, as well as his awareness of the ingredients that make up the various work environments, make it clear that it is the counselor who is best equipped to make certain decisions about appropriate vocational areas. The mystique of the psychotherapist should not blind the counselor to the fact that it is he, and not the therapist, who is the expert with regard to the world of work. The therapist's input can be very helpful, but in exploring vocational areas, the counselor's detailed knowledge of the entire range of daily activities involved in doing a job supplies the essential material needed to make a choice.

Furthermore, determining whether work with things is more indicated than work with people, determining the client's tolerance for noise, confusion, or distraction, and sorting out other work issues, are all part of the initial evaluation period. Before a career selection is made, the counselor has at his disposal various tools for further classification. Vocational tests are used in this process. Workshop evaluation is an excellent method for learning more about the client's reaction to different work requirements. The counselor's educated review and analysis of the client's employment history reveal a wealth of useful material. Many of these activities, carefully supported, can be started at very early stages in the client's recovery process.

There is not, as is widely believed, a clear relationship between work capacity and degree of emotional recovery. Some of the sickest and most mentally disturbed persons are able to work, some marginally, some with a high degree of competence. Also, it is often assumed that achievement of a level of social skills high enough to get along with other people on some basis of reciprocity is necessary to remain on the job, but this is not necessarily the case. Some expatients can act appropriately within a structured work situation when cues are available to guide them, but they may be immobilized and confused by the lack of structure in a social situation. Others may achieve a high level of social skills but be unable or unwilling to work. The counselor, with his knowledge of job requirements, can make these determinations with his clients.

In assessment, counselors should be aware that, regardless of how severely ill the client appears to be, there is always an intact portion of the psyche to which the rehabilitation effort can be directed. The focus should be on the healthy portion, the strengths. When the healthy part of the personality is expanded, the person's functioning improves. Evaluation must be focused on reality factors (behavior rather than intrapsychic phenomena) and on changing behavior rather than on changing basic character structure.

Vocational evaluation may be concerned with either raising or lowering work goals, depending on emotional strength. Probably the greatest value of the assessment is that the counselor helps his client to judge where he can function comfortably. For example, a 39-year-old graduate accountant with a master's degree in business administration had had two psychotic episodoes before he was referred for counseling. He was in the acute ward at the time of referral. After a time, he was able to see and accept the fact that he could not tolerate responsibility. He lowered his goals and has been successfully working as a clerk in a cement factory for 3 years with no recurrence of illness.

Vocational aptitude and performance tests are an effective means of helping the client select an occupation, eliminate inappropriate ideas, and start to plan for training. However, anxiety preceding, during, and after the tests should be anticipated, and tests should not be considered until the patient is ready to face his strengths and weaknesses. Also, client and counselor must both clearly understand that tests are only useful as part of an appraisal. In general, tests furnish clues which may reinforce choices or open up new areas of vocational exploration; they cannot be expected to give definitive answers.

Interpretation of tests is highly sensitive, and information gained is best used by relating it to the client so that he can draw his own conclusions. The client has made himself vulnerable in taking tests, and their results may trigger strong emotional reactions. Lifelong ambitions may seem to be shattered by the results. For example, a client who has always dreamed of being a doctor may be facing scores that make it obvious to him that he rates lower than 90 percent of the individuals succeeding as doctors. The alteration in his self-image may profoundly upset him for some time. Before further planning can be done, a number of sessions may be needed to help him accept the reality of his capabilities.

Where the overall evaluation indicates potential for sophisticated achievement, careful plans need to be made. Most often it is imperative to set interim goals to be achieved one at a time rather than one far-reaching final goal. Mental health clients may be overwhelmed by such expectations.

Evaluation may serve another purpose for psychiatric clients by clarifying the appropriateness of an individual's present occuption so that the cause of emotional difficulty can be searched for elsewhere. For example, an electronics engineer was in treatment for acute anxiety which he related to his job. He was referred for vocational counseling to select another occupation. All indications pointed to electronics engineering being particularly right for this man. He and his therapist were subsequently able to conclude that he was displacing his anxiety and guilt about his delinquent son and other problems onto his job.

During the entire course of the evaluation and training period, the client should be encouraged to continue in psychiatric treatment. The vocational counselor can bring the reality of the client's work performance and problems and his vocational assets and liabilities into the sometimes unreal world of the mental health clinic to assist in therapy. Vocational goals can be related to treatment goals. The client gains by both, and his chances for being reintegrated into the community are enhanced considerably.

Placement and Followup

It is particularly important for the counselor to remain involved for a period of time after job placement of mental health clients. Contact should be maintained and support given for at least several months until the client is stabilized on the job. The initial period on the job is a highly critical time. For the client, failure at this time can be totally devastating because he may only now have allowed himself to believe that success in a job and "normal" living might be possible for him.

Work is an extremely therapeutic activity for the mentally disabled. Not only does work help them remain in the community and out of hospitals, but it makes their lives more meaningful. Employment contributes to their mental health by increasing their feelings of self-esteem, mastery, and control over their lives, and it often leads to their achieving independence. It is viewed by many persons as the only means of extricating themselves from the mental health system and shedding their identity as mental patients. Failure, therefore, has tremendous meaning, and the counselor must remain available to discuss and resolve problems that inevitably arise during the initial period of adjustment.

BIBLIOGRAPHY

Arieti S (ed): *The American Handbook of Psychiatry*. Ed 2, New York, Basic Books, Vols. 1-6, 1974-1975.
Essentially an encyclopedia of psychiatry which is useful for reference when an in-depth coverage of a subject is desired.

Coyle JT: Psychiatric drugs in medical practice. Med Clin North Am 61:891-905, 1977.
This article describes the indications for use, mechanism of action, and side effects for antidepressants, lithium, and the major tranquilizers. These are discussed as major groups rather than individually.

Doll W: Family coping with the mentally ill: An anticipated problem of deinstitutionalization. Hosp Community Psychiatry 27: 183-185, 1976.
This is a study of the families of 125 patients discharged from three state mental institutions to live at home. The emotional and social costs to the family, the lack of community services for support and relief of the families, and failure to monitor the patient-family situation are discussed.

Hersen M, Bellack AS: A multiple-baseline analysis of social-skills training in chronic schizophrenics. J Appl Behav Anal 9:239-245, 1976.
This article gives an example of a behavior modification program for teaching social skills to chronic schizophrenic patients. Techniques used include instruction, feedback, and modeling.

Lamb HR, Associates: *Community Survival for Long Term Patients*. San Francisco, Jossey-Bass Inc., 1976.
This book focuses on the treatment and rehabilitation of the long-term severely disabled psychiatric patient. It deals with the new problem confronting mental health and rehabilitation professionals as the result of the marked decrease in the use of State hospitals and the need to serve these patients in the community.

Lamb HR, Associates: *Rehabilitation in Community Mental Health*. San Francisco, Jossey-Bass Inc., 1971.
This book was written primarily for vocational rehabilitation professionals and focuses on the community rehabilitation of psychiatric patients. It includes chapters on rehabilitation counseling, the sheltered workshop, sheltered work placements, therapeutic housing, social rehabilitation, and evaluation.

Niewoehner GJ: Effects of group counseling on vocational decisions of workshop clients: An incidental finding. Rehabil Lit 34:235-236, 1973.
Psychiatric clients in a transitional rehabilitation workshop, referred for work evaluation and work adjustment training, were placed in either group or individual therapy sessions. Group counseling focused on whether the client behavior matched the demands of appropriate work situations, while individual therapy focused on vocational planning and assessment.

Redlich FC, Freedman DX: *The Theory and Practice of Psychiatry*. New York, Basic Books, 1966.
An excellent textbook of psychiatry which covers both the descriptive and psychodynamic aspects of mental illness.

Spiegler MD: classroom approach teaches patients independence skills. Hosp Community Psychiatry 24:216-221, 1973.
A brief description of a classroom approach to teaching psychiatric clients social skills, self-care, recreational, and vocation skills.

20 MENTAL RETARDATION

Andrew S. Halpern, Ph.D.

DESCRIPTION

Definition

Mental retardation is not a disease, nor is it a set of precisely defined symptoms. It refers to a *broadly* defined set of behaviors that are sufficiently ambiguous to prevent us from being totally confident about when it is appropriate to apply this label to a given individual. This ambiguity is particularly evident in the milder levels of mental retardation where an individual's behavior is judged to be "almost normal."

Many descriptions and definitions of mental retardation have emerged over the years. Common to most of these definitions has been a recognition that persons who are labeled mentally deficient or delayed or retarded are *socially* less competent than their peers. Mentally retarded persons often have a limited repertoire of available skills and minimal insight into the causes and consequences of their behavior. Even though the social behavior of mentally retarded persons is usually not deviant in a psychiatric sense, there has been an unfortunate historical tendency to further complicate the lives of retarded persons by mislabeling them "insane."

During the twentieth century, especially in the United States, the term "intelligence" changed in status from a metaphysical trait to a scientific construct, due largely to the invention of the "intelligence quotient." As intelligence testing became more and more prevalent, the IQ emerged as a major defining characteristic of mental retardation. Anyone with a measured IQ below 70 or 75 on a standardized test of intelligence was a very likely candidate for eventually being labeled mentally retarded.

These two criteria—deficits in adaptive behavior and intellectual subnormality—are the major components of the most widely accepted definition of mental retardation, which was offered by the American Association on Mental Deficiency (AAMD) in 1977:

> Mental retardation refers to significantly subaverage general intellectual functioning existing concurrently with deficits in adaptive behavior, and manifested during the developmental period.

In addition to these two basic criteria, the AAMD definition specifies that the condition must emerge during the "developmental period" if it is to be properly labeled mental retardation. Generally, but not always, this is interpreted to mean that onset occurs prior to age 18.

Having identified the components of this definition, it is equally important to recognize that both etiology and prognosis have been deliberately omitted from the definition. Both of these omissions have major implications for an understanding of mental retardation.

There are many known medical causes of mental retardation, including a variety of infections and intoxications, traumatic events, metabolic disorders, and chromosomal abnormalities. For example, rubella, lead poisoning, and phenylketonuria are known to cause mental retardation. Unfortunately, known causes account for less than 25 percent of those persons who are diagnosed as mentally retarded. In the remaining majority of cases, the precise etiology is unknown.

Many of the medical conditions that are associated with mental retardation also produce sensory, motor, metabolic, anatomical, and/or emotional abnormalities which further complicate the life of the affected person, usually requiring special management and care. A complete catalog of these conditions can be found in the 1977 revised edition of the AAMD *Manual on Terminology and Classification in Mental Retardation.*

Mental retardation of known medical etiology, such as lack of oxygen (perinatal anoxia) during childbirth, can sometimes be prevented. Many of the known medical causes of mental retardation, however, are not preventable at this time, such as trisomy of chromosome 21 (i.e., three, rather than the normal two, chromosomes) which results in Down's syndrome. Because of our generally limited knowledge concerning the causes and prevention of mental retardation, etiology is not mentioned in the AAMD definition.

Prognosis is another major dimension that was deliberately omitted from the AAMD definition. For many years prior to the middle of this century, people

265

had argued that mental retardation was "incurable." This belief was so strong that if a person was diagnosed as mentally retarded at one age and then later rediagnosed as not retarded, the original diagnosis was changed to read "pseudoretarded."

Most people now believe that incurability is a pseudoissue for at least two reasons. In the first place, since we know so little about the precise causes of mental retardation, it seems presumptuous to assume that nothing will ever be found that might alter the impact of these causes. In a completely different vein, we now know that retarded behavior can be modified and that behavioral expectations in society are culturally relative. This means that a person's behavior may change to the point where it is no longer considered to be retarded, or that the very same behavior may be viewed as retarded in one social milieu but not in another. For these reasons, prognosis was intentionally omitted from the AAMD definition.

Classification

Mental retardation occurs in varying degrees, ranging from mild impairment to a profound deficit in functional behavior. The current classification system of the AAMD specifies four levels of retardation: mild, moderate, severe, and profound. Each of these levels is described in terms of the two major components of the definition of mental retardation: intelligence and adaptive behavior.

Intelligence. Along the dimension of intelligence, the four levels of mental retardation are identified with reference to IQ scores. Although there are many tests on the market that can produce an IQ score, only *individually* administered *standardized* tests of known *reliability* and *validity* should ever be used for the purposes of classification. Standardization of a psychological test refers to *uniformity of procedures* in administration and scoring. This relates to the need for controlled conditions in all scientific observations. Test reliability refers to the *consistency and stability of scores* obtained by the same persons when retested with the same test or an equivalent form. Test validity refers to the degree to which a test actually *measures what it purports to measure*.

The two most widely used and accepted instruments are the Stanford-Binet and Wechsler Scales. Table 20-1 shows the level of retardation with reference to these scales. This table, which reflects the AAMD 1977 position, lists a Wechsler IQ of 55–69 as falling within the level of mild impairment. The AAMD definition of 1961 recognized an additional category of borderline impairment, which included a Wechsler IQ of 70–84.

The State/Federal program of vocational rehabilitation still uses the 1961 AAMD definition. For purposes of establishing eligibility in this program, a diagnosis of mental retardation is acceptable when the

TABLE 20-1
RELATIONSHIP BETWEEN IQ AND LEVEL OF IMPAIRMENT

LEVEL	OBTAINED INTELLIGENCE QUOTIENT	
	Stanford-Binet	Wechsler
Mild	68–52	69–55
Moderate	51–36	54–40
Severe	35–20	39–25 (extrapolated)
Profound	19 and below	24 and below (extrapolated)

individual's IQ does not exceed 84 (Wechsler scales), provided the coexistence of maladaptive behavior associated with subnormal intellectual functioning is established. With the mandate in the Rehabilitation Act of 1973 to afford service priority to handicapped persons with severe physical and mental disabilities, State vocational rehabilitation agencies have been expanding their efforts on behalf of the more severely mentally retarded. A significant number of those served are in the mild classification, however, in the belief that intervention by vocational rehabilitation is necessary if they are to achieve a satisfactory and lasting vocational adjustment in the community.

Adaptive behavior. The dimension of adaptive behavior does not yet lend itself to a satisfactory measurement criterion for classification. The Vineland Social Maturity Scale and, more recently, the AAMD Adaptive Behavior Scale have both been widely used to provide comparative scores of adaptive behavior. However, neither of these instruments, nor any other currently available, are sufficiently reliable and valid to generate precise psychometric scores that might be used to delineate the four levels of mental retardation. In lieu of such criteria, the AAMD has specified eight behavioral dimensions which comprise a developmental description of adaptive behavior:

1. Sensory-motor skills
2. Communication skills
3. Self-help skills
4. Socialization (ability to interact with others)
5. Application of basic academic skills in daily life activities
6. Application of appropriate reasoning and judgment in mastery of the environment
7. Social skills (participation in group activities and interpersonal relationships)
8. Vocational and social responsibilities and performance

For purposes of classification, *behavioral descriptions* are then provided for identifying different levels of retardation at different ages.

The AAMD *Manual on Terminology and Classification in Mental Retardation* includes behavioral descriptions along several dimensions to provide indicators of the four levels of retardation, depending upon the age at which the behaviors are exhibited. Table 20-2 is derived from these descriptions, and indicates the highest level of adaptive behavior exhibited by persons 15 years of age and older for the four levels of mental retardation—mild, moderate, severe, and profound.

Because the classification criteria for intelligence are quantitative and the criteria for adaptive behavior are qualitative, there has been an unfortunate historical tendency to focus only upon intelligence during the diagnostic process of deciding whether or not to label a person mentally retarded. Since a deficit in one area does *not* automatically predict or cause a deficit in the other, focusing only upon intelligence will greatly enhance the likelihood of making a diagnostic error. In all cases of psychological testing for diagnosis, the cautions listed on page 270 should be observed.

In recent years, the validity of IQ scores has also been subjected to severe criticism. This criticism arose out of the observation that, based on IQ testing, a disproportionately large number of black Americans and Chicanos have been labeled mentally retarded. Both the content and the statistical interpretation of most intelligent tests, however, do not take into account the differences in behavioral expectations that exist in the various subcultures within the United States. In order to compensate for this problem, Dr. Jane Mercer has recently published the System of Multicultural Pluralistic Assessment. This system utilizes both previously existing and newly developed instruments for measuring intelligence and adaptive behavior, with *separate* interpretative norms for Anglo, black, and Chicano subcultures. Whenever a person from a racial or cultural minority group is labeled mentally retarded, the principles and practices presented in Dr. Mercer's system should be examined and understood.

Another group of persons who may be subject to inaccurate or inappropriate testing are those who have recently left an institution for the mentally retarded. The experiences available in an institution are very restricted. Consequently, the actual intellectual abilities of institutionalized persons may be underestimated on IQ tests because they have not had the wide variety of learning experiences available to those living in the community.

The whole issue of "labeling" or classifying has been a topic of great interest during recent years. Opponents of labeling suggest that calling a person "retarded" is basically a harmful practice, since the bearer of such a label is often stigmatized and ostracized as a consequence of being so labeled. Those in favor of labeling counter with the observation that the availability of services for handicapped persons in our society is usually dependent upon documenting their handicap as a criterion for eligibility. Without some alternative method for determining eligibility, it

would appear that labeling will remain a "necessary evil" of the rehabilitation process. One way that counselors can soften this blow to a retarded client's self-esteem is by providing an opportunity for the client to ventilate and explore his feelings about the consequences of being labeled retarded.

Prevalence

The most commonly offered prevalence figure for mental retardation in the United States is 3 percent of the general population. Deviations from this figure are predictable along the three dimensions of retardation: level, socioeconomic class, and age.

Level of retardation. The distribution of mentally retarded persons across levels of retardation is far from equal. Approximately 85 percent of this population are mildly retarded (IQ 55 to 70), 12 percent are moderately retarded (IQ 40 to 55), and the remaining 3 percent are either severely or profoundly retarded (IQ below 40). Most of the known medical causes of mental retardation are associated with the low prevalence categories of moderate, severe, and profound retardation.

Socioeconomic class. More than twice as many mentally retarded persons are found in the lower socioeconomic class as in the middle and upper classes combined. Most of this inequity is found within the category of mild retardation. Thus, it would seem that while the medical causes of retardation strike without regard for family income or social position, the many conditions associated with poverty and poor education seem to result in a high risk of *mild* mental retardation. This interpretation must be carefully modified with a reminder about the large number of persons within racial and subcultural minority groups who have been misdiagnosed as mildly retarded.

Age. If one were to divide the general population into three age groups—below age 5, 5 to 18, and above age 18—the prevalence of mental retardation will usually be estimated at around 1 percent for each of the younger and older groups, and between 5 and 6 percent for the middle group. Fewer younger persons are diagnosed as mentally retarded because only the more severe levels of mental retardation tend to emerge during early childhood. A large number of persons are identified during school years, because low academic achievement is by far the major "symptom" which causes a person to be evaluated for suspected mild retardation. Once mildly retarded persons leave school, many of them disappear into the adult population where their social environment may not require academic skills for survival and/or contacts with social service agencies become less frequent, allowing them to hide from the stigma of being labeled, served, and consequently counted as being mentally retarded.

Periodically, these mildly retarded persons do

TABLE 20-2

HIGHEST LEVEL OF ADAPTIVE BEHAVIOR BY MENTALLY RETARDED PERSONS 15 YEARS OF AGE AND OLDER

	Mild	Moderate	Severe	Profound
Independent functioning	Exercises care for personal grooming, feeding, bathing, toilet; may need health or personal care reminders; may need help in selection or purchase of clothing.	Feeds, bathes, dresses, and grooms self; may select daily clothing; may prepare easy foods for self or others; may wash and/or iron and store own clothes.	Independent feeding except for cutting meat; can dress self; may tie shoes; bathes self with supervision; is toilet trained; washes face and hands without help.	Feeds self with spoon or fork, may spill some; puts on clothing but needs help with small buttons and jacket zippers; tries to bathe self but needs help; can wash and dry hands but not very efficiently; partially toilet trained but may have accidents.
Physical	Goes about local neighborhood in city or campus at institution with ease, but cannot go to other towns alone without aid; can use bicycle, skis, ice skates, trampoline, or other equipment requiring good coordination.	Good body control; good gross and fine motor coordination.	Can run, skip, hop, dance; uses skates or sled or jump rope; can go up and down stairs alternating feet; can throw ball to hit target.	May hop or skip; may climb steps with alternating feet; rides bicycle; may climb trees or jungle gym; plays dance games; may throw ball and hit target.
Communication	Communicates complex verbal concepts and understands them; carries on everyday conversation, but cannot discuss abstract or philosophical concepts; uses telephone; writes simple letters or orders but does not write about abstractions or important or current events.	May carry on simple conversations; uses complex sentences; recognizes words, may read sentences, ads, signs, and simple prose material with some comprehension.	May communicate in complex sentences; speech is generally clear and distinct; understands complex verbal communication including words such as "because" and "but." Recognizes signs, words, but does not read prose material with comprehension.	May have speaking vocabulary of over 300 words and use grammatically correct sentences. If nonverbal, may use many gestures to communicate needs. Understands simple verbal communications, including directions and questions. Some speech may be indistinct sometimes. May recognize advertising words and signs. Relates experiences in simple language.

SOURCE: Derived from Grossman, et al., *Manual on Terminology and Classification in Mental Retardation* (1973 revision).

TABLE 20-2 — *Continued*

	Mild	Moderate	Severe	Profound
Social	Interacts cooperatively or competitively with others and initiates some group activities, primarily for social or recreational purposes; may belong to a local recreation group or church group, but not to civic organizations or groups of skilled persons; enjoys recreation, but either does not enjoy or is not competent at activities requiring rapid, involved, or complex planning and implementation.	May interact cooperatively and/or competitively with others.	May participate in group activities spontaneously; may engage in simple competitive exercise games. May have friendship choices that are maintained over weeks or months.	Participates in group activities and simple group games; interacts with others in simple play and expressive activities.
Economic activity	Can be sent or goes to several shops to purchase several items; can make change correctly; does not use banking facilities; may earn living but has difficulty handling money without guidance.	May be sent on shopping errand for several items without notes; makes minor purchases; adds coins to dollar with fair accuracy.	May be sent on simple errands and make simple purchases with a note; realizes money has value but does not know how to use it (except for coin machines).	Not applicable
Occupation	Can cook simple foods, prepare simple meals; can perform everyday household tasks; as adult can engage in semiskilled or simple skilled job.	May do simple routine household chores.	May prepare simple foods; can help with simple household tasks; can set and clear table.	Not applicable
Self-direction	Initiates most of own activity; will pay attention to task for at least 15–20 minutes; conscientious about work and assumes much responsibility but needs guidance for tasks with responsibility for major tasks.	May initiate most of own activities; attend to task 15–20 minutes (or more); may be conscientious in assuming much responsibility.	May ask if there is "work" for him to do; may pay attention to task for 10 minutes or more; makes efforts to be dependable and carry out responsibility.	Not applicable

become exposed to the vocational rehabilitation process. Even though they have generally been able to blend into the general adult population, the counselor may find that they do have socialization problems which result in difficulties in obtaining and maintaining jobs. Thus, one of the major thrusts of vocational rehabilitation services for these clients might appropriately be personal adjustment training.

STANDARDS OF EVALUATION

Evaluation has played two vastly different roles in the lives of mentally retarded persons: diagnosis and classification for the purpose of *justifying* special treatment; and identification of specific abilities, needs, and/or interests for the purpose of *specifying* precise educational interventions. Unfortunately, our efforts and accomplishments in the first area have greatly exceeded those in the second area.

The results of psychological testing may be profoundly affected by the testing and analysis skills of the examiner. The counselor should therefore ensure that his mentally retarded clients are tested by an examiner skilled and experienced in working with the mentally retarded. In addition, the counselor should be aware that many psychological tests have been used inappropriately with mentally retarded persons. When this occurs, there are five major problems that interfere with a valid interpretation of test findings:

1. Test instructions and/or items may require reading skills beyond the ability of a retarded examinee.
2. Test instructions and/or items may use language and concepts beyond the comprehension of a retarded examinee.
3. Test norms may be developed without adequate representation of retarded persons in the reference groups.
4. Test reliability with retarded examinees is unknown.
5. Test validity with retarded examinees is unknown.

Of these potential problems, the issue of degree of validity is clearly the most critical. Table 20-3 presents a list of standarized tests that are widely used and/or known to have high validity with mentally retarded adolescents and adults.

The uses of intelligence tests and measures of adaptive behavior for the purposes of diagnosis and classification have already been discussed. In addition to the limitations of IQ testing presented above, it is important to realize that IQ provides little assistance in identifying the *specific* deficits that are in need of remediation. Other types of measures are required for this purpose. Adaptive behavior scores are somewhat more amenable than IQ scores for the purpose of prescriptive recommendations.

Independent Living Skills

There is a tremendous need for appropriate assessment tools that will help classroom teachers structure their teaching objectives and methods with mentally retarded students. This need is especially great at the secondary level where the academic focus shifts from basic tool skills (reading and computation) to social and prevocational development. Two appropriate standardized tests and a behavioral checklist that have been developed in this area are presented in table 20-3. Many more such tests should emerge in the future, especially as the techniques for creating good "criterion-referenced" tests become more and more sophisticated.

Vocational Interests

Two appropriate tests for measuring vocational interests of mildly retarded persons are identified in table 20-3. Their general format involves the presentation of pictures, rather than verbal descriptions, as test items. Although the tests were developed exclusively with samples of retarded persons, which certainly enhances their validity, there are three shortcomings that should be kept in mind:

1. The range of vocations presented in the test items is restricted to those jobs that are most typically held by retarded persons.
2. Separate tests were developed for males and females in a way that contributes to irrelevant sex-role stereotypes.
3. Vocational interests lack stability when the general range of a person's experience has been restricted. Since mentally retarded persons, almost by definition, are restricted in their range of experiences, their vocational interests during adolescence and early adulthood are particularly susceptible to change.

Vocational Skills

Evaluation of a client's vocational skills and/or aptitudes is frequently an important part of the total rehabilitation program individually designed for a client. Recent opinion strongly suggests that "work sample" evaluation is more likely to produce valid results than paper-and-pencil testing. Although available research results do not yet substantiate this claim, the work-sample approach to vocational evaluation still seems to be the most reasonable approach to follow while we await the outcomes of future validation studies.

In 1975, the Vocational Evaluation and Work Adjustment Association (VEWAA) defined a work sample as "a well defined work activity involving tasks, materials, and tools which are identical or similar to those in an actual job or cluster of jobs." The associ-

TABLE 20-3
STANDARDIZED TESTS FOR USE WITH MENTALLY RETARDED ADOLESCENTS AND ADULTS

Domain Measured	Test	Age Range	Level of Retardation
Intelligence	Stanford-Binet	2–adult	All levels
	Wechsler Adult Intelligence Scale	16–adult	All levels
	Wechsler Intelligence Scale for Children (revised)	5–16	All levels
Adaptive behavior	Vineland Social Maturity Scale	All ages	All levels
	AAMD Adaptive Behavior Scale	All ages	All levels
Independent living skills	Social & Prevocational Information Battery	13–adult	Mild
	Social & Prevocational Information Battery– Form T	13–adult	Moderate
	Camelot Behavioral Checklist	2–adult	All levels
Vocational interests	Vocational Interest & Sophistication Assessment	13–adult	Mild
	AAMD-Becker Reading Free Vocational Interest Inventory	13–adult	Mild
Vocational skills	MICRO-TOWER	13–adult	Mild
	Vocational Information & Evaluation Work Samples	13–adult	Mild
	Singer Vocational Evaluation System	13–adult	Mild

ation further suggests that work-sample evaluation should always be preceded by some degree of client training. In their words,

If a client does not perform adequately following standardized industrial instructions, it is necessary to determine what type(s) of instruction will facilitate his understanding of the task.... The evaluation of the client's ability to learn, their retention, and most efficient means of acquiring information are integral parts of the total assessment process.

There are many work-sample evaluation systems that have been developed during recent years. Only some of these systems conform to the recommendations of the VEWAA, particularly the recommendation to include training as part of the evaluation process. Three work-sample systems with potential validity for use with mildly retarded clients are listed in table 20-3.

Vocational evaluation systems for use with moderately, severely, or profoundly retarded clients are still in their infancy. Some truly outstanding work is beginning to emerge, however, which will be discussed below.

Limitations of Test Data

Psychometric and medical data are very important parts of the counselor's total evaluation of a mentally retarded client. Equally important, however, is the information regarding such factors as the client's living arrangements, support of family and friends, and his performance as observed by the counselor. All of this data and information must be taken together when the counselor develops an individualized rehabilitation program for each mentally retarded client.

Evaluation Resources Available

Rehabilitation "facilities," including sheltered workshops, are the most common resource available to rehabilitation counselors for the purpose of obtaining diagnostic evaluations of mentally retarded clients. In some locations, these facilities are directly managed by the State rehabilitation agency, although it is more common for these services to be purchased by the state agency. Additional common resources include public schools, diagnostic clinics supported by the State department of mental retardation, public health facilities, university psychology and special education clinics, and private licensed psychologists. The particular constellation of available resources and evaluation expertise varies greatly from community to community.

REHABILITATION POTENTIAL

For at least 50 years, research evidence has been available suggesting that most mildly retarded adults are capable of achieving independent or semi-independent community adjustment, including successful competitive employment. Records kept by the Rehabilitation Services Administration confirm these findings, as illustrated in table 20-4. Most of the retarded clients described in table 20-4 were mildly retarded. With the emphasis in rehabilitation now shifting toward the provision of services for more severely disabled persons, one might wonder about the rehabilitation potential of moderately, severely, and profoundly retarded adults.

Evidence from other sources strongly suggests that moderately, severely, and even profoundly retarded adults are indeed feasible candidates for productive employment. In 1955, one study reported that six moderately retarded adults were taught a number of work tasks, including manufacture of a television plug by soldering color-coded wires to correct terminals, and assembly of a bicycle pump which required nine manual operations with small parts. More recently, moderately retarded workers have been taught to assemble electrical relay panels (1967), television rectifier units (1967), and 14- or 24-piece bicycle brakes (1972), to use a drill press in the manufacture of pencil holders (1969), and to insert circuit components (1973). In a demonstration workshop currently operating at the University of Oregon, moderately, severely, and profoundly retarded persons have been taught to complete a 52-piece cam switch assembly which requires the use of 5 different hand tools, a 24-piece and a 26-piece printhead assembly for a labeling gun such as the kind used in many grocery stores, a 4-piece electrical cord assembly involving the use of 3 different hand tools, and a 6-piece battery pack assembly which requires soldering.

Results such as these strongly suggest that the vocational rehabilitation potential for moderately, severely, and profoundly retarded persons is *not* a question of *feasibility*, but rather a question of *practicality*. Given the correct approach to training, a sufficient amount of time, and suitable training resources, we *know* that these persons can be taught a surprisingly wide repertoire of useful vocational behaviors.

THERAPEUTIC APPROACHES

Followup studies of mentally retarded adults placed on jobs have been surprisingly consistent in identifying personal and social problems, rather than problems related to job tasks, as the primary reasons for losing a job. Some examples of these problem behaviors include not getting along with fellow employees and/or supervisors, inappropriate hygiene and grooming, personal or family problems that affect work behavior, inadequate transportation, inadequate housing arrangements, and inappropriate use of leisure time. The lesson to be learned from these studies is that mentally retarded persons, like most persons, are not likely to achieve satisfactory vocational adjustment unless their personal, social, and community adjustments are also satisfactory.

This means that the individualized rehabilitation program for many mentally retarded clients must include a variety of personal living and social skill objectives, as well as ultimate vocational objectives. Achievement of these nonvocational objectives may well be the major factor in determining the success of vocational experiences in sheltered or unsheltered work environments. In particular, vocational success may depend on establishing satisfactory independent or semi-independent living arrangements and providing training in self-help and personal care skills, monetary skills, and personal adjustment (including sexual adjustment, see chap. 21). Postemployment services are also necessary for many retarded clients.

Table 20-2 indicates the highest level of several areas

TABLE 20-4
OCCUPATIONS HELD BY REHABILITATED MENTALLY RETARDED
AND NONRETARDED CLIENTS IN 1969

Occupations	PERCENT DISTRIBUTION	
	Retarded (N=26,840)	Nonretarded (N=210,972)
Professional, technical, & managerial	1.0	10.1
Clerical	5.7	12.7
Sales	1.6	4.3
Service		
Domestic	4.2	4.6
Food & beverage preparation	5.1	12.8
All other service occupations	19.7	11.6
Agriculture	3.8	3.8
Industrial		
Skilled	5.0	9.1
Semiskilled	3.2	3.6
Unskilled	28.2	16.9
Homemakers	5.0	15.3
Unpaid family workers	3.5	2.1
Sheltered workshop workers	6.1	0.9

From *Statistical Notes: A profile of mentally retarded clients rehabilitated during Fiscal Year 1969.*
U.S. DHEW, SRS,RSA, No. 29, September, 1971.

of adaptive behavior usually found at the four levels of mental retardation. In observing a client, a counselor may find that the client performs at one level in most behavioral areas but at a lower level in others. The counselor might then consider a training program directed toward achievement of the higher level in those areas in which the client's performance is less than expected. The table may help identify those areas of behavior that can be improved by training and counseling.

Furthermore, careful evaluation of the client's background and previous training may suggest to the counselor that the client has not had optimal learning opportunities in most areas of adaptive behavior. Under these circumstances, training may well raise the client's overall level of functioning to a higher level.

Training programs which focus upon personal and social skills development for retarded adults are often very difficult to find. Most such services currently available are restricted to younger children. Sometimes "sheltered workshops" and "activity centers" offer appropriate programs under the label of "personal adjustment training." Community colleges in some states have recently begun to develop adult education courses for retarded persons. Parent training is also sometimes available through programs sponsored by public agencies dealing with developmental disabilities. An inventory of locally available programs and services can often be secured from either the State Association for Retarded Citizens and/or the State Developmental Disabilities Council.

Since 1970, there has been a strong political movement in the United States to remove as many mentally retarded persons as possible from large state institutions for relocation in appropriate community residences. The rationale for this movement comes from the philosophy of "normalization," which states that every handicapped person should live and receive services in the "least restrictive" environment possible. The counselor should keep abreast of this movement in his own community so that he is always aware of the development of new programs and/or facilities that may be appropriate for his mentally retarded clients.

The range of least restrictive living environments includes nursing homes, group homes or halfway houses, foster care, parental care, semi-independent apartment living, and totally independent living. These various living arrangements will provide different levels of custodial care, training opportunities, and emotional support to residents, depending not only upon the needs of residents but also upon the training and attitudes of support personnel. The policy goal of fostering the greatest possible degree of client independence is not always matched by the opportunities actually provided to a client in a given living arrangement. Rehabilitation counselors should examine this "least restrictive" dimension closely for each retarded client, both in terms of the *existence* and the *quality* of local options for living arrangements.

Retarded clients who have been recently released from institutions are likely to experience several problems of community adjustment that derive from their previous institutional isolation. Highly prevalent and persistent problem areas that have emerged from recent deinstitutionalization studies include money management and utilization of community resources. Ability to function independently or semi-independently is the central concern, which may well be addressed most effectively through the new independent living provisions of the 1978 Rehabilitation Act.

VOCATIONAL IMPLICATIONS

Since we now know that a vocational objective is feasible for a retarded person with any level of impairment, the rehabilitation counselor should consider five basic dimensions when developing an individualized rehabilitation program for a client:

1. Physical limitations or medical problems resulting from conditions that frequently accompany mental retardation; e.g., seizures, speech impairments, and motor impairments
2. Client skills and deficits in a variety of vocational and environmental areas and in adaptive behavior
3. Training opportunities available to the client
4. Environmental supports available to the client, including social skills training, living arrangements, transportation access, and leisure opportunities
5. Vocational opportunities available

Parts of many programs may be fundable from nonrehabilitation sources, including general education, special education, vocational education, Medicaid, Supplemental Security Income, and other State and Federal programs.

The development of an individualized written rehabilitation plan (IWRP) should almost always include the retarded client, even when parents or guardians are also involved. There is an unfortunate, although understandable, tendency to underestimate the ability of retarded clients to comprehend the nature and purposes of services that are offered. When this happens, retarded clients are treated inappropriately and unnecessarily as children.

Physical Limitations or Medical Problems

Most *mildly* retarded persons do not suffer from any unusual physical limitations or medical problems.

More severely retarded persons, on the other hand, may well experience such limitations or problems, almost always resulting from some kind of insult to the central nervous system. Cerebral palsy and epilepsy are frequent companions of mental retardation, causing seizures, speech impairment, and/or motor impairments. Anatomical abnormalities such as hydrocephalus may require surgical intervention, and metabolic disorders such as galactosemia may require special dietary control. The range of possible medical conditions is quite large, and if any of these conditions is present in a retarded client, it must naturally be addressed in ways that are discussed in other chapters of this textbook.

Chronic medical conditions such as those listed above, or others which may be associated with mental retardation, often require a client to exercise significant preventive health behaviors to maintain a maximum level of health. The mentally retarded client will not be as adept at protecting himself against complications caused by poor maintenance as a nonretarded person would be. The counselor should become aware of whatever health maintenance measures are required by any associated medical condition. For example, medications may be required, or specific clinic visits may have to be made. The counselor should include training and practice in carrying out these health maintenance measures in the individual rehabilitation program for the client with associated medical problems.

Evaluation of Client Skills and Deficits

The important issues with respect to client evaluation have already been presented earlier in this chapter. To summarize, client evaluations should include the following characteristics:

1. Only psychological tests with known validity for the mentally retarded should be used.
2. Evaluations should cover social and prevocational skills, as well as vocational skills.
3. When skill acquisition is being predicted, the testing format should permit the retarded examinee to *practice* the target skill during the course of evaluation.
4. Since the vocational interests of many retarded persons may not be stable, the results of interest tests should be used very cautiously in making placement decisions.
5. Vocational evaluation of retarded clients should incorporate work samples.

Training Opportunities

The availability of appropriate training opportunities is probably the most critical dimension to be considered when developing an individualized rehabilitation program for a mentally retarded client. Whether the necessary training is provided in high school, in a community college, in a rehabilitation facility, or in the home, the basic principles of effective training are deceptively simple and similar.

Mentally retarded persons learn most effectively when the instructional process is highly structured and direct. One of the best ways to accomplish this is within a "task analytic" framework, whereby the skills to be learned are broken down conceptually, before actual instruction, into a set of interrelated and sequentially presented component parts. Each step of the instructional process is then carefully monitored, and if the client fails to achieve "criterion" behavior at any step along the way, the process is immediately altered. With this kind of approach, failure is viewed as a characteristic of the trainer rather than the trainee.

The stunning results of vocational training with moderately, severely, and profoundly retarded persons described earlier were accomplished entirely within a task analytic instructional environment. Of course, these structured instructional environments have also been used very effectively with mildly retarded clients.

On the other hand, there have been many known instances in which "vocational training" for mentally retarded clients has involved very little real or effective instruction. Even though the *training* has been grossly inadequate, the *client* may still have been judged as incapable, thereby enhancing both that individual client's history of "failure" and the general stereotype of "another job for which retarded persons are not qualified." If a rehabilitation counselor can find and/or generate appropriate training opportunities for mentally retarded clients, the probability of success is quite high.

Environmental Supports

Many retarded persons must be *taught* how to function independently or semi-independently in their communities. Areas of potential concern include self-help and social skills within the client's residence, access to required community services, mobility and access to transportation, and opportunity to experience recreational and leisure activities. Family attitudes can also become a critical determinant of client success or failure, particularly for those clients who still live with their family of origin during adulthood. For example, over-protective parents may quickly neutralize the effects of training that is designed to foster client independence. In general, where suitable alternatives exist, it is preferable for adult clients not to live with their families of origin. The individualized rehabilitation program for a mentally retarded client should include reference to each of these areas of community and social adjustment, in addition to specific vocational objectives.

When dealing with potential employers of mentally retarded clients of an ethnic subculture, it may be necessary for the counselor to ensure that the employer understands that certain behaviors which may appear "abnormal" or "retarded" or otherwise inappropriate are actually normal and acceptable within the client's own subculture. Distinctions must be made between behavior consistent with different cultural norms and maladaptive behavior actually associated with mental retardation.

Vocational Opportunities Available

A rehabilitation program individually devised for a mentally retarded client should definitely contain vocational objectives which not only reflect his skill and behavior levels, but also job availability, including jobs than can be created. Clearly, a vocational objective is unlikely to culminate in successful employment, even for a very well-trained client, if jobs in the area for which the client is trained are generally unavailable. Within the context of available jobs, however, there is often a tendency to underestimate the vocational potential of mentally retarded clients, thereby unnecessarily constricting the pool of available opportunities. Table 20-4 above provides some idea of the wide range of jobs in which mildly retarded persons have been successfully placed. The more recent findings with moderately, severely, and profoundly retarded persons extend these horizons even further. It is important that clients be encouraged to attempt to achieve their maximum potential level of performance by taking occasional risks and sometimes failing and learning from the experience.

The rehabilitation counselor serves his mentally retarded clients best by avoiding the stereotypes that have tended to restrict their vocational opportunities. No a priori judgment should be made regarding what a client can and cannot do. A comprehensive evaluation must be completed before any decisions are made. Extended evaluation has often proven to be a valuable tool in vocational planning, particularly when an opportunity for some training is afforded during this period.

BIBLIOGRAPHY

Brolin D, Kokaska C: Critical issues in job placement of the educable mentally retarded. Rehabil Lit **35**:174–177, 1974.

Discusses some critical issues in job placement of the mentally retarded; for example, who should take responsibility for finding employment and the availability of sufficient employment opportunities for the retarded.

Browning P (ed): *Mental Retardation: Rehabilitation and Counseling*. Springfield, IL, Thomas, 1974.

This book contains an excellent collection of chapters

dealing with a wide range of principles, programs, and practices that are directly relevant to the rehabilitation counselor who works with mentally retarded clients. An extensive bibliography is also provided for those who wish to pursue specific topics in greater depth.

Cegelka PT: Sex role stereotyping in special education: A look at secondary work study programs. Except Child **42**:323–329, 1976.

A review of work-study programs for the retarded revealed that girls were not being admitted or, if admitted, were not receiving equal opportunities. This article should encourage counselors to consider inequities due to sex-role stereotyping when placing mentally retarded clients in training programs.

Conley RW: *The Economics of Mental Retardation*. Baltimore, Johns Hopkins University Press, 1973.

This book discusses the economics of mental retardation. Chapters cover the epidemiology, etiology, and effects of mental retardation, programs for the mentally retarded, and a benefit-cost analysis of mental retardation. Most of the available data at the time of publication is from 1968. The presentation is mostly in the form of statistics on large population groups and is not particularly useful for dealing with individual clients.

Grossman H (ed): *Manual on Terminology and Classification in Mental Retardation*. Amer Assoc on Men Def, Special Publication Series No. 2, 1973.

This manual provides basic information about the definition, classification, and etiology of mental retardation, along with some recommendations about statistical reporting and a glossary of terminology prevalent in the field. Rehabilitation counselors should find this book very useful as a basic reference text.

Hardy RE, Cull JG: *Modification of Behavior of the Mentally Retarded: Applied Principles*. Springfield, IL, Thomas, 1974.

This book describes methods used to modify behavior of the mentally retarded and gives some examples of the types of behavior changed with each of the various techniques.

MacMillan D: *Mental Retardation in School and Society*. Boston, Little, Brown, 1977.

Robinson N, Robinson H: *The Mentally Retarded Child*. Ed 2 New York, McGraw-Hill, 1976.

These two books are among the best of the many introductory textbooks that cover the entire field of mental retardation from a variety of perspectives and contexts. Anyone working with mentally retarded clients will benefit greatly from such a broad awareness.

Mercer J: *Labeling the Mentally Retarded*. Berkeley, University of California Press, 1973.

The cultural relativity of mild mental retardation is both documented and discussed in this excellent book. The prevalence and reasons for mislabeling persons mentally retarded are also presented. One of the major products emerging from this work is the System of Multicultural Pluralistic Assessment.

Moen M, Bogen D, Aanes D: Follow-up of mentally retarded adults successfully and unsuccessfully placed in community group homes. Hosp Community Psychiatry **26**:754–756, 1975.

Of 85 patients discharged from institutions 6 months prior to the study, 72 were found to be successfully placed and 13 were unsuccessfully placed and returned to the institution. The most common behavior problems in the unsuccessfully placed group are discussed.

Wehman PH: Toward a social skills curriculum for developmentally disabled clients in vocational settings. Rehabil Lit **36**:342–348, 1975.

Describes four levels of social skills needed by the developmentally disabled in vocational settings: (1) *personal care*, e.g., personal hygiene and table manners; (2) *primary interaction*, e.g., proper greetings, such as "hello"; (3) *vocational survival skills*, e.g., use of telephones and public transportation; (4) *advanced interaction skills*, e.g., problem solving and knowledge of whom to trust.

APPENDIX

REFERENCES FOR THE TESTS LISTED IN TABLE 20-3

1. Stanford-Binet
   a. Buros OK (ed): *Mental Measurements Yearbook*. Highland Park, NJ, The Gryphon Press, 7:426.
   b. Buros, op. cit. 6:536.
2. Wechsler Adult Intelligence Scale
   a. Buros, op. cit., **7**:429
   b. Buros, op. cit., **5**:414
3. Wechsler Intelligence Scale for Children (Revised)
   a. Petrosko J: WISC-R. Measurement and Evaluation Guidance, 7:265–267, 1975.
   b. Krichev A: A revision that really is—the WISC-R. Psychology in the Schools, 12:126–128, 1975.
4. Vineland Social Maturity Scale
   a. Buros, op. cit., 4:94.
   b. Buros, op. cit., 3:107.
5. AAMD Adaptive Behavior Scale
   a. Buros, op. cit., 7:37.
6. System of Multicultural, Pluralistic Assessment
   a. Mercer J: Cultural diversity, mental retardation, and assessment. In Mittler, P. (ed): *Research to Practice in Mental Retardation,* Vol. I. Baltimore, University Park Press, 1977, pp. 353–362.
7. Social and Prevocational Information Battery
   a. Buros, op. cit., Volume 8, in press.
   b. Johnson, O: *Tests and Measurements in Child Development: Handbook II,* Vol. I. San Francisco, Jossey-Bass, 1976, pp. 274–275.
   c. Halpern A., et al.: Measuring social and prevocational awareness in mildly retarded adolescents. Amer J Ment Defic, 80:81–89, 1975.
8. Social and Prevocational Information Battery - Form T
   a. Irvin L, et al.: Assessing social and prevocational awareness in mildly and moderately retarded individuals. Amer J Ment Defic, 82:266–272, 1977.

b. Halpern A: Measuring social and prevocational awareness of retarded adolescents and adults. In Mittler, P.
(ed): *Research to Practice in Mental Retardation,* Vol. II.
Baltimore, University Park Press, 1977, pp. 395–402.

9. Camelot Behavioral Checklist
a. Foster RW: *Camelot Behavioral Checklist.* Camelot Behavioral Systems, 1974. P.O. Box 607, Parsons, KS 67357.

10. Vocational Interest and Sophistication Assessment
a. Buros, op. cit., **7**:1039.
b. Parnicky JJ, Kahn H, Burdette AB: Standardization of
the VISA (Vocational Interest and Sophistication Assessment) technique. Amer J Ment Defic, **75**:442–448, 1971.

11. AAMD—Becker Reading Free Vocational Interest Inventory
a. Parnicky JR, Presnall DM: Interest inventories and the
retarded. Rehabilitation Counseling Bulletin, **20**:118–
128, 1976.

12. MICRO-TOWER
a. Loeding D: Micro-Tower. ICD Rehabilitation and Research Center, 340 East 24th Street, New York, NY
10010.

13. Vocational Information and Evaluation Work Samples
a. Vocational Information and Evaluation Work Samples.
Vocational Research Institute, Jewish Employment and
Vocational Service (J.E.V.S.), 1913 Walnut Street, Philadelphia, PA 19103.
b. A Comparison of Seven Vocational Evaluation Systems.
Materials Development Center, Stout Vocational Rehabilitation Institute, University of Wisconsin-Stout
Menomonie, WI 54751.

14. SINGER Vocational Evaluation System
a. A Comparison of Seven Vocational Evaluation Systems.
Materials Development Center, Stout Vocational Rehabilitation Institute, University of Wisconsin-Stout,
Menomonie, WI 54751.

21 SEXUAL ADJUSTMENT TO CHRONIC DISEASE AND DISABILITY

Theodore M. Cole, M.D.
Sandra S. Cole, B.A.

DEFINITION OF SEXUALITY

Each time a rehabilitation counselor opens a case with a new client, many human issues may emerge. Sexuality is one of them. However, not until the decade of the 1970's did the behavioral and emotional aspects of sexuality become an acceptable area for client-counselor interaction. Before then, almost all professional journal articles about sexuality dealt with medical and reproductive aspects. In the last few years, publications, conferences, seminars, and general awareness of the role of sexuality in the overall rehabilitation process have finally established sexuality as a legitimate health concern for physically disabled men and women.

Not everyone agrees that sexuality is as important an issue as other problems facing the recently disabled adult. Some professionals believe that the immediate post-trauma hospitalization period is too early for the disabled person to be concerned with sexual issues. Hospitalized disabled patients participating in two studies considered sexual function least important when compared to other physical functions, such as ambulation, transfers, and bowel and bladder function.

However, if sexuality is regarded as sex organ function, or if conclusions are drawn on the basis of surveys of hospitalized persons who are still in the early stages of disability adjustment, the broader and deeper meaning of sexuality may be overlooked. Sexuality is more than genitality or sex acts. It is reflected in all that a person is and does, and it may take years to adjust sexually after onset of a severe disability. Sexuality can be broadly thought of as an avenue towards intimacy.

Intimacy is of vast importance to people and everyone is capable of it, able-bodied or disabled, young or old, married or single. It is the isolation from intimacy that is frightening. Problems may arise when health care providers and/or patients equate intimacy with sex acts. If, in order to spare themselves discomfort, they avoid discussing sexuality, they may lose a natural avenue to understanding and talking about intimacy. The result may be to isolate the disabled person even further, producing fear and more disability. Health providers should understand that adherence to a limited, genital concept of sexuality may exclude those whose physical disabilities have caused their genitals to be lost, damaged, or denervated. Similarly, if sexuality is restricted to interaction between partners, then widows, widowers, and the unmarried may be overlooked. Or, if sexuality is confined to heterosexual intercourse, other aspects of sexual expression may be restricted as, for example, solitary masturbation or homosexuality.

When intimacy is achieved between two people, it's a very special relationship. It's the feeling of mutual comfort, acceptance, and trust, whether together or apart. It's the many things they do for each other and have together that are exclusively theirs. It's the ability to be unguarded and to expose their "bad" as well as "good" points with a feeling of safety.

The ways in which two people express their intimacy are legion. Intimacy is the eye contact that says, when others are talking, "I know how you're feeling about what we are hearing." It's the comment made in public with special meaning for only the two. It's a touch or a hand hold, a hug or a kiss for no special reason other than contact. It's sitting and lying together and talking, or saying nothing with comfort and ease, for the warmth and closeness it provides. It's expressed in private jokes, pet names, carefree giggles, and gentle caresses. Intimacy is always sexual but not necessarily genital. Intimacy may include intense expressions of body and genital contact, however comfortably achieved, in an atmosphere of open communication. Fulfillment of intimacy is not limited to the orgasm of sexual intercourse.

Comfort or discomfort with intimacy may influence how one person interacts with another, how clients work with staff, or how a person interacts with his sexual partner. In order to have a healthy capacity for intimacy, one must have a healthy self-image. Healthy sexuality, in turn, is a part of a healthy self-image.

There is strong evidence that there is a distinct relationship between self-esteem and sexuality in the able-bodied as well as the physically disabled. A positive

compensatory mechanisms for re-entering the world self-esteem may enhance a client's ability to develop following disability.

It is assumed that successful work leads to increased self-esteem. A client will probably continue in a work activity which has produced increased self-esteem. Such activities will benefit the client and may lead to a decreased willingness to accept the dependent role. In the case of a physically disabled person, this may lead to a decrease of complaints and of need for outside medical support.

Similarly, the achievement of intimacy with a partner may lead to increased self-esteem and may further encourage the individual to continue other activities, such as employment. These activities may not only satisfy self but may also decrease feelings of castration, and result in less social withdrawal and therefore less need for outside social support. The result is a reduced social and dollar cost to society. Activities deliberately designed to increase a client's self-esteem thus may produce decreased utilization of health care resources and reduced costs for society in general.

Journals for professionals and periodicals circulated to disabled persons are now emphasizing that sexual rehabilitation should be expected from health professionals and institutions. Institutional prohibitions which, until recently, have discouraged intimacy between clients and their spouses are giving way. In some locations, privacy rooms are now available within the institution so that residents can use them with their partners for intimate exchange, which may or may not include sexual activity. Perhaps one day sexuality will be recognized as a part of living which many adults desire at intervals and around which much of their lives and activities are intertwined.

SEXUAL DYSFUNCTION IN THE NONDISABLED

Sexual dysfunctions are best understood in context of the full sexual response cycle. The revolutionary work of Masters and Johnson identified four phases of this cycle.

The *excitement phase* begins for either sex when something sexually stimulating (for that individual) occurs. The excitement stimuli may be psychological and/or physical in nature. During this phase, both males and females will show increased muscle tension, heart rate, and blood pressure, and heavier breathing. As the stimulation continues, penile erection occurs in the male and vaginal lubrication in the female. If the stimuli are withdrawn or cease to be effective, the next phase will not occur and the body will begin to relax and return to a nonaroused state. If, however, excitement continues, the plateau phase is reached.

The *plateau phase* is a more advanced or accelerated excitement phase, occurring just prior to orgasm.

Maximum vasocongestion of the body, including the primary sexual organs, occurs. Again, if stimulation is ineffective or withdrawn, the body will show a gradual reduction of muscle tension and other physiological phenomena that are part of this phase. With effective stimulation, the third phase will be entered.

Once started, the third phase, *orgasm*, progresses if no psychic or physical discomfort accompanies it. It usually lasts only a few seconds. Males usually ejaculate and experience rhythmic contractions of penile and perineal muscles, while females experience rhythmic contractions of the vaginal and perineal muscles. Immediately after orgasm, there occurs a refractory period, during which further arousal will not occur. This may be as brief as several minutes or as long as many hours, depending upon such factors as the age of the individual and the intensity of sexual arousal. It is not uncommon for females to be able to achieve several orgasms in succession, with very brief refractory periods at the end of each. Although some males are reported to be multiply orgasmic, most do not experience this phenomenon.

The fourth phase is *resolution*. After orgasm and cessation of further stimulation, the body returns to a relaxed state.

Many people think of lack of orgasm as the only definition of sexual dysfunction but, as this description of the sexual response cycle indicates, sexual dysfunction can occur during the excitement and plateau phases of the cycle and thus prevent orgasm from being reached. Educating persons about the phases, training them to be comfortable with themselves during the excitement and plateau phases, and/or therapy concerning sexuality *in toto* can produce highly positive rehabilitation effects for disabled and nondisabled persons alike. This is true even for those disabilities where orgasm, as described, does not occur.

Although sexuality, intimacy, and genital function can be separated, they are often interconnected. It is helpful, therefore, to define the more common genital dysfunctions so that it can be understood how they can cause or be caused by personal or interpersonal difficulties. It must be kept in mind that the genital aspects of sexual function have an impact upon the total personality. Changes in genital function will almost always create alterations in the personality structure of the individual.

Female Sexual Dysfunction

Preorgasmia. Women who have never experienced an orgasm by any means are considered preorgasmic. In able-bodied women, the roots of preorgasmia are often found in their religious upbringing, family environment, or sometimes in an early sexual trauma, such as molestation or rape.

One of the most effective modalities for treatment is

a women's therapy group in which all the members are preorgasmic. The therapist tries to help the women "give themselves permission" to be sexual, to explore, accept, and be comfortable with their bodies. They are taught about masturbation, their own anatomy, and their own individual sexual responses.

A second effective method for treatment is couple counseling, which focuses on mutual body pleasuring and development of a trusting sexual communication. Therapy may include resolution of a power struggle between the couple related to assigned roles. The main objective of treatment is to reduce the woman's involuntary inhibition of her orgasmic response and to help her achieve her first orgasm, often through masturbation.

Secondary nonorgasmia. Secondary nonorgasmia in able-bodied women is often situational. Women who experience orgasm with masturbation or a partner's digital stimulation but not with intercourse are included in this group. Also included are women who experience orgasm with some partners but not with others, women who experience physical orgasm but do not experience a psychological component, and women who experienced orgasm during an earlier part of their life but not now.

Treatment by sex counseling often focuses on the same issues that preorgasmic women find important. However, there may be more emphasis upon the meaning of intimacy, relationships, and sexual flexibility, and less on behavioral objectives, such as orgasm through masturbation.

Dyspareunia. Women who experience disabling pain during intercourse are considered to have dyspareunia. Prior to counseling, the woman should receive a thorough medical examination to exclude organic causes of pain, such as injury to the vagina, venereal disease, lack of vaginal lubrication, atrophy of the vaginal tissues, an intact hymen, abnormalities or disease of the internal sexual organs, or hemorrhoids. Before treatment is begun, a thorough sexual history is important to exclude a traumatic sexual event early in her life which may have precipitated sexual anxiety.

In the absence of medical disease, treatment focuses on helping the woman accept herself and her participation in a trusting, intimate relationship free from concern over power and control. Treatment often involves exploring the meanings sex may have for the woman.

Sexual aversion. Women who are repulsed or terrified by sex are considered to have sexual aversion. Etiological factors may include one or a combination of the following: doubts about her own sexual adequacy; over-reaction to body odors, penis size, or semen; an early traumatic sexual experience; or extremely prohibiting religious views, leading to feelings of guilt and shame regarding sex. Sexual aversion is often found in a woman whose partner is impotent or ejaculates prematurely.

Successful treatment of sexual aversion includes increasing the woman's flexibility, expanding her sexual meaning system, and enhancing the couple's sense of themselves as sexual persons. Much attention is paid to "giving the couple permission" to act and think sexually. Therapy can be carried out in women's groups or in couple counseling.

Vaginismus. Vaginismus occurs during attempted penile penetration and is defined as an involuntary spasm of the muscles on the pelvic floor which surround the outer one-third of the vagina. Muscle spasms frequently produce pain if penetration is achieved. Etiologically, this dysfunction is also associated with sexual fears and anxiety about intercourse, which may include fantasies of damage done to the vagina if intercourse occurs. The cause in some women is found to be lack of self-acceptance, a low capacity to develop a sexual relationship, inability to trust a partner, religious prohibitions, or previous sexual trauma. In this dysfunction, as in dyspareunia, a thorough medical examination must be done to differentiate phobic avoidance of intercourse from a medically treatable condition.

If no medical treatment is indicated, the therapist focuses on training the woman to dilate her own vagina with progressively larger dilators introduced under her own control. The partner often assists in the therapy. The woman is also taught relaxation exercises and is given information to dispel sexual myths and misconceptions. Frequently, therapy has to include work on trust and intimacy issues within the relationship. Vaginismus is sometimes associated with impotency in the male partner, whose successful treatment may ameliorate the woman's symptoms.

Male Sexual Dysfunction

Premature ejaculation. An able-bodied man who reaches ejaculation before he may wish is said to ejaculate prematurely. This is one of the most common sexual dysfunctions of men and is one of the easiest to treat successfully. Generally, there is no relationship between premature ejaculation and specific sexual conflicts or psychopathology.

Treatment often focuses on teaching the man to develop more successful communication with his partner in order to control the amount of sexual stimulation he receives in the process of intercourse. Behavioral techniques, such as manually squeezing the penis to reduce erection and delay ejaculation, have also been used successfully. The man can be treated individually, in a men's group, or in couple counseling. The prognosis for cure is excellent.

Primary impotence. A man who has never been able to maintain an erect penis for sexual penetration is considered to have primary impotence. He may report nocturnal or morning erections or erections during masturbation. However, he is unable to achieve an erection for purposes of vaginal penetration. A physical examination is extremely important to eliminate the possibility of medical problems, especially if he is not experiencing nocturnal emissions or erections during masturbation. It is believed that anxiety, occurring at the time of sexual activity, disrupts the man's erectile response. The anxiety may be rooted in a sexual trauma in early life, male sex-role stress, feelings of inadequacy, or prohibiting religious or moral views.

Primary impotence is often treated in couple counseling, or in men's groups if a consistent sexual partner is not available. Treatment is designed to reduce anxiety by restoring the man's confidence in his own sexuality. The man's ability to "allow" an erection may be enhanced by encouraging him to have erections without the demand for sexual intercourse or ejaculation. If a man's confidence in his ability to have repeated erections can be gained, coitus may be possible.

Secondary impotence. Secondary impotence is seen in men who are able to achieve erections on some occasions but not on others. For example, erection may be possible during foreplay but may dwindle as coitus is attempted. Other men report the ability to achieve erections while clothed but lose their erections when the penis is exposed to a partner's view. Some men lose their erections when the partner assumes control over the sexual situation, whereas others lose the erection if the partner does not assume control. Some men report achievement of only partial erections, and others have erections with some partners but not with others. Causative factors include inopportune use of alcohol and drugs and all the possibilities mentioned under primary impotence, especially intimacy and relationship issues.

Treatment is similar to that for primary impotence, with special emphasis put on the couple's relationship. Reduction in alcohol or drug consumption is often indicated.

Retarded ejaculation. Men whose ejaculatory reflex is inhibited while erection remains intact are considered to experience retarded ejaculation. They may experience ejaculation through manual or oral stimulation by a partner but are unable to ejaculate while the penis is contained in the vagina. Etiologic factors often include guilt feelings surrounding sex generally or guilt feelings with specific sexual partners. Religious prohibitions, a previous history of a traumatic sexual event, fear of pregnancy in a partner, or homosexual/bisexual conflicts may also play a part.

Treatment focuses upon changing the association between ejaculation and negative consequences. When the man understands the psychic conflicts or phobic components associated with retarded ejaculation, treatment can be successful. Often treatment is provided in couple counseling or in men's therapy groups.

As this brief description of the more common sexual dysfunctions shows, the etiology is often related to dysfunctional sexual attitudes, behavioral problems, specific relationship problems, or early traumatic sexual experiences. However, none of them presuppose the presence of a physical disability as a causative factor or an initiating event leading to sexual dysfunction. Any of the above sexual dysfunctions can be seen in a physically disabled adult. In addition, the severely disabled may have sexual dysfunction induced by the disability itself. The counselor should therefore be acquainted with the ways in which sexual function may also be altered by disability.

While the above discussion largely referred to heterosexual dysfunction, the counselor should not lose sight of the fact that homosexuality as a preference exists amongst the nondisabled and the disabled populations. Data regarding the frequency of homosexual behavior amongst the handicapped populace are unavailable. However, the counselor should recognize that heterosexual, homosexual, and bisexual preferences exist in both the physically disabled and the able-bodied populations. Value judgments in this area are no more appropriate to the professional role than they would be in other personal areas. The counselor may wish to make referral for sexual counseling in instances where the client identifies problem areas and service needs. However, it would be inappropriate to refer a client on the basis of sexual preference alone.

SEXUAL DYSFUNCTION IN THE DISABLED

Classification of Severe Disabilities

Severe disabilities can be grouped into four categories with respect to sexual function. Placement in a category depends on the person's age at the time of onset and the progressive or stable nature of the disability.

Type I. Disabilities classified as Type I are those which begin at birth or before puberty and are nonprogressive, such as congenital brain injury, limb amputation in early life, congenital loss of sight or hearing, and mental retardation. Persons with these disabilities experience a lifetime of being different from their peers. The overly protective or guilt-laden attitudes of society or parents may have had an inhibiting effect upon these persons' psychosocial maturation. Experiences that are important to adolescence may be either unavailable or consciously kept from them. As a result, some may emerge from adolescence with maturational deficits, lacking certain social skills. They may find themselves in an adult world, wanting to be sexually sophisticated, but lacking the requisite education.

In particular, the mentally retarded can frequently benefit from a positive attitude toward sexuality. They experience a variety of sexual problems, the most serious of which is prejudice. Societal prejudice often relegates the retarded person to a subhuman or perennial childhood status, regardless of the person's level of function. This attitude often leads to suppression of the retarded person's sexuality and withholding of sexual education.

Despite recent conferences on the sexual rights of the retarded and a statement issued from the President's Committee on Mental Retardation in 1969 that "the retarded are due the same inalienable rights to life, protection of the law, dignity of person and opportunity as all other Americans," little progress has been made in developing working policies or programs in the sexual behavior area.

Many feel that the retarded are vulnerable to sexual abuse, while others see them as sexually dangerous to others because they lack control over their behavior. These points of view may apply to some retarded persons, but neither their vulnerability nor inappropriate sexual behavior will be overcome without education, training, counseling, and permission to be sexual beings. Rehabilitation programs are badly needed that will assist the retarded in gaining knowledge not only about genital function, masturbation, sex with or without marriage, birth control, childbirth, and parenthood, but also prostitution, homosexuality, venereal disease, sterilization, and sexual dysfunction.

Providing appropriate rehabilitation to a population whose intellectual abilities range from profoundly impaired to slightly impaired is tremendously complex. However, the rehabilitation counselor is most likely to encounter the more mildly retarded person who is trying to achieve an independent vocational and social life style. The counselor can increase the probability of successful independent-living rehabilitation by assessing the client's need for sex education classes, group discussion meetings, and counseling or psychotherapy programs.

Type II. Disabilities classified as Type II also begin before puberty and therefore may produce essentially the same effect on adult sexuality as Type I disabilities. However, they are progressive and the child can never be sure that his body will not become even more dysfunctional with time. Examples of these disabilities include juvenile rheumatoid arthritis, childhood-onset diabetes mellitus, muscular dystrophy, and cystic fibrosis. Because of the progressive nature of these disabilities, the clients may be regularly involved in medical treatment programs that require much of their energy. They may be left with a poor body image, a feeling of being sickly, and an unwillingness to regard their bodies as being able to provide sensual pleasure or themselves capable of achieving intimate relationships.

Type III. Disabilities classified as Type III are those which occur in adult life and are stable. Examples include traumatic spinal cord injury, amputation, and disfiguring burns. Persons so disabled can recall when they were "normal." This reference point may be helpful in their effort to re-establish their psychosexual identity. Further, they may already have learned the interpersonal skills necessary for the development of healthy adult sexual relationships. These skills may be modified and continue to serve them after they are disabled.

Type IV. Disabilities classified as Type IV are the degenerative diseases which will affect most adults who live to be old. They include, for example, degenerative heart disease, stroke, cancer, and chronic renal disease. Their onsets are often gradual and their course progressive, thus allowing for slow adjustment to the disabling process. However, like Type II disabilities, Type IV disabilities produce an unstable base from which clients can plan their lives. They, too, may find it necessary to invest considerable energy into maintaining their health, and they have great difficulty looking upon themselves as "well even though disabled."

With regard to mental illness, behavior displayed may vary dramatically. Any stereotyping of sexual dysfunction is therefore hazardous. The best assumption is that sexual preferences and functions vary widely for this group, just as they do within the nonhandicapped population.

Evaluation

All four types of sexual disabilities can be manifested as solitary or partnership problems, fertility concerns, or body-image issues. Therefore, depending upon the nature of the disablement, sexuality may be affected in the areas of masturbation, coitus, positioning techniques, sex-role stereotypes, procreational ability, or self-acceptance.

The duration of the disability often plays an important role in the client's awareness of a sexual concern or dysfunction. In a sample of recently hospitalized spinal cord injured patients, almost 50 percent believed that their sexual adjustment was good and only 9 percent rated it as poor at the time of discharge. However, a year or two later, as many as 38 percent stated that their sexual adjustment was now poor. This suggests an early lack of awareness of the changes that the physical disability produces in an individual's ability to perform sexually.

The work tolerance for many disabilities can be predicted by knowing the severity of the person's disability, his age, and his health status before the disability. Sexual activity is no different. Under usual circumstances, the cardiovascular stress of sexual intercourse does not exceed that caused by climbing two flight of stairs. However, if less stress must be recommended, the client can be assured that there remains, to the extent of one's imagination, a wide variety of sexual activities and techniques to enjoy. Or, if neuromuscular disorders limit mobility or postures, the client can be asked to explore the partner's willingness to assume responsibility for body positioning. Loss of finger dexterity may be compensated for by use of the mouth if both partners agree. Virtually no disability prohibits recumbency and closeness in bed. The overall benefits of seeing oneself as capable of giving and receiving sexual pleasure may far outweigh the risks to the body. On the other hand, the risks of foreclosing on the human need for intimacy may greatly overshadow the risks of physical harm resulting from intimate acts between two people who care for each other. It must always be kept in mind that intimacy and sexual contact do not require sexual intercourse or orgasm.

It is beyond the scope of this chapter to enumerate all of the sexual concomitants of the many disabilities that may affect men and women. However, the counselor should be aware of some of the physiological, psychological, and interpersonal alterations which may be imposed by the physical disability.

Medical evaluation. There are several resources to whom the counselor may turn when medical evaluation is needed for sexual dysfunction. A competent physiatrist, internist, urologist, gyne-cologist, or neurologist can obtain a proper medical history, perform an appropriate physical examination, and interpret the necessary laboratory reports. The physician has basically two tasks. One is to include or exclude treatable medical disease or impairment which may have an influence upon sexual function. The other is to diagnose medical causes for sexual problems which, even though not remediable by medical treatment, must be understood to facilitate adjustment and proceed with rehabilitation planning. The physician is most able to be helpful when the client and counselor can provide specific questions (e.g., ''Is there a medical cause for impotence?'' or ''Is there a medical reason why the client should not engage in sex acts such as intercourse or masturbation?''). The following discussion reviews the range of genital and reproductive impairments that may occur in the various disabilities.

At one end of the spectrum is loss of the genitals themselves, due to trauma or disease (usually cancer). Loss of part or all of the penis and testicles in the male can occur. In the female loss of the vulva, vaginal closure, uterus, ovaries, and the breast similarly can result in sexual dysfunction. In these more obvious situations, initiation of discussion of the meaning of these losses and the sexual adjustment problems they may be causing is important, since there may be a need for the client to explore the potential for an expanded view of sexual performance and gratification. Many persons who have lost their external genitalia continue to describe their sex lives as active and satisfactory. This suggests that if other aspects of the postdisability adjustment are adequate, sexual performance and gratification can be achieved.

Less vivid but still devastating dysfunctions can be seen in persons who lose sensation in their genitals due to metabolic diseases, such as diabetes mellitus, or nervous system diseases, such as multiple sclerosis and spinal cord injury. Not only may the individual receive less sensation, but physical orgasm may not occur, and potency and fertility may be lost in the male. Sometimes, a client may erroneously conclude that the loss of fertility and sensation is synonymous with the loss of emotional feelings and capacity for intimacy in general. They may withdraw behind a barrier of seeming indifference to sexual stimulation, forgetting that the largest part of their sexuality is in the psyche, not in the genitals.

The medical conditions that lead to loss of usual genital function are less dramatic than sensation losses but are sometimes equally dysfunctional. Examples include developmental or degenerative anomalies of the organs themselves or of the circulation supplying them. The male who is unable to achieve an erection due to insufficient blood supply may conclude that he is ''less of a man'' than he was before. Or the woman whose vagina has become damaged or obstructed by disease or injury may believe she is unable to perform as a female, even though her disability otherwise spares her entire body.

Some orthopedic or neurologically handicapping conditions may limit a person's sexual repertoire. Loss of joint mobility, as may occur in arthritis, multiple sclerosis, stroke, and cerebral palsy, may make traditional positioning for intercourse painful or impossible. Persons so affected may conclude that they can no longer engage in coitus. Some persons whose medical conditions cause their urine to drain from urethral catheters or ileostomies to collection bags may be unable to emotionally accept the appliances. Even the partners become convinced that the sex organs can no longer be used for pleasure. Approval of continued sexual desires and feelings, combined with sex coun-seling, may expand the client's concept of sexuality beyond genital function alone. With patience and support, clients and/or partners may be able to begin their adjustment as sexual persons. Then with specific help from a sex therapist who understands sexuality and physical disability, clients may begin to deal productively with this aspect of physical disability, which untreated may have the potential for creating severe conflict and often personality disorders.

Psychosocial evaluations. Psychological evaluations and decisions about whether a sex therapist should counsel alone with a client or with the client and his sexual partner together may be facilitated by resources generally available in all 50 states. One of these is the American Association of Sex Educators, Counselors and Therapists (AASECT) whose central office is at 5010 Wisconsin Avenue NW, Suite 304, Washington, DC 20016. Another is the local Planned Parenthood group listed in the telephone book. A third resource is the local or regional mental health center, which can be found through county medical societies or in local listings of social and health services. The primary professional disciplines offering sex therapy, depending on the local area, most often include psychologists, psychiatrists, physiatrists, urologists, gynecologists, neurologists, family medicine specialists, and social workers.

Sexual dysfunction following a physical disability may not be organically related to the disability. Some clients may attribute their sexual dysfunction directly to the physical disability and thus avoid having to deal with the psychological components of the disability. However, it is known that the psychological aspects of sexual dysfunction may be as disabling as the medical aspects. A case in point is vaginismus. A woman with multiple sclerosis and skeletal muscle spasticity may experience painful intercourse on the basis of involuntary contraction of the muscles of the pelvic floor, which she believes is caused by her spasticity. However, anxiety can greatly increase spasticity caused by central nervous system disease. In this case, relief of sex-related anxiety helps reduce her spasticity during intercourse and thus her vaginismus. The separation of medical from psychological influences will be necessary before useful therapy can commence.

Another example is spinal cord disorder which, in some men, would seem to explain the change in sexual function. However, with counseling and removal of sexual anxieties, genital function has improved. These cases suggest that sexual dysfunction may be a result of organic or psychological disorders or, as is probably true in the majority of instances, a combination of both. However, some persons are unwilling to accept their own adjustment problems as an explanation for sexual dysfunction. They would rather blame a medical problem over which they have no control. Referring such clients to a sex therapist may prove rewarding, since improved sexual functioning, as well as enhanced capabilities and general adjustment in other areas, may result.

Interpersonal evaluation. In addition to medical and psychological issues within the client, the sexuality of the spouse or partner must also be considered. The issues here can be understood in terms of interpersonal dysfunction. In these cases, a sex therapist may consider couple counseling essential to reduce sexual dysfunctioning. For example, an able-bodied spouse's sexual frame of reference to the partner may be dramatically altered by a disfiguring burn on the partner's face. Or a spouse whose partner has survived a life-threatening heart attack may consciously or unconsciously withhold sexual advances for fear that sexual activity may expose the partner to further risk. These conflicts can best be resolved by referring the couple to a qualified therapist for treatment as a sexual unit.

Other evaluation techniques. Self-disclosure is an important technique used in evaluation of sexual dysfunction in adults. Self-disclosure is the willingness to express one's own feeling about sexuality and does *not* imply disclosure of one's personal sexual activities. In this instance, the therapist may disclose that he of course has sexual feelings, that it is perfectly natural to have "turn-ons" and "turn-offs," and that sexual arousal may follow after a variety of simuli. It is important that a sex therapist not impose his values upon the client by advocating for or against certain activities or points of view. Self-disclosure may help the client feel that he is not the only person who is being asked to discuss this very private part of self.

The therapist should also convey the impression that the client has, of course, engaged in a number of sex-related activities. For example, consider the situation of a young man recovering from a crush fracture of the pelvis which has also caused injury to intrapelvic nerves and organs. In an attempt to learn the extent to which satisfactory sexual adjustment has been achieved and coitus or masturbation resumed, the client may be asked about the current frequency of these activities. By asking "how often" rather than "do you," the expectation is established that coitus and masturbation are normal activities for most people. It may then be easier for the client to talk about his attempts, rather than to hide them because he believes, for example, that masturbation is abnormal and he must not discuss it. Such approaches can bring out dysfunction problems that require additional referral and can provide valuable information through which a relevant plan of treatment can be developed by a sex therapist.

An honest and sharing discussion of sexuality may assist in breaking down the parent/child relationship which so often arises between the allied health professional and the client. In fact, honest and sharing discussions in almost any emotionally laden area may also assist in breaking down barriers that may exist. Sexuality, however, is a particularly powerful area because it is so personal. It is almost impossible to behave toward a client as if he were childlike and unable to perform if, at the same time, he is afforded the status of sexual respect. This means that the client should be given the expectation that sexual activity will take place in the future even if it presently is not occurring. If this is done in a supportive way, it can facilitate other areas of interaction between the professional and the client. If, on the other hand, "we" the professionals treat "them" the clients, a distance may be created which hampers the honest exchange inherent in personal adjustment counseling.

It is often very helpful to clients for the professional to have a small library of the various texts and pamphlets written for the consumer that deal with sexuality and illustrate the various approaches that can be taken and the devices available to enhance sexual function in disability. In addition, it may be appropriate to serve as an advocate for the client by helping him to find the financial resources to purchase equipment designed to create more effective sexual function. This service should be provided in the same straightforward and honest manner used in giving assistance to acquire equipment designed to facilitate physical mobility or ordinary activities of daily living.

SEXUAL COUNSELING

The opportunity for the client to enter into a discussion of sexuality should be integrated into other aspects of general counseling. If it is segregated and given separate handling, the message is conveyed that sexual function cannot be talked about openly or may not be appropriate for the disabled client. The counselor's uneasiness may cause the client to believe that there are "appropriate" and "inappropriate" questions to discuss. Depending upon what clients believe is appropriate, they may well not initiate questions regarding sexual issues which may be closely related to overall disability adjustment and in need of referral and treatment. In these cases, the counselor may lose a chance to be helpful. Counselors who initially feel awkward and uncomfortable using this permissive approach may wish to obtain additional training or supervisory assistance in this area. Also, practice will help to make the inclusion of sexuality as a "safe" topic for open discussion easier.

The degree to which a counselor predominantly concerned with vocational rehabilitation should become involved in the sexual adjustment of his client is a matter of debate. In instances where the nature of the disability has obvious and documented effects upon sexual functioning (e.g., spinal cord injury and multiple sclerosis), it would seem reasonable for the vocational counselor to place more emphasis upon this area. Even then, sexual function would be introduced in the context of other activities of daily living and not overemphasized. It is most likely that the counselor will obtain his evaluations through professional consultation and referral, rather than possess the training and time to conduct the evaluation personally. In any event, the interview must be adequately structured to allow for clients needing sex therapy services to surface those needs to the counselor. In fact, in cases where sexual dysfunction is so pronounced that it diminishes overall functioning and impedes vocational potential, the vocational counselor would be negligent if routine referral for appropriate sex therapy were not made.

Training and skill required to be an effective sex therapist will vary depending upon the intensity of involvement required to meet the objectives of the treatment plan. Some sex therapists have suggested a four-tiered scheme of involvement. The *first tier* is that level at which the therapist "gives permission" to the disabled person to have a sexual concern or dysfunction, or to bring it up and discuss it. It should be clearly indicated to the client that discussion of a sexual dysfunction or concern is appropriate and acceptable. This can be done by asking leading questions, initiating talk about sensitive subjects, or by simply listening to the spoken or body language of the client. All allied health professionals should be able to function at this level, with appropriate training and supervision. Not to do so may deny clients the opportunity to bring up the very real problems and concerns they may be facing so that appropriate referral for treatment can be made.

The *second tier* is the level at which the therapist provides limited information for general problem solving. Typically, the limited information is educational and nonpersonal and deals with the disability in a general sense. Most professionals may not be qualified to be involved beyond the second tier, and referral to a sex therapist should be made. Some, however, may have the special training required for the *third tier* of involvement, which is the level at which specific suggestions about sexual concerns and dysfunctions are provided. This implies that the therapist has taken a sexual history and is knowledgeable and trained in sexuality and the particular physical disability under consideration.

The *fourth tier* is the level of intensive therapy. This is provided by professionals who have been thoroughly trained in sex counseling and who also understand physical disabilities. Intensive therapy means exactly that. It often involves intrapersonal and psychological issues, and frequently requires relationship counseling. It goes well beyond providing an opportunity for discussion, limited information, or even specific suggestion. It implies a thorough understanding and training in psychodynamics, especially as they relate to sexuality. It also implies a thorough understanding of physical disability and rehabilitation and how the disabled person and his family may react to the disability within the context of a rehabilitation environment.

Professionals who might be expected to do intensive therapy would include those who have had formal training in sexual counseling as well as specific training in sexual adjustment therapy. These professionals are most commonly found in large rehabilitation or medical settings, but occasionally may be found in private practice as well. As described earlier, these therapists may be located through the American Association of Sex Educators, Counselors, and Therapists, local Planned Parenthood groups, or local or regional mental health centers and State psychological associations.

It is hoped that this chapter will encourage counselors to consider sexual adjustment as a significant element in the overall rehabilitation of the severely disabled. Not to do so may mean rehabilitation failures. The physical, psychological, social, and vocational rehabilitation of a client may often be incomplete without attention to the client's sexual adjustment as well.

BIBLIOGRAPHY

Anderson TP, Cole TM: Sexual counseling of the physically disabled. Postgrad Med 58:117–123, 1975.
Discusses the sexuality of spinal cord injured patients and explains the differences in responses of spinal cord injured persons compared to those of "normal" persons. Also discusses when sexual counseling should begin.

Annon J: The use of vicarious learning in the treatment of sexual concerns. In LoPiccolo J, LoPiccolo L (eds): *Handbook of Sex Therapy*. New York, Plenum Press, 1978.
A four-tiered hierarchical system of counselor-client interaction especially pertinent to sexual concerns but also useful for other personal counseling issues.

Cole TM: Sexuality and physical disabilities. Arch Sex Behav 4:339–403, 1975.
One of the early descriptive articles on sexuality and physical disability, including the classification and variety of disabilities and focusing especially on sexuality of the spinal cord injured.

Cole TM: Training for professionals in the sexuality of the physically disabled. In Pearsall and Rosenweig (eds): *Sex Education for the Health Professional*. New York, Grune & Stratton (in press).
A chapter in a book dealing with sexual training programs for health professionals.

de la Cruz FF, La Veck GD (eds): *Human Sexuality and the Mentally Retarded*. New York, Brunner Maxel, 1973.
Discusses the "normalization" philosophy in relation to sexuality. Contributors cover a wide variety of critical issues involved in granting freedom of sexual expression to the retarded.

Evans RL, Halar EM, DeFreece AB, and Larson GL: Multidisciplinary approach to sex education of spinal cord injured patients. Phys Ther 56:541–545, 1976.
Briefly explains what kind of evaluations should be done on a spinal cord injured patient prior to discussing sexual function. Discusses counseling and who should do it in a multidisciplinary setting. Advocates a team approach.

Hanson RW, Franklin MR: Sexual loss in relation to other functional losses for spinal injured males. Arch Phys Med Rehabil 57:291–293, 1976.

Results from a questionnaire administered to spinal cord injured males who were still hospitalized for the rehabilitation phase following acute spinal cord injury.

Kaplan HS: *The Illustrated Manual of Sex Therapy*. New York, Quadrangle Books, 1975.
Written both for professionals and couples, this book provides some counseling techniques used in various sexual dysfunctions. It also discusses the current trends in counseling.

Kent S: Coping with sexual identity crises after mastectomy. Geriatrics 30:145–146, 1975.
Short article dealing with some of the problems women face after having a mastectomy. Problems included those of body image and sexual relations. Prosthesis and support of the primary physician are important in patients' adjustment.

Labby DH: Sexual concomitants of disease and illness. Postgrad Med 58:103–111, 1975.
Discusses sexual activity after onset of cardiac disease, pulmonary disease, renal disease, diabetes mellitus, pelvic disease, and surgery.

Masters WJ, Johnson VE: *Human Sexual Inadequacy*. Boston, Little, Brown, 1970.
Explanation of relationship between sexual physiology and various sexual dysfunctions. Sex therapy experiences and techniques also discussed.
————: *Human Sexual Response*. Boston, Little, Brown, 1966.
Gives detailed description of male and female sexual physiology and response patterns.

Mooney TO, Cole TM, Chilgren RA: *Sexual Options for Paraplegics and Quadriplegics*. Boston, Little, Brown, 1975.
Discusses sexuality and sexual expression for physically disabled persons, focusing primarily on sexual alternatives for spinal cord injured males. Provides information on dealing with practical issues, such as catheters and leg bags, and some discussion of techniques for enhancing sexual interactions. Includes explicit photographs.

Scheingold LD, Wagner NN: *Sound Sex and the Aging Heart*. New York, Human Sciences Press, 1974.
Discussess sex and heart physiology. Offers some alternatives and suggestions for use with various cardiac conditions.

Spergel P, Rosenthal D, Albert BW: Sex—a rehabilitation issue: What priority and when? Abstract from Official Program of American Congress of Rehabilitation Medicine, San Diego, 1976. Arch Phys Med Rehabil 57:562, 1976.
Data on the importance of sexuality in comparison to other functional losses in a mixed group of hospitalized patients in the general rehabilitation service in Philadelphia.

Watts, RJ: Sexuality and the middle-aged cardiac patient. Nurs Clin North Am 11:349–359, 1976.
Discusses the sexuality of male cardiac patients. Kinds of activities, amounts of energy (MET's) used, and the appropriate time after onset of illness to begin these activities, along with some suggestions of things to avoid, are given.

22 CARDIOVASCULAR DISEASES

Henry L. Brammell, M.D.

INTRODUCTION

Cardiovascular diseases include those that affect the heart and those that affect the peripheral vascular system. The heart and blood vessels may be primarily attacked by these diseases or they may be secondarily affected as a consequence of another disease, such as diabetes (see chap. 24) or sickle cell disease (see chap. 27). The reader may wish to review the discussions of the normal function of the cardiovascular and pulmonary systems in chapter 3.

The major cardiac diseases covered in this chapter are atherosclerotic coronary heart disease, rheumatic heart disease, hypertension, and heart failure. Heart failure is discussed separately, even though it is actually a consequence of a specific underlying cardiac disease, because it is such an important source of disability and cause for job modification. The four individual discussions are preceded by a review of cardiac disease in general because of the many aspects that they all have in common.

The major peripheral arterial diseases discussed include the obliterative and arteriospastic disorders. Finally, the vein disorders — varicose veins and thrombophlebitis — are reviewed. As a group, these can be referred to as the peripheral vascular diseases, although often peripheral vascular disease is meant to convey peripheral arterial disease.

The reason for an extensive review of cardiovascular disease is clear. It is the leading medical problem in the United States both in terms of numbers affected and cost. The cost in the United States in 1977 was estimated at 26.7 billion dollars. This figure is the sum of the cost, in descending dollar amounts, of hospital and nursing home services, loss of productivity due to disability, physician and nursing services, and medication. The most costly disease is atherosclerotic coronary heart disease, the disease which causes heart attack and which affects at least four million citizens in the United States. Approximately 1,500,000 heart attacks occur each year, from which there are about 670,000 survivors. One third of these are under the age of 65 and hence are potential seekers of vocational services.

In the absence of significant physical or psychosocial disability, the younger survivors of heart attack remain at work. Many of those who are physically capable but do not return to gainful employment would profit from the services of a vocational rehabilitation counselor. The potential pool of these younger post-heart-attack clients is approximately 60,000 individuals. With national vocational rehabilitation rolls containing fewer than 5 percent of clients with cardiovascular disease (fewer than 10,000), the unmet need of persons with coronary heart disease is obvious. Furthermore, this sum does not include persons with other cardiovascular diseases, an additional 300,000 men and women, 75,000 of whom are under the age of 65.

The need for vocational services will surely increase with each passing year as medical advances continue to decrease death rates. The counselor's challenge is obvious: to keep this increasing number of productive post-heart-attack patients and other cardiovascular disease patients vocationally competitive.

Congenital heart disease is not specifically discussed in this chapter, for it is relatively rare, occurring in only 0.5 percent of live births, and therefore does not comprise a large portion of a counselor's cardiac caseload. A few remarks may, however, be of some interest. There are two major subgroups of persons with congenital heart disease, cyanotic and acyanotic. The cyanotic group have a blue color of the lips and nail beds, often die young, and have complex heart defects requiring early surgery to improve functional capacity and to extend life to vocational age. Acyanotic congenital heart disease is characterized by normal color of the skin and nail beds. The cardiac defects are less complex and more easily surgically corrected, resulting in excellent or even normal life expectancy and work outlook.

CARDIAC DISEASE IN GENERAL

Functional Disabilities

The client with cardiac disease whose condition is adequately controlled from a functional and symptomatic standpoint will not have performance impairment that will prevent him from handling various community environments. Specifically, there should be little, if any, impairment in ambulation and no impairment in eating, dressing, personal hygiene, or communication skills. In contrast to many disabled persons, the client with cardiovascular disease has a hidden disability, invisible to others. The hidden disability may pose problems for the client when performance expectations are high but cannot be met. Misunderstandings on the part of the supervisors, employers, neighbors, or family members are inevitable. These hidden disabilities in heart disease are those related to heart failure, pain, abnormalities of heart rhythm (cardiac arrhythmia), and psychosocial impairments.

Heart failure. One of the major causes of disability is heart failure, which is simply the inability of the heart to pump its blood adequately. This may occur in any form of heart disease. The reduction in the amount of blood pumped (cardiac output) produces symptoms of fatigue, lethargy, weakness, apathy, poor memory, and depression. The backing up of the blood and the resultant congestion of the lung produces the symptoms of an inability to lie flat because of shortness of breath, shortness of breath at rest or with exertion, sudden awakening in the middle of the night because of shortness of breath (paroxysmal nocturnal dyspnea), and cough. Heart failure is discussed in more detail on pages 303-304.

Pain. The major source of pain in cardiac disease is the heart. The usual cause of heart pain is an inadequate supply of oxygen to a portion of the heart muscle. When this occurs, the client experiences a discomfort in the chest called *angina pectoris*. This is usually located behind the breastbone and is described as a sensation of pressure, weight, tightness, constriction, or heaviness. It often radiates down the inner aspect of the left and/or right arm and through to the back or upward toward the jaw. Angina may be associated with shortness of breath, nausea, vomiting, and a cold, clammy sweat. Common precipitants include physical exertion, abnormalities of heart rhythm, cigarette smoking, exposure to cold air, and emotional upset.

Angina represents a transient imbalance between the oxygen supply to the heart and the demands of the heart muscle for oxygen. With an attack of angina, there is no damage to heart muscle and the client should be able to continue with usual activities after the pain has gone. Angina is commonly relieved by avoiding the factor which precipitated the pain and by taking nitroglycerine.

On occasion, the blood and oxygen supply to a portion of the heart muscle becomes so compromised or is lacking altogether that a segment of heart muscle dies. This is the process of *infarction* or *heart attack*. The pain of a heart attack is similar to that of angina pectoris, but it is much more severe.

From a vocational point of view, the most important pain is angina pectoris. It is the responsibility of the counselor, physician, and client to optimize the work environment by limiting or avoiding the particular activities that precipitate the individual client's angina.

Cardiac arrhythmia. Abnormalities of heart rhythm may decrease the total amount of blood that the heart pumps each minute, which in turn decreases the blood supply to any of the body's organs. As a result, many symptoms may occur, some of which are not obviously associated with the heart. Arrhythmias may be precipitated by exertion, emotional upset, certain medications, or by the underlying disease. Symptoms that may be associated with an abnormality of heart rhythm include palpitations, angina pectoris, heart failure, and neurologic symptoms.

Palpitation, an awareness of the heart beat, is experienced by fewer than 50 percent of clients with cardiac arrhythmias. However, palpitations remain an important symptom for treatment planning for those who can appreciate changes in their heart rhythm.

Angina pectoris can occur when the arrhythmia causes an inadequate flow of blood through the coronary arteries to the heart muscle, allowing the oxygen demand of the heart to exceed the oxygen supply.

Neurologic symptoms caused by the arrhythmias include faintness, fainting spells, focal or diffuse transient muscular weakness, and visual and speech difficulties.

Psychosocial impairments. Most of the major cardiac illnesses carry the threat of sudden death. The client lives with the knowledge that death can occur without warning at work, play, or rest. Fortunately, this knowledge does not usually cause disabling emotional problems. Most cardiacs are able to accept the threats of the illness and deal with them constructively. However, some degree of emotional upset and psychosocial impairment commonly occurs and must be dealt with in order to optimize the vocational as well as the medical outcome.

Emotional disability is particularly prevalent during and following an acute cardiac illness, especially heart attack. Approximately two-thirds of such individuals will have some disturbing emotional response, most commonly anxiety and/or depression. To some extent, the magnitude of the emotional response is a function of the client's personality. The person who was chronically dissatisfied, chronically depressed, hypochrondriacal, or hard-driving, time-conscious, and deadline- and goal-oriented is more apt to respond with a significant and possibly disabling degree of anxiety and/or depression. Although these personality types are often present, it should not be assumed that personality patterns are always the cause of persistent anxiety or depression following an acute cardiac illness. The response may indeed be due to real environmental problems. For example, the client may have substantial social or financial commitments and his ability to meet them may be severely compromised by his illness. When environmental causes are suspected, proper questioning by the counselor may uncover them. Referral to appropriate individuals or agencies can then be arranged, thus minimizing a substantial source of disability.

Regardless of personality type, being given a diagnosis of cardiac disease is often a crisis event and as such threatens many aspects of the client's life: job, income, pleasures, family, community ties, health, and, of course, life itself. The resultant fears can be very real.

In addition to fear, anxiety, and depression, another potential response to cardiac disease is denial. The client may deny the presence of illness, the importance of symptoms associated with the illness, or the existence of any resultant physical incapacity. Many rehabilitation workers have difficulty accepting denial as a client's defense mechanism, feeling that it reflects unrealistic expectations and a lack of understanding or adaptation to the limitations of the disease. On the other hand, denial may be an effective mechanism which helps the patient to cope with the stress of the illness and thereby reduce anxiety, deter depression, and control fear.

Response to an acute cardiac illness can be classified as aggressive, constructive, or regressive. This classification is particularly useful in assessing rehabilitation potential.

An *aggressive response* is characterized by a major amount of denial regarding the illness. These clients often tend to deny being ill or disabled in any respect. They will not be fearful, anxious, or depressed, and as long as there are not substantial complications of the illness, they will return to work at the earliest possible moment. Because of their degree of denial, they commonly do not follow medical advice and do not participate in their own care very well. They do not modify their activities, diet, smoking habits, body weight, and medications as may be recommended. Therefore, while their rehabilitation is quick, it tends to be frail and short-lived.

A *constructive response* is characterized by a realistic attitude toward the illness, its natural history, and what must be done to optimize short- and long-term health and vocational goals. These clients effectively "work through" the fear, anxiety, and depression associated with an acute illness, participate in their own care, follow instructions carefully, and generally do quite well.

A *regressive response* is characterized by an inability to cope with the realities of the disease. These clients become so distraught with the situation that even though they may be functionally capable of leading comfortable, productive lives, they are not emotionally able to do so. The rehabilitation potential for these individuals initially is poor. They form the core of the counselor's most difficult, challenging, and perhaps least successful efforts.

Rehabilitation potential. Generally, the natural history of cardiac disease is such that once the condition is stabilized, long-term vocational goals can be considered. The decline in functional capacity of cardiac patients is usually quite slow and can often be modified by properly timed surgery and adjustments of medications. Deviations from this general expectation of rehabilitation potential are reviewed in relation to the specific cardiac diseases.

Standards of Evaluation

A full understanding of the client and his rehabilitation potential requires that the counselor have access to and understand the meaning of certain basic medical information. This includes a complete *medical history* which contains the diagnosis, complications, medications, surgical procedures performed, and a comment regarding whether the illness is stable or unstable. A careful *physical examination* covering the heart, lungs, and peripheral vessels including both arteries and veins must be recorded. An *electrocardiogram (ECG)* and *chest X-ray* complete the basic minimum evaluation which should be performed by a cardiologist or an internist with special training in heart disease.

The ECG can indicate abnormalities of heart rhythm and provide evidence of heart damage, drug effects, or inadequate oxygen supply to a portion of the heart muscle. The chest X-ray may show evidence of pulmonary vascular congestion, dilatation and/or hypertrophy of any of the heart's chambers, primary lung disease, or fluid in the breathing spaces of the lung.

In many patients with cardiovascular disease, an *exercise stress test* should be performed in order to assess their functional capacity and provide a rational basis for activity counseling for work, play, and reconditioning. The exercise test has become an important clinical tool and its use is now widespread in cardiac rehabilitation as the single most important procedure available to assist in writing an individualized activity prescription. The counselor can use the information from the stress test to properly assess the client and his place in the world of work. The test, in particular, should be requested whenever a major job change is anticipated and before the client returns to work after an acute cardiac illness.

The test can be performed using either a bicycle ergometer or a motor-driven treadmill. It consists of several stages, each successively requiring increased work by the heart. The test is individualized and designed in such a way that a reasonable estimate of the energy required is known for each stage of the test.

The customary way to estimate energy cost of activities is to estimate the oxygen consumption required to accomplish a task. The basic metabolic unit for this estimation is called the MET. One MET is the amount of oxygen required by a person who is seated at rest doing nothing with either arms or legs. This amount is approximately 3.5 cc per kilogram of body weight per minute (cc/kg/min). Stages of the exercise test and many vocational, recreation, and reconditioning activities have been classified in terms of how many MET's, or multiples of the basic oxygen consumption at rest, are required.

There is no uniformly accepted method of performing a stress test, although in the United States almost all physicians utilize the treadmill. The amount of work done by the heart and the oxygen consumed when a person walks on a treadmill depends on the speed of walking and the "uphill grade" angle or the tilt of the treadmill. Each stage may require an increase in grade angle, an increase in speed, or both. The number of MET's required for each stage of any one test is known. The counselor can therefore learn the exercise level, and hence the job activity level, his client can achieve.

The exercise stress test should only be done with a physician present. Usually the patient is connected to an ECG machine while performing the test, and pulse rate and blood pressure are also monitored. Each stage of the test lasts 2 to 3 minutes and each subsequent stage immediately follows the previous one. The testing is stopped when the patient no longer is able to keep up with the treadmill or develops chest pain, or when the physician decides the ECG, pulse rate, and blood pressure levels suggest that too much work is being done.

Table 22-1 lists seven different stress test protocols in current use. The miles per hour and kilometers per hour speed and the grade angle for each stage of each test are given. Also contained in the table is the number of MET's each stage of each test requires. Thus, for example, a person who completes the last stage of the Bruce test (4.2 mi/h or 6.8 km/h at 16 degrees) can do activities that require 14 MET's. One who can achieve the fourth stage of the Naughton test (2.0 mi/h or 3.2 km/h at 10.5 degrees) can perform at the level of 5 MET's. Finally, table 22-1 also shows the equivalency of number of MET's with the Functional Classification of Cardiac Disease developed by the New York Heart Association. This functional classification, which is also in widespread use, is further described in table 22-2.

If a stress test device is not available to the attending physician or medical consultant, an estimate of the client's functional capacity can be made by the physician from the history, using the functional classification. It is important to emphasize that the functional capacity assessment is in terms of the *client's* usual level of activity, not that of the person making the assessment. "Ordinary" activity for the client should be assessed, keeping in mind that what is ordinary for one person may not be ordinary for another. It is best, of course, to have some objective

information regarding a client's functional capacity obtained from the stress test, but in the absence of objective guidelines, this subjective assessment should be made.

The counselor's procedure for using the results from the stress test for vocational counseling is quite simple. The test should indicate the highest heart rate that was safe for activity (clearance heart rate). If the clearance heart rate is not expressly stated on the report, the physician should be able to give the counselor this information. At the clearance heart rate, there was no angina pectoris, the ECG was normal, the blood pressure response was acceptable, and there were no heart rhythm abnormalities. Eighty-five percent of this heart rate is then calculated to provide a 15 percent safety margin. The stage at which the calculated heart rate occurred determines the MET level at which the client can safely perform. Table 22-3 lists the MET level requirement for a host of occupational and recreational activities. The counselor and client can both consult this table to determine what can be safely accomplished.

There are some potential limitations in transferring data from the exercise laboratory into the "real world." Such factors as emotional stress, work environment, and basic personality characteristics may require a scaling down of the level derived from the exercise data.

Emotional stress may be precipitated by dislike for the job, inability to get along with colleagues, a high level of job pressure and many deadlines to be met, an unpleasant work environment, and unfavorable attitude toward workers with disability, to name a few.

Work environment factors to consider include: temperature extremes which increase cardiac work and should be minimized or avoided; air quality, particularly if carbon monoxide is present, as it decreases the amount of oxygen available in the blood; and inclines to be negotiated, such as ladders, ramps, and steps, as they increase the cardiac work load.

Personality characteristics should also be considered. The client with an aggressive, attacking response may require a scaling down of the exercise test results, for such persons are inclined to expend more than the average number of MET's usually required to accomplish a specific task.

As part of the basic evaluation, many clients will have had *cardiac catheterization,* which provides the most definitive "hard" information about the heart's anatomy, heart function, and pressures within the heart chambers and vessels. This information is useful to improve the assessment of the client's prognosis, to decide on the proper form of therapy (medical or surgical), and to define the anatomy a surgeon would encounter should surgical therapy be selected.

In some clients, especially those in whom an abnormality of heart rhythm is suspected, a *continuous electrocardiogram* recording (Holter monitor) during

TABLE 22-1

COMMONLY USED TREADMILL EXERCISE PROTOCOLS

NO OF STAGES	Exercise Test	1	2	3	4	5	6	7	8	9	10	11	12	13	14	15
								MET's								
4	Speed mi/h (km/h)		1.6 (2.6)	1.6 (2.6)	1.6 (2.6)	1.6 (2.6)										
	Grade (degrees)		1.5	5.5	10	14										
7	Speed mi/h (km/h)		2.0 (3.2)	2.0 (3.2)	2.0 (3.2)	2.0 (3.2)	2.0 (3.2)	2.0 (3.2)	2.0 (3.2)							
	Grade (degrees) (Naughton)		0	3.5	7	10.5	14	17.5	21							
8	Speed mi/h (km/h)			2.5 (4.0)	2.5 (4.0)	2.5 (4.0)	2.5 (4.0)	2.5 (4.0)	2.5 (4.0)	2.5 (4.0)	2.5 (4.0)					
	Grade (degrees)			1.5	4.5	7.5	10.5	13.5	16.5	19.5	22.5					
10	Speed mi/h (km/h)			3.0 (4.8)	3.0 (4.8)	3.0 (4.8)	3.0 (4.8)	3.0 (4.8)	3.0 (4.8)	3.0 (4.8)	3.0 (4.8)	3.0 (4.8)	3.0 (4.8)			
	Grade (degrees) (Balke)			0	2.5	5	7.5	10	12.5	15	17.5	20	22.5			
11	Speed mi/h (km/h)				3.4 (5.4)	3.4 (5.4)	3.4 (5.4)	3.4 (5.4)	3.4 (5.4)	3.4 (5.4)	3.4 (5.4)	3.4 (5.4)	3.4 (5.4)	3.4 (5.4)	3.4 (5.4)	
	Grade (degrees)				2	4	6	8	10	12	14	16	18	20	22	
10	Speed mi/h (km/h)						3.75 (6.0)	3.75 (6.0)	3.75 (6.0)	3.75 (6.0)	3.75 (6.0)	3.75 (6.0)	3.75 (6.0)	3.75 (6.0)	3.75 (6.0)	3.75 (6.0)
	Grade (degrees) (Super Balke)						4	6	8	10	12	14	16	18	20	22
4	Speed mi/h (km/h)					1.7 (2.7)		2.5 (4.0)			3.4 (5.4)			4.2 (6.7)		
	Grade (degrees) (Bruce)					10		12			14			16		
			IV	III		II						I				

Functional Classification (New York Heart Association)

TABLE 22-2

FUNCTIONAL CLASSIFICATION OF HEART DISEASE CLIENTS AND CORRESPONDING ENERGY LEVEL
WHICH CAN USUALLY BE COMFORTABLY ACCOMPLISHED

Functional Class	Activity Limitation	MET's
I	No limitations; no symptoms with ordinary activity	7 & >
II	Slight limitation; comfortable at rest; symptoms with ordinary activity	5–6
III	Marked limitation; comfortable at rest; symptoms with less than ordinary activity	3–4
IV	Discomfort with any activity; may have symptoms at rest	1–2

SOURCE: New York Heart Association

normal work activities is useful. To accomplish this, the client has three or five electrodes attached to the chest. These electrodes are in turn connected to a small portable tape recorder which the client wears over the shoulder or around the waist. Study of the tape recording permits assessment of arrhythmias and other ECG changes for an improved understanding of the heart's response to specific vocational tasks and situations. This objective evaluation obtained under actual working conditions can be of great help to the counselor, the client, and the cardiologist.

In order to help the counselor obtain the necessary basic medical information about his cardiac client, a cardiac referral form (table 22-4) was developed at the University of Colorado Medical Center. The form has the advantages of brevity, yet the basic information required to make vocational decisions is present. The counselor can initiate the use of this form by sending it with a cover letter to the patient's physician or the VR medical consultant.

Total Treatment

Optimal treatment for clients with cardiovascular disease requires regular medical followup evaluation to detect changes in functional capacity and evidence of progression of the disease. The re-evaluations also allow for medication alterations to optimize function, decisions for surgery, if indicated, and making appropriate allied health referrals. The common drugs used in cardiac disease with their actions and common side effects are listed in table 22-5. Specific surgical procedures available to the patient with cardiac disease differ depending upon the specific disease.

For many clients, consultation with one or more allied health professionals may be helpful in ensuring a good vocational outcome. When the psychological responses of fear, anxiety, and depression are prolonged and affect normal day-to-day function, consultation with a clinical psychologist or psychiatrist may be helpful and necessary. An occupational therapist may be consulted to provide work-simplification techniques, both for home and for the job. The physical therapist may assist with the reconditioning program and provide specific exercises for improvement of joint mobility and specific muscle-group strength. The medical social worker may be very helpful to the client in solving acute social problems. A health educator in conjunction with the client's physician may prescribe and supervise a physical reconditioning program which improves functional capacity and endurance. Clients who are obese, diabetic, or have abnormalities of blood fats will benefit from consultation with a clinical nutritionist.

As long as the cardiac client remains stable, followup medical visits are scheduled every 6 to 12 months. Each visit includes a thorough cardiovascular history and physical examination and often an ECG, chest X-ray, and exercise stress test. In addition, the client is questioned for indications of nonmedical sources of disability (i.e., psychosocial and vocational problems) and appropriate referrals are arranged.

Vocational Implications

Since the sources of disability and effects of the disease on the body are much the same regardless of the cause of the cardiac problem, some broad generalizations can be made about specific aspects of work and the client with cardiac disease. The major areas to consider are educational requirements, aptitudes, interests, physical demands, and the environment in which the job is to be performed.

Education. Most clients with cardiac disease that is not accompanied by life-threatening complications (significant heart failure, life-threatening rhythm abnormalities, unstable chest pain) have a quite good long-range outlook. Therefore, if it appears that a change in vocation is necessary or desirable, long-term training plans can be made, including plans for completing a college education.

Aptitudes. Generally, the client with cardiac disease will have no changes in aptitudes and will not have disease-related impairments in intellect, learning

TABLE 22-3
APPROXIMATE ENERGY COST OF SOME COMMON VOCATIONAL AND RECREATIONAL ACTIVITIES

Sitting: light tasks (1.5 to 4.5 MET's)

Desk work, typing
Driving cars, trucks
Using hand tools, light assembly
Crane operation
Working levers
Playing cards, seated games
Machine sewing
Flying
Painting, recreational
Horseback riding, walk and trot
Golf cart, riding
Fishing from boat, seated
Riding mower

Standing: moderate tasks (2.5 to 5.5 MET's)

Standing quietly, working at own pace, light
    assembly or hand tools
Scrubbing, waxing, polishing
Assembly or repair of machine parts
Light welding, woodworking, interior carpentry
Power sanding
Stocking shelves
Light to medium assembly line work
Crank dollies, hitching trailers, operating large levers, jacks
Wiring house
Bricklaying, plastering, house painting, paperhanging
Hoeing, raking, weeding
Cleaning windows

Walking: light to moderate tasks (2.5 to 5.5 MET's)

Gas station attendant
Carrying trays, dishes, etc.
Walking to 4 mi/h (6.44 km/h) on level
Billiards, bowling
Fishing, bait casting and fly with waders
Shuffleboard
Volleyball, noncompetitive
Archery
Sail small boat
Dancing
Gardening
Golf
Tennis, doubles
Calisthenics
Making beds
Mowing lawns, cast or power unit
Table tennis

Standing and/or walking: heavy tasks (Average or range of MET's follows each task)	
Pushing or moving heavy objects— 75 lb (33.8 kg) or more, e.g., moving-van work	8.0
Cutting wood	
Power saw	2-4
Hand axe or saw	5-10
Digging, shoveling	4-8
Wheelbarrow	4-10
Plumbing	3-8
Snow shoveling	6-15
Lifting and carrying	
20-44 lb (9-19.8 kg)	4.5
45-64 lb (20.2-28.8 kg)	6.0
65-84 lb (29.3-37.8 kg)	7.5
85-100 lb (38.3-45 kg)	8.5
Pneumatic tool work	6.0
Skating, roller or ice	5-6
Badminton, competitive	5-7
Tennis, singles	6-9
Paddle ball, raquetball, squash, handball	7-15
Skiing	
Downhill	5-8
Cross-country	6-12
Water	5-7
Hunting	
Small game	3-7
Big game	3-14
Swimming	4-8
Jogging, running	7-15
Basketball	5-12

ability, verbal or numerical skills, form and space perception, eye-hand coordination, finger and hand dexterity, eye-hand-foot coordination, or color discrimination. Those aptitudes requiring physical stresses that exceed allowed limits should not be developed. The client with severe heart failure and a low cardiac output, and hence an inadequate blood supply to the brain, may have some difficulty in assimilating and retaining information, but these individuals are rarely candidates for vocational rehabilitation.

Interest. Cardiac disease does not usually modify the client's interest in work, play, home, or community activities. It is certainly desirable to encourage a full return to normal or customary aspects of living following resolution of an acute cardiac episode. Specific employment considerations, such as the need to deal with things and objects rather than people and ideas, personal interaction work as opposed to interaction with technical activities, organized activities versus

TABLE 22-4
UNIVERSITY OF COLORADO CARDIAC REFERRAL FORM FOR VOCATIONAL PLANNING

I.   Cardiovascular Data

    a. Specific diagnosis and dates of clinical events
    b. Pertinent history
    c. Physical findings and reports (BP, P, ECG, other lab)
    d. Medications
    e. Prognosis

II.   Functional Capacity

    a. Stress test results (if performed)
      Max HR and BP achieved
       % Estimated maximum HR achieved
      MET's
      Arrhythmias
      Symptoms
      Reasons for stopping
    b. Clearance MET level (MET's @85% of maximum tolerated or safe HR)
    c. Exercise prescription given
    d. Functional Classification

III.   Problem areas seen in relation to vocational planning

    a. Personality
    b. Psychosocial
    c. Physical

IV.   Vocational recommendations (Specific limitation, i.e., weight limits, hours, specific roles or
        tasks to be avoided, work environment, etc.)

    Date of release for work:

V.   Comments

abstract creative activities, prestige positions as opposed to production tasks, or working alone or in groups, are to a large extent not important considerations for the client with cardiac disease. Interest areas that require work loads exceeding a client's safe level should be discouraged.

As a rule, the client's response to stress and the amount and form of the stress on the job are key counseling considerations. Quite often, the cardiac client is a harddriving, deadline-oriented, competitive, and time-conscious individual who overcommits himself and is consequently anxious and frustrated. This type of personality, often called the *Type A behavior pattern*, is difficult to modify or control and requires a job situation that minimizes deadlines and quotas. The counselor may find it useful to visit the job site to observe the client at work to determine whether job modifications or a reduced activity prescription are required.

Physical demands. Before making some generalizations about the cardiac client and the physical demands of work, it is helpful to understand how the heart responds to different forms of muscular activity. Some activities may have to be avoided or their duration minimized to prevent a potential harmful response. The counselor should be able to identify the form of muscular exercise involved in various job tasks. He can then assist the client in minimizing those which cause symptoms or which are potentially dangerous. The three major forms of muscular activity to be aware of are aerobic, isometric, and isotonic exercise. Each produces a special cardiac response.

Aerobic exercise includes movements which are continuous and rhythmic. Common examples include walking, jogging, cycling, and swimming. These activities are performed with a consumption of increased amounts of oxygen. Individuals vary in their ability to take in and utilize oxygen, and each person has an individual maximum oxygen consumption capability.

In addition to increasing oxygen consumption, the heart rate increases to a maximal plateau that is related to age (i.e., maximum heart rate capability decreases with advancing age). Further, the systolic blood pressure (see chap. 3) increases with aerobic exercise, while usually the diastolic pressure remains the same or falls slightly. The cardiac output, the amount of blood the heart pumps in a minute of time, increases substantially as a result.

Aerobic exercise is the only form of exertion for which there is any evidence of a beneficial effect in patients with cardiac disease, especially those with coronary artery disease. Jobs which include aerobic

TABLE 22-5
SOME COMMON CARDIOVASCULAR DRUGS AND POTENTIAL SIDE EFFECTS

Drug	Purpose	Side Effects
Aldactazide	Antihypertensive diuretic	Drowsiness, nausea, vomiting, diarrhea, weakness, rash
Aldactone	Antihypertensive diuretic	Drowsiness, diarrhea, rash, impotence
Aldomet	Antihypertensive	Drowsiness, nausea, headache, weakness, vomiting
Aldoril	Antihypertensive	Drowsiness, rash, weakness, diarrhea
Apresoline	Antihypertensive vasodilator	Headache, vomiting, palpitations, diarrhea
Atromids	Lipid lowering agent	Nausea, vomiting, headache, fatigue
Cardilate	Vasodilator antianginal	Headache (usually temporary)
Chlorothiazide	Antihypertensive diuretic	Nausea, diarrhea, weakness, rash, dizziness
Coumadin	Anticoagulant	Excessive bleeding
Digitoxin	Digitalis preparation cardiotonic	Nausea, vomiting, arrhythmias
Digoxin	Digitalis preparation cardiotonic	Nausea, vomiting, arrhythmias
Diupres	Antihypertensive diuretic	Nausea, diarrhea, weakness, dizziness, rash, sedation, nasal stuffiness
Diurll	Antihypertensive diuretic	Rash, weakness, nausea, diarrhea, dizziness
Dyazide	Antihypertensive diuretic	Nausea, diarrhea, rash, dizziness, weakness, muscle cramps, dry mouth
Dyrenium	Diuretic	Nausea, diarrhea, weakness, headache
Esidrix	Antihypertensive diuretic	Rash, weakness, nausea, diarrhea, dizziness
Inderal	Antiarrhythmic antianginal antihypertensive	Fatigue, weakness, nausea, abdominal cramps, intensify asthma and heart failure
Isodordil	Vasodilator antianginal	Headache, flushing, dizziness, weakness, rash
Lanoxin	Digitalis preparation cardiotonic	Nausea, vomiting, arrhythmias
Lasix	Antihypertensive diuretic	Weakness, rash, nausea, diarrhea
Nitrobid	Vasodilator antianginal	Headache, flushing, lightheadedness, weakness
Nitroglycerine	Vasodilator antianginal	Headache, lightheadedness, flushing, weakness (transient)

TABLE 22-5 Continued

Drug	Purpose	Side Effects
Nitrol Paste	Vasodilator antianginal	Headache, flushing, lightheadedness, weakness
Norpace	Antiarrhythmic	Dry mouth, difficulty urinating
Peritrate	Vasodilator antianginal	Rash, headache, nausea
Quinaglute	Antiarrhythmic	Nausea, vomiting, ringing in ears, vertigo, visual disturbances
Quinidine	Antiarrhythmic	Nausea, vomiting, ringing in ears, vertigo, visual discrimination
Serpasil	Antihypertensive	Nausea, vomiting, diarrhea, rash, drowiness, stuffy nose

activity are particularly advantageous and should be encouraged.

Isometric exercise is muscular activity against a fixed, unmoving resistance. Hence there is minimal arm or leg movement even though muscles are contracting. It is sometimes termed static exercise. Common examples include the Charles Atlas dynamic tension program, exercise with the Bullworker device, doorway or desk exercise, working with the arms over the head (shoulder muscle isometrics), and carrying a bucket or suitcase (forearm isometrics).

The response of the cardiovascular system to isometric exercise is quite different from the response to aerobic stress. In isometric exercise, there is very little increase in heart rate, cardiac output, or oxygen consumed, but there is a very large increase in both systolic and diastolic blood pressure readings. This hypertensive response to isometric exercise is rapid in onset and is independent of the amount of muscle involved in the isometric stress. That is, the hypertensive response is just as strong with static exercise of the small forearm muscle (as in a handgrip) as it is to static exercise of the large muscles of the leg. In order for the heart to generate these very high pressures, the tension in the wall of the left ventricle rises considerably and with it the demand of the heart muscle for oxygen. If the client has a compromised blood supply to the heart, usually because of atherosclerotic coronary heart disease, oxygen supply to the muscle may not meet the demand and angina pectoris results.

Isotonic exercise is characterized by activities which maintain the same tone in a muscle through a full or partial range of joint motion. The activities are generally rhythmic and motion is continuous. Isotonic exercise is common in vocational tasks. The cardiovascular response to isotonic exercise is related to the resistance provided by the object moved. If there is low resistance, then the response is similar to aerobic exercise. If resistance is high, then the response is more like isometric exercise, that is, blood pressure rises.

Many jobs require a combination of aerobic, isometric, and isotonic exercise. From the point of view of the cardiac client, isometric and intense isotonic exercise should be minimized or avoided, and the amount of time spent in aerobic or low-intensity isotonic exercise optimized. If the cardiac client is taught to recognize isometric exercise and to avoid it, quite heavy work can often be comfortably and safely performed. For example, picking up and carrying a 50 pound sack in the arms would, if the distance carried is great enough, produce a substantial rise in blood pressure. On the other hand, if the client were to pick up the sack and immediately place it on a cart, then push the cart to the destination, the isometric response could be avoided. If a cart is not available, the client can be instructed to carry the sack on his shoulder rather than in his arms, a technique which also minimizes the isometric element.

Jobs are often classified as sedentary, light, medium, and heavy. Some brief comments regarding these work levels, the physical demands of each, and the ability of the cardiac client to adjust to these categories follows. It should be remembered that the client's ability to tolerate any level of work may be dependent on identifying and minimizing isometric stress, optimizing aerobic and low-level isotonic activity, and improving the work setting through work-simplification techniques. Most cardiac clients who have had an acute event, such as a heart attack, will be able to return to the pre-event employment. However, approximately one-third of these clients must have some modification in the intensity of daily job activities. Consultation with the client's physician will suggest what activities need to be modified. The counselor can then evaluate the specific daily job activities to determine modifications that are both necessary and still compatible with the worker's responsibilities.

Sedentary work requires lifting a maximum of 10 pounds (4.5 kg) of weight and tolerating modest walking, standing, or sitting requirements. Even Functional Class IV clients (see table 22-2) can generally perform sedentary tasks.

Light work requires lifting up to 20 pounds (9 kg) and may require substantial walking or standing. Work of this intensity is usually not a problem for the cardiac client.

Medium work requires an ability to lift up to 50 pounds (22.5 kg) with a usual requirement of 25 pounds (11.3 kg) combined with substantial walking and standing activity. This level of work can be tolerated by many cardiac clients as long as the lifting is intermittent and does not require carrying the weight for more than a few feet.

Heavy work requires lifting a maximum of 100 pounds (45 kg) with a usual lifting requirement of 50 pounds (22.5 kg). This level of work may be tolerated by some cardiac clients, but not by most, and should therefore generally be discouraged. *Very heavy work*, requiring a lifting maximum of greater than 100 pounds (45 kg) and a usual carrying capacity of 50 pounds (22.5 kg) as a routine job activity, should be avoided.

Environment. The environment in which the cardiac client performs his work may greatly affect his ability to succeed at a particular job. Extremes of temperature are cardiovascular stresses and should be avoided. The cardiac client therefore usually performs better at indoor work. Also, an environment with a high carbon monoxide level in the air should also be avoided because of the adverse effect on oxygen transport to the tissues. Most cardiac clients do not require a sheltered environment and are capable of working well in a competitive employment situation.

CORONARY HEART DISEASE

Disease Description

Coronary heart disease is the most prevalent and costly illness in the United States. Its exact cause is unknown, but several predisposing factors have been identified. The most important of these are a high level of cholesterol in the blood, hypertension, and cigarette smoking. Other risk factors include advancing age, male sex, physical inactivity, a Type A personality, obesity, high blood triglycerides (another fat element in the blood), diabetes, and a diet high in calories, fat, and refined sugars. In younger age groups, men are more apt to have coronary heart disease, and a family history of the disease is quite common.

Whatever the precise cause, the end result is the laying down of fatty material in the wall of a coronary artery. The process ultimately narrows the artery to such an extent that the oxygen demands of the heart muscle served by the artery cannot be met. When this occurs, the client experiences angina pectoris.

Angina pectoris is commonly relieved by rest and by nitroglycerine. Angina is transient, does not represent death of heart tissue, and hence is not a heart attack.

When a heart attack (*myocardial infarction*) occurs, the oxygen supply to a portion of heart muscle is completely interrupted and that portion of muscle dies. The pain of a heart attack is similar to that of angina pectoris but is much more severe. It is not relieved by nitroglycerine or rest and usually requires narcotics for relief. Other complications of coronary heart disease include sudden death, heart failure (see section below), and arrhythmias, in addition to angina pectoris and myocardial infarction.

Coronary heart disease often begins very early in life. Some early evidence of the disease has even been found in the arteries of infants. There is a long "incubation period" before the disease becomes obvious, usually in the fifth decade or later. However, coronary disease and heart attacks occur also in clients in their thirties and even twenties.

Once the diagnosis of coronary heart disease has been made, it can be assumed that the disease will be progressive, although the rate of progression may vary from client to client. If the only manifestation of the disease is angina pectoris, the average mortality is approximately 4 percent per year, and the average life expectancy from time of diagnosis is approximately 10 years.

The life expectancy of a client who has had a heart attack depends on the age of the client at the time of the heart attack and whether it was complicated by heart failure or life-threatening heart rhythm problems. In addition, the number of coronary arteries affected by the disease influences the outlook or prognosis for the client. This information is best obtained at cardiac catheterization.

Generally, the patient with stable coronary heart disease will have a slowly progressive course and may spend many years without symptoms or with stable symptoms. With proper management, angina pectoris and the symptoms associated with heart failure and arrhythmias may improve or be eliminated.

Functional Disabilities

Physical disabilities. The client with coronary heart disease may have no physical impairment, or he may be limited by exercise-induced angina pectoris, symptoms of heart failure (see below), or symptoms due to arrhythmias. Ambulation is limited only by the potential development of symptoms. All activities of daily living are usually comfortably performed and there are no limits regarding transportation or communication skills.

Psychosocial disabilities. The client with coronary heart disease must adjust to the reality that his illness is life threatening. As such, the diagnosis of coronary heart disease constitutes a crisis event in the client's life which threatens work, income, role at home and in the community, pleasures of all types, health, and longevity. Two-thirds of the clients who have had a heart attack will have some obvious degree of anxiety or depression. Fortunately for most clients, these responses are transient and there is no permanent effect on psychological or social functions. Family anxieties may also occur. They may contribute to less than optimum performance by the client and add to the stress factor.

Rehabilitation potential. The client's physician will generally be able to provide information regarding appropriate vocational goals. If the condition seems to be rapidly progressive and unstable, short-term (3 to 6 month) vocational goals are appropriate. On the other hand, if the condition is stable and uncomplicated, long-term goals (up to several years) can be identified. Training programs for the client with coronary heart disease should emphasize vocations that are not physically demanding so that possible progression of the disease and the development of new symptoms is less apt to compromise job performance and require retraining.

All comments made for cardiac disease in general with regard to standards of evaluation apply to the client with coronary heart disease.

Total Treatment

Optimum management of coronary heart disease includes identification and, if possible, modification of risk factors, medication to relieve symptoms, effective management of complications, and, when indicated, cardiac surgery.

Not all coronary heart disease risk factors can be modified. However, several of the more important factors can be detected and their impact on the natural history of the disease altered. Included in this group are cigarette smoking, hypertension, high blood cholesterol and triglyceride, physical inactivity, and obesity. In some clients with a Type A personality, behavior modification training may improve the stress response. Counseling and education of the patient's spouse to allay anxiety and promote active participation in the client's rehabilitation is also helpful.

Drugs used to manage angina pectoris include nitrates, both long- and short-acting, and a sympathetic nervous system blocker, propranolol (Inderal). The most commonly used short-acting nitrate is nitroglycerine, a small white pill which is dissolved under the tongue. It provides relief from angina pectoris in from 30 seconds to 3 minutes. In addition, nitroglycerine may be used prophylactically before an activity the client expects will produce angina. Nitroglycerine may cause side effects which some clients find disturbing. These include a feeling of warmth and flushing, an increase in heart rate, a pounding headache, and occasionally weakness and lightheadedness due to a drop in blood pressure.

Several long-acting nitrate preparations which are used to prevent attacks of angina work in much the same way as nitroglycerine. These preparations may be taken in one of a variety of ways: dissolved under the tongue, chewed, swallowed, or applied as a paste to the skin. They are all useful in preventing attacks of angina, especially when taken in combination with propranolol. When a combination of maximally tolerated doses of one of the long-acting nitrates and propranolol fails to provide adequate relief from angina pectoris, then coronary arteriography to determine the anatomy of the coronary arteries is indicated.

If coronary arteriography shows a localized narrowing, coronary artery bypass surgery is indicated. In this operation, a vein graft is used to bypass the obstruction. The surgery has been successful in relieving angina pectoris and permitting a return to a more normal level of activity for both work and play. It is yet uncertain whether coronary artery bypass surgery actually prolongs life.

Once the client's condition has stabilized, follow-up evaluations are usually scheduled at intervals from 3 months to 1 year. The appearance of symptoms suggesting heart failure, uncontrolled arrhythmias, or unstable angina pectoris are indications for an immediate re-evaluation.

Vocational Implications

Between 70 and 90 percent of clients who have had a heart attack are able to return to work, usually to the jobs they held prior to the attack. Of these, one-third will require some modification of the job tasks, such as less lifting or carrying and avoidance of emotionally stressful situations. Most clients following heart attack will be able to perform sedentary, light, and medium work in an environment where extremes of temperature are avoided. Specific vocational guidelines can best be reached by a coordinated plan developed by the rehabilitation counselor and the client's physician.

All the issues discussed earlier with regard to stress testing and the vocational implications of cardiac disease in general apply.

RHEUMATIC HEART DISEASE

Disease Description

Rheumatic heart disease appears in both acute and chronic forms. The acute form is seen only occasionally in adults. The acute disease (rheumatic fever) usually occurs between the ages of 7 and 12 and is caused by a reaction to one of the streptococcal bacteria. Main features of the acute illness include cardiac involvement which may affect the heart muscle, valves, and/or pericardium. Arthritis, skin rash, nodules under the skin, and involuntary motions of the extremities (chorea) may also appear. Acute rheumatic fever has a strong tendency to recur. Because it is not commonly seen in adults, it is not a major issue for the counselor and will not be discussed further.

Chronic rheumatic heart disease is of greater concern to the counselor. It characteristically follows the acute stage by one or more decades. Interestingly, at least half of the clients with chronic rheumatic heart disease will not recall or have knowledge of an episode of acute rheumatic fever. The major problem of chronic rheumatic heart disease is scarring of the heart valves (see chap. 3), resulting in narrowing of the valve opening (stenosis) and/or incompetent closure of the valve (insufficiency, regurgitation).

Stenosis of a valve creates resistance to emptying of the chamber behind the valve, causing the blood pressure to rise in order to pump enough blood through the smaller hole. Insufficiency increases the volume of blood which the chamber must pump since some of it gets pumped back through the valve that fails to close. The load imposed on the heart is therefore either a volume or a pressure load, which the heart can usually tolerate for many years by employing the mechanism of dilatation of the chambers and hypertrophy of the walls. The major valve problems resulting from chronic rheumatic heart disease are called mitral stenosis, mitral regurgitation, aortic stenosis, and aortic regurgitation. The tricuspid valve is occasionally affected and the pulmonary valve is rarely involved (see chap. 3).

Mitral valve stenosis occurs mainly in females and symptoms begin in the third to fourth decade of life. Symptoms of pulmonary vascular congestion occur because the obstruction causes blood to be backed up in the left atrium, pulmonary veins, and the lung. The main form of therapy for mitral stenosis is to surgically open the scarred valve, a procedure termed mitral commissurotomy. This operation may be repeated one or more times. The vocational outlook is quite good for the client with mitral stenosis, although the valve has a tendency to narrow again. Complications of mitral stenosis include abnormalities of heart rhythm, symptoms of both low cardiac output and pulmonary vascular congestion,

right ventricular heart failure, and formation of clots within the enlarged left atrium. Clots can break off and be discharged into the general circulation. These systemic emboli may lodge in the brain and cause stroke (see chap. 9), in the extremities and lead to amputation (see chap. 13), or in other body organs, particularly the kidney.

Mitral regurgitation permits the left ventricle to eject some blood back into the left atrium as well as forward into the systemic circulation through the aorta in the usual way. This places a volume load on both the left atrium and left ventricle. The client with mitral regurgitation usually has symptoms of heart failure which develop secondary to the regurgitation. Treatment of mitral insufficiency often ultimately requires surgical replacement of the mitral valve with a prosthetic valve.

Aortic stenosis places a pressure load on the left ventricle. Clients with aortic stenosis have symptoms of pulmonary vascular congestion, low cardiac output, fainting spells or near fainting spells, and occasionally angina pectoris when the stenosis becomes severe. Treatment of severe aortic stenosis is replacement of the aortic valve with a prosthetic valve.

Aortic regurgitation places a volume load on the left ventricle and the client has symptoms of pump failure. Treatment of severe aortic regurgitation is also prosthetic aortic valve replacement.

A heart valve scarred by rheumatic fever and an artificial valve are both subject to bacterial infection (bacterial endocarditis), a dangerous and life-threatening complication which is often insidious in onset.

Functional Disabilities

There are usually no physical impairments in the client with chronic rheumatic heart disease. The client can usually ambulate and accomplish ordinary personal care skills without problems. Similarly, there is no difficulty with communication or transportation. Valvular defects can, however, reach a point where exercise and activity tolerance levels are reduced. Psychosocial impairments do not usually result from chronic rheumatic heart disease because its slow development allows for continuous adaptation.

The counselor can usually set long-term vocational goals with the client. If there is a doubt about rehabilitation goals, the client's physician can indicate the appropriate timing based on anticipated course of the disease. Functional and vocational limitations of these clients can usually be delayed or reversed by surgical therapy.

Standards of Evaluation

The client with chronic rheumatic heart disease

must have regular medical followup visits to determine if there has been any progression, to adjust medical therapy, and to determine the best time to consider surgical therapy. Once surgery has been performed, the client will need regular visits to check on the level of anticoagulation of the blood, since most clients with a heart valve prosthesis must be on anticoagulants indefinitely. Anticoagulants inhibit clot formation on the artificial valve. In addition, functional capacity assessment and clinical evaluations to ensure proper functioning of the prosthesis are important. These visits will be scheduled every 6 to 12 months. Usual cardiovascular evaluation procedures, including ECG, chest X-ray, echocardiogram, and, on occasion, an exercise stress test are appropriate periodic tests. Cardiac catheterization is necessary when the physician needs to have direct evaluation of pressures and blood flow. These data help in making proper decisions regarding surgery.

There are no specific allied health professionals of special importance to these clients. The occupational therapist may help to ensure shop and home safety for the client whose blood cannot clot normally because he is on anticoagulants. This will minimize the likelihood of trauma and excessive bleeding.

Total Treatment

All persons with known rheumatic heart disease will be on continual prophylactic antibiotics, usually penicillin, for a variable period of time into the adult years. Drugs used in chronic rheumatic heart disease are the usual cardiac preparations and are given for the usual indications (see table 22-5). Many clients will be maintained on few or no drugs for many years. Others will have gradual progression of their valvular disease and will require cardiac surgery, either valve replacement or opening of a stenotic valve. The cardiologist and surgeon must decide on the best time for surgical therapy. If surgery is performed before there is much damage to the heart muscle, then hypertrophy and dilatation can be be largely reversed and the outlook for the client is good.

Almost all clients will take anticoagulant medication every day following replacement of a heart valve. This will require regular laboratory evaluation (at least weekly) to make sure that the level of anticoagulant is appropriate. Further, since individuals with rheumatic heart disease are susceptible to bacterial endocarditis, they all need antibiotic coverage before, during, and for a short time after dental manipulations and surgery or instrumentation on the genitourinary and lower gastrointestinal tract.

Medical followup evaluations are characteristically scheduled every 6 months to 1 year. Bacterial endocarditis must be sought at each followup visit.

Vocational Implications

The client with chronic rheumatic heart disease usually has no change in education, interest, or aptitude aspects of work. If the client is on anticoagulants, both he and the counselor must be aware of the necessity of avoiding trauma. The physical demands of work that can be met by a client with chronic rheumatic heart disease are largely a function of how well the pump can fucntion both before and after surgery. Clients who have had successful surgery can generally handle medium work and are often not limited by heavy work. There are no limitations on the type of motions involved (e.g., climbing and stooping) except for the occasional client who has residual discomfort at the site of a chest incision.

When dealing with the young client, the counselor should consult with the physician to determine whether functional deterioration over the next 10 to 15 years is expected. If it is, occasional rehabilitation planning that anticipates this deterioration may prevent the necessity for job change when it occurs.

HYPERTENSION

Disease Description

High blood pressure is one of the major medical problems in the United States. It is estimated that there are 25 million individuals with hypertension. It strikes all ages and both sexes, although blacks are more commonly affected than whites. Hypertension usually begins in adulthood and is detected at a routine medical evaluation. Patients with signficant high blood pressure are commonly asymptomatic until other organs become involved.

The cause of most hypertension is not known ("essential" hypertension). A small percentage of clients with this disease will have an identifiable cause, such as decreased blood flow to one or both kidneys. Certain hormonal diseases that induce hypertension and chronic kidney disease are often sought but not usually found.

Complications of high blood pressure include coronary heart disease, left ventricular heart failure, kidney failure, blindness (see chap. 29), and stroke (see chap. 9). The prognosis and course of the illness depend on early detection, adequate treatment, and careful followup. If these conditions are not met, then life-threatening complications may occur.

There are usually no specific physical or psychosocial impairments resulting from high blood pressure. Since prognosis of the client with hypertension is often good if he is on adequate therapy and is being followed closely, the counselor can usually plan for long-term vocational goals. High blood pressure is usually not a limiting factor in work unless job situations clearly increase the blood pressure.

Standards of Evaluation

The young hypertensive client deserves a full and careful medical evaluation to search for treatable forms of the disease. This evaluation will include studies of kidney, the adrenal gland, and other hormonal functions. It may involve hospitalization for diagnostic tests such as kidney biopsy, X-ray visualization of the blood supply to the kidneys (renal arteriography), and other sophisticated procedures.

The counselor should be aware of the importance of regular followup for the client with hypertension and should urge evaluation every few months if this has not been previously arranged.

Total Treatment

It is important to establish the cause of hypertension, institute therapy, and continue close followup evaluation indefinitely. If blood pressure becomes normal on therapy, it does not indicate that hypertension has been cured. Normalization of blood pressure on treatment therapy indicates only that treatment is effective and appropriate and should be maintained.

There are many drugs available for the treatment of high blood pressure. Dietary salt restriction may also be prescribed. Most clients will be receiving a diuretic and one or more additional drugs. Some of the stronger agents can cause impotence. Others can cause orthostatic intolerance, which is manifested by light-headedness, visual blurring, decrease in visual acuity, dizziness, or a near faint or actual fainting episode occurring with a rapid change in body position, usually from a stooping, bent over, seated, or lying position to standing.

Hypertension control requires daily medication. The counselor should ensure that his hypertensive clients are indeed taking their medications as prescribed and are getting their prescriptions refilled.

Vocational Implications

There are usually no training time intervals that the counselor need consider. For the occasional client who has a rapidly accelerating form of hypertension, short-term goals are best. Hypertension usually has no effect on the client's intellect, learning ability, verbal or numerical skills, coordination, or dexterity. One can generally permit the client to pursue virtually all interests. If, however, blood pressure is raised by emotionally stressful situations, these should be avoided.

The client with hypertension should avoid isometric activities because of the marked increase in blood pressure which they cause. Sustained lifting activities should be minimized. Also, in some clients, aerobic activities may be dangerous because in hypertension, the diastolic blood pressure will rise with aerobic activities.

The client with hypertension will have no problem with bending, stooping, and other body movements unless there are orthostatic symptoms resulting from medication. If such orthostatic symptoms develop, jobs requiring balancing and jobs involving the risk of falling and consequent serious injury should be avoided. The client can work either inside or outside. Temperature extremes are not usually a major consideration in uncomplicated hypertension.

HEART FAILURE

Disease Description

The development of heart failure and the symptoms associated with this condition have already been discussed (see p. 290). It may result from any form of heart disease and often represents a late stage when the heart's defenses against stress have been overcome. There are, however, acute forms of heart failure associated with an acute stress (e.g., heart attack or development of a severe abnormality of heart rhythm). These episodes of heart failure are often transient and may not have implications for work.

Shock due to heart disease is an extreme form of heart failure, with a poor near- and long-term outlook. Clients who have survived an episode of cardiogenic shock usually will have poor residual functional capacity, and job activities will often need to be severely curtailed.

Most episodes of acute and chronic heart failure can be modified with appropriate therapy, but unless the underlying problem is modified or removed, the course will be steadily downhill over one or more years. In some clients, heart failure will not be the cause of death. In others, a rapid progression of the underlying cardiovascular problem with heart failure can lead to physical incapacitation and death.

Functional Disabilities

The client with heart failure will usually have no problem with eating, personal care skills, transportation, or communication activities. Ambulation in many of these clients should be decreased because of shortness of breath brought on by physical activity.

There are usually no psychosocial impairments directly resulting from heart failure. However, in advanced disease, the same fears, anxiety, and depression common in coronary heart disease may exist if disease control is difficult. The outlook for the client with heart failure is generally guarded unless the cause of the failure can be removed. If this is not possible, medications can be given and the heart may adapt, permitting an acceptable level of function for an extended period of time. Clients who have an acute episode of heart failure may recover and do quite well. Those who have survived an episode of cardiogenic shock almost always have residual functional limitation and chronic heart failure. Under these circumstances the prognosis is guarded and short-term vocational training goals are appropriate.

Standards of Evaluation

When heart failure appears, most clients will have had a complete cardiovascular evaluation to identify the underlying disease. In addition, a decision will have been made or will need to be made by the client's attending physician as to whether the disease lends itself to surgical correction or not. Conditions that may be surgically approached include rheumatic valvular disease, coronary heart disease, congenital heart disease, and some muscle diseases of the heart. Conditions that are usually not surgically correctable include hypertension related to heart failure, end-stage rheumatic heart disease, coronary heart disease, and many primary diseases of the heart muscle.

Evaluation of the client with heart failure will include all of the tools available to the cardiologist, including electrocardiogram, echocardiogram, and heart catheterization. An exercise stress test is not a common evaluation procedure for the client in heart failure.

Total Treatment

Optimum medical therapy includes the use of diuretics to decrease the circulating blood volume. Diuretics cause loss of potassium into the urine, and the patient needs to replace this loss with potassium-rich foods or with potassium medicine. Digitalis is commonly given to increase the force of contraction of the failing heart. In addition, restriction of salt and fluids is often helpful. Recently, the long-acting blood vessel dilator preparations have been helpful in the management of heart failure. These medications decrease the resistance against which the heart must pump, thereby decreasing the work of the heart. All clients which chronic heart failure must be able to provide for adequate rest, both on the job and at home.

Chronic heart failure is monitored by regular followup visits to the physician, usually every 3 to 6 months and occasionally at longer intervals. Allied health professionals may be quite helpful in assisting with the management of the client with chronic heart failure. The clinical psychologist may help the client to cope better with changes in life style resulting from significant functional limitations. The vocational rehabilitation counselor and occupational therapist can assist with work simplification procedures that will be necessary as functional capacity decreases. The medical social worker is often helpful in aiding with family and financial concerns that develop when income drops because of a decrease in the client's productivity.

Vocational Implications

If heart failure is clearly established, the counselor should generally think in terms of medium-range training goals (i.e., up to 2 years) for the client. Occasionally, longer times may be considered, but these decisions should not be made without consulting the client's physician. Aptitudes are usually not affected by heart failure unless failure is very severe, in which case blood flow to the brain is decreased. Clients with heart failure may work well in groups and can perform abstract tasks well.

Emotional stress should be minimized and physical demands should be decreased as much as possible. Sedentary and light work are generally acceptable. Medium and heavier jobs are to be avoided. The client can usually bend, stoop, kneel, and balance without difficulty as long as the frequency of these activities is not too great and the load being handled is small. Climbing as a routine job activity is to be avoided but may be performed occasionally.

The counselor should direct the client toward indoor work where temperature is controlled, since temperature extremes may not be well tolerated. Humidity, noise, and vibration are usually not critical factors. Some clients may perform best in a sheltered competitive environment where the demands for a high quality product can be met but where the pressures of speed can be avoided. The client with heart failure often needs to be able to pace work activities during the day.

OBLITERATIVE ARTERIAL DISEASE

Disease Description

The major cause of obliterative arterial disease is atherosclerosis, the same process which involves the coronary arteries and causes coronary heart disease. Atherosclerosis most commonly involves the arteries of the abdomen (aorta, iliac) and the legs (superficial femoral, deep femoral, popliteal), and usually appears in mid to late adulthood.

Obliterative atherosclerosis (arteriosclerosis obliterans) is slowly progressive. Symptoms may be noted at rest or with exercise. With exertion, the client most commonly experiences weakness and a tight, cramping sensation in the muscle that is not receiving an adequate blood supply because of narrowing of the blood vessels. The discomfort noted with exertion is called *claudication* and may be felt in the calf, thigh, or buttocks, depending on which arteries are blocked (see table 3-6, p. 40). Symptoms at rest include numbness, tingling, and continuous pain, usually in the toes and feet. With severe disease, blood supply may be inadequate to maintain the nutrition of tissues, causing superficial ulcers and gangrene. Amputations are then required.

A less common but distinctive form of obliterative arterial disease is *Buerger's disease*, a nonatheromatous condition seen primarily in young men between the ages of 20 and 40 years. In contrast to obliterative atherosclerosis which involves medium and large arteries, Buerger's disease involves small arteries, and the hands as well as the feet are affected. Claudication of hands and feet occurs but calf claudication is rare. Fingertip ulcers may appear and necessitate amputations. Visual disturbances are common.

Functional Disabilities

Obliterative arterial disease may limit walking because of claudication. There is no loss of personal care skills unless fingertip gangrene occurs. Transportation and communication skills are unaffected. If visual problems occur, all the issues discussed in chapter 29 for cecutiency may apply. There are usually no psychosocial disabilities unless amputations are required (see chap. 13). The counselor can usually plan for long-term vocational goals, since limb loss rate in obliterative arterial disease is low, 2 percent per year in the client who does not have diabetes, and 7 percent per year in diabetic clients. As the disease progresses, planning that anticipates reduced leg exercise tolerance may need to be considered.

Standards of Evaluation

A careful history and physical examination is often all that is necessary to establish the diagnosis. Ankle blood pressure may be recorded before and after exercise and this is a useful method of following the course of the disease. X-ray studies of the artery (arteriography) are required to localize the segmental narrowings in obliterative atherosclerosis prior to surgery. This procedure is not required to make the diagnosis, however.

Total Treatment

Obliterative arterial disease is monitored clinically by changes in symptoms and evidence of poor skin nutrition. The post-exercise ankle blood pressure measurement is also helpful. Management includes exercise, weight reduction, meticulous foot care, and immediate care for all cuts and bruises. The client *must* stop smoking cigarettes completely. This, in fact, is the only known treatment for Buerger's disease, which is highly associated with the use of cigarettes. Surgical therapy is rarely required, but may include interruption of the sympathetic nerve supply to affected arteries (lumbar sympathectomy) or vein grafts which bypass the areas of obstruction to the arteries involved. If amputation because of gangrene is required, the issues discussed in chapter 13 apply.

Vocational Implications

Obliterative arterial disease has no specific impact on the client's educational goals or aptitudes. The counselor should channel the client's interest away from work in a cold environment. The client generally has no problem in dealing with people or with occupational stress, and may pursue concrete or abstract vocations. Walking and climbing may have to be minimized. The client with Buerger's disease which involves the hands may need to minimize dexterous hand work. The client can usually perform lifting tasks. Generally, there are no visual or auditory impairments. Clients should be guided toward indoor work and should avoid cool weather. Occupations that may involve trauma and skin damage, particularly in the lower extremities, should be avoided because the reduced blood supply interferes with wound healing.

ARTERIOSPASTIC DISORDERS

The two most important arteriospastic disorders are Raynaud's disease (or phenomenon) and livedo reticularis. *Raynaud's disease* and *Raynaud's phenomenon* are characterized by the sequence of pallor, blueness, and finally redness of an extremity, usually the hands, in response to cold or emotional stimuli. This condition is usually seen in women and begins in the late teens. It tends to involve both hands symmetrically. *Livedo reticularis* is recognized as a bluish mottling of the skin which gives it a "fishnet" appearance. Both of these conditions may be primary, that is, have no apparent cause, or secondary to another disease. The primary forms are benign, rarely lead to skin ulcers, and never are the cause of the client's death. The secondary forms are frequently serious and may have a fatal outcome. The counselor must know whether the condition is primary or secondary in order to make appropriate vocational plans.

There are often no physical or psychosocial impairments. Personal care skills may be affected if the client has ulcers on the fingertips. If the conditions are primary, the rehabilitation potential is excellent and the counselor can plan for long-term vocational goals.

Secondary forms will carry the prognosis of the underlying disease. The counselor should consult the client's physician to obtain this information.

The diagnosis is made by a careful history. An internist or peripheral vascular disease surgeon is the usual consultant. Extensive laboratory evaluation may be required to search for an underlying illness.

In primary forms, surgical interruption of nerves to the vessels (sympathectomy) has produced inconsistent results. Some medications have been reported to be of help. The management of secondary forms is the management of the underlying illness. The client with these conditions should be guided into positions that avoid prolonged exposure to cold. Indoor work is usually best, and generally a competitive industrial situation can be considered.

VARICOSE VEINS

Varicose veins are dilated, tortuous, superficial veins in which the valves that keep the blood returning toward to heart become incompetent. Veins of the lower extremities are usually involved. Varicose veins characteristically appear after the age of 20 and their cause is obscure, although hereditary factors are important. The client with varicose veins experiences feelings of heaviness and fatigue in the legs, which are particularly pronounced toward the end of the day. Edema of the foot and of the leg below the knee is usual. These symptoms are rapidly relieved by elevating the legs. The condition is slowly progressive.

There are usually no physical or psychosocial impairments and prognosis is good. Varicose veins is not a life-threatening condition and the counselor can plan for long-term vocational goals.

The usual management of varicose veins is to apply a close-fitting tailored compression stocking. It is rare for varicose veins to cause skin ulcers if the deep venous system is open. Occasionally, surgery to tie and strip out the superficial veins is required. There are no specific medications indicated that are of value.

The counselor should guide the client into positions that minimize the time spent standing stationary. Clients with varicosities are not limited by lifting requirements and may perform virtually all physical tasks. No environmental considerations are relevant.

THROMBOPHLEBITIS

Thrombophlebitis is an important acute disease of the veins characterized by inflammation and clotting. The involved veins, usually in the lower extremities, are commonly very tender. Usually no specific cause can be found, but injury, infection, and chemical irritation should be sought. Predisposing factors to thrombophlebitis include severe illness, immobilization, heart failure, any surgery, and severe trauma. Thrombophlebitis usually occurs in the deep veins of the legs and abdomen. If it is unrecognized or if treatment is delayed, clots can break off, float to the right heart, and lodge in the pulmonary arteries (pulmonary emboli) to cause a lung infarction.

The *post-phlebitic syndrome* is a late complication of one or more episodes of deep thrombophlebitis with resultant chronic venous occlusion and destruction of the valves in the veins. Ultimately, the patient with the post-phlebitic syndrome will have swelling of the limb and rupture of superficial veins which leads to pigmentation, scarring of the tissue under the skin, and ulcers. The patient will complain of swelling and extremity pain which is worse at the end of the day. The condition is progressive and can be only temporarily arrested. Unlike occlusive arterial disease, this condition does not lead to amputation. There are usually no psychosocial impairments. The client can accomplish personal care skills without difficulty and the counselor can plan for long-term vocational goals.

The diagnosis of thrombophlebitis and post-phlebitic syndrome is made on the basis of the history and the physical examination. If the diagnosis is in doubt, a venogram is indicated. Ultrasound tests of blood flow in the veins are also helpful.

The major form of therapy for post-phlebitic syndrome is a tailored pressure stocking which the client must always wear when on his feet. When possible, the feet should be elevated. If the client develops ulcers, bed rest, elevation, and perhaps skin grafting (see chap. 32) are employed.

In acute thrombophlebitis, hospitalization, bed rest, elevation, and anticoagulant agents are used. If pulmonary embolization occurs more than once, the inferior vena cava (see chap. 3) may be tied off to prevent a clot that may break off from reaching the lung.

The client with the post-phlebitic syndrome should be guided into positions in which he is not on his feet for long periods of time, and he may need to be in a job situation where his feet can be elevated for a time in the middle of the day.

SUMMARY

These discussions of the diseases of the cardiovascular system will hopefully assist rehabilitation counselors to take up the challenge that exists. In particular, the underserved population of those disabled by cardiac disease can well benefit from imaginative vocational planning. The exercise stress tests and the known demands of many occupational endeavors provide the means for quantitative assessment and specific recommendations.

BIBLIOGRAPHY

Brammell HL, McDaniel J, Niccoli SA, Darnell R: *Cardiac Rehabilitation: A Handbook for Vocational Rehabilitation Counselors.* An overview of cardiac rehabilitation geared to the vocational rehabilitation counselor with a special interest in cardiac clients. Available from the University of Colorado Medical Center, Box C-242, 4200 E. Ninth Ave., Denver, CO, 80262, from State rehabilitation agencies, or from RSA.

Cay EL, Vetter NJ, Phillips AE: Practical aspects of cardiac rehabilitation: Psychosocial factors. G. Ital Cardiol 3:646, 1973.

An excellent paper dealing with psychosocial issues following heart attack.

Gutmann MC, Benson H: Interaction of environmental factors and systemic arterial blood pressure: A review. Medicine 50:543–553, 1971.

Review of the relation of elevated blood pressure to rapid cultural change, urbanization and urban life, socioeconomic mobility, necessity for continuous behavioral adjustments, stress, and physiologic mechanisms.

Jenkins CD: Recent evidence supporting psychologic and social risk factors for coronary disease. N Eng J Med 294:1033–1038, 1976.

A review of the literature, 1970–1975, on psychosocial variables associated with coronary disease. Discussion centers on the "coronary-prone behavior pattern—Type A."

Kjøller E: Resumption of work after acute myocardial infarction. Acta Med Scand 199:379–385, 1976.

Review of a study of 644 patients discharged from a Coronary Care Unit in Denmark in a 3-year period. Factors influencing return to work are discussed.

McDaniel JW: *Physical Disability and Human Behavior.* Ed 2, Pergammon Press, New York, 1976.

An overview of psychological considerations in disability.

Naughton JP, Hellerstein HK (eds): *Exercise Testing and Exercise Training in Coronary Heart Disease.* Academic Press, New York, 1973.

A good overview of many aspects of exercise and cardiac rehabilitation.

Niven RG: Psychologic adjustment to coronary artery disease. Postgrad Med 60:152–157, 1976.

This article reviews some common factors and problems associated with adjustment to coronary artery disease during the chronic adjustment phase of the disease (after the disease has stabilized). Describes signs and symptoms that require immediate attention.

Schiller E, Baker J: Return to work after a myocardial infarction: Evaluation of planned rehabilitation and of a predictive rating scale. Med J Aust 1:859–862, 1976.

Review of a study of cardiac rehabilitation after myocardial infarction in men of working age. Describes factors used to predict return to work and the factors actually found at 6-month followup to have influenced return to work.

23 PULMONARY DYSFUNCTION

Ben V. Branscomb, M.D.

INTRODUCTION

The chronic pulmonary diseases represent the third largest group of diseases resulting in total disability awards under the Social Security system, exceeded only by the cardiovascular and renal diseases. Annually, the deaths attributable to chronic obstructive pulmonary diseases (COPD) are approximately equal to the number of deaths from motor vehicle accidents plus the total American deaths in the Vietnam conflict. Furthermore, most victims suffer from significant impairment for many years. Chronic pulmonary problems thus represent a major challenge to the vocational counselor. In the majority of chronic pulmonary disorders, a reasonable level of comfort and physical activity, including gainful employment, can be achieved.

In this chapter, COPD, asthma, occupational lung disease, and cystic fibrosis are discussed. COPD is extensively presented. The others share many features in common with COPD, and hence their understanding requires first an understanding of COPD. Chapter 3 should be reviewed for an appreciation of normal respiratory and cardiac function.

CHRONIC OBSTRUCTIVE PULMONARY DISEASE

Disease Description

The two principal chronic obstructive pulmonary diseases are chronic bronchitis and emphysema. *Chronic bronchitis* is characterized by chronic inflammation of the bronchial tubes, with increased quantities of mucus and mucus-secreting cells. These secretions cause obstructions of the small and medium-sized bronchioles (see chap. 3). The obstruction traps air (gas) and hence interferes with expiration. A cough results in an effort to clear the secretions, and expectoration therefore occurs. The presence of secretions and the obstruction can be heard with a stethoscope (rales) and shortness of breath occurs on exertion.

Emphysema is a destructive process involving breakdown of the alveolar walls (see fig. 3-28, p. 43),

with enlargement of the alveoli. Breakdown of alveolar walls interferes with the elastic recoil of the lung on expiration, obstructs the airways, and traps air in the alveoli. The diagnosis of emphysema requires proof that the aveolar walls are destroyed. It is difficult to diagnose, except by inference, without direct examination of the lung tissue itself.

When breakdown creates large air sacs, the term *bullous emphysema* is used. It indicates destruction of lung in especially large areas, often the size of an orange or larger. These bullae are seen as large air holes or cysts on the chest X-ray. Occasionally, the process can involve the entire upper half of both lungs, which seem to have "disappeared" on the chest X-ray. This is called the "disappearing lung syndrome." Persons with bullous emphysema often have excellent function in remaining portions of the lung and can be quite active in spite of the spectacular X-ray appearance.

Chronic bronchitis is the usual cause of emphysema. Consequently, it is customary to use the term "COPD" to refer to both, without regard for the fact that bronchitis usually has reversible features and emphysema does not. When the term "COPD" is used in the remaining discussion, it means either bronchitis or emphysema. Whenever a comment is specific only for one of the two, the disease name is used.

Although there is much overlap, COPD patients have been conveniently divided into two groups, often identified by the British colloquialisms "blue bloaters" and "pink puffers".

"Blue bloaters" (in English slang "to bloat" means "to spit") include those patients who are characterized by the production of mucus, a conspicuous cough, expectoration, and wheezing. The mucus obstructs air flow to many undamaged areas of lung. When venous blood from the right heart passes through these normal lung areas, oxygen cannot be picked up because there is no "fresh" air. Blood returning in the pulmonary vein to the left heart is therefore low in arterial oxygen tension or pressure (PO_2). Although such persons are rarely actually *blue* (cyanotic), this word refers to the usually low PO_2. To counteract the reduced oxygen, these patients develop increased red blood cell concentrations (polycythemia).

"Blue bloaters" have frequent exacerbations and remissions of symptoms because of the variability in the amount of mucus. The reduced oxygen requires that the heart work harder to pump more blood in order to move oxygen to the tissues. Patients can therefore develop a chronic low-grade congestive heart failure (see chap. 22) which is usually well tolerated.

A "pink puffer" tends to be a "dry" patient, with little or no mucus. Widespread alveolar wall breakdown (emphysema) is dominant. Because the destruction of the alveoli includes destruction of their surrounding capillaries, the blood passes mostly to the more normal lung areas. Therefore, the blood which does pass through the lung tends to come in contact with air, even though much lung may be destroyed and there may be a considerable increase in blood pressure in the right heart (pulmonary hypertension). The arterial oxygen content, as a result, is typically normal or only minimally reduced. Thus the patients are "pink." The word "puffer" refers to their greater shortness of breath (dyspnea). Because of the widespread alveolar damage, the loss of elastic lung recoil is extensive. Expiratory obstruction is severe and dyspnea is intense.

The clinical course for the "pink puffer" is more stable than for the "blue bloater." Exacerbations and remissions are not likely. Once respiratory failure or right ventricular heart failure occurs, treatment is less successful, since there are fewer factors that can be reversed.

Etiology. By far the most important cause of emphysema is chronic bronchitis. Emphysema also results from other severe chronic pulmonary diseases, such as occupational pneumoconiosis, asthma, cystic fibrosis, Boeck's sarcoid, and severe thoracic spine curvatures.

It is well established that cigarette smoking is the major cause of chronic bronchitis. Cessation of smoking is regularly followed by marked reduction in symptoms of COPD, including reduction or total cessation of cough and expectoration and improved physical activity. Although there is a small minority of persons with COPD who have never smoked, cessation of smoking represents the major opportunity for prevention and treatment and cannot be overemphasized. Unquestionably, many unknown factors determine why some nonsmokers develop emphysema, why COPD is more common in males than in females, even with the same smoking and occupational exposure, and why the rate of progression varies so greatly from person to person. Air pollution has also been reasonably well established as a causal factor. It can induce acute exacerbations in COPD patients and deaths in those persons who have a limited pulmonary reserve.

Signs and symptoms. COPD is usually diagnosed in the fifth or sixth decade. Commonly, moderate or severe loss of lung function is present at the time of diagnosis. This delay in diagnosis is explained by the fact that normal persons have approximately twice the lung function needed for even heavy physical exercise. Further, many persons, including those engaged in physically demanding occupations such as mining, never engage in activities sufficiently demanding to require an abnormal breathing effort. In addition, the cough and expectoration which often precedes the shortness of breath by 5 to 20 years is often dismissed as normal (e.g., "just a smoker's cough"). Cough is never "normal." If it is recurrent or persistent for several weeks, it always requires study, not only for COPD but for the possibility of cancer, tuberculosis, and other diseases.

Cough is the predominant symptom of chronic bronchitis. The diagnostic criterion often used is the presence of cough the first thing in the morning or off and on during the day for most days out of the week for 2 months during 2 or more years. The mucus produced is ordinarily clear or white. Small amounts of blood are sometimes produced. This finding always requires further study for cancer and other disorders.

The lung becomes progressively vulnerable to attacks by bacteria and viruses because of the thick secretions, ineffective cough, and swollen, inflamed bronchial membranes. Two or more prolonged "heavy chest colds" a year are typical, and in some persons infection is almost continuously present. During infection, the person becomes more short of breath and produces larger quantities of usually gray or yellow sputum.

Pathology. Obstruction of the bronchioles is the result of several factors. As already discussed, increased volumes of thick mucus and inflamed, irritated, and swollen bronchial walls are contributory. In addition, *bronchospasm* is an important factor. Bronchospasm refers to constriction of the muscles surrounding the bronchial tubes (see chap. 3). Some degree of bronchospasm may always be present, with a superimposed severe constriction of the muscles during exacerbations. The degree of bronchospasm is highly variable. There is none in the small number of patients with "pure" emphysema—persons whose changes are confined to destruction of alveolar walls. In other persons with COPD, bronchospasm may be so conspicuous that the term "chronic asthmatic bronchitis" is used, since bronchospasm is the main component of asthma.

Emphysema itself is an additional cause of obstruction and, because obstruction from this cause cannot be reversed, it becomes the factor that limits maximum physical activity. The obstruction in emphysema occurs as a result of changes in the alveolar walls.

A fine network of elastic fibers normally lines the alveoli and extends through the entire lung. These elastic fibers keep the walls of the bronchi apart, maintaining an adequate diameter for air passage. During inspiration, when the chest becomes larger and the elastic fibers are stretched, the walls of the bronchi are pulled further apart. During expiration, bronchial diameters reduce.

In emphysema, the ruptured or destroyed alveolar walls and the resulting destruction of elastic tissue removes the mechanism by which the airways are normally held open. Consequently, the airways are only open at fullest inspiration when the remaining tissues are on maximum stretch. Indeed, as the disease progresses, many areas will not open at all. The patient therefore tends to breathe with his chest in a fully inflated position (barrel chest). With expiration, the collapsing airways produce the characteristic wheezing.

When such a patient attempts to exhale more rapidly by contracting his chest muscles to compensate for the missing elastic recoil, the pressure inside the chest increases. This increased pressure tends to collapse the walls further. Consequently, obstruction is more severe with rapid breathing than with slow breathing. Inspiration effort remains relatively normal because the added negative pressure in the chest during inhalation tends to pull the walls of the bronchi apart.

At first, obstruction in COPD is present only during episodes of increased bronchial inflammation, such as occur with infections or exposure to irritating dusts or fumes. Gradually, obstruction becomes continuous, with superimposed increased obstruction during exacerbations. After a further lapse of time, a gradually increasing component of irreversible obstruction results from emphysema superimposed on the potentially reversible bronchitic obstructive processes.

As COPD advances, the patient experiences progressively increased difficulty eliminating secretions. Obstruction interferes with the rapid expiration required for effective coughing. Consequently, the cough is frequent and harassing and there are often protracted spells (paroxysms). At first, dyspnea occurs only with heavy exercise, but subsequently it occurs with milder exercise. Ultimately, it occurs even during speaking and at rest.

Oxygen lack itself, except at high altitudes where arterial oxygen levels are low, is rarely the cause of dyspnea. Shortness of breath is predominantly the result of the increased effort required to breathe with obstruction present.

Typically, the disease extends for many years, often 10 or 15, after significant symptoms appear. In early stages, arterial blood gas concentrations frequently remain normal. As the condition progresses, the PO_2 may be somewhat reduced at rest but improves with exercise. This improvement is due to better ventilation of the partially obstructed lung during the deeper breathing of exercise. In late stages, usually when the obstructive problems are severe, the PO_2 is low at rest and falls with exercise because oxygen is used up faster than it is taken in. Exercise capacity is usually very limited in such persons.

The normal resting oxygen concentration (tension) is approximately 100 mm Hg for a 20-year-old subject. It drops to approximately 70 mm Hg at age 70. A moderate reduction of this PO_2 value below that expected for a person's age may indicate that disease is present.

Arterial carbon dioxide concentration (tension, PCO_2) is another measure that is used to monitor COPD. The normal PCO_2 remains at approximately 40 mm Hg throughout life. PCO_2 is usually normal until very late in the disease and may rise only in terminal patients. Elevation of PCO_2 values means obstruction is severe and too much air is trapped in the alveoli. The carbon dioxide produced by the various body tissues therefore cannot be exhaled and eliminated.

Complications. The major complication of chronic bronchitis is, of course, emphysema. Other complications of COPD include recurrent infections, pneumonia, heart failure, and respiratory failure. Death occurs most often as a result of respiratory failure, often associated with an acute infection. Less frequently, death occurs from cardiovascular complications such as arrhythmias or pulmonary embolus (see chap. 22), both of which are increased in persons with severe COPD.

Infections frequently begin as viral "colds" which descend into the chest and commonly evolve into bacterial infections. In other persons, bacteria are the initial offenders. The most common organisms are pneumococci and the influenza bacillus. In moderate or severe COPD, chest infections are often life threatening.

Right ventricular congestive heart failure, often called *cor pulmonale*, is frequent in severe COPD. It is manifested by ankle edema, reduction in exercise tolerance, and rapid heart rates. It develops because many capillaries in the lung are destroyed in COPD. The resultant low oxygen tension in areas of lung which are obstructed stimulates a reflex constriction of the small pulmonary arteries. Consequently, the resistance to blood flow through the lung is increased. In order to drive the blood through this increased resistance, the right ventricle is forced to generate an abnormally high pressure. The demand for increased cardiac output during exercise causes an additional increase in pulmonary artery pressure. This continued stress on the right ventricle leads to its failure. Right ventricular failure is often present for many years. Moderate physical activity, including employment, is compatible with this complication under medical treatment.

Respiratory failure is a late development in which the delivery of oxygen to the tissues is greatly impaired. Typically, the PO_2 is below 50 mm Hg. When the

PCO_2 is greater than normal, the patient may be said to be in respiratory failure. Respiratory failure usually implies an imminent risk to life and generally requires hospitalization, often in an intensive care unit. Many patients who reach such a level of severe respiratory impairment may die should a lung infection or any other crisis occur. If, however, treatment succeeds, even such persons may live for several years and enjoy many worthwhile, though extremely limited, activities. At this point, such activities only rarely include gainful employment. This is an important concept because it underscores the value of maximum medical and rehabilitation treatment for the very severely impaired.

Functional Disabilities

Physical disabilities. The earliest manifestations of COPD, cough and expectoration, limit activities only as a result of the negative impact on others, including an employer or co-workers. Subsequently, dyspnea becomes the limiting impairment. A number of years may elapse before dyspnea is sufficient to limit walking on the level and the requirements of moderate and sedentary activities. In time, however, dressing, bathing, and even speech cannot be accomplished without distressing air hunger.

Driving is possible with severe COPD, although walking to and from the car may be difficult. Stair climbing is restricted in moderate disease, and hurrying up even minimal grades is usually impossible. In contrast, level walking and seated activities in which hands, arms, and shoulders are used are acceptable.

There are some patients with COPD who remain astonishingly active physically in spite of severely reduced oxygen tensions and chronically elevated carbon dioxide levels. For example, a person with a PO_2 of 60 mm Hg, and a PCO_2 of 80 or 90 mm Hg may be able to walk several blocks slowly, drive an automobile, and remain at work at a sedentary occupation. Such patients emphasize the fact that the arterial blood gas values alone cannot adequately define disability.

Psychosocial disabilities. Dyspnea is a frightening and distressing symptom. Consequently, fear must frequently be allayed. Depression is also frequent and focuses on the loss of valued activities, the loss of a previously cherished image of vigor and health, and the conviction that there is an inexorable downhill course. Many patients are unaware of the improvement possible through medical and rehabilitation measures and this contributes to the depression.

Often the patient's spouse fails to understand the seriousness of the patient's impairments and may react with unconscious hostility to his limitations. In other couples, the spouse is overly protective and this results in excessive dependency, inactivity, and diminished socialization. Anxieties, fears, and misconceptions are common among many of the other family members as well.

Rehabilitation potential. The client's rehabilitation potential may be greatly enhanced by medical treatment. If the medical consultant states that treatment has not been optimal, the complete rehabilitation plan should include an evaluation of the client's response to medical treatment. This response will vary depending on disease factors, patient compliance, and the practical availability of medical care in a particular community setting. After a 2 to 3 month period of active medical treatment, appropriate vocational goals can be perceived.

Medical considerations in planning the rehabilitation program include the following: What environmental limitations exist? Of what severity and duration may periodic exacerbations be anticipated? Excluding exacerbations, what is the client's capacity for exercise? Will his functional capacity decrease with time and at what rate?

The rate at which function will decrease or exacerbations and complications increase is an important consideration. The rate of deterioration is extremely slow in persons with moderate disease and well-controlled reversible factors. In general, a reasonably stable patient with moderate disease might safely expect employment to be possible for 5 years or more. In severe COPD, 1 or 2 sedentary years would be more likely. Periodic exacerbations and continuation of smoking significantly reduce the outlook. If the option of a sedentary occupation is available, such employment would be wise even in mild to moderate disease, especially in young persons, since one does not know the prognosis and a sedentary job might continue 4 to 5 years longer than one requiring more activity.

Standards of Evaluation

Medical evaluation. The history and physical examination should be carried out by a specialist in internal medicine or medical pulmonary diseases. The counselor may have to ask the physician to provide the specific information he needs. This includes precise descriptions of the nature, frequency, periodicity, and circumstances under which symptoms are experienced and the probable future frequency of exacerbations of the disease. The counselor should ask whether the medical examination was carried out on a typical day or one on which the patient felt particularly ill or well. He should learn from the physician, in general terms, the proper treatment and, specifically, whether the client is currently receiving optimum treatment. The physician should also be able to estimate the patient's probable future symptoms and exercise capacity, based on optimum treatment reasonably available to him. Sufficient history and physical and laboratory findings should be included in the report so that another physician reading it would reasonably be expected to arrive at the same conclusions. Attention should also be directed toward impairments which may be reversible.

A chest X-ray and spirogram (see below) are required. Provision should be made for obtaining further tests, such as the frequently needed arterial blood gas studies. Lung volume tests and observation of the patient during exercise are frequently needed. The consultant can explain the meaning of all laboratory studies to the counselor and client.

The *chest X-ray* is essential to eliminate cancer, tuberculosis, and other serious problems. The chest X-ray may further show the changes associated with bullous emphysema. In many persons with COPD, the X-ray is completely negative. Therefore, it has very low diagnostic reliability in COPD and little or no value in estimating a client's functional capacity and rehabilitation potential.

The *spirogram* measures several factors. One is the maximum volume of gas that can be inspired and expired. This is the vital capacity, or VC (see p. 44 and fig. 3-31). Also important is how fast the total forced expiratory volume (FEV) is exhaled. The volume exhaled during forced expiration during the first 1, 2, and 3 seconds (FEV_1, FEV_2, FEV_3) is measured. In addition, the maximum voluntary ventilation (MVV) is also measured. This records the maximum volume of air the subject can breathe in 12 seconds, breathing in and out as rapidly and forcefully as possible. Multiplying this measure by five yields the MVV in liters of air per minute.

The VC and FEV are reduced in obstructive disease, but other chest diseases also reduce them. The timed FEV's primarily reflect obstruction and thus are the physiological hallmark of COPD. The MVV is influenced by a number of factors, including the patient's ability to sustain a maximum breathing effort over time. Many physicians find the MVV useful in estimating physical capacity because it combines a number of the elements required for breathing during work.

Since the spirogram requires maximum patient performance, it is only valid when cooperation is complete. The technician must be able to transmit to the patient by description and demonstration the level of effort required. The test should be carried out three or more times using an apparatus which records a permanent tracing. Study of the record not only documents the test but also can disclose irregularities indicating an unsatisfactory test. Since many inadequate devices are on the market, the apparatus should be one of the types approved by the Disability Determination Unit of the Social Security

Administration. The best value obtained from the patient is reported, not the average of the three or more tests.

Arterial oxygen and carbon dioxide blood gases determinations and lung volume measurements should be obtained on persons with moderately severe or severe symptoms. The physician and the counselor should both observe the patient during level walking or stair climbing. Highly motivated, lean persons accustomed to physical activity sometimes perform surprisingly well, whereas sedentary and obese persons perform poorly. The observer notes whether the patient's complaints and pulmonary function studies are consistent with his apparent exercise capacity and he can check for malingering, exaggeration, or understatement of symptoms.

Psychosocial evaluation. A clinical psychological assessment may be in order to determine whether the extent of the patient's fear, anxiety, and depression is sufficient to interfere with planning. A social worker can identify any family problems created by the disease, and can also assess the level of the family's understanding of the disease.

Total Treatment

Medical management. Although there is no cure for COPD, many symptoms can be managed with considerable effectiveness. The most important element in management is the ready access of the patient to an interested, skillful physician. An exacerbation may mean that maintenance treatment must be changed. Therefore, medical contact during an exacerbation is essential. The physician will attempt to define reversible factors, identify irreversible ones, and develop a plan of treatment for both.

The team approach, using respiratory therapists, respiratory care nurses, physical and occupational therapists, and psychologists, has demonstrated value. The rehabilitation counselor is also an important member of this team and can contribute much to the patient's quality of life. Each patient must be considered individually, and rigid programs in which the patient interacts unselectively with a series of allied health professionals is inappropriate and expensive, especially if careful medical supervision is lacking.

Oral bronchodilators are administered to treat bronchospasm. Theophylline (aminophylline) is a common first choice. If spasm is insufficiently controlled, a drug from the class of substances resembling epinephrine (adrenergic drugs) is commonly added. Examples are metaproterenol and turbutaline.

Aerosols can be used to deliver adrenergic drugs directly to the lungs. The patient inhales a mist containing the medication, which is blown into the mouth through a handbulb or compressor-powered devices called nebulizers. Aerosols may be used by patients with only rare and mild bronchospasm or for the occasional quick relief of spasm by patients already receiving full doses of the oral preparations. Unfortunately, because of convenience and immediate sense of relief, they are often overused and can become, like cigarettes, an additional source of bronchial irritation.

Steroid therapy can produce striking improvement in bronchospasm and bronchial inflammation. There are, however, side effects from these cortisone-like preparations when overused. They should be reduced or discontinued as soon as practical, using the other medications for maintenance therapy.

The side effects of steroids include osteoporosis of the vertebral bodies with collapse, resulting in severe pain; activation of latent diabetes or tuberculosis; general muscular weakness; and serious peptic ulcer. Persons receiving 15 mg or more of prednisone are at risk of developing these complications and must, in particular, avoid too much trauma to their bones. Despite these complications, steroids are invaluable for overcoming exacerbations of inflammation and bronchospasm, and some patients can only be managed when these drugs are used continuously.

Beclomethasone is an inhaled corticosteroid hormone which produces no systemic side effects and is consequently a useful means of achieving steroid benefits without complications. It provides the benefit equivalent to only about 10 mg of prednisone.

Cessation of smoking is of great therapeutic value in managing excessive secretions. Within a week, secretions diminish and improvement continues for 6 months or longer. Continued smoking counteracts an otherwise therapeutic regimen. Bronchodilators and antibiotics, when indicated, are also used to manage excessive secretions.

Physical measures are also helpful in eliminating secretions, and their systematic use is an important component of the total program of bronchial hygiene. These measures require considerable patient education. Usually they are initiated by a physical or respiratory therapist, who also subsequently checks the patient's progress. After training, these measures can often be carried out by the patient alone or with the assistance of a family member. The physical measures include postural drainage, chest percussion, and expulsive coughing. For *postural drainage*, the patient lies over the side of the bed or across a stack of rolled-up blankets to allow gravity to assist in the elimination of sputum. *Chest percussion* consists of tapping the chest with moderate vigor. The resulting vibrations assist in liberating retained secretions. *Expulsive coughing* is performed either in the seated position or during postural drainage. The patient exhales several times completely and forcefully without coughing. The objective of these complete expirations is to force the mucus toward the upper part of the airway. The patient then takes a deep breath and coughs forcefully to expel the secretion.

High fluid intake is important to prevent dehydration, and may also make the secretions more liquid. The patient's home and work environment should not be extremely dry, since this increases the thickness of the sputum. The patient may inhale saline or water aerosols from two to four times a day to deliver humidity directly to the lung. An ultrasonic nebulizer is a device which administers the smallest water particles in the largest volume. It is expensive, must be carefully cleaned to avoid deposition of bacteria into the lung, and should be used only when it is demonstrated to be superior to other methods.

Intermittent positive pressure breathing (IPPB) is a technique using a machine to assist inhalation. When the patient inhales through a mouthpiece, the device delivers air under pressure. Thus it assists in deep inspiration but does not affect expiration. The device can simultaneously deliver water or bronchodilator from a nebulizer. IPPB is often beneficial for hospitalized patients but probably should be used only rarely by outpatients. The patient must be instructed in proper cleaning of all inhalation equipment, since these devices can serve as a source of infection.

Exercise below and up to the point of moderately severe dyspnea is beneficial in COPD, except when uncontrollable heart failure is present. Systematic exercise can gradually increase tolerance for the exercise itself and hence for other spontaneous activity. Exercise does not improve specific lung function, but it does improve the performance of the muscles so that more exercise can be accomplished with the same level of pulmonary impairment. It is likely that regular exercise also results in a behavior modification. The person becomes adapted to the sensations of difficult breathing and learns to accept them without fear or anxiety, thereby gaining an improved life style.

Graded exercise programs, often called reconditioning exercises, should be under direct medical supervision, since marked oxygen deficiency during exercise, unacceptable heart failure, a tendency to arrhythmias, or a risk of myocardial infarction represent contraindications. Portable oxygen or oxygen from a long tube is sometimes used during reconditioning exercises.

Oxygen is required by some patients with COPD, even though shortness of breath is largely due to the mechanical effort of moving air rather than oxygen lack. Sometimes oxygen is given before, during, or after heavy exercise to patients who otherwise would be totally housebound and able to walk less than 200 feet. Some patients who have a sufficient ventilatory capacity to be able to sustain moderate exercise are unable to do so because they have exceptionally low oxygen levels and hence benefit from oxygen. Small amounts of oxygen breathed continuously from a portable device can keep such persons active.

Unfortunately, some persons obtain oxygen and use it frequently even though dyspnea is not the result of oxygen lack. Anxious persons may become emotionally crippled by the fear of leaving the oxygen source. Oxygen use requires careful supervision and instruction and under no circumstances should it be used without arterial blood gas monitoring.

Antibiotics are frequently used in COPD during intercurrent infections. A sputum culture for type of organism should be obtained if there is suspected infection. Tetracycline or ampicillin are commonly used antibiotics. The patient may be taught to recognize the signs of infection early and take antibiotics without consulting the physician. Prophylactic antibiotics are sometimes prescribed for patients who have frequently recurring infections. They take the antibiotics, for example, during alternate weeks during the winter cold season as a preventive measure.

Digitalis preparations and diuretics are usually used if heart failure is present, as described in chapter 22. Most patients with COPD and right ventricular failure have significantly reduced arterial oxygen concentrations. Consequently, oxygen may be an important part of the treatment of heart failure. Heart failure can usually be successfully managed while maintaining physical activity in all but the most severely impaired persons.

Psychosocial treatment. The education of both patient and spouse is an integral part of the comprehensive treatment program. Emphasis is placed on the nature of the disease process, how to use different medications, the desirable level of activity, how to maintain good health care, recognition and management of infections, control of smoking and adverse environments, and physical measures.

In addition to education, psychological counseling can further help alleviate fear, anxiety, and depression. The concept of goal identification and incremental progress toward the goal removes uncertainty. Social casework counseling with the entire family can help them sort out and solve problems generated by any required reduction in the patient's social roles.

Vocational Implications

The client must receive regular ongoing medical treatment for the rest of his life if employment achieved is to be sustained. When planning with a new client, the counselor may prefer an extended evaluation if the client has not yet had intense treatment and maintenance. A higher level employment goal may result.

Cough and expectoration may, as a cosmetic impairment, preclude some jobs requiring close interpersonal interaction. The counselor should be guided by the client's past history and the consultant's predictions regarding absenteeism. The amount of pulmonary function loss is not itself a predictor.

"Blue bloater" type clients are most prone to periodic exacerbations, and hence absenteeism, usually resulting from infection, bronchospasm, or excessive fatigue. If COPD is only moderately severe (i.e., the client can climb two flights of stairs without becoming exhausted and the

FEV_1 is 2 liters or more), absenteeism is not likely to be a problem. A client with severe disease (i.e., one who can climb only one flight of stairs and whose FEV_1 is 1 liter or less) will probably require some accommodation for absenteeism due to exacerbations.

The client's usual exercise capacity is evaluated primarily by the history, pulmonary function studies, and results of exercise treatment after a total program is initiated. Slow walking on the level is often practical when stair climbing, running, and any rapid exercise are precluded. An individual limited to slow walking on the level can usually not carry objects, even those weighing only 5 pounds. On the other hand, clients able to climb only one flight of stairs and whose FEV_1 may be 1 liter can often use the arms and shoulders effectively for a full 8-hour shift if they remain seated. Cab driving or operating an industrial sewing machine may be quite suitable for such persons. Homemaking, requiring the use of arms and shoulders while standing or walking, probably would not be suitable.

A resting PO_2 below 60 mm Hg or one which falls by 10 mm with exercise usually permits only sedentary employment. There are many jobs and other activities that are largely sedentary but require occasional greater levels of activity. For example, a seated occupation may require a walk to the mailroom or carrying 10 pounds 200 feet 3 times a day. If this produces moderately severe dyspnea, the job may nevertheless be acceptable if exercise can be followed by a few minutes of recovery while seated, if this short-time activity is modified to be performed by others, or if objects can be moved on a rolling cart.

It is important for the client, the workers around him, and the employer to realize that moderately severe shortness of breath does not damage the patient. It only makes him feel uncomfortable. They must know that, in fact, it is desirable for persons with COPD to exercise daily to the point of moderate discomfort, except for those with profound oxygen lack or uncontrolled heart failure.

All of the above indicate the crucial necessity of analyzing *all* the physical demands, both usual and intermittent, of a potential job. The physician can help the counselor best when specific questions are raised. Sheltered workshops, job stations, or other work sampling techniques under observation can help in such an evaluation.

Where a potential job has occasional demands beyond the patient's capacity, job restructuring is helpful. It is usually easier to do this for a trusted employee already on the job but experiencing difficulty than attempting restructuring with new placements.

The most important vocational determinant is the level of exercise at which the client experiences distressing dyspnea. The following general guidelines are illustrative, but it must be remembered that there is a great variation in the exercise tolerance of persons with similar medical findings, and that selecting a job with low physical demands is a wise concession to possible future progression of the disease.

Even with cough and expectoration, if the client has a normal spirogram and normal resting and exercise blood gases and can climb four flights of stairs without distressing dyspnea, heavy work or very heavy work is acceptable.

If the FEV_1 is 3 liters, the MVV 90 liters per minute, and the client can climb three flights of stairs without significant distress, medium work should be possible.

If the FEV_1 is 2 liters, the MVV 60 liters per minute, and two flights of stairs can be climbed with perhaps heavy breathing but no severe distress, light work should be acceptable. Substantial homemaking and domestic activities are usually possible.

An FEV_1 of 1 liter, an MVV of approximately 30 liters per minute, and stair climbing limited to one flight will usually permit sedentary work including light housekeeping. Below this level, intermittent homebound employment and totally sedentary sheltered workshop work would represent optimistic goals.

If stooping and kneeling are required, if the PO_2 is 10 mm below normal at rest or falls with exercise, if portable oxygen is used, or if there is evidence of impaired cardiac function in spite of treatment, a job one or two levels less demanding than those described above should be selected. Extremes or sudden changes in temperature, occupations requiring exposure to adverse weather conditions, extremes of dryness or humidity, and atmospheric dusts and irritating gases should be avoided. If the client has significant ongoing infections or if two or more chest colds per year are anticipated, his future employment should be free from exposure to adverse weather conditions, smoke, fumes, and dust. When infection is the major factor in spite of good management and when there is no way to avoid outdoor employment, moving to a warmer, drier climate is occasionally recommended. This usually entails significant financial and social hardship, and medical benefits are usually not large. If the client continues to smoke, environmental manipulations are almost superfluous.

If a client is breathing oxygen continuously from a portable device, the employer should be informed. Although oxygen is not explosive, it should not be used in immediate proximity to flames, smoking, or highly flammable substances.

ASTHMA

Disease Description

Asthma, sometimes called reversible airway obstruction, is characterized by bronchospasm, edema of the bronchial walls, infiltration of the bronchial wall with eosinophil cells, and production of excessive mucus. Commonly, the term "bronchospasm" alone is used when all four processes are taking place, since they occur simultaneously and respond to the same treatment.

Asthmatic attacks, or paroxysms of bronchospasm, may last from minutes to hours and then subside completely. Occasionally, particularly with infections, an attack can last days or weeks (status asthmaticus) and rapidly debilitate a patient because of fatigue, loss of sleep, and poor nutrition.

In an asthma attack, there is acute airway obstruction. Shallow rapid breathing with cough, wheezing, dyspnea, and often thick sputum result. In more severe or advanced cases, the attacks are superimposed on a continuous, less severe bronchospasm.

About half the attacks develop during childhood, but the disorder can begin at any age. About 15 percent begin after the age of 40. One-third of children with asthma outgrow the disorder, and in one-third, the problem becomes very infrequent and mild during adulthood. However, the remaining one-third have lifelong manifestations.

The course of the disease is variable from patient to patient and in any one patient. Often several months of frequent attacks alternate with similar periods of relative freedom. When poorly controlled and severe, asthma may ultimately lead to emphysema. When frequent lung infections are also present, the condition of chronic asthmatic bronchitis, which is indistinguishable from COPD, may develop.

In a minority of cases, the stimulus that triggers bronchospasm can be traced to pollen, mold, dust, food, aspirin, or some substance to which the patient is allergic. If so identified, the condition is called allergic asthma. In nonallergic asthma, the stimulus is difficult to identify. In some it is a respiratory infection; in others, exercise or bouts of deep breathing may precipitate an attack. Cigarette smoke, air pollution, nonspecific dusts, and fumes also induce attacks in many nonallergic asthmatics. Emotional stress has also triggered attacks.

Functional Disabilities

No activity is possible during an attack. The process of breathing nearly totally consumes the patient's energies. Except for slow walking or simple sitting, not much can be done. Lying down, eating, and even dressing may require energies not available to the patient. Between attacks, however, the patient usually has perfectly normal functional abilities. If there has been progressive loss of lung function with emphysema or chronic asthmatic bronchitis, then limitations as discussed for COPD may be present between attacks. The severity of the handicap is therefore dictated by the frequency and length of attacks, as well as the level of functioning between attacks.

If the asthma seen in an adult originally developed during childhood, psychological and social disabilities may be present similar to those discussed for hemophilia (see chap. 26) and sickle cell disease (see chap. 27). Frequency of attacks, school and parental responses, and the total treatment received in childhood influence the degree of such disabilities. Factors to consider are inadequate basic education, delayed social maturation, reduced experiences, impoverishment of interpersonal skills, passivity, dependency, denial, lack of self-confidence, and depression.

Rehabilitation potential is governed largely by control of frequency and length of attacks and the breadth of precipitating factors. For some, goals established can include long-term training and education. For others, only a short-term service program may be indicated.

Standards of Evaluation

Medical evaluation is essentially the same as described for COPD. In addition, careful review and perhaps skin testing by a specialist in allergies is included to identify any specific allergens to be avoided.

Clinical psychological review of educational achievement and personality patterns for those with childhood-onset asthma is helpful for planning. In the young adult where significant parental contact remains, social service review of prior and current relationships may suggest conflicts in need of resolution. Where emotional stresses are contributory to a precipitation of attacks, social and psychological review may help identify them.

Total Treatment

Medical treatment is directed at symptomatic relief of an attack, control of identified precipitating factors, and maintenance medication to inhibit an attack if the patient is exposed to the triggering stimulus.

Acute attacks rarely require hospitalization. Patients may be trained to abort an attack themselves. Self-administration of oral or injectable bronchodilators may be approved by the patient's physician. Others may need to go to their physician or a hospital emergency room for acute treatment. Continuous oral bronchodilators to suppress attacks, with additional medication to be used at the earliest onset of wheezing, is conventional. Status asthmaticus usually requires hospitalization.

Identification and avoidance of allergens, nonspecific irritants, and other circumstances shown to induce attacks is beneficial. Part of the treatment may be a series of hyposensitization "shots" for those patients who, by history and skin testing, demonstrate allergy. The selective use of bronchodilators, antibiotics, steroids, and physical measures are as described for COPD. Medication adjustments as the seasons, environments, and attack frequency change usually require medical follow-up at 2-month intervals.

In some instances, as dictated by the psychosocial evaluation, ongoing contacts with a psychologist and social worker may be beneficial. As discussed above for COPD, when multiple professionals are involved, mutual communication and integration of the various treatment approaches is essential.

Vocational Implications

For clients who have significant chronic airway obstruction or who overlap with the spectrum of COPD, the job with the most uniform irritant-free environment and the least physical demands is desirable because of the possibility of later progression. Most asthmatics who have little or no continuous obstruction and two to four attacks a month are capable of medium work. Except for persons with mild attacks responding well to treatment, abrupt temperature changes, exposure to outdoor weather, dusts, and heavy industrial pollution should be avoided. The acceptability of occasional absenteeism and freedom from environments which induce attacks or predispose to respiratory infection are frequent vocational requirements.

Industrial asthma refers to a form of the disease in which a particular occupation seems to induce the asthma attack in the worker. Meat packing, baking, and exposures to certain fibers and agricultural products are examples. When a relationship between symptoms and a particular job is clearly documented, a job change is necessary.

Persons with severe and frequent asthma attacks may successfully engage in moderate work if the work does not directly initiate the attacks and if absenteeism can be accommodated. In this group, sheltered work may be necessary.

The counselor's approach involves the same considerations described for COPD. However, asthmatics are frequently younger than clients with COPD and, while individual attacks are more severe, remission is more complete. Environmental considerations discussed earlier are particularly important, since bronchial irritation and infections not only induce attacks, but tend to predispose asthmatics to COPD.

Conflicts may occur between interests and aptitudes and the environments that must be avoided. In such situations, exploration of new interests and generation of new skills will tax the counselor's ingenuity. For clients whose attacks are well controlled, and who have demonstrated effective monitoring of their own health and good attention to their medication and physician's recommendations, the counselor can comfortably consider long-term goals. These may include extended education, particularly if early education was impoverished, and extensive vocational training. Selection of employment possibilities may require that the counselor interact with the client's physician to ensure that a particular environment is suitable.

It may be useful to contact an employer regarding restructuring a client's job to avoid even occasional exposure to a particular irritating environment. Expected length and frequency of absenteeism as a result of attacks may need to be communicated to a potential employer to avoid later problems. Both employers and co-workers also need to understand that an attack, while debilitating, is rarely, if ever, life threatening. Such knowledge is necessary to allay their own fears should they have occasion to witness an attack.

OCCUPATIONAL LUNG DISEASE

Disease Description

Many occupational fumes and dusts are irritating to the nasal and respiratory membranes, especially in smokers and persons with COPD. Other compounds, including oxides of nitrogen, beryllium, cadmium, and other metals, and chemicals encountered in rubber and plastic industries, cause inflammation and scarring (fibrosis) of the lung in persons continuously exposed.

Another disease, *hypersensitivity pneumonitis,* also induces lung inflammation and scarring. It is caused by a specific organic substance to which the person has become sensitive. The disease is often identified by the occupation in which it occurs. For example, "farmer's lung" and "mushroom picker's lung" are caused by a particular fungus associated with moldy hay and mushrooms, respectively.

Proteins in an industrial product itself can incite the disease. Thus, "fish meal lung" and "furrier's lung" exist. Of the many fungi capable of inducing hypersensitivity pneumonitis, only one, *Aspergillus fumigatus,* actually infects, grows, and reproduces in the host.

Hypersensitivity pneumonitis is characterized by cough, wheezing, and dyspnea on exposure, followed by progressive fibrosis and a clinical course resembling COPD. The worker must be removed from the exposure.

Byssinosis is caused by compounds in cotton fibers capable of inducing an asthmatic reaction in some workers. Initially, there is a characteristic history of symptoms occurring only on the first day of the work week. Over an extended period, the illness develops into chronic asthmatic bronchitis if exposure is not controlled.

Another family of lung diseases, the *pneumoconioses,* consist of localized scarring in the lung caused by deposits of certain dusts. The most important of these diseases are coal worker's pneumoconiosis, asbestosis, and silicosis. Most workers exposed to any of these dusts do not develop occupational lung disease. Individual predisposition and the intensity and duration of exposure are important factors. Smoking is especially important as a predisposer in pneumoconiosis. Indeed, the duration of smoking is several times more significant than the duration of underground mining in the development of respiratory symptoms in coal miners.

There is a long time interval between the onset of the disease and the development of chronic pulmonary problems in occupational lung disease. In byssinosis it is 10 to 20 years. Coal worker's pneumoconiosis and silicosis usually require 20 years or more for the development of X-ray changes, although some show up after 10 years of very heavy exposure.

The impairments, clinical manifestations, and complications resemble those seen in COPD. After removal from the offending substance, hypersensitivity pneumonitis should subside completely or continue as a form of COPD, depending on the stage of the disease. Pneumoconioses are frequently diagnosed by X-ray at a time when pulmonary function is normal or slightly reduced. Unless scarring is severe or unless there is significant COPD, progression may not occur or may be extremely slow.

The same evaluation methods used in COPD apply to the occupational lung diseases. Blood tests and reproduction of the symptoms by a test exposure demonstrate the altered immune state in hypersensitivity pneumonitis. The chest X-ray has more significance in the pneumoconioses than in COPD because widely scattered small scarred areas and other changes are visible and hence useful for the diagnosis.

In addition to cessation of exposure, all the factors noted for treatment of COPD usually apply for the occupational lung diseases.

Vocational Implications

The guidelines suggested for COPD are also appropriate for occupational lung diseases. Vocational planning is based on pulmonary function studies and symptoms. The many years of client exposure required before disability occurs brings such persons into vocational rehabilitation late in their vocational careers. For the pneumoconioses, it may be in the fifth or sixth decade. While their prior work history is generally good, it is usually limited in breadth, and many of these workers are poorly equipped by education, skills, and social factors for transfer into other occupations.

The legal implications of pneumoconiosis often generate severe obstacles to vocational rehabilitation. For example, the current policies governing compensation in coal worker's pneumoconiosis may result in a worker with normal pulmonary function studies and a negative X-ray being declared totally disabled. The fear of liability by employers often limits job opportunities, and financial considerations influence the motivation and cooperation of the worker.

CYSTIC FIBROSIS

Disease Description

Cystic fibrosis is a hereditary disorder in which many mucus-secreting organs in the body are damaged by an abnormal, thick mucus which blocks glands and ducts and leads to degeneration and scarring of the organ. Although "advertised" mostly as a disease of the lung, the damage is most apparent in the pancreas. Pancreatic involvement leads to severe progressive chronic malnutrition and growth retardation. Constipation, diarrhea, and excess fat in the stools are associated.

Excessive dense mucus in the small bronchi leads to a severe progressive chronic bronchitis, fibrosis, and emphysema. Although other structures are involved, such as the entire intestinal tract, the clinical course is largely determined by the severity of the involvement of the pancreas and the bronchopulmonary system.

In spite of treatment, most patients die during infancy or childhood. Rarely, patients survive past the age of 20. Death results from malnutrition, intestinal or biliary obstruction, respiratory failure, almost continuous suppurative pulmonary infections, and pneumonia. Wheezing, dyspnea, greatly reduced exercise tolerance, multiple medical visits, and short stature are common. In some patients, the problems are primarily respiratory and all the issues associated with COPD are generally applicable. However, in cystic fibrosis, progression is more rapid and difficult to control, and the thick, frequently infected mucus which cannot be effectively cleared is a constant problem. In milder cases, the disease may involve primarily the pancreas and gastrointestinal system. With less respiratory disease, these patients can survive into adulthood.

Diagnosis is established by a positive family history and typical findings on the history and physical examination. Cystic fibrosis is strongly suggested if the sweat sodium and chloride concentration is greater than 60 mg per liter in children and above 80 mg per liter in adults. Careful medical evaluation is necessary to rule out COPD, chronic pancreatitis, congenital or acquired defects in the immune system, cirrhosis, and gastrointestinal diseases resulting in malnutrition, all conditions with greater treatment possibilities than cystic fibrosis.

The evaluation, therefore, should include sweat sodium and chloride determination, sputum examination, pulmonary function studies, arterial blood gases, chest X-ray, immunoglobulins, and blood and stool examinations to demonstrate failures in digestion and absorption of nutrients.

A clinical psychologist can assist in evaluating and planning an educational program for an ill and often homebound child. The social worker is usually required to evaluate the impact of the child's illness on the vocational capacity of the parents.

The pulmonary manifestations require intermittent or continuous antibiotics, the frequent use of humidity aerosols, postural drainage and other mechanical measures to eliminate secretions, and sometimes bronchodilators. Many patients are occasionally or continuously enclosed in high humidity tents. Pancreatic enzymes taken by mouth are usually required. A high-calorie, high-protein, low-fat diet is used, with additional vitamins A, D, and K and sometimes additional salt. Nutrition can be controlled in the 20 percent of patients with normal or only moderately impaired pancreatic function.

Avoidance of respiratory infections and adverse environments is essential. Heat must be avoided because it results in excessive and occasional fatal loss of salt through the sweat.

There are many hospitalizations. In between hospitalizations, home management is expensive and complicated by the use of aerosol generators, tents, and frequent medications. These problems, plus the emotional ones related to the gravity and progressive nature of the child's illness, impact heavily on the parents, requiring counseling and ongoing support. Prolonged institutionalization of the child may even be required.

Vocational Implications

Usually, vocational rehabilitation is directed primarily at the parents and will consist of medical assistance, visiting homemakers, visiting nurses, and homebound care programs so that the parents' employment can be maintained and their financial burdens reduced. Support services to the parents is a concept that can be considered so that their child's disability does not interfere with their own vocational stability.

The median age of survival is now 17 years. Fifty percent of patients therefore are over 17 at the time of death. Increasing numbers of patients are thus surviving into adulthood, and in the future, as treatment techniques improve, more will enter the employment market. For those with mild and stable pulmonary involvement and reasonably good nutrition, 5 years of homebound or sheltered employment might be a reasonable goal.

BIBLIOGRAPHY

Agle DP, Baum GL: Psychological aspects of chronic obstructive pulmonary disease. Med Clin North Am 61:749–758, 1977.
   This article describes some of the psychological aspects of COPD. Although written for physicians, the information could help a counselor in considering types of employment for clients, primarily with regard to level of adjustment to the disability and ability to cope with anxiety and depression.
Barstow RE: Coping with emphysema. Nurs Clin North Am 9:137–145, 1974.
   A description of the sick role and the coping mechanisms most commonly used by emphysema patients.
Dyksterhuis JE: Vocational rehabilitation of chronic obstructive pulmonary disease patients. Rehabil Lit 33:136–138, 1972.
   This article primarily deals with the vocational evaluations of 147 patients. The major factors affecting the probability of vocational success are discussed.
Hodgkins JE, et al: Chronic obstructive airway diseases: Current concepts in diagnosis and comprehensive care. JAMA 232:1234–1260, 1975.
   A well-documented, broad summary of COPD.
Morgan WK, Seaton A: *Occupational Lung Diseases.* Saunders, Philadelphia, 1975.
   Occupational pulmonary diseases are thoroughly discussed in this small volume.
Murray JE (ed): *Lung Disease: State of the Art, 1975–1976.* New York, American Lung Association, 1977.
   This is a state-of-the-art review of asthma.

Petty TL, Branscomb BV, Farrington JF, Kettel LJ, Lindsmith LA: Community resources for rehabilitation of patients with chronic obstructive pulmonary disease and cor pulmonale. Circulation 49:A-1 to A-20, May 1974.

Several different types of rehabilitation programs, each operating in a different community setting, are described. (Note:A-1 to A-20 follow the advertising section at the end of the journal.)

Rosenlund ML, Lustig HS: Young adults with cystic fibrosis. The problems of a new generation. Ann Intern Med 78:959–961, 1973.

Because more cystic fibrosis patients are living to adulthood, the authors began a group counseling program for teenage patients and their families. This article discusses some of the most common problems encountered.

Wood RE, Boat TF, Doershuk CF: Cystic fibrosis. Am Rev Resp Dis 113: 833–878, 1976.

All aspects of the disease are covered, including cystic fibrosis in adults.

24 DIABETES MELLITUS

Leona V. Miller, M.D.

DISEASE DESCRIPTION

Diabetes mellitus, a chronic disorder of metabolism that affects all body systems, was recognized as early as 2000 B.C. Although the incidence varies in different ethnic groups and cultures, it is found in all parts of the world.

It has been estimated that as many as 10 million Americans may be directly affected by this disease. A report from the National Commission on Diabetes states: "The average American born today has a better than one-in-five chance of developing diabetes unless a method of prevention is found." Although there is no cure for diabetes, effective (though not complete) treatment exists.

Diabetes is primarily a disease of the insulin-producing cells of the pancreas. The consequent insulin deficiency results in impaired utilization (metabolism) of carbohydrates, fats, and proteins. In particular, the carbohydrate metabolism deficiency results in a defective ability to utilize glucose. Hence, the level of glucose in the blood is abnormally high *(hyperglycemia)* and glucose spills into the urine *(glucosuria)*.

There are two main classes of diabetes, the adult (maturity)-onset type and the juvenile-onset type. The majority of diabetics have the maturity-onset type. Only 5 percent of the total diabetic population have juvenile-onset diabetes.

The maturity-onset type of diabetes develops in middle age or later years. In the early stages of the disease, referred to as "chemical" or "latent" diabetes, the patient may be asymptomatic. An abnormal blood sugar may be found on hospitalization for an unrelated cause or during a routine physical. In the more advanced stages, the patient may either present with the symptoms of urinary frequency (polyuria), excessive thirst (polydipsia), or excessive hunger (polyphagia), or with blurred vision. The need to excrete excess sugar causes the polyuria and results in the patient being excessively thirsty. Since the sugar that is lost means lost calories, polyphagia results, and the patient tends to eat more to compensate for the lost

calories. Nevertheless, weight loss may ensue. In the obese patient, this weight loss may not be obvious or may be mistakenly attributed to diet. The blurred vision is due to fluctuations in blood sugar that cause lens changes. All these symptoms are usually reversible. At the time the diagnosis is made, patients with advanced diabetes often already have circulatory or neurologic complications.

Juvenile-type diabetes manifests itself in infancy, adolescence, or young adulthood. However, it can also occur in the older person, and the maturity-onset type can occur in children. The diagnosis of juvenile-onset-type diabetes is generally not difficult. The onset is abrupt, with symptoms of weight loss, polyuria, polydipsia, or polyphagia. Juvenile-type diabetic patients generally have an absolute lack of insulin and are prone to develop ketoacidosis and diabetic coma (see below) if they are not treated appropriately with insulin. Their diabetes is the most difficult to control and they often develop vascular complications 15 to 20 years after onset.

Etiology

While the exact etiology of diabetes is not known, there is good evidence that persons who develop the disease have a genetic predisposition. Diabetes occurs more frequently in siblings of diabetic patients and more often when both parents are affected. The maturity-onset-type diabetes has a strong genetic component. When one identical twin develops maturity-onset diabetes, 90 percent of the time the second twin will also develop the disease. On the other hand, in juvenile-type diabetes, the second twin develops the disease only 50 percent of the time. Genetic factors are obviously not the sole cause, for if they were, then both identical twins would develop diabetes.

Corticosteroid therapy, oral contraceptives, and pregnancy also influence the onset of diabetes in susceptible individuals, and there is some evidence to suggest that certain types of viral infections may produce the disease, although this is not yet certain. Further, diabetes may be an autoimmune disease, that is, the body's immune system treats the insulin-producing cells as a foreign tissue and makes antibodies against them, hence impairing their ability to produce insulin.

Finally, certain disease states cause diabetes in the absence of genetic susceptibility, namely: (a) pancreatic disorders, such as pancreatitis (an inflammation of the pancreas), surgical removal of the pancreas, and hemochromatosis (a disease that causes liver cirrhosis and pancreatic cell destruction); and (b) disorders of other endocrine glands, such as pituitary tumors, adrenal tumors or hyperplasia, and hyperthyroidism.

Pathology

The pancreas, which lies in the upper part of the abdomen, is the site of pathology in diabetes. The pancreas has two main functions and sets of specialized cells. One set secretes enzymes into the gastrointestinal tract to assist in the digestion of carbohydrates, proteins, and fats and is not altered in diabetes. The other set, the *islets of Langerhans*, is responsible for the secretion of the hormones insulin and glucagon. It is these cells that are impaired in diabetes.

Insulin is secreted primarily in response to the concentration of glucose in the blood. The normal response of the pancreatic cells to glucose consists of an initial rapid release of preformed insulin, followed by a slower release of newly formed insulin. When the disease is fully developed, both phases of insulin secretion may be impaired or absent.

While defective insulin secretion is thought to be the primary disorder in diabetes, there is some experimental evidence to indicate that the hormone glucagon may also contribute to the disordered metabolism. The action of glucagon is the opposite of the action of insulin. Glucagon normally stimulates glucose production and is secreted when the blood glucose falls, or when there is stress or increased need for glucose, as in the exercising muscle. Glucagon is normally suppressed by elevated blood glucose levels. In diabetes, this appears not to be the case.

The major metabolic function of insulin is to aid the body in storing fuel. Insulin does this by stimulating withdrawal from the blood and subsequent storage of carbohydrates (glucose) in muscle and liver, of fats in adipose tissue, and of proteins in muscle. Further, insulin inhibits the breakdown of these fuels from storage sites. When insulin secretion is impaired, ingested glucose is not stored, and glucose that is stored is released into the blood stream. This causes the blood glucose to rise. As a result, the amount of glucose in the blood increases (hyperglycemia) and is greater than normal even in the early morning before breakfast (fasting state), as well as 2 to 3 hours after a meal (postprandial).

If the diabetes is severe and the patient has no insulin secretion whatsoever, the body will be unable to handle fats and proteins properly. Weight loss occurs, and if the disease state goes unrecognized and untreated for a period of time, *ketoacidosis* may develop.

In ketoacidosis, the body begins to break down fats for fuel because there is no insulin to metabolize glucose. When an excess of fatty acids are broken down, the body's capacity for metabolizing these breakdown products (ketones) is exceeded. The ketones then circulate in the blood and cause derangement of the body's acid/base balance. Ketones are also excreted in the urine (ketonuria).

The high blood glucose level in ketoacidosis causes increased urination (diuresis), dehydration, loss of electrolytes, and, in severe cases, peripheral circulatory failure. The increased ketone level in the blood and resulting acidosis causes vomiting, further loss of electrolytes, and further dehydration. The patient may lose consciousness (diabetic coma).

The onset of ketoacidosis is gradual. Symptoms develop over days or even weeks before the patient becomes drowsy and loses consciousness. Symptoms include thirst and polyuria, fatigue, weight loss, possible vomiting and abdominal pain, overbreathing, and finally coma. The patient's skin and mouth will be dry, his face may be flushed, and his temperature may be low.

Ketoacidosis may occur in the known diabetic who is poorly controlled or is under stress from infection, trauma, surgical procedures, heart attack, stroke, or severe emotional stress. Pregnant diabetic patients may also develop ketoacidosis if not carefully controlled. Ketoacidosis is a life-threatening situation. It requires hospitalization and treatment with insulin, intravenous fluids, and electrolytes.

Hypoglycemia, also called insulin reaction, is a complication of insulin therapy and should not be confused with hyperglycemia. It occurs when the patient's blood sugar level becomes too low for the amount of insulin he has taken. The onset of hypoglycemia is rapid and is caused by insufficient carbohydrates in the diet, delayed meals, or prolonged or unusually strenuous physical activity. The signs and symptoms are many and varied, but usually include one or more of the following: intense hunger, sweating, palpitations, inability to concentrate, unsteadiness, double vision (diplopia), and a tingling sensation in the mouth and lips. The patient may be pale and may have a raised pulse rate. He may become excited, nervous, irritable, or confused, or he may be unusually aggressive or affectionate. If hypoglycemia is severe, there may be temporary weakness of one or both extremities on one side of the body (monoplegia or hemiplegia), or the patient may lose consciousness.

Complications

The major complications of diabetes involve the circulatory and nervous systems.

Circulatory system. For reasons not yet clear, diabetes can induce sufficient narrowing of the arterial blood vessels to produce thrombosis. Involvement of the major arteries (macroangiopathy) may result in heart attacks (myocardial infarctions), strokes, and gangrene of the more distal parts of the lower extremities, necessitating amputations below or above the knee. Complete discussions of these complications are found in chapters 22, 9 and 10, and 13, respectively. Small-vessel lesions (microangiopathy) lead to renal failure (see chap. 25) and retinopathy which may cause blindness (see chap. 29).

Nervous system. Diabetes, again for reasons not yet clear (possibly vascular and possibly related to carbohydrate metabolism), can also cause peripheral neuropathy (see chap. 7). The neuropathy may involve the autonomic nervous system and cause gastrointestinal dysfunction such as diarrhea, constipation, nausea, or vomiting. Male patients with autonomic dysfunction frequently develop sexual impotence. Further, a low blood pressure while standing (postural hypotention) may produce dizziness and even faints while the patient is erect. A disturbance in bladder function may also occur.

Neuropathy of the somatic nervous system (p. 101) may induce weakness or paralysis of isolated peripheral nerves, including the cranial nerves. More commonly, a sensory loss peripherally (e.g., hands and feet), with or without weakness, occurs. Loss of sensation may lead to joint deformities through overuse, and foot ulcers through failure to detect a sore. Foot ulcers and circulatory system insufficiency can jointly contribute to gangrene, infection, and lower limb loss. The problem is compounded by the fact that wound healing is deficient in diabetic patients.

While there is still controversy whether good blood sugar control can delay or prevent the circulatory and neurologic complications, every effort is made by most physicians to maintain control.

In addition to these major complications, vaginal and urinary tract infections may also occur. These are stimulated, in part, by sugar in the urine, since sugar is a good culture medium for bacteria.

Prognosis

The prognosis for the diabetic is dependent on a number of factors, namely, the age of onset, the duration, the type of diabetes, and the degree of control of blood sugar.

While the circulatory complications are related to the duration of disease in juvenile-type diabetic patients, some patients remain free of complications for 30 to 40 years. Unfortunately, it is not possible at this time to predict which patients will develop complications. For the maturity-onset diabetic, the circulatory sequelae that lead to heart attacks, stroke, and loss of lower limbs are the most important. Until these develop, the maturity-onset diabetic is often remarkably symptom free.

The life expectancy of patients with diabetes mellitus is approximately one-third less than that of the general population. The life expectancy for the blind diabetic, however, is approximately 5 years. In 1975, there were 38,000 deaths directly attributable to diabetes. Since diabetes is often a contributory rather than the primary cause of death, many authorities believe that under-reporting of deaths due to diabetes occurs. Cardiovascular and cerebrovascular complications are the common causes of death in diabetics.

FUNCTIONAL DISABILITIES

Physical Disabilities

The diabetic patient who is knowledgeable about the disease, is under optimal management, and has been found on physical examination to have none of the long-term complications described, can generally be estimated to be free from physical disabilities for a minimum of 5 to 10 years. He is not likely to come to the attention of a rehabilitation counselor unless psychological or social problems are significantly interfering with function.

In the later years, should small-vessel problems develop, vision may deteriorate until blindness ensues. In addition, the patient may develop renal disease that leads to renal failure. Both disorders are often present at the same time. Further, diabetic patients who are blind often also have neuropathy, with loss of sensation in their fingers, making it difficult or impossible for them to learn Braille, and sensory loss in the lower limbs, making it more difficult for them to learn blind ambulation.

If the larger vessels are sufficiently involved to cause stroke, myocardial infarctions, and amputations, the physical disabilities are as reported in chapters 9, 10, 22, and 13 respectively.

Psychosocial Disabilities

There is no specific psychosocial problem that exists in all diabetic patients. Some patients find it emotionally difficult to accept the diagnosis, the dietary restrictions, the daily urine testing, and the injections. Their compliance with good management may be poor and they may have frequent hospitalizations for uncontrolled diabetes and hypoglycemia.

The restrictions imposed by diabetes are particularly disturbing to the child or adolescent. The disease tends to make them dependent on their parents, often at a time when they are striving to become independent. This may heighten the conflict with parents, and under these circumstances, the disease may be used as a weapon against the parents. They may miss meals, ingest increased amounts of carbohydrates, or refuse to test their urine.

Both children and adults with diabetes may become excessively dependent on other family members. This dependence restricts their activity, and their reluctance to be away from home or to make new friends interferes with education, extracurricular activities, and job opportunities.

The young child or adolescent with mild hypoglycemic episodes may become a behavior problem, have temper tantrums, or experience difficulty in concentrating on school work.

The diabetic patient who develops a serious compliction (e.g., blindness, stroke, or amputation) often is depressed, may be suicidal, may refuse to make plans for the future, and may not cooperate in a rehabilitation program. During this period, the patient requires strong support from family, friends, and health care professionals. If the depression is prolonged, psychiatric counseling may be necessary.

Rehabilitation Potential

The diabetic patient *with no complications* may be seeking vocational rehabilitation because he may be engaged in work that has become dangerous due to hypoglycemic reactions, or because control of his diabetes may be difficult due to irregular working hours and meal times, causing his physician to recommend employment changes. As previously discussed, these patients may be free of complications for a number of years, and long-range vocational goals may be planned.

Diabetic patients with either impending blindness (proliferative retinopathy) and/or renal failure generally have a reduced life span, and therefore short-term goals for retraining should be sought. The patient with neuropathy, but otherwise free of long-term complications, has a better prognosis, and longer-term goals are appropriate. One- to two-year goals may be undertaken by the client who has had a myocardial infarction and is free of angina or other complications.

The patient who has had a foot or leg amputation secondary to large-vessel disease generally has significant widespread vascular disease, and life expectancy is therefore lessened. Short-term goals should be undertaken. If the amputation was done primarily for infection, and large-vessel disease is not a major problem, life expectancy may not be lessened, and 1 or 2 years of training may be undertaken. More than 50 percent of patients who have one limb amputated for vascular disease will have the other limb amputated within 5 years.

STANDARDS OF EVALUATION

Medical Evaluation

The diabetic patient should have a thorough medical history, with particular attention paid to onset of diabetes, type and duration of therapy, onset of complications, reasons for any hospitalizations, and a thorough review of symptoms relating to diabetes and other body systems. This is best performed at a diabetes center or by an internist with special interest and training in diabetes. The patient should have a complete physical examination, with particular emphasis on the following areas.

Eye. A complete eye examination should be performed, including tonometry to determine if glaucoma is present, and a funduscopic examination to determine if retinopathy exists. Nonproliferative retinopathy does not carry a poor prognosis, but if proliferative retinopathy is present, the patient must be referred to an ophthalmologist. It is this type of retinopathy that leads to blindness, if untreated.

Circulatory system. Peripheral pulses should be checked carefully. If the patient suffers from cramping of the legs on walking a short distance (intermittent claudication) or rest pain, and the femoral and popliteal pulses (see p. 304) are diminished, the patient should be referred to a vascular surgeon.

Nervous system. When peripheral neuropathy is present, the patient will have loss of sensation, particularly light touch and temperature. Deep tendon reflexes at the ankle and knee will be diminished, position sense will be impaired, and weakness may be present. A patient with these symptoms should be referred to a neurologist.

Skin. The feet should be evaluated for calluses or fungal infections. If these are found, the patient should be referred to a podiatrist for further care.

Kidney. If renal disease is present, the patient may require evaluation by a nephrologist.

Nutrition. If diabetes control is poor or if obesity exists, the patient may need to be referred to a dietician for dietary instructions.

Laboratory Tests

The diagnostic tests should include: yearly chest X-ray; ECG (yearly in patients who have had diabetes for 10 to 20 years, or in middle-aged or elderly patients); serum BUN or creatinine to evaluate renal function; 24-hour urine for protein to evaluate renal function; serum albumin (low albumin indicates presence of renal or liver disease); serum cholesterol and triglyceride (if elevated, special diet and/or stricter control of blood sugar is required; elevations may aggravate vascular problems); and frequently fasting and postprandial blood sugars to monitor control of diabetes.

The main test to corroborate the diagnosis of diabetes is the glucose tolerance test (GTT). In this test, the patient, while in a fasting state, swallows 100 grams of glucose in liquid form. His blood sugar level is measured just before the glucose meal and 1, 2, and 3 hours later. If the blood sugar value exceeds certain values in some or in all four specimens, the diagnosis is determined. Table 24-1 indicates the highest values accepted as normal for plasma glucose and whole blood glucose. The arbitrary number of points given if these values are exceeded is also given. A total of two points, however obtained, usually means diabetes is present.

Psychosocial Evaluation

Evaluation by a social worker and/or psychologist will identify problems of emotional instability, excessive dependency, or denial of the disease. Any of these problems may cause the patient to be in poor control through failure to follow instructions regarding diet, exercise, or medication. Referral for psychological counseling may be appropriate where these problems exist.

Because the diabetic carries a great deal of responsibility for the control of his own disease, his knowledge of diabetes and self-management should be evaluated. If his knowledge is deficient, he should be referred back to his physician or to a diabetes center for appropriate education.

An educational and vocational history should also be obtained. Where the patient's education was restricted because of medical needs or social withdrawal during the school years, academic achievement testing by a clinical psychologist may be useful.

Male patients who are impotent should be evaluated by a psychologist to determine whether the sexual dysfunction is psychological rather than organic, and to identify family problems and depression caused by the patient's impotence. If the problem is clearly organic, the patient should be referred to a urologist for consideration of a penile implant.

TOTAL TREATMENT

The treatment of diabetes involves four major areas: (a) education in self-care, self-monitoring of disease, and medication administration; (b) maintenance of appropriate diet, alone or with diabetic agents; (c) medications (oral agents or injectable insulin); and (d) the management of complications.

Education

All diabetic patients require instructions in diet; general hygiene, with particular attention to foot care; home urine testing for sugar or ketones; and recognition and treatment of hypoglycemic reactions from too much insulin. Patients who are taking insulin also require instruction and demonstration of proper syringe preparation and injection.

Diet

All diabetic patients should be prescribed an American Diabetes Association (ADA) diet. If weight reduction is necessary, the diet should also be restricted in calories. The diet prescribed must be appropriate for the age and activity of the patient. The contents of the diet are 50 percent carbohydrate, 30 percent fat, and 20 percent protein. In addition to the patient, the person actually preparing the meals must also understand the diet.

TABLE 24-1
GLUCOSE TOLERANCE TEST*

Time	Plasma Glucose (mg/100ml)	Whole Blood Glucose (mg/100ml)
Fasting	125 (1 point)	110 (1 point)
1 hour after glucose ingestion	195 (½ point)	170 (½ point)
2 hours after glucose ingestion	140 (½ point)	120 (½ point)
3 hours after glucose ingestion	125 (1 point)	110 (1 point)

*Standardization of the oral glucose tolerance test. Report of the Committee of Standards of the American Diabetes Association. Diabetes 18:299–307, 1969.

The diabetic patient does not have to purchase special foods, and, except for the portions prescribed, the diet is appropriate for all family members. Maturity-onset patients are often obese and may be controlled on a diet regimen alone. Many, however, also require oral hypoglycemic drugs or insulin for control of blood sugar.

Medications

The patient may require oral hypoglycemic agents or insulin. If the patient has had recent weight loss, is pregnant, or tends to spill ketones in the urine, insulin is preferred. Though controversy exists regarding use of oral agents, many patients are still treated in this manner.

The oral agents now in use are the sulfonylureas. Elderly patients who are symptomatic (e.g., spilling sugar in urine) are best treated with the short-acting agent tolbutamide. This agent does not often cause hypoglycemia. It may be used as well in middle-aged diabetics.

Acetohexamide and tolazamide are somewhat longer acting, and many diabetics are treated with these agents. The longest acting agent is chlorpropamide. This medication need only be taken once a day. Chlorpropamide can induce hypoglycemia and low sodium in the blood. Therefore, patients taking this drug must be carefully followed.

Juvenile-onset patients and maturity-onset patients who are ketosis prone or have renal or cardiac complications should be treated with insulin. The patient may be prescribed a long-acting medication (generally NPH or Lente insulin) once a day, or a combination of insulins (NPH or Lente plus a short-acting insulin, CZI) once a day.

The amount and type of insulin is selected and monitored on the basis of urine sugar testing carried out by the patient at home, and both fasting and postprandial blood sugars tested by the physician.

Home urine testing is quite simple. A drop of urine on a special paper tape (e.g., Diastix) is all that is necessary. The color change occurring in the tape is compared to a color chart. Different colors indicate, in a relative way, the amount of sugar in the urine (e.g., 1^+, 2^+, 3^+, 4^+). Large-size tapes and color charts (Mega-Diastix) are available for diabetics with severe visual impairments. Ketones in the urine can also be tested with special paper tape (e.g., Ketostix) in a similar way.

Occasionally, a somewhat more complex home urine testing procedure which is more quantitative will be prescribed (e.g., Clinitest). Measured amounts of urine and water are placed in a test tube. A tablet is added, which makes the liquid "boil." The color of the liquid after the boiling stops is compared with a color chart to indicate the amount of glucose in the urine.

A new tactile urine testing procedure has been developed for blind diabetics (touch fermentation test). Urine is mixed with bakers' yeast in a test tube, which is then capped with a rubber protector. If there is glucose in the urine, the yeast will cause it to ferment and release carbon dioxide gas. This will inflate the rubber. The blind person can feel the gas pressure under the rubber if the test is positive. A second test tube containing urine and a glucose tablet is used as a control.

In many diabetic patients, particularly the middle-aged or elderly, it may not be possible to attain blood sugar levels close to the normal range (60 to 130 mg%). Fasting blood sugars up to 150 mg% and postprandial blood sugars up to 250 mg% may be acceptable.

In young patients, generally every effort is made to keep the blood sugar as close to the normal range as possible. Since absolute normal blood sugars are difficult to attain in all patients without precipitating hypoglycemia reactions, fasting blood sugars in the range between 100 and 130 mg%, and 3-hour postprandial blood sugars in the 130 to 180 mg% range, are acceptable. The major problems relate to maintenance of a balance between insulin, diet, and exercise. Young diabetics are encouraged to participate in regular school activities and extracurricular sports. However, they must be taught to take extra carbohydrates and to decrease their dose of insulin when engaging in moderate to heavy exercise. Meals cannot be delayed or missed or hypoglycemia will be precipitated.

Even the well-controlled diabetic may occasionally have an episode of hypoglycemia if a meal is delayed or missed or if there is unexpected physical exertion. The confusion, delayed reaction time, or loss of manual dexterity which may occur during such an episode is rapidly reversed by ingestion of sugar in any form.

Management of Complications

The combination of macrovascular and microvascular disease in the lower extremity, coupled with sensory loss, frequently leads to foot ulcers, gangrene, and amputation. To prevent these complications, special care must be taken of the feet, and special shoes may have to be prescribed.

The diabetic patient with lower limb amputations can be taught to ambulate (see chap. 13). Care must be taken, however, to ensure that the prothesis fits properly, as the sensory deficit in these patients does not alert them to pressure points that may produce ulcerations.

The diabetic patient with a cardiac disease or a

cerebrovascular accident can be managed as the nondiabetic patient with similar complications (see chaps. 22, 9, and 10).

VOCATIONAL IMPLICATIONS

Aptitudes

The diabetic client who is free of complications and is maintained in good control has no diminution of motor and mental skills. The client with peripheral neuropathy may have problems sensing texture or handling small objects, but motor coordination is generally not affected.

Depending on the area of the brain involved, the client who has had a stroke will have varying difficulties with motor and mental skills. The blind diabetic who has not suffered a stroke can be expected to have no reduction in mental capacity.

Interest

The diabetic who has no complications may generally pursue any activity of interest. However, any work or play that might be dangerous if sudden hypoglycemia were to develop is to be discouraged if the client's blood sugar is not easily controlled. Such things as motorcycle riding, driving an automobile, flying, scuba diving, and work around heavy machinery, on ladders, or at construction sites should only be permitted if the client's physician feels that the diabetes is sufficiently stable. Also because of the possibility of hypoglycemia, a diabetic taking insulin should probably not work entirely alone. Further, jobs requiring irregular working hours and meal times should be discouraged.

Physical Demands

The diabetic with no complications may engage in any type of physical activity, dependent, of course, on his strength. However, the physical exertion required by a job should not vary from day to day. The following types of diabetic clients should not engage in medium to very heavy work: the middle aged; the cardiac; those taking insulin who are subject to hypoglycemia; and those with vascular disease, neuropathy, or impaired vision. The client with severe neuropathy of the lower extremities may not be able to engage in light work if it entails too much standing or walking. The client with neuropathy involving the hands should not work where thermal or chemical burns might occur. Occupations involving an unusual injury hazard should be avoided because of the difficulty in wound healing associated with diabetes.

Environment

The client with uncomplicated diabetes generally can work in any environment that is not unsafe for workers in general. The client with neuropathy, cardiac disease, or vascular disease should not work in unprotected outside areas where dampness, cold temperatures, extreme heat, or abrupt temperature changes can occur. These may have an adverse effect on circulation. In addition, the hands and feet of a diabetic client with neuropathy may be insensitive to heat and cold and must be protected from burns and frostbite.

BIBLIOGRAPHY

Alexander RW, Tetrick L, Friedman GJ: Physicians' guidelines for the diabetic in industry. J Occup Med **16**:802–803, 1974.
    Short article giving physicians' guidelines for the control of diabetics. Includes guidelines for job placement restrictions and a short summary of work attendance.
Cohen EB, Mastbaum L: Employment for patients with diabetes. Minn Med **57**: 241–244, 1974.
    This short article briefly describes the employment of diabetics with regard to absenteeism, education, driving, the kinds of limitations placed on employment, and work records. Emphasizes individual evaluation.
Cull JG, Hardy RD (eds): *Counseling and Rehabilitating the Diabetic.* Springfield, IL, Thomas, 1974.
    An easy-to-read book covering the management, medical, and psychosocial aspects of juvenile-onset diabetes. Includes several case studies.
Education and Management of the Patient with Diabetes Mellitus. Elkart, IN, Ames Company, Division of Miles Laboratories, Inc., 1973.
    This monograph is based on material presented at a conference in 1972, "An Interdisciplinary Approach to the Education and Management of the Patient with Diabetes Mellitus." It was prepared to enable health professionals to plan and execute diabetes patient education programs. Contains useful information on techniques to motivate the patient in self-care, and outlines the tasks of the professionals and the responsibilities and tasks of the patients. It also contains a bibliography of educational materials for patients and professionals.
Ellenberg M, Rifkin H (eds): *Diabetes Mellitus: Theory and Practice.* New York, McGraw-Hill, 1970.
    Many authors from all over the world have contributed to this textbook that details the biochemistry, pathology, new research advances, and treatment of diabetes and its complications. In addition, there are excellent chapters on psychiatric aspects of diabetes, employment, insurance, and summer camps for children.
Fajans SS, Sussman KE (eds): *Diabetes Mellitus, Diagnosis and Treatment,* Vol. III. New York, American Diabetes Association, 1971.
    Up-to-date book that summarizes what is new in research and therapy of diabetes mellitus.

Guthrie DE, Guthrie RA: Diabetes in adolescence. Am J Nurs **75**: 1740–1744, 1975.

In general terms, this article discusses the problems adolescent diabetics and their parents face in accepting diabetes. No solutions are offered.

Marble A, White P, Bradley RF, Krall L (eds): *Joslin's Diabetes Mellitus*. Ed 11, Philadelphia, Lea & Febiger, 1971.

This comprehensive textbook on diabetes mellitus represents the cooperative efforts of clinicians and researchers associated with the Joslin Foundation. They have had extremely extensive experience caring for the diabetic patient. Covers in detail pathophysiology, etiology, treatment, and complications. Excellent reference for students interested in diabetes. Contains a comprehensive bibliography.

Moore RH, Buschbom RL: Work absenteeism in diabetics. Diabetes **23**: 957–961, 1974.

One hundred and eight employed diabetics were compared to an age-matched control group for an average of 4 years. A similar absenteeism rate was found for both groups. Other studies have not used an age-matched control group.

Travis LB: *An Instructional Aid on Juvenile Diabetes Mellitus*. Galveston, University of Texas Medical Branch, 1973.

This monograph was designed for children with diabetes mellitus but it has been used successfully in teaching adult patients, medical students, nurses, and other persons involved in caring for or interacting with diabetic persons. It contains excellent pictures and diagrams on metabolism, urine testing, insulin, hyperglycemia, management, and diet. Recommended for anyone working with diabetics, as it will assist them in answering questions posed by the patient.

25   END—STAGE RENAL DISEASE

Alvin E. Parrish, M.D.

DISEASE DESCRIPTION

Kidney disease offers a unique situation in rehabilitation. Medical advances in the last 20 years now make it possible to maintain life in individuals who would otherwise have died of kidney failure, using two modalities: the artificial kidney, by a technique known as hemodialysis, and kidney transplantation, using either kidneys from living, related donors or from fatal accident victims (cadaver donors). Associated with this ability to prolong lives, sometimes up to 10 or more years, is the problem and necessity of returning these individuals to a useful life. Vocational rehabilitation is especially important for these patients because they need to regain their ability to care for themselves and return to productive work.

According to a Department of Health, Education, and Welfare survey ending June 30, 1976, there are 25,000 patients undergoing maintenance dialysis in the United States. There are at least that many in Western Europe. This number is growing at a rate of 5,000 to 10,000 patients per year and is rapidly resulting in a major economic problem, due to the high cost of maintaining a patient on dialysis.

Normal Kidney Function

The kidneys are essential in maintaining the homeostasis of the body. They regulate the composition and volume of body fluids by conserving essential substances and water and maintaining the body's acid-base balance, and also detoxify and excrete noxious, foreign, or nonessential materials through the process of urine formation. In addition, the kidneys are associated with other functions, such as blood pressure control, red blood cell formation, and the metabolism of insulin and other substances.

Each kidney contains approximately one million functional units called *nephrons* (fig. 25-1). Each nephron consists of a *glomerulus, a Bowman's capsule,* and a *renal tubule*. A glomerulus is a cluster of capillaries. It is partially encased by the Bowman's capsule, which extends to form the renal tubule. The renal tubule itself is closely surrounded by capillaries.

The first step in the process of urine formation is *glomerular filtration*. The blood enters each of the glomeruli through a single *afferent arteriole*, and flows through the capillary cluster within the glomerulus. With each passage, about one-fifth of the blood plasma water plus solutes (such as urea, creatinine, glucose, and sodium) filters through the walls of the capillaries into the Bowman's capsule. Subsequently, this filtrate passes into the renal tubule. Blood cells and blood proteins are too large to pass through the glomerular filter. The blood components that were not filtered leave the glomerulus through the *efferent arteriole*, which branches into a second set of capillaries that surround the renal tubule (the *peritubular capillaries*).

The second step in the process of urine formation is *tubular reabsorption and secretion*. In the renal tubule (a complex structure), vital substances, such as glucose, water, and amino acids, are *reabsorbed* from the original filtrate back into the blood via the peritubular capillaries. At the same time, substances that need to be removed from the blood, such as toxins and metabolic endproducts, which did not all pass through glomerular capillary walls, are *secreted* by the peritubular capillaries into the filtrate in the renal tubule. Reabsorption and secretion occur in all portions of the renal tubule by osmosis, diffusion, and active transport. The filtrate, which is now called urine, leaves the renal tubule and enters a *collecting tubule*. The collecting tubules join increasingly larger tubules. Eventually, all final tubules discharge urine into the renal *pelvis* from which it passes down the ureter into the bladder, where it is stored until eliminated during urination.

Kidney Failure

When the kidney fails, one or all of its functions fail. Early manifestations of kidney failure may be so slight as to go unnoticed. Usually, they result from a decrease in the glomerular filtration and tubular secretion processes, leading to a decrease in concentration of noxious substances and hence an increase in urine flow (polyuria), especially at night (nocturia), in order to remove solutes. Later, an elevated blood pressure may develop. Still later, the filtering process fails further, so

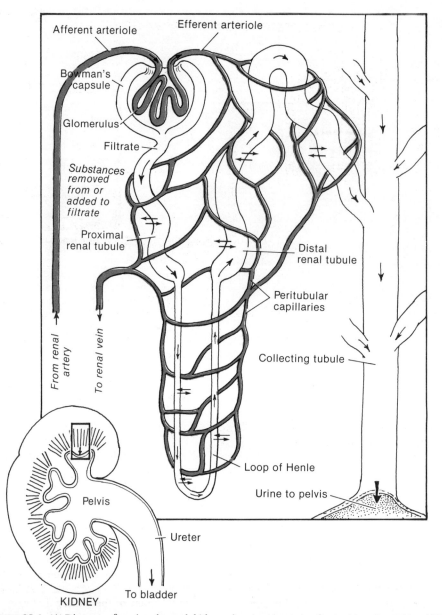

FIGURE 25-1. *(A)* Diagram of section through kidney showing that urine formed is collected in pelvis and transmitted to bladder by the ureter. *(B)* Diagram of single nephron. Fluid filtrate that has passed through walls of the capillaries in the glomerulus is collected in Bowman's capsule and funneled into proximal and then distal renal tubules. In the tubules, various substances are removed or added to the filtrate by the peritubular capillaries. The distal tubule conducts urine into a collecting tubule, which receives urine from several nephrons before discharging into pelvis.

that not even water is filtered well. Urine volume then decreases and the condition of *uremia* is present. At this stage, dialysis or transplantation becomes necessary because there is no longer an effective means of removing toxic substances as fast as they are produced.

The glomerular filtration rate (GFR) is the amount of filtrate passed through the glomerular capillary walls per minute. It is usually estimated by determining the amount of creatinine, a metabolic endproduct, that is discharged into the urine per minute. Since the concentration of creatinine in the filtrate is almost the same as in the blood, the volume of filtrate passed can be calculated as follows:

$$\text{GFR} = \text{amount of filtrate per minute } \frac{\text{(ml)}}{\text{(min)}} = $$

$$\frac{\substack{\text{amount of creatinine} \\ \text{excreted in urine per} \\ \text{minute}} \quad \text{(mg/min)}}{\substack{\text{concentration of} \\ \text{creatinine in blood} \\ \text{serum}} \quad \text{(mg/ml)}}$$

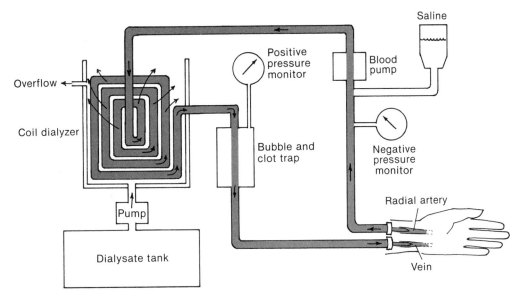

FIGURE 25-2. Schematic diagram of a renal dialyzer. "Waste" blood from the radial artery is pumped through coils with cellophane walls, which are embedded in renewable dialyzer fluid. Waste products pass through the coils' walls into the dialyzer fluid, which is discarded. Before "clean" blood is returned to the vein, it passes through a trap for removal of bubbles and clots. Pressure gauges and saline connection ensure that the volume of blood leaving the artery equals the volume returning to the vein.

If kidney damage occurs, then filtering decreases and the GFR decreases. Further, in kidney disease, creatinine itself is not excreted well so that the concentration of serum creatinine increases. Table 25-2 (see p. 334) demonstrates the classification of renal function based on GFR and serum creatinine. If serum creatinine exceeds 8 mg/100 ml (mg%) and/or GFR is less than 10 percent of normal, then dialysis is usually required.

Artificial Kidney

The procedure of hemodialysis is dependent on the fact that when two solutions are separated by a semipermeable membrane like cellophane, water and its dissolved contents will diffuse through the membrane until both solutions are of the same concentration.

The cellophane used in the artificial kidney (fig. 25-2) allows water, various salts, urea, creatinine, and other substances of small molecular weight to diffuse through it, but prevents larger things like blood cells, bacteria, viruses, and blood proteins from doing so, much like the filtrate passing through the walls of glomerular capillaries. Blood from the patient is pumped through a tube of cellophane surrounded by a water solution of salts (the dialysate) resembling the normal salt concentration of human plasma. Impurities in the blood, as well as many normal blood constituents, diffuse through the cellophane into the surrounding solution, which is then discarded. The blood, after passing through the cellophane tube, is returned to the patient. The use of this technique on a regular basis allows an individual with kidney failure to clear his blood of impurities and survive.

Etiology

Table 25-1 lists a variety of diseases of the kidney which may result in end-stage renal disease. Kidney disease may affect any age group. Some forms may be inherited and others, even though not inherited, may have onset in childhood. The most common kidney diseases are those related to high blood pressure (hypertension), polycystic disease of the kidney, and glomerulonephritis. The symptom complex exhibited by patients with end-stage renal disease is the same without regard to the basic kidney disease, and the actual cause of the kidney disease is usually of secondary importance, except in a few instances, such as diabetes or lupus erythematosus.

Diabetes, through its effect on the vascular system, may involve the kidney sufficiently to cause kidney failure. The prognosis is usually worse than in other forms of kidney failure because of the vascular complications affecting other systems (see chaps. 3, 13, and 24). Similarly, lupus erythematosus involving the kidney also has a poor prognosis because of the involvement of the basic disease in other body systems.

End-stage renal disease may develop rapidly, as occurs in rapidly progressive glomerulonephritis, so that treatment with the artificial kidney is begun soon after the initial onset of renal disease. The onset of kidney failure more frequently does not occur until years after the beginning of kidney disease. In inherited diseases of the kidney, such as polycystic disease, renal failure may not begin until the individual is in his 30's or 40's.

Signs and Symptoms

The term *uremia* is used to describe the clinical symptoms of end-stage renal disease. Since uremia is a generalized metabolic abnormality, these symptoms usually involve all systems of the body. Symptoms and signs may include decreased urine output, anemia, osteoporosis, heart failure, ulcers, bleeding from the stomach, mouth, or rectum, loss of appetite, lethargy, nausea, vomiting, swelling of the legs or entire body, loss of memory, difficulty in concentrating, peripheral neuropathy with weakness and sensory loss, sexual dysfunction, and occasionally, coma and convulsions.

The earliest signs of kidney failure are often an inability to concentrate and a shortened attention span. As a result, individuals with failing kidneys who have jobs that require mental rather than physical exertion may quit their jobs to take less exacting ones or be fired for their inability ot keep up with their work before it is recognized that kidney failure is the cause. As kidney failure becomes more severe, physical impairment becomes more predominant, with increasing inability to eat, weight loss, weakness, and easy fatigability. It is then that the individual whose occupation requires more physical activity begins to have difficulty and may lose or quit his job.

Of the various signs and symptoms, anemia, osteoporosis, and peripheral neuropathy require special attention.

Anemia. Anemia is a usual finding in uremia and is the result of the diseased kidney's inability to produce erythropoietin, the hormone necessary for blood formation. The anemia seems to be an important part of the physical weakness that accompanies kidney failure, but not the only cause.

Blood transfusions help but have the added risk of further depressing blood formation and of transmitting hepatitis. Type B infectious hepatitis appears to be transmitted by blood from infected individuals or carriers, and therefore may follow blood transfusion. It can also be transmitted by contact with the blood or secretions of infected or carrier patients and therefore can even spread in a dialysis center from patient to patient and to staff. Consequently, nephrologists tend to give as little blood as possible.

Peripheral neuropathy. Involvement of nerves in the hands and feet due to uremia may eventually lead to peripheral neuropathy with weakness and loss of sensation in the arms and legs. Subsequent paralysis may be so severe as to make the individual bedridden. Involvement of the autonomic nervous system (see p. 28) may lead to diarrhea, fainting on standing, and sexual impotence.

Except for adapting to the disability of hand or leg

TABLE 25-1
USUAL DISEASES RESULTING IN KIDNEY FAILURE

Glomerulonephritis	37%*

Vascular disease
    Nephrosclerosis
    Malignant hypertension
	24%

Interstitial nephritis
    Pyelonephritis
    Analgesic abuse
    Drug toxicity
	15%

Diabetes	7%
Polycystic disease	7%
Other congenital diseases	2%
Other diseases	8%

* Incidence at George Washington University Medical Center

weakness, no specific treatment exists, although neuropathy is inclined to clear with dialysis or transplantation.

Hyperparathyroidism and osteoporosis. In kidney failure, the parathyroid glands become overactive. These glands, located in the neck, normally help to control phosphate and calcium in the blood and bone. When they become hyperactive, there is a loss of calcium from bone (osteoporosis) and deposition of calcium in places other than bone, including the skin. This increased parathyroid gland activity, together with the failure of the body to utilize vitamin D properly, subsequently may lead to bone pain and, occasionally, bone fractures. Deposition of calcium in the skin seems to be associated with intense itching.

The treatment of this secondary hyperparathyroidism is the removal of part or all of the glands. Prevention of this complication is difficult but is partially aided by aluminum hydroxide taken orally to reduce blood phosphorus.

FUNCTIONAL DISABILITIES

Functional disabilities in patients with renal failure can be quite variable. A classification system established by the American Heart Association is shown in table 25-2. This table is very useful in categorizing the functional problems associated with renal disease, and can serve as a useful guide for counselors.

This classification divides patient evaluation into three categories: (a) Symptoms (Roman numerals); (b) Renal function (letters); and (c) Performance (Arabic numerals). Each of these is divided into five or six levels of increasing severity of impairment. Thus, an asymptomatic individual with good function and no physical impairment would be classified as class I-A-1, whereas a comatose person with no kidney function would be class V-F-5. This classification is being used by more and more nephrologists, and receiving a patient with such a classification will help the counselor determine the degree of disability. Most patients who require dialysis or transplantation will be class III-E-3 or greater.

For the most part, the consideration of rehabilitation begins once hemodialysis with the artificial kidney is started. Most patients receiving maintenance dialysis will be classified no better than II-F-1 or II-F-2.

Physical Disabilities

An individual with peripheral neuropathy may have problems in walking due to "foot drop." Stair climbing and balance may also be impaired. Grip strength and hand skills, such as writing, may be affected. Paralysis of one or both hands is occasionally seen. With adequate dialysis, the patient's condition may improve, but this may require months to accomplish and recovery may be incomplete.

The presence of anemia impairs the individual's ability to perform physical activities, with the degree of disability related to the severity of anemia. It is not unusual to see blood counts reduced 50 percent or more in renal failure anemia. Affected individuals become short of breath with minimal exertion and often complain of weakness, easy fatigability, and lack of stamina, requiring them to be more sedentary.

Intellectual Disabilities

Uremia, through mechanisms which are at present unknown, may interfere with the function of the brain. As a result, uremic patients may find concentration and prolonged mental effort difficult. This is almost always associated with either inadequate dialysis or no dialysis at all, and is usually quickly corrected by treatment with the artificial kidney.

Psychosocial Disabilities

Pre-existing problems, such as marital discord, are usually magnified by maintenance dialysis. The patient's spouse may be unable to adapt to the problems of end-stage renal disease and the marriage may disintegrate. The patient's family may desert him, refusing to take him home even when he is capable of caring for himself. They may even refuse to allow him to go to limited-care centers for hemodialysis or accept a kidney transplant.

In some reported groups of patients, the amount of emotional adjustment was related to IQ, with poorer adjustments occurring in those individuals with lower IQ.

Individuals with end-stage renal disease frequently show signs of psychological disturbances as a result of the disease and its treatment. The management of patients with kidney failure includes intensive medical care, close association with nurses and doctors, and loss of large amounts of time while receiving dialysis. This degree of care extends over a period of months or years and usually for the rest of the patient's life. As a result, the patient may display defense mechanisms and develop varying degrees of dependence, feelings of uselessness, hostility, and depression. The manifestations of these disturbances may take a number of forms.

Defense mechanisms. The most common defense mechanism is *denial*, the patient's failure to recognize the fact that he is ill at all. Another frequently observed mechanism is *projection*; the individual ascribes symptoms to others and can talk about these, but he cannot comfortably discuss his own symptoms. He may also become overly concerned with the minutia instead of the major problems (*displacement*). Finally, he may behave in a manner opposite to his true feelings (*reaction formation*). He may hate the doctor but be congenial and cooperative. This mechanism may need psychiatric help if it is sufficiently exaggerated.

Dependence. It is very easy for a critically ill person to come to depend on family members and medical personnel for both physical and emotional support. This is normal to a degree but can become so extreme that the person loses motivation to do anything for himself, including caring for his personal hygiene. This is most apt to happen to individuals with low-paying jobs, and is often augmented by the fact that his medical care is supported by Federal, State, or private agencies. The individual may quit his job or ask for retirement, sometimes without telling the medical staff. Once he has started this pattern, it may be impossible to change it and he becomes entirely dependent on his family and the medical staff.

Feelings of uselessness. The physical disabilities accompanying kidney failure, the necessity for frequent dialysis, and the attentiveness of the family and medical and social personnel often make the patient feel as if he no longer has any useful role in life. Impotency in males and physical weakness augment this.

Hostility. Individuals with chronic kidney failure may express their frustration with their debility by becoming hostile to the personnel trying to help them. This may take the form of noncompliance with medical management and include over-consumption of liquids or foods they should avoid, failure to take medication, or failure to show up for dialysis. Hostility is occasionally manifested as open aggression. It may result in the individual having multiple complaints about personnel, the dialysis center, or his family. It may also result in reaction formation, as above.

Depression. Depression may be exhibited as a part of all of the above and as a lack of motivation. The patient begins to realize the future implications of his disease, that he will be under some sort of treatment for

TABLE 25-2

CRITERIA FOR EVALUATING SEVERITY OF ESTABLISHED RENAL DISEASE

Classification of Signs and Symptoms by Severity

Class I: Requires (a) plus one or more of (b) through (f):
  (a) No symptoms directly referable to renal disease
  (b) Fixed proteinuria (> 200 mg/24 hours)
  (c) Repeatedly abnormal urine sediment or bacteriuria in properly obtained urine specimens
  (d) Demonstrable radiographic abnormality of the upper GI tract
  (e) Hypertension attributable to past or active renal disease
  (f) Biopsy-proven parenchymal renal disease

Class II: Any two or more of the following:
  (a) Symptomatic because of symptoms directly referable to kidney (e.g., hypoproteinemic edema, dysuria, flank pain, renal colic, nocturia)
  (b) Radiographic evidence of osteodystrophy
  (c) Stable anemia attributable to renal disease
  (d) Metabolic acidosis attributable to renal disease
  (e) Severe hypertension (diastolic BP > 110 mm Hg)

Class III: Any two or more of the following:
  (a) Symptomatic osteodystrophy
  (b) Symptomatic peripheral neuropathy
  (c) Nausea and vomiting without primary GI cause
  (d) Limited ability to conserve or excrete usual dietary load of sodium and water; tending to sodium depletion, dehydration or congestive heart failure
  (e) Impaired mentation attributable to renal disease

Class IV: Any two or more of the following:
  (a) Uremic pericarditis
  (b) Uremic bleeding diathesis
  (c) Asterixis and severely impaired mentation, with or without convulsion
  (d) Hypocalcemic tetany

Class V: Coma

Classification of Renal Functional Impairment

Primary	*Secondary*
Class A: GFR normal	Serum creatinine normal 0.6–1.3 mg% *
Class B: GFR still > 50% of normal	Serum creatinine normal to 2.4 mg%
Class C: GFR 20–50% of predicted normal	Serum creatinine 5.0–7.9 mg%
Class D: GFR 10–20% of predicted normal	Serum creatinine 8–12 mg%
Class E: GFR < 10% of predicted norrmal	Serum creatinine > 12 mg%
Class F: GFR < 5% of predicted normal	

*mg% means mg/100 ml serum

Performance Classification

Class 1: Capable of performing all usual types of physical activity

Class 2: Unable to perform the most strenuous of usual types of physical activity for that particular patient, e.g., sports activity, fast walking, running, shoveling, lawn mowing

Class 3: Unable to perform all usual daily physical activities on more than a part-time basis, e.g., household duties, employment, driving an automobile, playing with children

Class 4: Severe limitation of usual physical activity; may need assistance for some facets of self-care, e.g., shaving; mentation may or may not be impaired

Class 5: Semicoma or coma

SOURCE: Council on the Kidney in Cardiovascular Disease, American Heart Association

the rest of his life, and that this treatment will seriously interfere with his usual life style.

Psychological and social counseling and/or psychiatric treatment may be indicated when the above emotional difficulties become extreme.

Rehabilitation Potential

Patients falling into a classification of II-F-3, 4, or 5, or worse (table 25-2) have sufficient disability to require rehabilitation efforts. The first requirement in the reversal of disability is either adequate hemodialysis or kidney transplantation, plus maximal control of the ancillary diseases, such as heart disease, hypertension, and infection. The goal of medical treatment is to advance the patient to the levels of performance class 1 or 2. Once at that level, vocational rehabilitation and a return to a useful life can commence in earnest.

Individuals in class II-F-1 or II-F-2 can usually return to their previous life style. Those who had sedentary jobs or did not undertake strenuous activities prior to becoming ill can most likely return to them, even if they are in performance class 2. If, however, their activities require more physical activity than they are capable of, their life style or occupation will need to be changed. Appropriate vocational counseling and possibly retraining then become critical to success.

In performance classifications 1 and 2, the psychosocial problems noted above become predominant and may significantly interfere with rehabilitation. In addition, previous work experiences, intelligence level, and the possibility of secondary gain all influence the degree of return to normal life that can be achieved.

Secondary gain may be an important factor in rehabilitation failure. It may be to the patient's advantage to remain on dialysis and reject the potential "cure" of a transplant if he gains the support of his spouse in a faltering marriage. Prolonged illness may be of economical benefit to the patient. He receives his medical care and may receive financial assistance sufficient to allow him to support his family without working. If the patient is a wife or child, the family may receive funds in excess of their ordinary income. Often, especially in low-paying jobs, it may seem more "worthwhile" for the patient to receive a disability retirement rather than to continue working. This removes all further incentive and attempts at rehabilitation fail.

STANDARDS OF EVALUATION

For the proper assessment of the status of an individual with renal disease, an accurate diagnosis must be made. It is important to recognize that some causes of kidney failure are reversible and a long and complicated program of dialysis or transplantation may not be necessary. Such diseases as vasomotor nephropathy (also called acute tubular necrosis, lower nephron nephrosis, hemoglobinuric nephrosis, shock kidney), obstructive uropathy, acute glomerulonephritis, and acute pyleonephritis (see glossary) are reversible in most instances, leading to either complete or almost complete recovery in less than 6 months.

The most common methods for evaluating individuals with kidney disease are:
1. Careful history and physical examination
2. Urinalysis with special attention to the urinary sediment and protein content
3. X-ray, either an intravenous pyelogram or a retrograde pyelogram
4. Kidney biopsy
5. Creatinine clearance

All of these studies are usually performed under the direction of the nephrologist or internist, who should remain the primary physician. Any problems suspected later by the counselor or others should be referred to this physician.

The clinical course of the illness usually helps to distinguish reversible from nonreversible disease. The individual who has been ill for some time most likely will show a course progressing to uremia over a period varying from months to years. X-ray and/or biopsy may be helpful in determining the cause of uremia, but biopsy may not be necessary. The degree of uremia is usually estimated by measuring the patient's blood urea nitrogen (BUN) or creatinine.

The sudden appearance of uremia without a previous history of known kidney disease requires more careful medical evaluation. Intravenous or retrograde pyelography are almost essential to establish the diagnosis and prognosis. Consultation with a urologist is essential where obstruction to urine flow is suspected. Once it has been determined that the individual has end-stage renal disease, the degree of functional impairment can be further defined by kidney function tests and by evaluation of physical, psychosocial, and vocational capabilities.

The most useful kidney function tests are the glomerular filtration rate (GFR) of the kidney and measurements of the creatinine concentration in the blood. Both serve as a basis for the classification of renal function seen in table 25-2.

Before entering into a dialysis or transplant program, the individual should be futher evaluated as follows:

1. A psychologist or psychiatrist familiar with the problems of end-stage renal disease should interview the patient. The Wechsler Adult Intelligence Scale (WAIS) or the Minnesota Multiphasic Personality Inventory (MMPI) may be helpful.

2. A social worker's evaluation of the family structure, housing, and finances is critical. The latter is of special importance, since under Public Law 92-603 most persons can have their medical expenses paid by

the Social Security Administration if this is applied for properly.

3. A vocational evaluation that includes current employment requirements, employer attitudes, prior job history, and education is necessary to assist in planning.

4. A neurological evaluation that includes nerve conduction velocity measurements may be helpful.

5. A dietary evaluation and consultation with the patient and his family, unless a regular diet is allowed, may ensure patient compliance.

If, in the course of these evaluations, significant psychiatric, neurological, or other medical problems are discovered, the patient should be seen in consultation by the appropriate specialists, who may include a urologist, psychiatrist, and/or transplant surgeon. Again, these studies and consultations should be arranged by the primary physician, usually the internist or nephrologist.

Finally, all of the information gathered by the various specialists should be discussed by the physicians, nurses, social workers, and counselors to develop a plan for the management of the patient's problems. Most of these steps in evaluation are now required by Federal regulation (see bibliography) and are in operation at approved end-stage renal disease treatment centers.

TOTAL TREATMENT

Hemodialysis

In most instances, a single session of dialysis takes 3 to 6 hours, 2 to 3 times a week, and is done either at home or in a dialysis center. It is both possible and practical to train patients and their families to carry out the dialysis procedures in their homes. It works best when the patient himself carries out most of the work involved, using his family only for added help. Using this method of management, the overall cost of dialysis is reduced and a degree of flexibility for the patient is possible. The total time involved is about the same as in center dialysis but the procedure can be done at night or on weekends, allowing the patient to be free during the day for employment. In some instances, it is possible to utilize technicians to help with home dialysis. This frees the family from responsibility but increases the cost and reduces the flexibility of home dialysis.

Blood from the patient to be dialyzed can be obtained in several ways. The two most common are by means of an *arteriovenous fistula* or an *arteriovenous shunt*. The former is the most commonly used and the most satisfactory for prolonged use. The surgeon constructs the fistula by connecting an artery, usually in the forearm, to a vein in the same area under the skin. After a period of time (2 to 8 weeks) the vein becomes enlarged and carries a high volume of blood.

Large-bore needles can then be inserted into the vein to draw and return blood to the patient.

The arteriovenous shunt is similar, except that plastic tubes are permanently placed in the artery and vein, brought through the skin to the outside, and connected together. Dialysis is then accomplished by connecting the plastic tubes to tubes leading to and from the artificial kidney.

There are many modifications of these surgical techniques, including the use of dacron tubes or vein grafts from the patient. The procedures for establishing "blood access" are a cause of additional disability among patients with end-stage renal disease. The techniques, while usually very succesful over long periods of time, may have complications that further compound the disability, namely, hemorrhage, infection, and clotting.

Dialysis reduces the level of blood urea nitrogen and creatinine in the blood but rarely brings them to normal levels (BUN 10–15 mg% and creatinine 0.5–1.0 mg%). The BUN and creatinine levels of a patient on dialysis are not maintained at a constant level but show wide variations, being highest in concentration just before dialysis.

There is no reliable method of determining the adequacy of dialysis at present except the general assessment of the patient's condition. This is quite unsatisfactory and usually requires months of observation to evaluate. Individuals with inadequate dialysis usually have multiple complaints and problems. Since many of their problems are related to central nervous system involvement, nothing can be done until their dialysis is improved.

Once a patient has started on a dialysis program, he runs about a 15 percent chance of dying during the first year. A yearly patient loss rate of 15 percent follows.

Mortality is also dependent on the patient's other diseases. Hypertension, unless it can be controlled, lupus erythematosus, and diabetes all decrease the life expectancy. Diabetes nearly doubles the mortality rate during dialysis and after transplantation over that of nondiabetic individuals.

A well-motivated individual usually does well. One who appears to lack motivation, does not follow medical advice, does not take his medication, and overindulges in food or fluids usually has a much shortened life expectancy. Morbidity may range from almost zero upward, and about 10–12 percent of patients on hemodialysis seem to be hospitalized at any one time.

Complications related to hemodialysis further increase the amount of time devoted to the treatment of kidney failure. The major complications that can arise from the procedure are:

1. Shunt and fistula problems
2. Septicemia and endocarditis
3. Pericarditis and pericardial tamponade

4. Peripheral neuritis
5. Autonomic dystonia
6. Post-dialysis neuropathy
7. Dysequilibrium syndrome
8. Intracranial bleeding
      Stroke
      Subdural hematoma
9. Endocrine failure
10. Heart failure
11. Suicide
12. Homicide
13. Hyperparathyroidism

Problems stemming from the use of arteriovenous shunts are the most frequent complication and often result in hospital admission, leading to loss of time from work. Shunts are prone to infection and may lead to the presence of bacteria or their toxins in the blood (septicemia) and inflammation of the inner wall of the heart (endocarditis). Other ''accesss'' techniques are less subject to this, but any may become infected and produce symptoms resembling endocarditis.

Pericarditis and pericardial effusion are serious and potentially fatal complications occurring in inadequately dialyzed patients. The management includes increased dialysis time and, in some instances, surgical treatment with the formation of a hole (''window'') in the pericardium to allow the fluid to drain into the pleural space (see p. 44).

A common complication of dialysis is the inability to sleep. This may seriously interfere with the patient's job and is difficult to treat.

The counselor may detect, during his contact with the patient, the development of new complaints or the recurrence of old ones. If this happens, the primary physician should be notified so that he can treat or ameliorate the problem as soon as possible.

Another approach to dialysis, peritoneal dialysis, does not involve direct access to the blood. In this technique, the dialysate is infused directly into the abdominal cavity and the waste products diffuse into the fluid from the many capillaries in the lining (peritoneum) of the abdominal organs. Dialysate is then removed from the abdominal cavity and discarded. This technique can also be used at home.

Kidney Transplantation

Except in identical twins, the success of transplantation of human kidneys is totally dependent on the degree to which the body's ability to recognize and destroy anything foreign to itself is suppressed. Currently, the management of this immunological process is fraught with numerous hazards.

Prior to transplantation, it is necessary to determine the recipient's tissue type and blood group. It is currently thought that the more identical the donor and recipient, the better the chance for a successful transplant. Although there are more than 40 tissue antigens related to transplant rejection, the chances for a successful transplant are favorable if there is a good match between donor and recipient in only 4 of these. If there is no match at all, the chances for survival of the kidney are poor. In addition, the blood types must match.

Living-related donors are best, with survival rates of the transplant about 85 percent per year. These donors are usually parents or siblings of the patient, and after the tissue and blood typing of these relatives, the patient receives the best match available, assuming, of course, the potential donor agrees.

If the patient is to receive a cadaver kidney, his tissue and blood types are entered in a center or regional computer memory and each time a donor kidney becomes available within the cooperating area served by the computer, the tissue type is matched and the best recipient is determined. The kidney is then shipped on ice or on a perfusion pump to the transplant center and the patient receives the kidney. Cadaver donors with good tissue matching provide a transplant survival rate of about 70 percent per year.

After transplantation of the kidney, usually just under the skin into the groin area, the major treatment effort is to keep the recipient's body from destroying the transplant. This is accomplished by the use of drugs that interfere with the body's ability to react and destroy foreign material. The drugs most frequently used are azathioprine (Imuran) and steriods (usually prednisone). X-radiation may be used, and sometimes antilymphocyte serum is used to destroy blood lymphocytes which could destroy the transplant.

If a transplant is successful, the recipient has a chance of returning to a relatively normal life with no physical restrictions. Rehabilitation, however, may be difficult because of the preceding long period of debility associated with renal failure and requires an aggressive effort to succeed.

The complications of transplantation include rejection, infection, hemorrhage, and leakage of urine. Most serious of these is rejection, which occurs in almost all transplanted patients (except those with transplants from identical twins) after a varying period of time. Treatment following transplantation is directed at preventing or at least delaying rejection. Since in all but identical twins rejection eventually occurs, transplantation at the present time can be considered only as a temporary measure.

The drugs used to delay rejection act by depressing the body's ability to fight infection, leading to the second important complication of transplantation. Infection may be produced by any micro-organism, even those not ordinarily associated with disease in man, and treatment may be difficult and prolonged.

A successful transplant may result in many months or years of a reasonably normal life or may produce many months of hospitalization because of the complications, with an increased incidence of death. In the event of failure of the transplanted kidney, the patient returns to hemodialysis. One can expect more problems of depression and difficulties in rehabilitation after transplant failure.

Psychosocial Treatment

Usually about 1 to 2 weeks after dialysis has begun, the individual has returned sufficiently toward normal that the counselor should begin active support of the patient to prevent, as much as possible, the development of the psychosocial problems previously mentioned. Several things may help to prevent these problems.

1. The patient needs much emotional support from the counselors, social workers, physicians, nurses, and family, and may require repeated explanations of the goals of treatment and expected recovery before he is convinced that success is possible.

2. The family, especially the spouse, needs to be supported to achieve the belief that the patient can return to a more normal life.

3. The attitude of the staff and the counselor needs to be oriented to the return of the patient to an activity spectrum close to his former life style. The emphasis here should be for the patient not to give up his job if he has one, and to begin to plan for work that draws on prior skills, education, and experience.

4. If possible, the employer should be enlisted to directly reassure the patient that he will have his former job or a related job when cleared for work by the treating staff.

5. A meeting between the patient and another individual with end-stage renal disease who has made a successful recovery should be arranged, for it may be of inestimable value.

6. Sometimes, giving a depressed individual small tasks to do—helping other patients, for example—may help develop the attitude that successful performance is still possible.

VOCATIONAL IMPLICATIONS

Individuals with end-stage renal disease may have both mental and physical problems, even though they are receiving treatment with regular maintenance dialysis, and may continue to have these problems after kidney transplantation. Vocational rehabilitation in end-stage renal disease begins once treatment for kidney failure has been started. It can only become effective when medical treatment has improved the individual's physical status so that he is essentially independent in his personal care, and must be accompanied by a positive attitude that the individual will return to an active, productive life. Rehabilitation

needs to be undertaken aggressively with speed, sympathy, and encouragement.

Maintenance Dialysis Clients

Education. Retraining of these clients is frequently necessary, especially those whose previous occupation involved heavy manual labor. Retraining should be limited to that requiring minimal time. Three months is ideal and a year is maximum. More than this may be unattainable and probably in all but very special circumstances should be discouraged.

Aptitudes. Inadequate dialysis may result in the individual continuing to have impaired intellectual ability. This will manifest itself in decreased attention span and decreased ability to concentrate, which may adversely affect his learning ability. Retraining in highly complicated fields, therefore, is probably not indicated, although occasionally a highly motivated person with above-average intellectual abilities can succeed in overcoming these problems.

Physical demands. Individuals receiving treatment with intermittent hemodialysis almost always have severe physical limitations. Primarily, these are due to (a) the presence of blood "access," usually in an arm or leg; (b) persistent anemia; and (c) residual symptoms and possibly neuropathy.

In general, occupations requiring sedentary work produce no problems. Most clients can engage in light work, provided that the maximum physical requirements do not extend over prolonged time periods. Within the constraints of dialysis time, clients should be able to work full time. The majority of clients experience difficulties in undertaking medium work, but occasionally someone who has remained in good physical condition can continue to do this. Heavy work and very hard work, as a general rule, are impossible for these clients.

The type of blood "access" may limit the individual's ability. A shunt in an arm or leg prohibits the use of that extremity for all but the simplest and lightest of work. Shunts also must be protected from infection, and immersion in water must be avoided. A fistula, including one made with various types of grafts, limits the use of the extremity to a lesser degree. The major limitation is that the blood flow to that extremity should not be restricted. The ability to carry objects may therefore be limited. Fistulae are not as prone to infection as shunts and can be immersed in water.

Peripheral neuropathy, although usually not a major problem in adequately treated patients, may occasionally interfere with occupations requiring the use of the legs to operate machinery. Clients with peripheral neuropathy will usually be limited to sedentary work because of leg weakness. In extreme instances, peripheral neuropathy may occasionally interfere with the ability to use the hands (usually both), but this is unusual. Adequate dialysis, or even kidney transplantation, may not improve this disability.

Environment. Individuals with end-stage renal disease almost always have heat intolerance. Most do not perspire normally, some not at all. Occupations requiring exposure to heat of any sort, indoors or out, should be avoided. Exposure to cold, wet, or humid conditions should not produce problems, nor should noise, vibrations, fumes, gases, dust, or poor ventilation.

Kidney Transplant Clients

Once a successful transplant is done, many of the problems interfering with work disappear. Intellectual ability returns, shunt and fistula problems are gone, and anemia and symptoms of uremia disappear. Physical ability improves but may not return to its predisease level. The danger of infection, however, increases. Clients should not be placed in environments where infection could occur. Physical exertion should be such that the transplanted kidney is not exposed to injury. Since it is usually placed in the groin, excessive bending should probably be avoided.

Unfortunately, not all kidney transplants are successful. Some may result in only incomplete return to normal. Such individuals will continue to have impairment of their performance ability, similar to that which existed before the transplant. Many of these individuals, in addition, suffer profound depression because of the failure to return to a near normal life. These persons require emotional support from all who contact them.

BIBLIOGRAPHY

Abram HS: The psychiatrist, the treatment of chronic renal failure, and the prolongation of life: II. Am J Psychiatry **126**:157, 1969.
This is a very good description of the emotional problems occurring in patients with renal disease.

Calne R: *A Gift of Life: Observations on Organ Transplantation.* New York, Basic Books, 1970.
A somewhat simplified approach to transplantation.

Dansak DA: Secondary gain in long-term hemodialysis patients. Am J Psychiatry **129**:352–355, 1972.
The author describes the various secondary gains and the complications these produce.

De-Nour AK, Czaczkes JW: Personality factors influencing vocational rehabilitation. Arch Gen Psychiatry **32**:573–577, 1975.
This is a predictive study of 50 male renal disease patients who underwent a psychiatric examination to assess their predialysis work history, satisfaction with work, sick role, and dependency needs. The influence of these factors on vocational rehabilitation after dialysis is discussed.

Federal Register **40**(127):27781–27793, 1975.
These are the basic rules for dialysis and transplant centers.

Goldberg RT: Rehabilitation of patients on chronic hemodialysis and after renal transplantation: A comparative study. Scand J Rehabil Med **6**:65–69, 1974.
A comparative study of the vocational rehabilitation of patients awaiting transplant, after transplant, and on long-term hemodialysis. Factors such as predisability interest patterns, work values, education plans, and interest in maintaining employment are discussed.

Goldberg RT: Vocational rehabilitation of patients on long-term hemodialysis. Arch Phys Med Rehabil **55**:60–65, 1974.
Vocational plans, work interests, and values prior to chronic renal failure were assessed to determine the consequences of long-term hemodialysis on vocational plans and employment in 27 men. Vocational rehabilitation of patients on home, overnight, and center dialysis are compared, and factors in satisfactory adjustments are discussed.

Hampers CL, Schupak E, Lowrie EG (eds):*Long-term Hemodialysis: The Management of the Patient with Chronic Renal Failure.* Ed 2. New York, Grune & Stratton, 1973.
This is a basic medical textbook covering hemodialysis.

Moore FD: *Transplant: The Give and Take of Tissue Transplantation.* New York, Simon & Schuster, 1972.
A review of transplantation, including ethical and moral issues.

Najarian JS, Simons RL (eds): *Transplantation.* Philadelphia, Lea & Febiger, 1972.
This is a basic medical-surgical textbook describing the techniques and problems associated with kidney transplantation.

Yadav RV, Marshall VC, Johnson W, Mathew TH, Kincaid-Smith P: Cadaveric renal transplantation: long-term survival. Med J Aust **1**:729–733, 1972.
A study of the survival rate, rehabilitation, return to work, restoration of well-being, sexual activity, and adjustment to financial, social, and family stresses in patients with cadaveric kidney transplantation.

26 HEMOPHILIA

Shelby L. Dietrich, M.D.

DISEASE DESCRIPTION

The hemophilias are a group of congenital, inherited disorders in which a blood coagulation factor does not function. Normally there are 13 coagulation factors in the blood. These factors are special proenzymes which are capable of changing to active enzymes. When a blood vessel is damaged, the collagen in its walls is exposed. Platelets adhere to the collagen and build up a ''plug'' to momentarily stop the blood flow, but platelets alone cannot contain the flow indefinitely. Simultaneously, by an unknown mechanism, one or more of the coagulation factors in the blood are ''activated'' from their inert state. This initiates a complex sequence of reactions involving the other coagulation factors one after the other. The final step is the conversion of fibrinogen in the blood into fibrin strands which interact with the platelets to form the mature clot. Repair of the vessel wall requires first that a clot be formed. If one of the coagulation factors is missing, the sequence of reactions is incomplete and fibrin cannot be produced. Therefore, a clot is not formed and bleeding continues or resumes.

Two of these blood coagulation factors, factor VIII and factor IX, are involved in the two main types of hemophilia. Hemophilia A, also known as classical hemophilia or factor VIII deficiency, is the most common, accounting for 75-80 percent of hemophiliacs. Hemophilia B, also known as Christmas disease or factor IX deficiency, is seen in approximately 19 percent of hemophiliacs. There are approximately 25,500 persons in the United States with either hemophilia A or hemophilia B. The incidence is 25.8 cases per 100,000 males. Ninety percent of this population is under age 25, with a median age of 11-1/2 years. Therefore, many hemophiliacs are either first coming into or are in the early stages of their vocationally productive years.

The remainder of the patients belonging in this group have much rarer disorders, such as von Willebrand's disease, which is a combination platelet defect and factor VIII deficiency, or other rare coagulation factor deficiencies, namely factor VII, factor X, or factor XI deficiency.

Etiology

Even before the laws of Mendelian genetics were known, hemophilia was recognized in ancient writings as a sex-linked disease. The gene controlling factor VIII and factor IX production is located on the X chromosome, and therefore the disease is transmitted by the mother to her male offspring. The carrier mother may also transmit the defective gene to female offspring, who will be carriers of this disorder. Male hemophiliacs, genetically, will have all carrier daughters and all normal sons. Families of males affected with either factor VIII or factor IX deficiency will demonstrate approximately the same degree of severity in all affected persons. Von Willebrand's disease may be found in either sex and is transmitted in an autosomal, dominant gene. The degree of severity may vary from one family member to another.

Pathology

The hemophiliac who lacks one of the essential coagulation factors does not bleed more profusely than the normal person but continues to bleed because of the inability of the body to form a clot. The clinical severity of the disorder depends generally upon the degree of deficiency of the specific coagulation factor. The amount of coagulation factor VIII or IX in the blood of normal persons is variable. The amounts cluster about a mean value, which is taken as 100 percent. Thus, some normals may have greater than 100 percent activity of the factor and of course some may have less. Normal ranges of these factors may therefore be from about 50-150 percent or more. Persons with values from 30-50 percent may be carriers of hemophilia or have a very mild form of the disease. Such persons need to be very carefully evaluated. Below about 30 percent, the lower the value, the more severe the disease.

Spontaneous hemorrhage occurs most frequently in the patient with less than 1 percent of factor VIII or IX (severe hemophilia). Patients with moderate hemophilia (1–5 percent of normal factor VIII or IX level) rarely have spontaneous hemorrhage but will

341

experience significant hemorrhage after minor trauma. Mild hemophiliacs (with factor VIII or IX levels greater than 5 percent but less than 50 percent of normal) may have no spontaneous bleeding but will usually bleed extensively at trauma or surgery. Hemophiliacs do not bleed excessively from superficial cuts or lacerations. However, they may be subject to internal bleeding from the gastrointestinal tract or kidneys, or into the soft tissues of the pelvis.

Complications

Severe hemophiliacs manifest the most striking and difficult complication of this disease by their tendency to suffer recurrent bleeding into joints (*hemarthroses*) without antecedent or specific trauma. Patients often give a history of awakening in the morning and finding a swollen, painful knee or elbow (fig. 26-1). Because of this tendency to recurrent hemarthroses, the hemophiliac has a strikingly high incidence of degenerative joint disease resulting from the vicious cycle of bleeding, immobilization, muscle weakness and atrophy around the joint, and rebleeding into the same area. This ultimately results in degeneration and destruction of articular cartilage and bone. It is hoped that modern treatment will prevent much of the joint disability now found in approximately 75 percent of adult hemophiliacs. For unclear reasons, another complication is an increased incidence of hypertension in adult hemophiliacs.

Prognosis

The person born with hemophilia will remain a hemophiliac throughout his life. The severity of his disease as measured in the laboratory by coagulation factor assay will remain unchanged. The type and specific nature of clinical problems presented by an individual patient will depend largely upon the patient's age, degree of established joint disease (arthropathy), and other complicating medical or emotional problems.

Twenty-five years ago, hemophilia was considered a disease of young persons because so few patients lived into adult years. With modern treatment methods, this situation has drastically changed. One may now expect most hemophiliacs to survive well into adult years, including their productive work years, and to approach a normal life expectancy. However, patients will require treatment throughout their lives for bleeding problems, as well as other incidental medical problems. Hemophilia is best considered a chronic, but not necessarily fatal disease for which effective, though temporary, corrective treatment is available, including reconstructive or corrective orthopedic surgery.

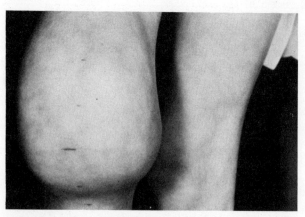

FIGURE 26-1. Knee joint of hemophilic patient with recent hemarthrosis. In addition to swelling, pain is also present.

FUNCTIONAL DISABILITIES

Physical Disabilities

The most common physical disabilities found in hemophiliacs are: limited joint range of motion, limited mobility, and chronic pain as a result of hemophilic degenerative arthropathy involving one or more peripheral joints (fig. 26-2). Hemophilic arthropathy is similar to any severe degenerative disease in that the patient may have chronic pain, restricted range of motion, or restricted ability to climb steps or perform heavy manual tasks. Prolonged standing or sitting may also be difficult for some patients. The functional disabilities of hemophilic arthropathy most closely resemble the problems found in adults with rheumatoid arthritis (see chap. 14).

Very few adult hemophilic patients will have significant impairment in their skills or activities of daily living or in their ability to drive a car, although a few severely affected adults may require automobile hand controls. Occasional hemophilic patients may require the use of assistive devices, such as canes, elbow splints, knee splints, or ankle supports, for varying periods of time to facilitate ambulation and upper extremity activities.

Psychosocial Disabilities

Psychosocial disabilities of hemophiliacs arise from a complex interplay of physical, mental, and social factors. The unstable and unpredictable nature of the day-to-day existence of the hemophiliac who is unable to predict or, in many cases, control when a bleed may occur sometimes leads to an attitude of apathy and apparent lack of motivation in seeking educational or vocational skills. If also coupled with parental overprotectiveness and extreme curtailment of activities during growth, social and psychological

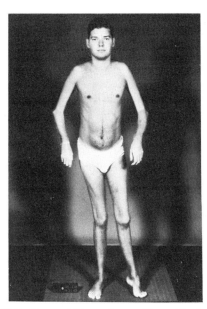

FIGURE 26-2. Hemophilic patient with residuals of prior hemarthroses into elbows, hips, and left ankle. The subsequent joint damage (arthropathy) has produced limited full elbow straightening (extension), stooped posture from loss of hip extension, and the ankle deformity shown.

maturation may be delayed and the patient may become excessively dependent. Such persons may even be referred to as having passive-dependent personalities.

Parents often still exert considerable influence on their hemophilic sons when they have reached vocational age. If the parents have not worked through their own feelings of concern and guilt and continue to promote their son's dependency, vocational plans may be sabotaged.

Some hemophiliacs, especially during adolescence, find acknowledgement of the association between trauma and a bleeding episode too threatening. They cope with this anxiety by denying the existence of their disease. This denial is often expressed by repeated risk-taking behavior. When such behavior continues into the early adult years, it is clearly inappropriate and represents maladjustment.

Many adult hemophiliacs may have suffered from disrupted or incomplete education resulting from bleeding problems that occurred in childhood and caused prolonged or frequent absence from school, with subsequent academic retardation. Those patients who participate in self-infusion on the home program of concentrate administration (described under Total Treatment) are now able to some extent to prevent bleeding problems at their very onset and to have more control over their school or work attendance.

Rehabilitation Potential

Most patients with hemophilia present excellent

potential for rehabilitation since the disease in itself is not fatal, adequate medical treatment may prevent many of the crippling medical problems associated with this disease, and most patients have good motivation toward future work or vocational placement. Whatever functional disabilities the patient has at the time of the initial application and medical evaluation, though not curable, nevertheless are not inexorably progressive. Long-term planning for vocational services is appropriate for most hemophilic patients.

It must be understood that hemophilic patients cannot be considered "rehabilitated" in the sense that problems presented have been dealt with and a permanent solution found. Hemophilia is an inherently unstable, though not necessarily progressive, disease state. Should progressive joint deformity or other unforeseen medical factors alter the patient's functional status, then he may again become a candidate for rehabilitation and vocational guidance services.

STANDARDS OF EVALUATION

Medical Evaluation

Diagnosis of hemophilia is usually made at birth of a male infant by analysis of umbilical cord blood when a positive family history of hemophilia exists. If the diagnosis is not made in this manner, prolonged bleeding from circumcision, multiple bruises, or prolonged superficial bleeding from facial or tongue lacerations usually leads to the diagnosis being made by the time the child reaches 1 year of age. The precise diagnosis of these diseases is made in the laboratory by a hematologist who performs a battery of coagulation tests, including specific factor assays, platelet function tests, and tests for inhibitor (or antibody) to factor VIII or IX.

When the client appears for vocational rehabilitation assistance, the diagnosis has already been made, and the client knows he has hemophilia. If at this time a hematologist is not actively involved in his continuing care, this needs to be established first. In addition to being able to advise the counselor and the client regarding the client's needs and restrictions, the hematologist can provide genetic couseling to the client about future children. The hematologist probably would also make contact with other relatives with regard to carrier status and genetic counseling.

A complete medical evaluation, either by the hematologist or an internist, will include history, physical examination, radiographs (X-rays) of previously involved joints, and other pertinent laboratory tests. In particular, close scrutiny is indicated to detect hypertension.

Evaluation of the joints is usually performed by an

orthopedist and physical therapist. The orthopedist performs a complete musculoskeletal examination of the patient, reviews radiographs of peripheral joints, including the hips, and arrives at an orthopedic diagnosis and treatment plan for the individual patient.

The physical therapist measures the patient's joint range of motion, evaluates mobility and activities of daily living, and makes recommendations to the physician for further treatment, if indicated by the findings. If at all possible, the musculoskeletal examination and evaluation should be performed by orthopedists and physical therapists familiar with the problems of hemophilia.

In hemophilia centers with experienced nurse specialists or nurse coordinators, a nursing assessment will be performed to determine the patient's life style, previous and present use of plasma concentrates, appropriateness for participation in a self-infusion program, and general understanding of the disease. If the patient is already on self-infusion, the nurse specialist or coordinator will supervise this program by maintaining close personal contact with the patient by telephone and by periodic nursing assessment visits. The nurse will also check the patient's records of his self-treatment for completeness, accuracy, and indications of bleeding patterns for further intervention or change in treatment.

Particularly for those patients with severe joint problems affecting ambulation, transfer skills, personal hygiene, and dressing activities, it is useful to obtain assessments by a physiatrist within a rehabilitation team setting where medical, social, psychological, and vocational problems can be simultaneously evaluated.

Psychosocial Evaluation

A social casework evaluation should be performed to determine the patient's access to appropriate treatment, his willingness to be treated, and his comprehension of the need for treatment. Because of the unpredictable nature of hemophilia and bleeding episodes, it is essential that patients be treated adequately and promptly for bleeding problems so that they may maintain their functional status and participate in either school or work. In addition, the social worker will assess the impact of the disease on the patient and his family and evaluate other factors in the patient's life, such as school and/or family problems. Counseling of the parents may be appropriate if they continue to encourage excessive dependency in the patient which interferes with vocational planning.

If medical needs, such as physician visits, hospitilization, or bed rest periods, occupied enough of the patient's time during the preteen and teenage years to cause social or academic difficulties, personality assessment and academic achievement testing by a clinical psychologist may be useful. Psychological and/or psychiatric assessment is also important for patients who seem to have passive-dependent personalities or engage in repeated risk-taking behaviors.

TOTAL TREATMENT

Optimum medical treatment for the patient with hemophilia consists of providing him with an adequate supply of his deficient blood coagulation factor at the time of a bleeding episode, combined with medical supervision by a knowledgeable team of physicians. All hemophilia patients need an individualized treatment program with appropriate medical and orthopedic evaluations to determine the proper course of therapy.

Treatment of hemophilia changed radically in the 1960's when the development of cryoprecipitate and plasma concentrates made therapy for the first time effective, reasonably accessible, and convenient for the patient. The technical development which led to this marked improvement in treatment efficacy was the ability to isolate and purify factor VIII and IX concentrates from human plasma. Previously, ordinary transfusion of plasma was the only available means of replacing the patient's deficient clotting factor. Fresh or fresh-frozen plasma is still used for replacement therapy, but its use is limited by the ability of the circulatory system to handle large quantities of fluid.

Cryoprecipitate is produced by rapid freezing and slow thawing of plasma. The precipitate thus formed is rich in factor VIII. Therefore, it can only be used for replacement therapy in hemophilia A. Cryoprecipitate can be prepared relatively easily and inexpensively by blood banks.

Higher concentrations of both factor VIII and IX are produced commercially as *plasma concentrates* by utilizing other precipitation methods. The concentrates can be given to the patient in a quantity adequate to raise his deficient factor VIII or IX level to hemostatic levels (30 to 50 percent of normal) and maintain that level, if necessary, by vein infusion every 8 to 12 hours at the time of a bleed. The infusion itself takes 20 to 30 minutes. Plasma concentrate replacement therapy restores the patient's blood clotting mechanism to normal for only a limited period of time, since the half-life of factor VIII measures 8 to 12 hours in the body and the half-life of factor IX measures 12 to 24 hours (table 26-1). The amount of factor VIII or IX concentrate to be infused is based on the patient's body weight and the nature of the bleeding problem.

Most hemophiliacs who undergo surgery require infusion of concentrate every 12 hours for 2 to 3 weeks following surgery. Since the amount of factor VIII or

TABLE 26-1
THE HEMOPHILIAS

Diagnosis	Deficiency	Genetics	Treatment
Hemophilia A (Classical hemophilia)	Factor VIII (also called antihemophilic factor or AnF) Severe < 1% Moderate 1–5% Mild > 5%	Sex-linked (X) recessive	Fresh-frozen plasma Cryoprecipitate Factor VIII concentrates
Hemophilia B (Christmas disease)	Factor IX (also called plasma thromboplastin component or PTC) Severe < 1% Moderate 1–5% Mild > 5%	Sex-linked (X) recessive	Fresh-frozen plasma Factor IX concentrates
Von Willebrand's disease	Factor VIII (variable) plus platelet dysfunction	Autosomal dominant Varying degrees of expressivity	Fresh-frozen plasma Cryoprecipitate

IX used is a function of both body weight and the severity or nature of the bleeding problem, it is apparent that severe bleeding problems, increased body weight, or both, will necessitate higher doses of factor concentrate with a concomitant increase in cost. Although the exact price of factor VIII or IX concentrate varies from hospital to hospital, the general range is $40 to $60 per vial.

In general, treatment for bleeding into a joint involves replacement therapy and immobilization of the affected joint for several days. If the joint is painfully distended, replacement therapy is continued and the patient may require short-term hospitalization. The affected joint is splinted, but the splint is removed daily for a period of cautious physiotherapy to maintain range of motion.

For minor surface wounds, replacement therapy may not be required. Often a pressure bandage will be sufficient treatment. Oral lacerations, however, require vigorous replacement therapy until the wound is healed.

Treatment of the rarer factor deficiencies and von Willebrand's disease will not be detailed here except to state that fresh-frozen plasma can be used in treatment of all these deficiencies with moderate success.

Home treatment has become an established part of medical care of hemophiliacs and is supervised both by individual physicians and hemophilia treatment centers nationwide (fig. 26-3). Criteria for selection of patients for home treatment include severe factor VIII or IX deficiency, accessible veins, and absence of medical complications. A most important additional criterion is motivation and willingness on the part of the patient and family to undergo an intensive period

of instruction in techniques of concentrate reconstitution and venipuncture, as well as instruction in the theoretical and medical areas of evaluation of hemorrhages. The number of training sessions required will vary with the ability of the parent, patient, or wife to learn the necessary techniques. Six 1-hour sessions are sometimes sufficient. More may be necessary and a certain amount of reinstruction may be required.

The interrelationships among family members should also be taken into account. Home therapy may be contraindicated when the family relationships promote the patient's inactivity and passivity, because home therapy may intensify, rather than diminish these tendencies. Where psychological problems within the family are not present, however, home therapy may diminish feelings of helplessness, fear, anger, and anxiety, and promote independence and the satisfaction of being able to take an active role in medical care.

The availability of home treatment is particularly important for those in school or at work, since the ability to treat hemorrhages promptly often prevents absence from school or work. Further, because treatment of hemorrhages is not delayed, orthopedic problems may be less frequent. All patients on home treatment programs of self-infusion should be followed carefully by a knowledgeable physician or hemophilia center with *mandatory re-examination and re-evaluation at yearly intervals* or more often if indicated.

The patient's use of plasma factor concentrates should be determined by his medical condition rather than by his ability to pay for these costly products. Patients who have either no third-party payer or inadequate third-party insurance often neglect treatment or undertreat their acute bleeding problems, thus hoping to decrease the expense of their disease. Although there may be short-term savings in such an approach to treatment, the long-term effect appears to be increased incidence of severe joint arthropathy, an unmeasurable increase in pain and suffering, and a deleterious effect upon the patient's overall rehabilitation potential.

Part of each patient's total treatment program is an intensive exercise program which is both preventive and rehabilitative in nature. Patients who maintain physical fitness even in the presence of hemophilic arthropathy are usually able to engage in more active school or vocational activities and have fewer problems with mobility and daily living. For some patients, a course of physical therapy, either as an inpatient or as an outpatient, combined with intensive medical treatment, may result in significant improvement in arthritic symptoms and improved muscular strength. Often stronger muscles may give better joint protection.

Certain patients with moderate to far-advanced degenerative joint or extremity changes are candidates for reconstructive orthopedic surgery, including hip or knee joint prosthetic replacement, to decrease pain. Total joint replacement in a hemophiliac is a major hematologic, medical, and surgical undertaking and should be performed only in institutions equipped with experience, personnel, and adequate plasma concentrates to perform such surgery.

Anti-inflammatory drugs and drugs for joint pain (analgesics) play a significant but secondary role in the management of hemophilic problems. Aspirin-containing compounds must be avoided because they interfere with platelet function.

It must be stressed that the medical and orthopedic care of the hemophilic patient is never "complete" in the usual sense of this word. Medical and orthopedic treatment is an ongoing, life-long process for these patients, and adequate medical care is the foundation for effective educational and vocational planning.

Under recent Federal legislation, comprehensive hemophilia treatment centers have been established in various parts of the United States. A directory of these centers and services is available from the National Hemophilia Foundation (see bibliography).

VOCATIONAL IMPLICATIONS

Education

Hemophilic clients may manifest academic retardation because of excessive or repeated school absence. Educational goals certainly need not be time-limited for hemophilic clients but should be determined by the individual's abilities and interests.

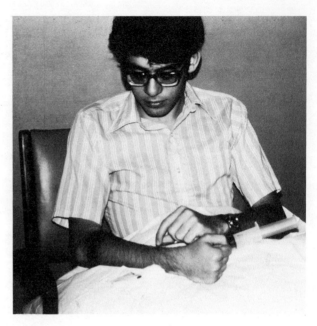

FIGURE 26-3. Hemophilic patient inserting needle into vein at home for infusion of plasma concentrate.

Aptitude

Data from the Los Angeles Orthopaedic Hospital Hemophilia Center compiled in 1968 on 78 hemophilic clients, aged 16 to 50, all of whom were given the Weschler Adult Intelligence Scale, revealed a full-scale mean score for this group of 116.7. In contrast, 78 clients, aged 7 to 20, given the Wide Range Achievement Test, showed the group placed in the 78th percentile in reading, the 38th percentile in spelling, and the 46th percentile in arithmetic. Inferences from these data suggest that school absenteeism was reflected in the unexpected low arithmetic and spelling scores. Other tests used were the Strong Vocational Interest Blank and the Minnesota Multiphasic Personality Inventory (MMPI). The mean of the standard scores in the Strong Vocational Interest Blank for the Masculinity-Femininity Index indicates typically masculine interests. On the MMPI, neither the adolescent nor the adult showed any major disturbance.

Information on aptitudes, interests, education, and rehabilitation counseling are best summarized by quoting from Taylor in *Comprehensive Management of Hemophilia* (p. 142):

Improved medical procedures have greatly improved the probability that hemophiliacs can carry out training programs and comply with the physical demands of their jobs. Furthermore, legislation in many states allows the working hemophiliac to qualify for state funds to pay for the major portion of the cost of medical care and specifically for plasma concentrates. Thus, hemophiliacs in these states who are now recipients of SSI benefits should have an incentive to seek employment.

Physical Demands

Physical demands of any specific job must be evaluated in terms of the individual orthopedic and medical characteristics of the client in question. In general, most clients with hemophilia are able to cope with occupations or jobs demanding sedentary work, light work, and occasional medium work. Obviously, potentially hazardous occupations should be avoided. It should be kept in mind that the major joint involvement in hemophiliacs is usually in the lower extremities, with the upper extremities relatively little affected.

Clients requiring analgesic medication for their joint problems may suffer some decrease in coordination or mental alertness. Job requirements must, of necessity, be considered in light of the individual client. There are no environmental restraints or restrictions on the hemophiliac's ability to work.

An important function of the rehabilitation counselor is the interpretation to the prospective employer of the medical aspects of hemophilia and the need for both therapeutic and preventive treatment. The counselor may also dispel many commonly held misconceptions among the lay public about the disease. It must be remembered that the younger client group has enjoyed the benefits of improved treatment, including self-infusion. As this group enters the job market, fewer and fewer orthopedic difficulties and physical limitations should be found and hemophiliacs will increasingly be able to compete on an equal basis. However, modern treatment has not made the hemophiliac "normal," and rehabilitation counseling and guidance must be based on an understanding of the medical problems present and the need for life-long medical care and surveillance.

BIBLIOGRAPHY

Agle D: Psychological factors in hemophilia—the concept of self care. Ann NY Acad Sci **240**:221–225, 1975.
A short review of the psychological factors associated with hemophilia is presented. Self-hypnosis is mentioned as a possible method of reducing anxiety and tension and thus the frequency and severity of bleeding episodes. Both the psychological benefits and the potential risks of home therapy are discussed.

Boone DC (ed): *Comprehensive Management of Hemophilia.* Philadelphia, F.A. Davis, 1976.
This multiauthored book, written by the members of the Hemophilia Center staff at Orthopaedic Hospital, covers all aspects of medical, hematologic, orthopedic, and psychosocial problems affecting the hemophiliac. It is an excellent basic reference for all those concerned with the care of the hemophiliac.

Gilbert MS, Aledort LM (eds): Comprehensive care in hemophilia: A team approach. Mt. Sinai J Med NY **44** (3), 1977.
This publication presents in clear and understandable style the experiences of the hemophilia team from Mt Sinai and New York Hospital, New York. The chapter on psychosocial aspects of hemophilia is particularly comprehensive.

Hilgartner MW (ed): *Hemophilia in Children. Progress in Pediatric Hematology and Oncology.* Vol. 1. Littleton, MA, Publishing Sciences Group, 1976.
Authoritative, scientific review of clinical and laboratory aspects of hemophilia covering problems of adults as well as children.

Jones P: *Living with Hemophilia.* Philadelphia, F.A. Davis, 1974.
This informative book, which is intended for the patient or family, is most helpful in learning to cope with the day-to-day problems and emergencies presented by hemophilia.

Kasper CK, Southgate MT: Clinical grand rounds: The many facets of hemophilia. JAMA **228**:85–92, 1974.
This article presents an excellent example of the team approach to treatment and rehabilitation. Included are reports on the history and present status of a single hemophilic patient from each member of the team: hematologist, orthopedic surgeon, radiologist, pathologist, nurse coordinator for home therapy, psychiatric social worker, and vocational rehabilitation counselor.

Katz AH: *Hemophilia: A Study in Hope and Reality.* Springfield, IL, Thomas, 1970.
The author was one of the pioneer investigators and authors in the field of vocational and rehabilitation counseling of hemophiliacs and details his experiences in this study.

Katz AH: Vocational problems in hemophilia. Ann NY Acad Sci **240**:246–254, 1975.
The several factors contributing to the vocational difficulties of hemophiliacs are discussed. Importance of early involvement of the vocational counselor is emphasized.

Levine PH, Britten AF: Supervised patient management of hemophilia: A study of 45 patients with hemophilia A and B. Ann Intern Med **78**:195–201, 1973.
This article presents the results of a one-year study of 45 hemophilic patients participating in home therapy. Data on absenteeism, days hospitalized, outpatient visits, and health care costs were compared with similar data from the previous year.

National Hemophilia Foundation, 25 West 39th Street, New York, NY 10018. Phone: (212) 869-9740.
The National Hemophilia Foundation has available a number of excellent informative pamphlets on various aspects of hemophilia, as well as information regarding the Federally funded hemophilia treatment centers and other treatment facilities.

Vogel JM: *How to Live with Hemophilia.* New York, Interbook Inc., 1973.
This easy-to-read book is written for the family and friends of hemophiliacs. It describes in simple terms what hemophilia is and how it affects the daily living of a person with hemophilia. Inheritance and treatment are also included.

27 SICKLE CELL DISEASE

Cage S. Johnson, M.D.

DISEASE DESCRIPTION

Sickle cell disease is a complex and multifaceted problem that may affect any of the body systems. Because of the many possible manifestations of the disease, no two patients will be exactly alike, thereby making it difficult, if not impossible, to categorize patients for rehabilitation purposes. Each case must be assessed on an individual basis. Because of the many misconceptions about sickle cell disease, an extensive discussion of the disease and its effects is presented as an introduction to the subject. For the vocational counselor, an understanding of the basic dynamics of the disease is essential for the complete evaluation of affected individuals.

Sickle cell disease gets its name from the special shape of the red blood cell that develops in this disorder. An understanding of the normal red blood cell and the structure and function of hemoglobin is therefore necessary.

Normal Red Blood Cell

The normal red blood cell (rbc) is a highly specialized component of the blood whose sole purpose is the delivery of oxygen from the lungs to the tissues. During its journey through the vascular system, oxygen is bound to the protein hemoglobin (Hb). The process by which the Hb is able to bind and release oxygen at the appropriate moment has been the subject of scientific research for many years and is still not completely understood.

The rbc, like other cells, has a double-layered membrane, one layer of protein and one of fat (lipid). This membrane has three unusual properties: (a) it is very pliable, or deformable, and hence is able to squeeze through the small capillaries of the vascular tree, which are less than half the width of the cell; (b) the inner surface of the rbc membrane is sticky, so that small tears can be resealed; and (c) instead of being round, the cell is pinched in on the sides (fig. 27-1) to allow oxygen to easily diffuse into the cell at the lung alveoli (see chap. 3, p. 43).

The rbc has no nucleus and therefore cannot renew its components as it ages. Consequently, it has a

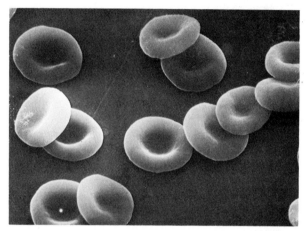

FIGURE 27-1. This scanning electron photomicrograph of normal red blood cells (magnified x6,000) shows the round cell without a nucleus and the disc-like shape with pinched-in sides. Inside are the millions of hemoglobin molecules. (Courtesy of Richard F. Baker, Ph.D., University of Southern California School of Medicine, Los Angeles, CA)

limited life span. The rbc is produced from nucleated precursors in the bone marrow and is released into the circulation, where it resides for 120 days. At the end of this period, the aged rbc's are destroyed. New cells are manufactured continuously in the bone marrow to replace the old ones. Every day about 1 percent of the total rbc's in the body are replaced. New cells are called *reticulocytes* and can be recognized under the microscope by special staining techniques.

Normal Hemoglobin

Dissolved in the water inside each rbc are 280 million molecules of Hb. Each Hb molecule is made up of four protein chains of atoms (*globins*; fig. 27-2). Attached to each globin is a specific ring of atoms (protoporphyrin) containing an iron atom. The protoporphyrin-iron complex is called *heme*; hence, the name given to the entire molecule, hemoglobin. Oxygen is bound to each iron atom of heme. The globin chains function to (a) make heme soluable in water; (b) protect the site of oxygen attachment from destruction; and (c) give Hb the property that allows

349

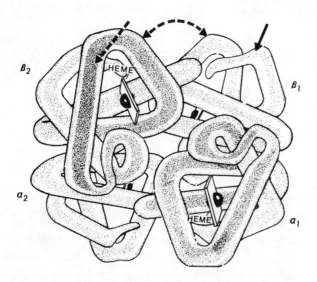

FIGURE 27-2. Schematic conception of the hemoglobin molecule, showing the four globin chains, **α**₁ and **α**₂ on the bottom and **β**₁ and **β**₂ on the top. The rectangle represents the heme and the black ball depicts the iron atom. Heme is enclosed in a pocket formed by the folding of the globin chains. Oxygenation of the molecule occurs at the iron atom. In hemoglobin S, the amino acid substitution occurs at the solid arrow on the **β**₁ chain and the dashed straight arrow on the **β**₂ chain. The curved dashed arrow shows the areas where the beta chains move closer together during oxygenation.

oxygen automatically to be bound in the lungs, where oxygen pressure is high, and released in the tissues, where oxygen pressure is low.

In man, there are four different globin chains that can be mixed together to make a Hb molecule: alpha chains with 141 amino acids, and beta (fig 27-3), gamma, and delta chains, each with 146 amino acids. The sequence of amino acids in the beta, gamma, and delta chains is very similar.

Each globin chain is wrapped tightly around its heme, forming the ''pocket'' that protects the heme (fig. 27-2). As the molecule picks up oxygen, the beta chains move closer together and the heme pockets open slightly, allowing the oxygen molecule to enter the pocket. When oxygen is given off at the tissue level, the beta chains move apart, closing the heme pocket. This process is repeated continually throughout the life of the rbc.

When rbc's are destroyed, mostly in the spleen, the globins are broken down into their individual amino acids, which recycle to make new proteins. Similarly, the iron is recycled to make new Hb. The protoporphyrin ring changes to bilirubin, a yellow pigment, which is excreted by the liver into the gallbladder to form bile. Bile is secreted into the small bowel where it facilitates the digestion and absorption of fats in the diet.

There are three types of normal hemoglobin. Each is composed of different combinations of globin chains.

1. *Hb A* has two alpha chains and two beta chains and makes up 97 percent of adult Hb.
2. *Hb A₂* has two alpha chains and two delta chains and makes up 3 percent of adult Hb.
3. *Hb F*, or fetal Hb, has two alpha chains and two gamma chains and comprises 80 percent of the Hb in newborn infants.

At 3 months of age, gamma chain production is replaced by beta chain production, so that Hb F is gradually replaced by Hb A. Hb F is usually less than 1 percent of the total Hb after 1 year of age.

Hb production is genetically controlled. The genes on the maternal and paternal chromosomes each control half of the Hb production. The genes for alpha chains are located on one pair of chromosomes, while the beta, gamma, and delta chain genes are on another pair of chromosomes. Each globin chain gene ''instructs'' the rbc to make a specific globin chain by controlling the sequence of amino acids. The globin chains are matched with a heme and then made into a Hb molecule when the four chains join together.

Abnormal Hemoglobin

The cause of sickle cell disease is genetic. It derives from the presence of gene mutations which produce abnormal hemoglobins. In the United States, most cases of sickle cell disease occur among Afro-Americans. About 1 in 12 blacks carries the Hb S gene (*sickle cell trait*). If two gene carriers marry, each child they have has one chance in four of inheriting the disease. Altogether, about 1 in every 500 black children has one of the sickle cell diseases. The sickle cell gene is not confined to blacks. It is also carried by some people of Arabian, Greek, Maltese, Sicilian, Sardinian, Turkish, and southern Asian ancestry. Many scientists believe that the abnormal gene arose in these populations as protection against malaria.

Over 200 different abnormal Hb's have been discovered to date. Most of these are extremely rare. Only three of them are associated with most sickle cell disease problems.

1. *Hb S* is the most common of the abnormal hemoglobins. In Hb S, the gene controlling beta chain production inserts the amino acid valine in position #6 instead of glutamic acid (fig. 27-4).
2. *Hb C* is the second most common abnormal hemoglobin. In Hb C, the gene controlling beta chain production inserts the amino acid lysine for glutamic acid in position #6 (fig. 27-4).
3. *Thalassemia* is a different type of Hb mutation. Here, the gene is normal with regard to amino acid sequence but the rate of globin chain synthesis is reduced. In *alpha thalassemia,* alpha chain synthesis is impaired, and in *beta thalassemia,* the beta chain synthesis is impaired.

The presence of most abnormal Hb's is readily

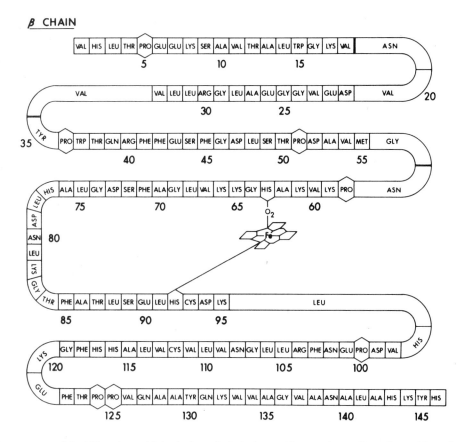

FIGURE 27-3. The sequence of the 146 amino acids in the beta chain is shown. The numbers refer to the position of a particular amino acid. The heme is shown between histidines at positions 63 and 92, and the position of oxygen between the #63 histidine and the heme is shown. Only 19 amino acids are used in making globin chains: ala=alanine, asn=asparagine, asp=aspartic acid, arg=arginine, cys=cystine, gln=glutamine, glu=glutamic acid, gly=glycine, his=histidine, ile=isoleucine, leu=leucine, lys=lysine, met=methionine, phe=phenylalanine, pro=proline, ser=serine, thr=threonine, trp=tryptophan, tyr=tyrosine, val=valine.

ascertained by a laboratory test called *electrophoresis* (fig. 27-5). In this technique, an electrical current is passed through a solution of Hb. The Hb's migrate toward the positive or negative pole, depending on the overall electrical charge of the molecule. Many, but not all, of the abnormal Hb's have an electrical charge different from normal Hb and can be separated and identified by this procedure. The others require special techniques for identification.

The Sickle Phenomenon

Sickle cell disease gets its name from the characteristic sickle shape that the rbc assumes when Hb S is present. During deoxygenation at the capillaries, the abnormal valine in the beta 6 position (fig. 27-2) becomes attracted to an adjacent Hb molecule and forms a bond with that molecule. As more and more bonding occurs, a tubular crystal is formed (fig. 27-6) that grows the entire length of the cell and distorts the cell membrane into the characteristic sickle shape (fig. 27-7).

When the cell is reoxygenated in the lungs, the crystals disperse and the cell returns to the rounded shape. After several passes through this sickle-unsickle cycle, the membrane becomes permanently deformed and rigid. This rigid, fragile cell is called the *irreversibly sickled cell.* The membrane has become so stiff that the cell will neither sickle on deoxygenation nor become rounded on reoxygenation. *This rigid, irregularly shaped cell is believed to be responsible for all of the problems caused by sickle cell disease.*

The irreversibly sickled cell is so fragile that it is easily destroyed as it passes through the blood vessels, curtailing its life to 8 to 15 days rather than the normal 120 days. The bone marrow must increase rbc production drastically in order to keep up with the rate of destruction. But even at maximum output, the marrow is unable to manufacture enough cells to maintain normal levels. A severe anemia (hemolytic anemia) due to the rapid destruction of cells results. Further, rbc cell rigidity inhibits passage through the capillaries. The irreversibly sickled cell may become wedged in a capillary and block the passage of blood. A gradual buildup of sickled cells in the blood vessels occurs until a portion of the circulation is completely cut off.

The part of the body supplied by the occluded vessels therefore receives no further blood (ischemia). The consequences of a blocked blood supply are several. In particular, ischemia may produce pain from lack of oxygen, and ischemic tissue may undergo necrosis (infarction), with subsequent healing by scar tissue formation (fibrosis). Any organ may be involved in this process. The degree of pain or organ damage is related to the size of the vascular area involved and the degree and duration of the ischemia. Some episodes, called *crises,* last only hours with little tissue damage, while others may last days to weeks with major organ damage.

Although the exact cause of sickle crises is not known, certain factors have been shown to have a contributory role. Lack of oxygen has the major role. Infections, dehydration, excessive blood acidity (acidosis), and exposure to extremes of temperature all may precipitate a crisis. Actually, almost any kind of mental or physical stress has been known to precipitate a crisis.

Sickle cell disease is the term used to refer to that group of genetic disorders of Hb synthesis which have the following characteristics:

1. The determination of the presence of Hb S by electrophoresis and the demonstration of the sickling phenomenon from a blood sample under the microscope
2. The laboratory signs of a chronic hemolytic anemia
3. A characteristic clinical picture for each type, with recurrent crises and frequent infections

Three major types of sickle cell disease exist: sickle cell anemia, hemoglobinopathy SC, and sickle thalassemia. Although other types do occur, they are very rare.

Sickle Cell Anemia (SCA)

SCA is the most common and most severe form of sickle cell disease. In SCA, both the maternal and paternal beta globin genes possess the Hb S mutation. The Hb in the blood is therefore 80–90 percent Hb S.

The hemolytic anemia is usually evident by age 4 to 6 months, although symptoms usually do not begin until age 1-1/2 to 2. The anemia is severe, with Hb levels in the range of 6–9 gm/100 ml (normal 14 gm/ 100 ml) and occasionally as high as 11 gm/100 ml. The patients with SCA have frequent painful crises during childhood, usually with infections. Peak mortality due to serious infections occur in the period from 2 to 5 years of age. During adolescence, there is a reduction in the frequency of crises and infections, and a quiescent phase of the disease is often seen.

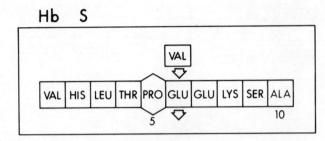

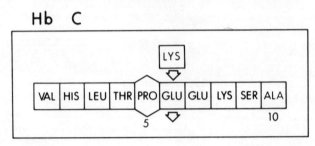

FIGURE 27-4. The first 10 positions in the beta chain are shown. In Hb S, the glutamic acid in position 6 is replaced by valine, and in Hb C by lysine.

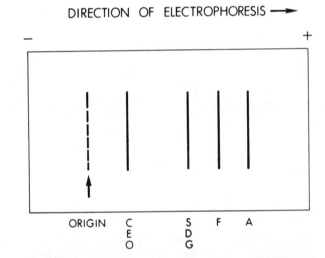

FIGURE 27-5. Hemoglobin electrophoresis on cellulose acetate is schematically shown. A solution of hemoglobin has been placed at the point marked origin; electrical current has been applied to the solution, and the hemoglobins have migrated according to the overall electrical charge on the molecule. Hb A moves close to the positive (+) pole with Hb F slightly behind. Hb S, D, and G, and Hb C, E, A₂ and O migrate together at positions closer to the negative (−) pole. Hemoglobins that migrate together on this type of electrophoresis can be separated by altering the voltage, degree of acid concentration, or supporting material.

Growth in those with SCA is usually delayed so that they are smaller than other children of the same age. Puberty and the prepubertal truncal growth spurt are also delayed so that about half of all patients have a

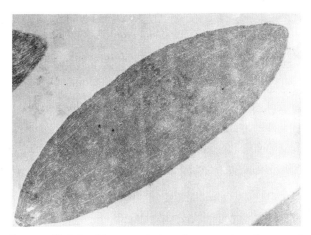

FIGURE 27-6. In this transmission electron microphotograph (magnified x43,000) of a section through a sickled cell, the tubular crystals of sickled hemoglobin are seen running across the length of the cell. These distort the cell into the characteristic sickled shape. (Courtesy of Richard F. Baker, Ph.D., University of Southern California School of Medicine, Los Angeles, CA)

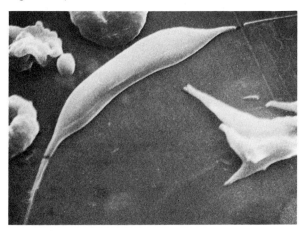

FIGURE 27-7. Compare the appearance of this cell with figure 27-1. This scanning electron microphotograph (magnified x4,000) shows cells from a patient with sickle cell anemia which have been deoxygenated. The cells then assume bizarre shapes, as in the cell in the lower right corner. The large cell in the center shows the classical "sickled" shape for which the disease was named. In this instance the cells have been exposed to a small amount of oxygen just before the picture was taken. The right side of the "sickled" cell has begun to return to the disc shape (as in fig. 27-1). The tapering needles of membrane on each end of the cell have broken off during this early phase of the reoxygenation process. As a result of the "sickle-unsickle" cycle, the red cell membrane becomes damaged, leading to the consequences of sickle cell disease. (Courtesy of Richard F. Baker, Ph.D., University of Southern California School of Medicine, Los Angeles, CA)

"typical" tall, thin appearance with disproportionately long limbs.

The spleen is enlarged from birth until age 7 or 8. At about this time, as a result of recurrent sickling episodes producing infarction and fibrosis, the spleen gradually shrinks away (autosplenectomy).

During late adolescence and early adulthood, the frequency of crises increases, although there is wide variation in disease manifestations from patient to patient. After years of uncontrolled sickling, the effects of recurrent occlusion of the blood vessels with ischemia, infarction, and fibrosis are seen in the form of chronic organ damage. For example, the kidney is often damaged, but any organ in the body may be affected. In the adult, management of the effect of organ damage may become the major issue.

Serious infection remains a problem throughout the course of the disease. In adults, mortality is most commonly due to infection or chronic renal failure (see chap. 25). There is no peak mortality period in adulthood as there is in childhood, and the overall life span for adults with SCA has not been defined. *Many patients now survive into middle age and beyond.* Thus, for any single individual with this disease, ultimate prognosis cannot be predicted.

While almost all patients with SCA are diagnosed during childhood, a few patients who do not have any crises or infections are not diagnosed until adolescence or adulthood. These patients may remain entirely free of symptoms for long periods. Although the variation in the degree of illness is perhaps greater than in any other chronic disease, most patients settle into a pattern during adulthood with regard to the frequency of crises. When this pattern is broken, there is usually an identifiable reason which, when alleviated, allows the patient to return to his basic pattern.

Hemoglobinopathy SC

Hemoglobinopathy SC results from the inheritance of one beta globin gene with the mutation Hb S (fig. 27-4) and the second beta globin gene carrying the mutation Hb C (fig. 27-4). Therefore, Hb S and Hb C each make up about 50 percent of the Hb in the blood. Some confusion in terminology can occur because the abbreviation "SC disease" is used both to refer to hemoglobinopathy SC and also as an abbreviation for "Sickle Cell Disease," the general term that covers all forms.

Hemoglobinopathy SC is about one-third as common as SCA. The hemolytic anemia is evident by 6 months of age, but typically symptoms are not present until adolescence or early adulthood. Unlike SCA, the diagnosis is in most cases not made until later in life. The anemia is milder than that of SCA, with Hb levels of 10 to 12 gm/100 ml or more. The spleen is enlarged throughout life in most patients, and crises and infections are less frequent than in SCA. Capillary plugging sufficient to produce death of bone (aseptic necrosis), such as in the head of the femur, and also disease of retinal blood vessels (sickle retinopathy) are perhaps more common than in SCA.

More importantly, mortality in this form of disease differs from that in SCA. Death in childhood is very rare. Peak mortality occurs in the 40 to 60 age group, with death usually due to complications of arteriosclerotic heart disease rather than complications of sickle cell disease. The disease is unpredictable in its manifestations, but is generally less severe than SCA.

Sickle Thalassemia

Sickle thalassemia results from the combined inheritance of Hb S and beta thalassemia. In the severe form, the beta globin production is completely suppressed. In the mild form, beta chain production is only partially suppressed. In an effort to compensate for the missing beta chains, delta and gamma chain production increases slightly, leading to elevated Hb A_2 and F levels in the blood in both the mild and severe forms.

The severe form of sickle thalassemia results in a blood picture similar to SCA. The blood contains 70–85 percent of Hb S, 5–20 percent of Hb F, and greater than 4.5 percent of Hb A_2. Hb levels are 9–11 gm/100 ml. This form of sickle cell disease is very similar to SCA in its onset, course, and prognosis. The spleen may be enlarged throughout life or may disappear. Prior to the advent of techniques to measure Hb A_2 levels, these patients were usually diagnosed SCA. This confusion often still exists.

The mild form of sickle thalassemia yields blood that is 50–70 percent Hb S and 10–30 percent Hb A. Hb A_2 and F levels are elevated. Anemia is mild with Hb levels of 10–12 gm/100 ml or higher. The spleen is usually enlarged throughout life. The onset, course, and prognosis of mild sickle thalassemia is similar to that of hemoglobinopathy SC.

Because of the presence of Hb A on electrophoresis, this condition is often confused with sickle cell trait (see below). The presence of hemolytic anemia, splenic enlargement, and crises enables the distinction to be made easily.

Other Variants

Combinations of one gene for Hb S and another alpha or beta chain mutant, such as Hb D, E, O, and G, are rare. The severity of these hemoglobinopathies depends upon the degree to which the variant Hb participates in the sickling process. In some of these combination hemoglobinopathies, the disorder is essentially benign, like sickle cell trait, whereas in others it may be as severe as SCA.

Sickle Cell Trait

Individuals with sickle cell trait have received one gene for the abnormal Hb S and one for the normal Hb A. Fifty-five to sixty percent of the Hb is A and 40–50 percent is Hb S. The Hb A_2 and F levels are normal. The red blood cells of such individuals can be made to sickle in the test tube, so these individuals do meet the first criterion for sickle cell disease. However, there is no anemia in sickle cell trait, as rbc survival is normal. Furthermore, these individuals do not have recurrent crises or frequent infections. Although under unusual circumstances sickle crises have been seen in persons with sickle cell trait, this is the exception rather than the rule. Sickle cell trait is therefore not considered a disease. Crises can be seen in individuals with sickle cell trait when there is severe lack of oxygen, as might occur in severe pneumonia, while under anesthesia, or when flying at high altitudes in unpressurized aircraft.

The hemoglobin concentrations found in the three main types of sickle cell disease and in sickle cell trait are summarized in table 27-1. Normal hemoglobin concentrations are also shown for comparison.

Complications

In addition to the multiple problems that can occur as a result of the abnormal hemoglobin, patients with sickle cell disease are also subject to the other diseases that afflict mankind. Care must be taken to avoid attribution of all of the signs and symptoms in an individual patient to the sickling process, overlooking the possibility of another illness contributing to the picture. This concept must be kept in mind when evaluating a patient with sickle cell disease, and emphasizes the individualized approach to each situation in determining whether a condition is actually a complication of the primary disease.

The complications of sickle cell disease include chronic hemolytic anemia, sickle cell crises, recurrent infections, and chronic organ damage. These complications are most frequent and most severe in patients with SCA, but there is marked variability in all forms of the disease. Some patients with SCA can be described as mildly affected, while some patients with the milder forms of the disease may be severely affected.

Chronic hemolytic anemia. The rbc survival is shortest in SCA and somewhat longer in the other forms. This explains why the anemia is more severe in SCA. The rbc precursors in the bone marrow increase markedly in number and the bone marrow space therefore enlarges. Increased rbc production is reflected in an increased number of reticulocytes in the blood. As the marrow space enlarges to accommodate the increase in rbc production, the bones become thinner. The remodeling of bone in this fashion may produce marked protrusion of the jaw (prognathism) and the tower skull deformity. Prognathism produces malocclusion of the teeth and may predispose to early tooth decay and gum disease.

The rapid destruction of the rbc's produces large

TABLE 27-1
HEMOGLOBIN CONCENTRATIONS IN
VARIOUS CONDITIONS

Condition	Hb A	Hb A$_2$	Hb F	Hb S	Hb C
Normal	97%	3%	<1%	...	...
Sickle cell anemia	...	3%	8–15%	80–90%	...
Hemoglobinopathy SC	...	...	2%	49%	49%
Sickle thalessemia, severe	...	>4.5%	5–20%	70–85%	...
Sickle thalessemia, mild	10–30%	>4.5%	5–20%	50–70%	...
Sickle cell trait	55–60%	3%	1%	40–45%	...

amounts of bilirubin faster than it can be converted by the liver into bile. Thus, the level of bilirubin in the blood is two or three times normal and imparts its yellow color to the eyes and skin as *jaundice*. The large amounts of bilirubin processed by the liver and stored in the gallbladder tend to form *gallstones*. Although virtually all patients develop stones, not all patients have symptoms from them requiring surgical removal of the gallbladder.

Since anemia reduces the oxygen-carrying capacity of blood, to deliver adequate amounts of oxygen to the tissues the blood either must be pumped faster than normal, or more oxygen than usual must be removed per unit of blood. Both of these compensatory mechanisms come into play in sickle cell disease. The required faster pumping of blood increases the workload on the heart and lungs and leads to easy fatigability, difficult breathing on exertion (exertional dyspnea), lightheadedness, and reduced exercise tolerance. The degree of symptoms is proportional to the degree of anemia. The extraction of more oxygen from the red cell in the capillaries aggravates the sickling phenomenon and may lead to more vessel plugging in crises.

Sickle cell crises. Four kinds of sickle cell crises occur: (a) vaso-occlusive; (b) aplastic; (c) splenic sequestration syndrome; and (d) hyperhemolytic. By far the most common is the vaso-occlusive, or "painful," crisis. In this type, the "crisis" refers to episodes of pain severe enough to require medical attention.

The *painful crisis* has a sudden onset, may last from 3 or 4 days to 2 weeks, and may be localized to one area of the body or may be generalized. The pain is deep-seated and of an aching quality. Commonly, an obvious precipitating stress is not identified. While there is significant discomfort due to these crises, they are never fatal unless accompanied by some other complication. Vaso-occlusive crises are frustrating for both patient and physician. Repetitive crises are emotionally exhausting, as the patient must constantly face the prospect of yet another episode.

In the *aplastic crisis*, the precursor cells that produce rbc's in the marrow are destroyed by an unknown mechanism. Consequently, the level of Hb in the blood falls rapidly to dangerously low levels. This complication is often seen in a viral infection which, in itself, may not be severe enough for the patient to seek medical attention. The very low Hb, however, requires rapid attention. Deaths from aplastic crisis occur when it is not recognized and treatment is delayed.

In one form of aplastic crisis, widespread sickling occurs in the bone marrow, with destruction of the marrow. In this situation, the bone marrow heals by fibrosis (myelofibrosis). The loss of marrow space then limits maximum rbc production, adding another cause of anemia to the chronic hemolysis from sickling.

In the *splenic sequestration syndrome*, infection causes the spleen to enlarge rapidly. The rbc's are trapped in the enlarged spleen and removed from the circulation faster than they can be replaced. The Hb level therefore falls precipitously. This combination of abrupt worsening of the anemia with severe bacterial infection is the most common cause of death in childhood. Adults are rarely affected because of autosplenectomy. This complication is common only in SCA.

In the *hyperhemolytic crisis*, an abrupt worsening of the chronic hemolytic anemia occurs due to infections, certain drugs, or toxins. Again, Hb levels fall faster than rbc's can be manufactured, and the steady state is upset. Because most of these episodes are mild, with Hb levels dropping only a small amount, this complication is frequently overlooked and only severe cases are noted by the physicians caring for the patient. It is perhaps the least reported complication of the disease.

Infections. Bacterial infections are a major cause of morbidity and mortality in sickle cell disease. The frequency of these infections ranges from 25 to several hundred times that of the general population.

Although the exact reason for the increased susceptibility to infection is poorly understood, a contributing factor is the damage or loss of the spleen. In young children in particular, the damaged spleen is unable to perform its functions of clearing the bloodstream of bacteria. A further contributing factor is that ischemic tissue may provide a portal of entry for bacteria and a site for infectious organisms to grow easily. If bacteria get into the bloodstream (septicemia), the course of the disease may be measured in hours from the onset of symptoms to death. Meningitis, another life-threatening condition, also occurs at a rate much greater than that in the general population.

After age 5 or so, multiple exposures to infectious agents lead to the development of bloodstream antibodies which can contain infections, and the role of the spleen is diminished in importance. After this time, the incidence of septicemia and meningitis declines, while high attack rates for the more localized infections (pneumonia, pyelonephritis, osteomyelitis) continue.

Chronic lung disease. Pulmonary involvement in sickle cell disease is common. Pneumonia, the most common complication, accounts for over 20 percent of all hospital admissions and occurs in all age ranges. Resolution is slow over 10 to 14 days despite adequate antibiotic therapy.

Vaso-occlusion of pulmonary blood vessels by sickled cells results in *pulmonary infarction*. Signs and symptoms are similar to those of pneumonia, and it is difficult to differentiate between these two entities even with special tests. Infarction may also result from fat embolism. Fat from infarcted bone marrow releases from the marrow space into the circulation and lodges in the lungs. Fat embolism is more common in hemoglobinopathy SC than in other forms of sickle cell disease. Coma and severe oxygen deficiency (hypoxia) are the major symptoms.

These pulmonary insults result in scarring of the lungs, which can be seen on the chest X-ray. Eventually the patient may develop pulmonary hypertension. The reduced pulmonary function, like that of chronic obstructive pulmonary disease (see chap. 23), produces lowered arterial oxygen levels and tends to aggravate the sickling process.

Chronic heart disease. An enlarged heart (cardiomegaly) and heart murmurs are almost universal features of sickle cell disease because of the anemia. In this condition, the chest X-ray shows the mild cardiac enlargement. The electrocardiogram frequently shows various conduction abnormalities and evidence of large ventricles (ventricular hypertrophy). Sickling in coronary arteries (see p. 39) may produce sufficient fibrosis of the heart muscle to result in cardiac insufficiency. Subsequent reduced cardiac output lowers arterial oxygen levels and aggravates sickling.

Chronic bone disease. One of the more important physical impairments in sickle cell disease results from involvement of the bones and joints by the vaso-occlusive process. *Bone infarcts* (aseptic necrosis) involving the small bones of the hands and feet are common in children but heal without residual deformity. In older patients, the crucial sites of involvement are the heads of the femur and humerus and the thoracic and lumbar vertebrae (see chap. 3). Other bones are frequently affected but usually heal without long-term disability. Following infarction, repair is accomplished by resorption of dead bone and then by new bone formation.

During the acute phase of a bone infarct in the femur, severe pain prevents ambulation. During repair there is no pain. Thus, if the bone infarction is not detected, continued weight bearing produces fragmentation and collapse of the infarcted bone sufficient to produce a severe degenerative osteoarthritis (see chap. 14) and a serious ambulation problem. Unfortunately, the diagnosis is usually not made until the late stages of the process.

Acute *arthritis*, usually of the large joints, due to infarcts in the joint capsule, can also occur. This condition is marked by severe pain, swelling, and redness about the joint.

Further, since infarcted bone is an excellent culture medium for supporting bacterial growth, *bone infection* (osteomyelitis) is a frequent complication of sickle cell disease.

Chronic central nervous system damage. Meningitis of sufficient severity to produce *inflammation of the brain* (encephalitis) may cause permanent central nervous system damage. Occlusion of the tiny vessels supplying the carotid artery leads to thrombosis of the carotid system and subsequent *stroke*. CNS infarction may also result from fat emboli. *Cerebral hemorrhage* is often seen, due to rupture of the infarcted vessels. Stroke and meningitis are primarily found in the very young child, while cerebral hemorrhage is seen in all age groups. All of the long-term disabilities discussed in chapters 9 and 10 may result from one of these episodes.

Chronic eye disease. Sickle cell *retinopathy* is more commonly found in those with hemoglobinopathy SC or sickle thalassemia than in those with SCA. The disorder begins with an infarction of the retina which then stimulates new blood vessel growth into the vitreous cavity (see chap. 29). There are no symptoms until these abnormal vessels bleed or cause retinal detachment and hence decreased vision.

Chronic kidney disease. Chronic renal failure is the second most common cause of death in the adult population. The kidney is particularly susceptible to sickling and hence to infarction. Fat emboli may also induce kidney infarction. The infarcted kidney becomes unable to conserve water and large urine volumes result. Consequently, the patient must continuously drink large amounts of fluids to prevent dehydration, which can aggravate sickling. A bloody urine (hematuria) may also occur.

Increased fluid intake and large urine volumes are actually found in all patients with sickle cell disease and often in those with sickle cell trait, even in the absence of gross kidney failure. Ordinarily this is of little consequence to the patient unless free access to water is impaired.

Kidney infarctions are also common. It is the combination of many infarcts and chronic infection which may produce slowly progressive *chronic uremia*. If renal function rapidly deteriorates, dialysis may be required (see chap. 25).

Liver disease. Cirrhosis of the liver is a rare complication of sickling because of the regenerative capacity of the liver. More commonly, accumulation of iron in the liver (hemisiderosis) is seen, due to iron overload from frequent transfusions or long-term iron therapy.

Leg ulcers. Leg ulcers are seen in most patients with SCA during the young adult years. They are less common in the other variants of sickle cell disease. Ulcers are due to infarcts in the skin and are found around the ankles. They enlarge slowly, are difficult to heal, and are aggravated by prolonged standing in one position. Recurrences may be prevented by fitted elastic stockings.

Priapism. Priapism is a painful, persistent erection due to massive sickling in the penis. Prolonged priapism frequently results in impotence because of scarring of the erectile mechanism. Libido and ejaculation are unimpaired.

FUNCTIONAL DISABILITIES

Physical Disabilities

In general, the patient with sickle cell disease has little physical impairment aside from the reduced exertional capacity and fatigue due to the anemia. Clearly, during sickle cell crises, pain may indeed inhibit function. Chronic problems with ambulation, transfer skills, eating, dressing, communication, or other activities of daily living may be found if some of the organ system complications have occurred. The potential breadth of these disabilities and their treatment are similar to those discussed in chapters 9, 10, 14, 22, 25, and 29.

Psychosocial Disabilities

Because sickle cell disease is an incurable lifelong disorder, psychosocial function is a critical aspect of evaluation and management. Potential areas of concern begin early in the course of the disease because of frequent illnesses and the need for medical attention both in crises and during symptom-free periods. Sibling rivalry may be a particular problem because the child with sickle cell disease may require a disproportionate share of the parents' time and attention. Parental guilt over the genetics of the disease or fears of recurrent illness or early death lead to overprotectiveness. Further, because of the patient's large urine volumes, the family may have to deal with enuresis and its obviously disruptive influence.

The child with sickle cell disease may cope with subtle pressure by developing a pattern of dependency and withdrawal that may persist throughout life. On the other hand, the child may utilize manipulative behavior based on the frightening aspects of the disease as a means of dealing with stress. These problems must be dealt with calmly, providing consistent reassurance and support and avoiding reinforcement of negative behavioral mechanisms.

Because of recurrent hospitalization, these youngsters have difficulty in school performance. Fortunately, many areas have volunteer organizations that supply tutorial services to maintain education during periods of illness. Obviously, poor academic performance due to frequent absences can become self-perpetuating. The child's sense of self-worth may be threatened. This situation can become frustrating enough that the youngster drops out of school, thereby limiting his future vocational potential.

Delayed growth and puberty development can be extremely critical during adolescence. These aspects of the disease can contribute, via peer pressure or ridicule, to anxiety and a poor self-image. Impotence as a complication of priapism has an obvious negative effect on self-image and interpersonal relationships.

The stresses of the disease due to the unpredictability of crises, the real possibility of serious organ damage or early death, and the inability of the individual to exert any influence on the course of the disease often result in feelings of hopelessness, poor self-image, and severe depression. The patient's attitudes are shaped by internal factors, including the degree and accuracy of his knowledge and understanding of the disease, and external factors, including the quality of medical care and the attitudes and support of medical professionals, family, and the community.

The prospect of sudden death is real; it is aggravated by the widely circulated but inaccurate notion that all patients with sickle cell disease die by age 20. When this false information is added to the knowledge of a continuing physical disability in the form of a chronic illness, the patient has little motivation to plan for a future, not only in terms of self-support, but even in view of any future life at all.

These features of the illness tend to produce a passive-aggressive personality, severe dependency, anxiety, depression, and self-pity, and frequently result in problems with alcoholism, drug abuse (particularly narcotics), and occasionally suicide.

Rehabilitation Potential

Assessment of rehabilitation potential is perhaps the most difficult aspect of sickle cell disease. The prognosis is extremely uncertain, due to the possibility of fatal infection occurring at any time. However, this is not too common. Only 15 percent of patients followed in the hematology clinic at the University of Southern California during the past 20 years have died; about half of these deaths were due to infection. The second most common cause of death was chronic renal failure. These two conditions accounted for more than 60 percent of the deaths. The remainder of the mortality was due to a wide variety of illnesses not necessarily related to the hemoglobinopathy and thus not crucial to the rehabilitation aspect.

Those patients with chronic renal failure are best evaluated as described in chapter 25. Rehabilitation goals will be limited by the degree of disability and the prognosis as determined by a period of observation. The likelihood of renal disease entering an accelerated phase is always present and makes short-term vocational goals more realistic. Exceptions may be made for those with mild impairment of renal function who have been stable for enough time to indicate a more remote chance of progression.

In the absence of renal disease, the potential for rehabilitation should be evaluated in view of the complete unpredictability of chronic organ damage occurring at a later time. Pulmonary, cardiac, bone, or eye disease may not be present initially but may become evident and require periodic reassessment of vocational status during the time of rehabilitation counseling and planning.

It must be continually kept in mind that the majority of individuals with sickle cell disease are mildly affected, do not develop serious disability, and live long, productive lives. Rehabilitation potential should be assessed in view of this majority of patients who are functioning well, rather than the minority who are severely affected by sickle cell disease. Whether the severity of disease in terms of the degree of chronic complications influences prognosis has not yet been determined. Therefore, the major emphasis should be placed on long-term goals, recognizing the possibility of decreasing function over time.

STANDARDS OF EVALUATION

Medical Evaluation

Evaluation of the patient with sickle cell disease includes a careful history detailing the frequency, duration, and location of crises, the severity of any chronic complication, the pattern of serious infections, and the previous need for transfusion therapy. This information will document the pattern and severity of the disease. Physical examination should record evidence of pulmonary, cardiac, and other organ dysfunction. Baseline laboratory tests should include a complete blood count, a urinalysis, tests of renal and liver function, chest X-ray, and electrocardiogram.

Frequent pneumonia and/or pulmonary infarction might require specific pulmonary function testing and blood gas analysis. The presence of unusual murmurs or signs and symptoms of cardiac failure might require extensive cardiologic evaluation with echocardiogram or catheterization. Aseptic necrosis may need evaluation by the orthopedist, physiatrist, or physical therapist. Involvement of other organ systems by the chronic complications of sickle cell disease requires complete evaluation by the appropriate medical specialist.

The physician or specialist conducting the evaluation may provide better information to the counselor if specific questions or vocational problems to be addressed are provided. In all instances the evaluation and care of the patient must be directed and coordinated by the hematologist or internist who has the responsibility for primary care. Such a physician can serve also as the initial contact for a patient seeking genetic counseling for family planning.

In view of the multifaceted nature of sickle cell disease, the counselor should ensure that his client has a specific ongoing relationship with a physician or center skilled in the evaluation and management of sickle cell disease. Personal communication by the counselor with the medical consultant during the evaluation phase can greatly aid program planning.

Psychosocial Evaluation

The potential educational and psychosocial disabilities that may accompany sickle cell disease suggest that evaluation by a clinical psychologist or psychiatrist to assess educational achievement levels, personality, and emotional maturity is indicated. Evaluation by a social worker to help assess family interaction and social maturation can also be very helpful in suggesting appropriate management of the counseling process.

TOTAL TREATMENT

Since there is no cure for sickle cell disease, its treatment is basically one of control of the various complications already enumerated. Further information can also be found in the chapters that deal with specific disabilities related to the various organ systems that may be involved.

Chronic Hemolytic Anemia

Rapid rbc loss will require blood transfusions and hospitalization. To ensure rbc production, a well-balanced diet including adequate protein, fats, and other nutrients is essential. Iron is essential for Hb production, and the body rigidly conserves this mineral. Since anemia from any cause increases iron absorption from food, and since transfusion therapy adds to the iron supply, rarely are patients with sickle cell disease iron deficient, and iron therapy is contraindicated. Excess iron is toxic to many tissues, and iron therapy can be harmful when administered for long periods in these patients.

Other essential elements of rbc production are vitamin B_{12} and folic acid. Vitamin B_{12} body stores are high in relation to daily requirements, and this vitamin is recycled by the body after use. Thus there is no need for B_{12} therapy. On the other hand, folic acid stores are small relative to daily requirements, and many studies of sickle cell patients have shown low folic acid levels in the blood. Folic acid supplements are therefore frequently used in the treatment of sickle cell disease to ensure adequate amounts for the accelerated rbc production.

In addition, transfusion therapy may be necessary prior to surgery to reduce anesthetic risk, in serious infections to increase oxygen-carrying capacity, or whenever rbc production is transiently limited.

Sickle Cell Crises

Vaso-occlusive crisis. Aggressive treatment of any precipitating factors, such as infection, while maintaining comfort is the primary approach of any treatment. Unfortunately, no satisfactory treatment exists for shortening the duration of these crises, despite all of the knowledge concerning the properties of Hb, because no drug is known which will *safely* reverse sickling, although oxygen is given and may reduce further sickling. Pain relief usually requires narcotics, and fluids are given by vein to reverse any degree of dehydration. Acidosis, when present, is reversed with alkalinizing solutions, and the patients are kept warm and rested until the crisis passes. Careful identification of the precipitating factors may decrease frequency of crises if they can be avoided.

Aplastic crisis. Transfusion support and aggressive treatment of the infection associated with the destruction of rbc precursors in the bone marrow is necessary until the marrow recovers (about 10 days).

Since severe deficiency of folic acid limits rbc production and may lead to an aplastic crisis-like situation, folic acid supplements are usually given to prevent a crisis.

Splenic sequestration syndrome. As in the aplastic crisis, treatment is directed at the infection which is causing the spleen to enlarge rapidly. The anemia is supported by transfusions.

Hyperhemolytic crisis. Treatment consists of removing the offending toxin or drug or aggressive treatment of the infection causing the crisis, while supporting the anemia with transfusion therapy.

Infections

Although antibacterial therapy of infections is usually successful when treatment is begun early, doses must be higher than those usually given. Furthermore, the response to treatment is frequently slower in these patients, so that hospitalizations and convalescence are generally longer.

If bacterial septicemia occurs, immediate institution of antibiotics and supportive transfusion are crucial for a successful outcome. But even in the best of situations, therapeutic failure is high because of the rapidity with which these infections spread.

Chronic Lung Disease

Because of the high incidence of secondary infection, treatment for pulmonary infarction is the same as for pneumonia, with fluids, expectorants, and antibiotics, usually penicillin. Supplemental oxygen is given in high concentration and monitored by analysis of concentrations of oxygen and carbon dioxide in the arteries, both for prevention of further sickling and to overcome the impairment of oxygen transfer across the infected or infarcted lung segments. Transfusion is frequently necessary to improve oxygen-carrying capacity.

In severe pulmonary infarction, the technique of replacement of nearly all the blood (exchange transfusion) may be employed to prevent further sickling. In this procedure, transfusion is alternated with blood letting (phlebotomy) until the patient's rbc's have been nearly replaced by rbc's containing only normal Hb A. When this has been accomplished, sickling with vaso-occlusion is essentially impossible, due to the dilution effect of the normal rbc's. Because of the risk of transfusion reactions, hepatitis, and other complications of multiple transfusions, this therapy is reserved for severe sickling episodes only.

Treatment of fat embolism syndrome is primarily supportive, with oxygen, fluids, and transfusion.

Chronic Heart Disease

Treatment of cardiac insufficiency with digitalis and salt restriction is beneficial. Diuretic therapy may aggravate sickling by dehydrating the patient and must be carefully monitored. Transfusions may be necessary to reduce cardiac workload. Intracardiac angiography, if necessary, must be preceded by exchange transfusion to avoid acute deoxygenation by the dye injection. This is one of the rarest complications of sickle cell disease but, when present, produces significant functional impairment.

Chronic Bone Disease

Treatment of aseptic necrosis, when diagnosed early, consists of avoiding weight bearing until healing is complete. In the late stages, analgesics for pain control and supportive devices are used. If symptoms are not controlled, insertion of an artificial hip joint may be necessary. This condition may be aggravated by heavy lifting, especially when the spine or hips are involved, so that X-ray evidence of changes in these bones should alert the counselor to steer the patient into more sedentary occupations.

Sickle cell arthritis responds to rest and analgesics within 10 to 14 days and leaves no residual joint impairment. Treatment of osteomyelitis involves long-term antibiotic therapy and surgical removal of infected bone.

Chronic Central Nervous System Damage

Exchange transfusion may be of benefit in the acute phase of a stroke syndrome caused by CNS infarction. Otherwise, the treatment of the consequences of stroke are as in chapter 9.

Chronic Eye Disease

All patients with hemoglobinapathy SC or sickle thalassemia should have periodic ophthalmologic examinations to detect the presence of the proliferative vessels in the vitreous cavity. At the early stages of the process, laser treatment (photocoagulation) of the abnormal vessels can prevent bleeding and retinal detachment. In the later stages, removal of the vitreous (vitrectomy) or scleral buckling may be necessary to preserve vision. Scleral buckling is a surgical procedure to correct retinal detachment. The posterior part of the sclera (see p. 47) at the position of the retinal detachment is buckled inward to bring it close to the detached retina. This is usually followed by a diathermy or laser technique to fuse the retina back onto its surface. Scleral buckling must be preceded by exchange transfusion to prevent ischemia and infarction of the anterior cavity of the eye and resulting shrinkage and wasting of the eyeball (phthisis bulbi). The poorly deformable sickle cells in the capillaries of the choroid are unable to squeeze past the area of the buckle into the anterior cavity of the eye and must be replaced by more normal cells to maintain a healthy ciliary body and iris (see p. 47).

Leg Ulcers

Most leg ulcers respond to medicated leg wrappings, but occasionally bed rest, transfusion, or skin grafting is necessary to heal a chronic ulcer. Fitted elastic stockings may prevent recurrence.

Priapism

Initial treatment of priapism consists of moist heat, sedation, and removal of the sickled blood from the penis by insertion of large needles. Transfusion may be beneficial. Other surgical measures for relief of priapism have a high rate of subsequent impotence. Artificial erectile protheses have been developed for the treatment of impotence.

Psychosocial Disabilities

During vocational counseling, ongoing therapy by a clinical psychologist or psychiatrist may be recommended if evaluation indicated that treatable maladaptive behavior patterns have developed. Similarly, if evaluation indicates family social problems amenable to treatment, an ongoing case-work relationship between a social worker and the client, family, or both may be considered.

VOCATIONAL IMPLICATIONS

For sickle cell disease, the major vocational considerations will be in the area of physical demands because prolonged strenuous exertion is not possible for most clients, due to the anemia and reduced exertional capacity. In addition, excessive exertion and the resultant fatigue may precipitate a painful crisis. Fortunately, most clients have defined their intrinsic physical limits by the process of trial and error over the years and will be able to detail quite specifically for the counselor the types and duration of physical activities of which they are capable. Furthermore, each client may be able to delineate the types or duration of certain activities which are likely to produce symptoms.

Almost all clients will be capable of sedentary and light work, and most will be capable of medium work. Those with major neurological handicaps or joint limitations due to aseptic necrosis may be able to perform sedentary work only, depending on the degree of functional capability. Assessment by a physical therapist or, more directly, a sheltered work evaluation may be necessary to clearly define the work capacity of these individuals.

Some individuals with mild anemia and near normal exertional capacity will be capable of heavy work. Most of these will be clients with hemoglobinopathy SC or sickle thalassemia but will include a few with SCA. Few clients will be able to perform very heavy work.

Heavy lifting may aggravate early aseptic necrosis, particularly of the spine and hips, while prolonged standing may aggravate or initiate leg ulcers. The risk of these two complications, while not an absolute caveat, should be considered by the counselor, and, when possible, the client should be steered into work situations where the need for heavy lifting and prolonged standing are less.

The tendency to automatically consign individuals with sickle cell disease to the most sedentary positions is unreasonable and should be avoided. This attitude has been prevalent for many years and fails to recognize the wide variability in the degree of anemia, frequency of symptoms, and functional impairment. Imposition of arbitrary restraints on those with sickle cell disease may produce justifiable resentment, since the clients are generally well aware of their physical limitations. The expression of negative attitudes will be counterproductive to the goals of rehabilitation.

Other physical skills demanding fine motor coordination, such as climbing, balancing, bending, reaching, and fingering are only likely to be impaired in those with neurological dysfunction or joint disease. These factors should be evident in the history and physical examination, and appropriate evaluation by a neurologist, physiatrist, or physical therapist can define the vocational potential for these individuals. Impairment of visual acuity due to retinopathy may be present and require evaluation during the counseling and planning phase of rehabilitation.

Environmental factors are extremely important in the determination of work capacity because of their effect on the frequency of crises and infections. Exposure to hot, humid environments is unwise because of the extra stress on the heart and the reduced exertional capacity in this disease. However, some clients may be able to tolerate such conditions. Exposure to cold, moist environments must be avoided since this potentiates sickling in nearly all clients and thus tends to increase the frequency of crises or the risk of infection.

All clients with sickle cell disease must be placed in situations where there is free access to water or other fluids so that dehydration does not occur and precipitate crises. Further, their high urine output requires ready access to restrooms.

Naturally, occupations in which there is an abrupt change in oxygen level are unsuitable for clients with this disorder because of the effect of oxygen on sickling.

When all these environmental factors are taken into account, inside work is obviously preferable to outside work for clients with sickle cell disease. The prohibition on outside work is relative and not absolute, and other factors, such as aptitude, training, geography, and climate may favor outside work. In making this decision, the counselor may be guided by the client's knowledge of his own capabilities, based on previous exposure to situations likely to be encountered in a given occupation.

Clients with a history of frequent pneumonia or evidence of chronic pulmonary impairment as a result of frequent pulmonary insults may be sensitive to noxious fumes, high dust exposure, and poor ventilation. These situations may produce acute symptoms with difficult breathing or may increase the risk of infection due to irritation of the lung tissues.

In general, vocational goals should not be time limited for clients with this disease. As discussed under rehabilitation potential, the prognosis is uncertain because of the risk of sudden death but this risk is small and should not overly influence decisions regarding specific training objectives.

Because of negative attitudes instilled in these clients early in life, educational opportunities may have been sacrificed to the expectation of early death. Since the misconception that those with sickle cell disease are not expected to attain adulthood is so prevalent, no efforts are expended to prepare these individuals for the activities of adult life, particularly in the area of vocational planning. All who work in the field know of tragic cases where youngsters were advised to drop out of school, despite good academic achievement and motivation, since there was no need for them to make plans for a future that would not come to be. This tendency to promote low levels of academic achievement and lack of skills and preparation for adult life is a major problem for workers in the field, and much effort is aimed at reversing this trend. Therefore, many of these individuals may need further education or specific training to reach vocational readiness.

One area of need that is not well appreciated is vocational counseling in job interview situations, appropriate grooming and dress, and handling of application forms. These individuals are not likely to have received this type of information prior to referral for vocational counseling.

For most clients, aptitudes are not affected by the disease. Those with neurological handicaps from stroke or meningitis may have diminished intellectual and fine motor skills, while those with aseptic necrosis of joints may have impaired dexterity. Those with retinopathy may have impaired eye-hand-foot coordination. Combinations of the various complications of the disease may exist in a single individual and multiple impairments may be present. The history and physical examination should delineate these for the counselor.

In sickle cell disease, the environmental and physical demands are most important in determining the area of vocational guidance. The education, aptitudes, and interests of the client have less direct bearing on this decision. In the area of interest, the disease has no effect on whether the client will function better when dealing with abstract versus concrete situations, nor whether technical versus interpersonal relationships predominate.

However, stress may present a problem to these

individuals. Why stress affects the disease is not understood, but it has been known to precipitate painful crises.

The subsequent loss of time from work when crises occur is one of the major obstacles to employment. Crises may occur frequently during the training or probationary period because of stress, and the client may utilize his sick time allotment too quickly. This latter situation may abruptly increase the level of anxiety if the individual fears he may lose his job if he becomes ill again. Thus, the client may have severe difficulty in keeping a position once hired. For these reasons, persons with sickle cell disease are reluctant to disclose the nature of their illness, and fear of discovery adds further to the stress. Therefore, less stressful situations, smaller stages of incremental goals, proper support by the counselor, and some employer preparation are more compatible with the disease. For the same reasons, situations where performance is measured in prestige and esteem are generally more appropriate, since emphasis on production may increase the fear of illness and subsequent failure to meet quotas.

Although sickle cell disease seems to present many impediments to successful vocational counseling and employment performance, one must realize that the majority of persons with this disease do not suffer from the myriad problems described here. Rather, they generally function well, are without severe impairment, and are infrequently hospitalized because of crises. Most of them are presently gainfully employed without disclosing the nature of their illness. Although they fear discovery, they have made successful adjustments to the situation.

It is the minority of patients who are frequently ill and disabled because of sickle cell disease who will be the primary recipients of vocational rehabilitation. In the hematology clinic at the University of Southern California, some 35 percent of patients are responsible for 75 percent of the total hospital admissions for this disease. It is this latter group and those just entering the job market who will need rehabilitation services, not the 65 percent who are functioning well. Successful rehabilitation for this group will be difficult but rewarding for all concerned.

Not all clients with sickle cell disease can be placed in full-time competitive employment. For some, the physical disability due to neurological or other handicaps may necessitate placement in sheltered workshops only. For an unfortunate few, the severity of the disability will not permit any kind of employment, and social, cultural, or recreational activity may be all that is possible.

BIBLIOGRAPHY

Cerami A, Washington E: *Sickle Cell Anemia*. New York, The Third Press, 1974.
This easy-to-read book describes the medical aspects of sickle cell anemia and the related hemoglobinopathies. Information is included on genetics and treatment, along with a brief discussion of the sickle cell controversy in the U.S. and a description of the disease in Africa.

Diggs LW: Sickle cell crises. Am J. Clin Path **44**:1-19, 1965.
This is the classic description of sickle cell crises and chronic complications by one of the foremost authorities in the field.

Kumar S, Powars D, Allen J, Haywood LJ: Anxiety, self-concept, and personal and social adjustments in children with sickle cell disease. J. Pediatr **88**:859-863, 1976.
This article describes a study of the personal, social, and overall adjustment of a group of adolescents with sickle cell disease compared with a group of adolescents with no chronic disabilities.

Powers DR: Natural history of sickle cell disease: The first ten years. Sem Hematol **12**:267-285, 1975.
This article describes the clinical and demographic features in 422 cases of sickle cell disease in Los Angeles. Emphasis is placed on the differences between adults and children with the disease, particularly with regard to morbidity and mortality.

Serjeant GR: *The Clinical Features of Sickle Cell Disease*. Amsterdam, North Holland Publishing Co., 1974.
This text describes the natural history and clinical features of 438 cases of sickle cell disease in Jamaica. There are good descriptions of the types of crises and the chronic complications of the disease and of the clinical differences between the types of sickle cell disease. Emphasis is placed on the large number of cases over age 30, in which the disease appears more benign than usual, and implications for a longer life expectancy are discussed.

Sinnette CH, Gillman RA: Vocational rehabilitation and sickle cell anemia. Urban Health **3**:38-41, 1974.
This is a description of the method of vocational rehabilitation used at the Harlem Hospital Sickle Cell Center in New York. There is a brief discussion of the disease and the major problems in this area. Realistic rehabilitation goals are well outlined, and methods of achieving these goals are discussed.

Whitten CF, Fischoff J: Psychological effects of sickle cell disease. Arch Intern Med **133**:681-689, 1974.
This article contains a complete delineation of the effects of the disease on psychosocial functioning in childhood, adolescence, and adulthood. The role of the family and the community is discussed, as are the effects of fear, anxiety, and knowledge of the disease on the individual. The positive and negative effects of legislation are considered, and methods of dealing with some of these problems are presented.

28 CANCERS

John E. Healey, Jr., M.D.
Jack Zislis, M.D.

DISEASE DESCRIPTION

The significance of the cancer problem is reflected in the estimate of 690,000 new cancer cases for the year 1977 in the United States. This figure is exclusive of carcinoma in-situ of the uterine cervix (40,000) and non-melanoma skin cancer (300,000). In addition, there are over 2 million individuals living today who have survived 5 or more years.

A 5-year survival rate is a measure of the percentage of patients alive at the end of this arbitrary interval of observation after the date of diagnosis. This rate assists in evaluating the efficacy of treatment and provides a sound base for therapeutic planning for cancer patients. A majority of the patients who have survived 5 or more years are still in need of rehabilitation services.

Cancer covers the entire age spectrum from childhood to old age. Although cancer is much more frequent in the adult population, it is responsible for more deaths in the 3-to-14-year-old group than any other disease. The estimated incidence of new cancer cases for 1977 reveals little difference between male and female. Cancer may affect every part of the body.

Cancer is a costly disease. The Health Insurance Institute statistics for 1974 show that the average *per day hospital costs* were $127.00. This would mean that a hospital stay of 28 days would cost a family or an individual $3,515.00. This figure does not include physician's fee for service, drugs, home nursing, or sick room equipment. The average length of hospitalization for initial cancer treatment varies from 12 to 16 days in specialized cancer centers.

What is not apparent is how cancer influences the earning power of those affected either directly or indirectly. It has been estimated that, including loss of earnings, the total cost of cancer in the United States amounts to over $18.9 billion a year.

Pathology

The basic difference between normal cells and cancer cells is the manner of their growth. Normal body cells grow in a coordinated and controlled manner. There are times when this "normal" growth

pattern may be triggered to go beyond its normal rate of growth, as in the case of a normal pregnancy, the repair of tissue injuries, or the replacement of blood loss. This proliferation of growth is always controlled, and once the end point is reached, the growth pattern reverts to normal.

Cancer cells, on the other hand, once triggered by whatever causative factors, continue to multiply beyond normality, overpowering the growth-control mechanism and resulting in an uncontrolled *localized* cellular mass. This mass of cells may compress, become invasive, and destroy adjacent normal tissues. These cancer cells, by further proliferation, may invade blood vessels or lymphatics and spread to distant parts of the body. At these points, secondary cancerous deposits (*metastases*) develop which further invade and destroy the cellular structure of whatever organ or site they select.

A *tumor* is a growth of new cells that proliferate without control and serve no useful function. It is therefore called a new growth, or *neoplasm*. Some neoplasms, such as fatty tumors (lipomas), are *benign* and remain at the site of origin. Others are *malignant* growths (i.e., cancers) and spread by *direct invasion* into adjacent tissues or *metastasize* by way of lymphatics (see p. 40) or blood vessels to other anatomic sites in the body.

Cancer cells are classified into two main *histological types*. Malignant cells may be *well differentiated*, i.e., retain their identifiable characteristics, or they may be *anaplastic*, i.e., lose their normal appearance. The latter type usually implies a less favorable prognosis. The histological types are determined by microscopic examination of tissue from the tumor.

Cancer is not a single disease entity but a group of more than 100 different diseases. The term *carcinoma* refers to those cancers arising from epithelial cells. Examples of such tissues are cellular linings of body organs, body cavities, skin, and glandular tissue, such as breast or prostate. A malignant *melanoma* is a form of carcinoma that arises from pigment-producing melanin cells. The primary site is usually the skin. Cancers arising from connective and supporting tissue, such as bone, cartilage, nerve, and

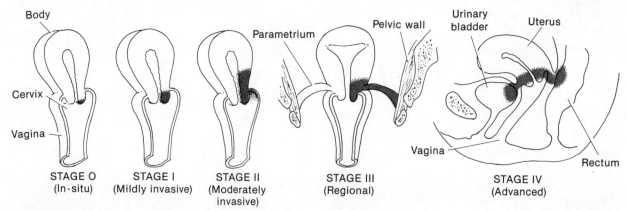

FIGURE 28-1. Staging of cancer of the cervix of the uterus.

fat, are referred to as *sarcomas*. *Lymphomas* are malignant disorders characterized by lymph node enlargement and include Hodgkin's disease, lymphosarcoma, reticular cell sarcoma, and giant follicular lymphoma. *Leukemias* are malignant transformations of the white blood cells. These malignant cells infiltrate into the bone marrow or other body tissues, such as the spleen and/or lymph nodes, and circulate in the blood. The leukemias are divided into two basic categories, acute and chronic. The *acute* type usually occurs in young individuals, and is characterized by the presence of very bizarre and immature cells. In the *chronic* type, which usually occurs at an older age and is less virulent, the cells are much more mature.

Stages of Cancer

Cancer begins as an abnormal proliferation of cells. While these proliferating cells still remain at the site of origin, they are *localized* and are termed *in-situ cancers*. These in-situ cancer cells may penetrate the lining tissue and invade the underlying tissue. Although still localized, such cancers are now regarded as *invasive*.

These localized cancers may extend to regional lymph nodes (see p. 41) draining that specific anatomic site. This stage is referred to as *regional* involvement. Regional cancer, if not treated, may eventually spread to other parts of the body. This latter stage is then termed *advanced* or *disseminated* cancer.

For some cancers, staging is more specific. This can best be exemplified by the staging of cancer of the uterine cervix (fig. 28-1). *Stage 0* (in-situ cancer) is limited to the epithelial lining of the cervix. This stage is 100 percent curable. When the cells invade deeper tissue but remain confined to the cervix, the cancer becomes *Stage I* (mildly invasive). When the cell growth extends into the body of the uterus or upper vagina, it is regarded as *Stage II* (moderately invasive). *Stage III* (regional) cervical cancers involve the structures of the

pelvic wall, and *Stage IV* (advanced) implies that the tumor has extended to other body sites, such as the rectum, urinary bladder, or other body sites outside of the pelvis.

These stages constitute the *clinical staging* of cervical cancer and should not be confused with classification of cervical smears obtained by the Papanicolaou technique (Pap test). Five classes of cervical smears are described by this test: *Class I* smears are normal and contain no abnormal cells; *Class II* smears contain cells that are atypical for the cervix; *Class III* smears contain cells frankly abnormal in size, shape, and organization; *Class IV* smears contain cancerous cells which are not invasive (Stage 0 above); *Class V* smears contain cancerous cells which are invasive (Stage I above).

Signs and Symptoms

Since there are so many types of cancer, a complete discussion of all the signs and symptoms is impossible. The American Cancer Society has, however, established seven warning signals:

1. Change in bowel or bladder habits
2. A sore that does not heal
3. Unusual bleeding or discharge
4. Thickening or lump in breast or elsewhere
5. Indigestion or difficulty in swallowing
6. Obvious change in wart or mole
7. Nagging cough or hoarseness

Etiology

Because of the variety of cancers, it is unlikely that a single causative factor will ever be identified. It is becoming increasingly apparent that more than one factor must occur coincidentally to convert the normal cell into a "cancerous" cell.

With two exceptions, cancer is not hereditary. Familial polyposis of the colon, a precursor of cancer, is indisputably hereditary, and retinoblastoma, a

TABLE 28-1
COMMON OCCUPATIONAL CARCINOGENS

Agent	Organ Affected	Occupation
Wood	Nasal cavity and sinuses	Woodworkers
Leather	Nasal cavity and sinuses, urinary bladder	Leather and shoe workers
Iron oxide	Lung, larynx	Iron ore miners, metal grinders & polishers; silver finishers; iron foundry workers
Nickel	Nasal sinuses, lung	Nickel smelters, mixers, & roasters; electrolysis workers
Arsenic	Skin, lung, liver	Miners; smelters; insecticide makers & sprayers; tanners; chemical workers; oil refiners; vintners
Chromium	Nasal cavity and sinuses, lung, larynx	Chromium producers, processers, & users; acetylene and aniline workers; bleachers; glass, pottery & linoleum workers; battery makers
Asbestos	Lung	Miners; millers; textile, insulation & shipyard workers
Petroleum, petroleum coke, wax, creosote, anthracene, paraffin, shale, and mineral oil	Nasal cavity, larynx, lung, skin, scrotum	Workers in contact with lubricating, cooling, paraffin, or wax fuel oils or coke; rubber fillers; retort workers; textile weavers; diesel jet testers
Mustard gas	Larynx, lung, trachea, bronchi	Mustard gas workers
Vinyl chloride	Liver, brain	Plastic workers
Bis-chloromethyl ether, chloromethyl methyl ether	Lung	Chemical workers
Isopropyl oil	Nasal cavity	Isopropyl oil producers
Coal soot, coal tar, other products of coal combustion	Lung, larynx, skin, scrotum, urinary bladder	Gashouse workers, stokers & producers; asphalt, coal tar, pitch workers; coke oven workers; miners; still cleaners
Benzene	Bone Marrow	Explosives, benzene, or rubber cement workers; distillers; dye users; painters; shoemakers
Auramine, benzidine, alpha-Nephthylamine, beta-Nephthylamine, magenta, 4-Aminodiphenyl, 4-Nitrodiphenyl	Urinary bladder	Dyestuffs manufacturers & users; rubber workers (pressman, filterman, laborers); textile dyers; paint manufacturers

SOURCE: National Cancer Institute

tumor of the eye in children, occurs with a suspicious frequency in some families.

Cancer is not a contagious disease. Although *virus-like* particles have been linked to certain tumors, their etiological role is still very speculative.

Chronic irritation has long been recognized as a predisposing factor. Examples of this factor are: cancer of the lip in pipe smokers; melanoma arising in a mole located in a friction zone of a brassiere, belt, or suspenders; and cancer of the cervix in women with chronic inflammation of the cervix (cervicitis).

Precancerous lesions are benign lesions which may undergo malignant change. Examples include leukoplakia of the oral cavity (a buildup of cells into thick, whitish plaques); pigmented moles; polyps of the colon and rectum (elongated growths arising from the intestinal wall); neurofibromatosis (multiple benign nerve tumors which can be associated with growth disturbances, skeletal defects, and mental retardation); and senile keratosis (lesions of the skin seen in older persons, associated with chronic ultraviolet exposure).

Exposure to known carcinogens is regarded by many as the major causative factor in cancer. Major emphasis is now being directed toward the identification of certain environmental factors by epidemiological statistics of cancer. Recently, an increase in tumors of the thyroid gland has been recognized in patients who received, years ago, X-ray therapy for acne, hypertrophy of the tonsils or adenoids, sinusitis, and tinea capitis, a fungus infection of the scalp. *Smoking* has been clearly associated with the development of lung cancer. Table 28-1 identifies certain cancers known to be associated with specific carcinogens.

Prognosis: General

Cancer has always been regarded in a very fatalistic manner by the laity, allied health professionals, and physicians alike. In the early 1940's, only one of every four cancer patients survived for 5 years or longer. There was no effort to rehabilitate them, except for an occasional laryngectomy patient who was given instructions in esophageal speech. The prevailing feeling was that the cancer patient had no rehabilitation potential and all such efforts would be a waste of time and energy.

It is interesting, however, that such an attitude does not prevail in regard to the patient who experiences a myocardial infarction, even though 35 percent of these patients do not survive more than 1 month after their first attack. Nor does this fatalistic feeling hold true for stroke patients, of whom 50 percent will die within 1 year of the initial seizure. Thus, it is not simply the fear of death that accounts for this attitude. It is the image of disfigurement, disability, abandonment, and lingering and painful death.

In the 1950's, survival rates in cancer began to change. Great advances were made in the various diagnostic techniques, refinements were made in surgical treatment, new radiation therapy modalities were developed, and chemotherapeutic drugs (anticancer drugs) were being developed. Physicians began to realize that all three disciplines—surgery, radiation therapy, and chemotherapy—should be considered in treatment planning.

It was the passage of the National Cancer Act of 1971 that brought to the forefront the rehabilitation needs of the cancer patient. The last of the seven objectives of the National Cancer Program read: "To restore patients with residual deficits as a consequence of their disease or treatment to as nearly a normal functioning state as possible."

Unfortunately, we hear only of the failures of cancer treatment and the mortality rates of different cancers. We hear little of the successes of cancer treatment. Actually, the 5-year survival rates for some cancers have increased significantly in the past 10 years and have leveled off for most cancers. The overall incidence of cancer has slightly decreased over the past 25 years, particularly in cancers of the rectum, esophagus, stomach, and uterus. Figure 28-2 illustrates the changes in 5-year survival rates in some anatomic sites over the past 10 years. These changes are a reflection of the tremendous advantage of the multidisciplinary approach in treatment planning among specialists in surgical oncology, radiation therapy, and medical oncology.

By far the majority of people today regard all cancer as a progressive disease. This statement is true if definitive treatment means are not entertained. The goal in cancer treatment, as in the treatment of any other chronic disease, is to "control" that disease. With proper treatment, if diagnosed prior to its dissemination throughout the body, cancer need not be a progressive disease. It is, however, unpredictable. This is particularly true in patient response to anticancer drugs (chemotherapy). Some will respond in a remarkable manner, others will not.

Many cancers are curable, especially skin cancers. Treatment, however, may produce cosmetic defects which require either plastic surgery or other reconstruction rehabilitative procedures (see chap. 32).

Prognosis: Individual

It is almost impossible to cite specific prognostic criteria for any single cancer patient. First, as already alluded to above, cancer is a group of over 100 different diseases. Prognosis depends upon several factors, particularly the stage of the disease at the time of diagnosis, the histological type, and the anatomic site.

Stage. The stage of the disease is the most significant factor affecting prognosis, regardless of the anatomic site or histological type. The earlier the diagnosis of any cancer is made, the better the possi-

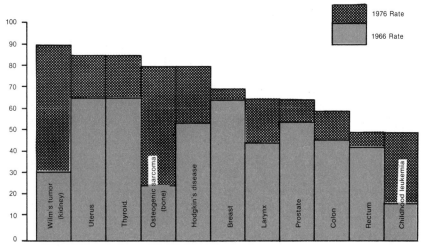

FIGURE 28-2. Five-year survival rates for each of several tumors. Note in particular the large gains made for Wilm's tumor (kidney), osteogenic sarcoma, and leukemia.

bility for a cure. The more advanced the stage at the time of diagnosis, the poorer the prognosis. As a general guide, cancers in Stages 0, 1, and 2 (in-situ, mildly invasive, and moderately invasive) are curable. Cancers in Stage 3 (regional) are controllable. For cancers in Stage 4 (advanced), no real control is possible.

Histological type. It would be impossible for us to discuss the various histological types of tumors as related to the prognosis of the referred potential client. There is, however, a real relationship. For example, a chondrosarcoma of bone whose cells are well differentiated has a much better prognostic outlook than does a Ewing's tumor of bone whose cells are anaplastic. Again, the counselor must depend upon the opinion of the medical consultant or, preferably, upon the primary physician for this phase of evaluation.

Anatomic site. Prognosis also varies depending on the anatomical structure of the body involved. A patient who has skin cancer certainly has a greater survival potential than one who has lung cancer. Likewise, a patient who has a bone cancer requiring amputation of an extremity has a greater rehabilitation need than a patient who has a hysterectomy for uterine cancer.

FUNCTIONAL DISABILITIES

Comprehensive care of the cancer patient must focus attention on the effects of the disease process as it modifies the patient's functional status in broad categories of activity. The multidisciplinary evaluation of the patient's functional assets and limitations is essential to coordinated planning for his future.

The functional limitations associated with specific cancers can only be discussed in a general way. Table 28-2 provides a general guide to functional limitations often associated with cancers involving nine anatomical regions. Functional level will, of course, also be affected by the course of the disease, the

patient's age, and psychosocial factors.

A description of specific tasks a patient cannot accomplish is a valuable tool for the professional working with the patient. Whenever possible, however, limitations should be converted to a description of the patient's residual assets and the positive orientation of tasks the patient *is* able to accomplish.

The diversity of cancer is such that all organs, structures, and systems are potentially vulnerable. Intrinsic growth properties are characterized by considerable variability in cellular proliferation, invasiveness, dissemination, and response to treatment. Structure and function usually go together. Therefore, when evaluating the patient's functional status, it is essential to determine both the region or anatomical structure of the body that is affected and the type of tumor. Cancers of nine anatomical sites are discussed here.

Breast Cancer

Breast cancer which results in the surgical removal of the breast has the shock impact of body-part loss. In addition to the cosmetic problem presented by the loss, the sexual connotations of the breast may result in psychosexual adjustment problems. Some surgical or radiation treatments of breast cancer will diminish the lymphatic system's function of draining fluids from the upper extremity and may result in *lymphedema*. Dependent upon the degree of swelling, stiffness of the shoulder and particularly of the hand may follow, thus limiting arm reach and hand dexterity. Similarly, dependent upon the extent of surgery and/or radiation therapy to the axillary area, weakness and pain may affect the involved shoulder, restricting mobility.

Limitation in activities of daily living, i.e., grooming, bathing, toileting, and dressing, plus reaching overhead and behind, may be associated with

TABLE 28-2

GUIDE TO POTENTIAL FUNCTIONAL LIMITATIONS OF CANCERS AND THEIR IMPROVEMENT WITH REHABILITATION

(x indicates functional limitation; y indicates improvement potential)

Functional Activities	Breast	Head & Neck	Musculoskeletal: Upper	Musculoskeletal: Lower	Colorectal Digestive	Leukemia Lymphoma	Nervous System: Brain	Spinal Cord: Paraplegia	Spinal Cord: Quadriplegia	Peripheral	Lung	Genito-urinary	Skin
Transfers				x		x	x	x	x	x			
Standing				x		x	x	x	x	x			
Ambulation	x			x		x	x	x	x	x			
Toileting	x			x	x	x	x	x	x	x		x	
Bathing	x	x		x	x	x	x	x	x	x	x	x	
Grooming	x	x	x			x	x	x	x	x	x		
Dressing	x	x	x	x		x	x	x	x	x	x		
Feeding		x	x			x			x	x			
Driving	x	x	x	x		x	x	x	x	x			
Public Transportation				x			x	x	x	x			
Speech		x					x						
Writing			x				x		x				
Psychological-Sexual	x	x	x	x	x	x	x	x	x	x	x	x	x
Social Adjustment	x	x	x	x	x	x	x	x	x	x	x	x	x
Cosmesis	x	x	x	x	x							x	x
Level of Independence Improved by Rehabilitation	y	y	y	y	y	y	y	y	y	y	y	y	
With training	y	y	y	y	y	y	y	y	y	y	y	y	
With orthotics-prosthetics	y	y	y	y	y	y	y	y	y	y		y	
With adaptive aids	y	y	y	y	y	y	y	y	y	y		y	

the restriction of shoulder and arm mobility. Ability to carry moderate to heavy objects may be impaired if the pectoralis major muscle has been removed during surgery. Driving a car without power steering or automatic transmission may be limited by shoulder and arm pain, swelling, and mobility restriction.

Head and Neck Cancer

Treatment of cancers involving the head and neck regions is usually associated with multiple functional problems. Radical neck surgery results in paralysis of muscle groups innervated by cranial nerve XI (see p. 24) which are important in head movement and shoulder-girdle function. Resulting postural changes in the shoulder may be evident. Limitations in reaching, moderately heavy lifting, and grooming activities can be expected to accompany the shoulder girdle restriction.

Disfigurement is inherent in surgical procedures such as removal of an eye, nose, ear, jaw, tongue, cheek, palate, or maxilla. The loss of an eye would result in an impairment of depth perception and some visual field deficit which, in turn, may limit safe driving. Severe limitation or total absence of speech is a result of surgical resection of part of the tongue and/or laryngectomy. Associated problems will occur in areas of feeding, chewing, swallowing, salivary control, and tracheostomal care.

Inseparable from the obvious cosmetic defects related to the treatment of these cancers are the profound psychological implications. Reactions of mourning, self depreciation, and depression may lead to withdrawal from all social contact.

Musculoskeletal Cancer

In musculoskeletal cancers, amputation of an extremity is a frequent outcome. With regard to functional problems, the same descriptions that characterize amputations from causes other than cancer are applicable (see chap. 13).

However, the amputee cancer patient has additional special problems. First, the site of the amputation for cancer tends to be at a higher level and frequently may be a hip disarticulation, hemipelvectomy, or forequarter (interscapular-thoracic) amputation; second, the use of chemotherapy and local radiation can lead to skin and tissue changes affecting the stump. These important differences combine to make prosthetic fitting and successful utilization of the prosthesis a special, but not insurmountable, challenge.

Digestive Tract Cancer

Cancer of the colon, rectum, and the various digestive organs frequently requires major resections that necessitate the diversion of bowel excretions via a colostomy or ileostomy (see glossary). Fear of social embarrassment, odors, leakage, and clothing bulges may cause the patient to withdraw from social and vocation participation, and may become the source of psychosexual maladjustment.

Leukemias and Lymphomas

The leukemias and lymphomas are characterized functionally by general weakness and a limited tolerance for stress and activities requiring energy expenditure. Further, the patient may be especially vulnerable to pathologic fractures of bone from trauma ordinarily not damaging.

Central Nervous System Cancer

Cancer of the central nervous system results in functional limitations determined by the site of the lesion. For example, a spinal cord tumor may cause spinal cord damage, and a brain tumor may mimic a stroke syndrome. The range of problems may therefore be the same as those discussed in chapters 5, 9, and 10.

Lung Cancer

In lung cancer, functional limitations are far outweighed by high mortality and short life expectancy. Surgery to remove cancerous lung tissue may be associated with postoperative limitations of pulmonary function and impairment of the mechanics of breathing due to chest wall resection. Postoperative local pain may cause restricted movement of the shoulder girdle, leading to postural disturbances and limited mobility of the shoulder and upper arm which impede dressing, bathing, and grooming activities. Remote effects of certain lung cancers can cause neuromuscular disorders associated with weakness and incoordination.

Genitourinary Cancer

In genitourinary cancer, surgical removal of the urinary bladder requires the construction of a "bladder" from the intestines (ileal conduit or loop) which opens through the abdominal wall where the urine is collected in a special bag glued to the skin. Functional problems include skin irritation, leakage, cosmetic concerns with the appearance of the opening, odors, and psychosexual problems.

Skin Cancer

Skin cancer is usually not associated with functional problems when treated prior to local invasion by the cancer, although a cosmetic problem may remain.

TABLE 28-3
FACTORS IN REHABILITATION POTENTIAL ASSESSMENT FOR CANCER PATIENTS

Positive (+)	Questionable (?)	Negative (−)
Cancer completely irradicated	Prevailing statistical information indicates that the specific cancer has a high incidence of metastasis and/or shortened life expectancy	Cancer not completely removed
No local spread		Cancer shows local spread
No regional lymph node spread		Cancer shows regional lymph node spread
No evidence of distant metastasis (e.g., to other organs or bones)	Duration and degree of response of the cancer to, for example, chemotherapy or radiation therapy is uncertain, although some remission is noted	Evidence of distant metastasis to organs or bones
Cancer remission by chemotherapy or radiation therapy	Patient participating in rehabilitation program	Cancer not responding to chemotherapy or radiation therapy
Functional losses are temporary		Functional losses are permanent
Patient has been made independent through rehabilitation		Maximal functional independence not achieved
Good adjustment to disability		Poor adjustment to disability and not amenable to psychological counseling
Strong family support		Little or no family support

However, if the cancer has spread locally into neighboring tissues, the extensive surgery and/or radiation therapy required may result in cosmetic and functional deficits depending on location. Functional deficits associated with metastasis also depend upon the target organ or structures affected (table 28-2), as is true for all tumors.

REHABILITATION POTENTIAL

Vocational planning for the cancer patient requires the counselor to assimilate many areas of information about the tumor itself, the region of the body involved, the magnitude of the patient's functional limitations, his success in a physical restoration program, and his motivation, family support, and psychological adjustment. In addition, information relative to work demands, employer attitudes, and the patient's education, work history, aptitudes, and interests must all be synthesized to formulate the most meaningful vocational plan. Table 28-3 is presented as a guide to help the counselor ask the appropriate questions, collect significant data, and weigh the important variables.

There are no absolute answers, no guarantees to reinforce the "best" vocational decision. Utilizing table 28-3 as a guide, the counselor should be able to determine the appropriate emphasis on short- vs. long-term planning. If the information collected regarding a given cancer patient consistently falls in the Positive (+) column, long-term planning is feasible. If information describing the patient consistently falls in the Negative (−) column, limited goals would seem justified. When data describing the patient appears in the middle, Questionable (?) column, a gray area characterized by unknowns is implied. Emphasis on short-term goals with frequent reassessment of the patient's status would be indicated.

When information describing the patient falls in more than one column, a mixed profile of the patient emerges. The counselor must examine the data and assign priority weights to the variables about which data is available. When vocational decisions must be made for the mixed-profile patient, those variables relating to the status of the patient's cancer as it affects his morbidity and life expectancy must be weighted more heavily than such factors as family support and adjustment to disability.

In vocational planning and goal setting with the cancer patient, the counselor must be sensitive to the multidimensional impact of cancer on the patient and his family. Psychosocial adjustment and vocational planning are dependent on each other, and rehabilitation potential is maximized when help with coping is offered to the patient and his family.

STANDARDS OF EVALUATION

When a cancer patient is referred to a vocational counselor for acceptance as a client in the pretreatment or immediate post-treatment period, the counselor should consider certain disease criteria. He should carefully examine the medical record for information concerning the anatomic site, the histological type, and the stage of the disease. Often the referral will be made months or even years after the primary treatment has occurred. In such cases, the counselor must be aware of what constitutes proper followup of the cancer patient. He usually can obtain this from his medical consultant or from an oncologist.

An important factor that must always be considered is the fact that one cannot "categorize" a cancer patient regarding his prognosis. *The patient that a counselor is evaluating may be the one individual in five who falls into the 20 percent survival category rather than the 80 percent mortality rate* of a particular type of cancer. The vocational counselor must, therefore, create close communication with the referring physician to ascertain the true disease status and prognosis of that particular patient.

Evaluation of Initial Treatment

Diagnosis is, in most cases, determined by removal of the involved tissue and examining it under the microscope. Oncologists all agree that initial treatment planning after diagnosis is vital to successful control of cancer. It has become evident that multidisciplinary treatment planning is by far the most effective approach. This means that the surgeon, radiation therapist, and medical oncologist must all be involved in such planning. Ideally, a cancer treatment team should also include other professionals (social worker, nurse oncologist) able to assess for functional, psychosocial, and potential vocational problems to stimulate appropriate referral during and after initial treatment. Early detection of real or potential rehabilitation problems leads to earlier solutions and less disability.

Evaluation of Followup Management

As with other chronic diseases, continued followup examinations of the cancer patient are imperative if the disease is to be controlled. Some cancers can be cured by the initial treatment, but because of the possibility of *recurrence* or the appearance of metastatic lesions which were not apparent at the time of the initial diagnosis (*occult metastasis*), frequent followup of these patients is essential. The earlier a metastatic lesion is detected, the better the chance of control if such lesions are localized.

At times, a progressive cancer can go into a stage of *remission*. This is particularly true in those patients receiving radiotherapy, chemotherapy, or immunotherapy. Followup is important in these patients to detect, as early as possible, any *exacerbation* of disease.

Continued followup of the cancer patient is also important, since patients who have been cured of their first cancer have a greater risk of developing a second primary cancer than persons who never have had a cancer.

During the first year after initial treatment, patients should receive followup examinations every 1 to 3 months. During the next 4 years, they should be examined every 3 months, and in the next 5 years (6 to 10 years after initial treatment), every 6 to 12 months. After 10 years have elapsed since initial treatment, followup examinations may no longer be necessary.

Evaluation Tests

Patient evaluation in the initial treatment period can be readily obtained from review of the medical records. For patients referred months or years following their definitive treatment, evaluation is dependent upon the followup records. It may be advisable that a psychological evaluation be performed on all patients, since practically all cancer patients have need of such counseling. Further, a complete review of the social and family situation for problem detection should be performed.

TOTAL TREATMENT

Today it is recognized that the optimum treatment of cancer is best attained by a multidisciplinary approach to treatment planning. This approach requires the planning input from the surgical oncologist, medical oncologist, and radiation therapist. It may be decided that, for a particular tumor, a single modality of treatment, whether surgery, chemotherapy, or radiation, is all that is required. In another case, a combination of any or all of these modalities of treatment may be indicated.

Whatever modality is used in the treatment of the cancer patient, certain deficits may occur which prevent the patient from carrying out his everyday activities. These deficits may be physical, psychological, social, or vocational. When a physical deficit is present, the other problems may be greatly magnified. On the other hand, if the patient's psychological, social, or vocational problems are overlooked, his physical restoration may be hindered. It is therefore important to treat the patient within the context of all possible rehabilitation problems.

The achievement of total treatment is best carried out in medical centers where the concept of the Tumor Board or Tumor Clinic conference has developed. Such centers ensure an appropriate multiprofessional medical input. Where they also include other professional personnel sensitive to rehabilitation problems, a treatment plan or a total assessment can be achieved into which the counselor can interject the various aspects of his vocational plan as appropriate.

Surgery

Surgery is the most effective means of cure if the cancer is diagnosed early, particularly before regional invasion. This requires not only removal of the tumor, but also a wide margin of surrounding tissue. Such curative resections by surgery often require the interruption of the respiratory, digestive, or urinary tracts, resulting in the necessity for rehabilitative adjustments on the part of the patient. In addition, nerve elements must be removed in certain instances in order to remove the primary tumor. Such procedures may involve parts of either the central or peripheral nervous system.

Some tumors previously deemed inoperable by surgical criteria can now be converted into operable lesions by the use of preoperative irradiation of the tumors or by the administration of chemotherapeutic drugs. By these means, the tumor is reduced to a size which enables the surgeon to remove it successfully.

Because of the enthusiasm resulting from preliminary reports regarding the beneficial effects of chemotherapy, there has been a trend toward less radical surgery for cancer than in the past.

Radiation Therapy

There are three forms of radiation therapy: X-rays, radium, and artificial radioactive isotopes. *X-rays* are electromagnetic waves ranging in strength from thousands to millions of volts. *Radium*, a radioactive element that occurs in nature, emits alpha particles, beta particles, and gamma rays. *Radioactive isotopes* are produced artificially in an atomic reactor and also release beta particles and gamma rays.

Methods of delivery. Radiation therapy may be delivered as *external radiation* or *internal radiation*. External radiation may be delivered by low voltage or orthovoltage X-ray machines. Such machines have little penetrative power and are therefore used on superficial lesions, such as those on the skin. Generators that produce voltages of more than 800 kilovolts (kv) are called suprovoltage machines. The most common of the latter are the cobalt 60, the cesium 127, the linear accelerator, and the betatron.

Internal radiation using radium or radioactive isotopes may be used to treat a lesion by directly implanting these materials into the tumor (*interstitial therapy*) or by placing them into a cavity containing or adjacent to the tumor (*intracavity therapy*). Other isotopes may be administered orally or intravenously (*systemic therapy*).

Principles of radiation therapy. The use of radiation in the treatment of cancer is based on the fact that cancer cells are more sensitive to these various rays than are normal tissue cells. The principle of radiation therapy is to deliver the dosage that will destroy the cancer with the minimum damage to surrounding normal tissue. Such an achievement is dependent upon several factors: (a) the radiosensitivity of the tumor cell (lymphocytes, bone marrow cells, germ cells of ovary and testis, and epithelial cells are the most sensitive,

whereas muscle and nerve tissue are the least sensitive); (b) the stage of the tumor (small lesions respond much more rapidly than large tumors); and (c) the tissues involved (the more accessible the tumor, the better the response; for example, skin vs. bone).

Radiation may be the curative treatment of choice in a small portion of cancer cases and may also be used as a curative treatment in combination with surgery and/or chemotherapy. It is also utilized for symptom control (palliative treatment) in patients with recurrent or progressive disease or for relief of pain.

Complications. As with other treatment modalities for cancer, certain side effects may occur with radiation. These effects may be local or systemic. One major systemic effect is *radiation sickness*, which occurs immediately following treatment and is temporary, treatable, and extremely variable from patient to patient. It is characterized by nausea and vomiting, loss of appetite, weakness, and profuse perspiration. Another systemic effect is the *depression of the bone marrow*, resulting in a lowering of the red and white blood cell production. This effect is more serious, since the patient then is more susceptible to infection. Transfusions and antibiotics may be necessary.

Local side effects include *skin reactions*. Precautionary care measures should be prescribed to the patient. Particularly, heat applications of any form are to be avoided (except showers and baths, of course). *Mucositis*, an inflammation of the epithelial lining of the digestive tract, is another complication and may cause diarrhea. *Radiation fibrosis* of normal soft tissue in the radiation area, such as in lung or nerve tissue, may produce serious rehabilitation problems.

Chemotherapy

Within the past 10 years, the number of effective "anticancer" drugs has increased from 17 to 44. Initially, these drugs were administered only to those patients with advanced cancer. Today, however, chemotherapy is used as an adjuvant modality with surgery and/or radiation therapy, and a small percentage of tumors may be cured by chemotherapy alone. These drugs are given by either the oral, intravenous, or intramuscular route, and frequently a combination of these drugs is used (multiple-drug regime).

Principles of chemotherapy. As in radiation therapy, the principle of chemotherapy is the effective destruction of the rapidly growing tumor cells with the minimum effect upon normal body cells. Because they attack the cells, the drugs are sometimes called cytotoxic. Since chemotherapy is given systemically, this goal is much more difficult to achieve. The chemical effect of these drugs upon the cellular growth mechanisms of cell mitosis and RNA, DNA, and protein synthesis is beyond the purpose of this discussion. Suffice it to say that all the available drugs act upon certain phases of the cell cycle.

Complications. Anticancer drugs act upon the most rapidly growing cells of the body. The most active, of course, are the cancer cells. Unfortunately, certain normal cells of the body, such as the bone marrow, the cells lining the entire alimentary tract, and the hair follicles, grow rapidly as well.

The effect upon the bone marrow cells is the most serious complication. The white-cell counts can be reduced to such a level that infection may be a life-threatening situation, even requiring the patient to be temporarily placed in a germ-free environment. The platelet cells of the body may also be markedly reduced, resulting in bleeding episodes. The effect upon the cells lining the alimentary tract may result in severe gastrointestinal disturbances or oral or pharyngeal infections. The effect on the hair follicle cells frequently results in loss of hair, but this can easily be remedied by the fitting of a wig. In addition, cytotoxic drugs may increase the risk of infection, predispose to malignancy, and increase mutations in offspring. Many patients tolerate these drugs extremely well; others, however, given the same drug or drugs in the same dose, may experience these side effects.

Rehabilitation Treatment

The psychological, social, and vocational problems of the cancer patient requiring rehabilitation intervention procedures differ very little from those of any other disabled individual. The major difference is the presence of the fear of disease progression. Similarly, the physical restorative problems require the same physical therapeutic measures required of other physically limited individuals. The rehabilitation potential of patients whose cancer has been controlled is probably greater than that of other chronically handicapped groups.

The total treatment of the cancer patient, then, may include surgery, radiation therapy, or chemotherapy, or a combination of these modalities, plus rehabilitation treatment. The bottom portion of table 28-2 indicates that the functional limitations listed can be improved with training and, in most cases, also with prosthetic or orthotic devices and adaptive aids.

A useful resource is the local clubs, sponsored by the American Cancer Society, for patients who have already gone through many aspects of cancer treatment. These organizations are often quite helpful in facilitating the adjustment of new cancer patients. In particular, the Reach for Recovery club for mastectomy patients, the International Association of Laryngectomees, a club for those who have had their vocal cords (larynx) removed, and the Ostomy Rehabilitation Program, a club for those with intestinal cancer, have been very helpful.

VOCATIONAL IMPLICATIONS

The goal of successful employment for the cancer client will require cooperation and coordination among many professionals. Each client presents a differing set of needs that will be met by a different program of services. The counselor is challenged to confront comprehensive problems and effectively deal with multifaceted solutions.

After rehabilitation potential has been established, specific vocational choices can be evaluated with regard to physical and environmental job demands, and the client's education, aptitudes, and interests in correlation with his disease status.

The time limits of educational and vocational training programs for cancer clients are linked to morbidity and life expectancy prognostications (see table 28-3). A return to the client's former employment should be explored, particularly if long-term training and education are not feasible. It would seem good general practice for the counselor to establish an early contact with the client's former employer to determine potential re-employment possibilities. If the client has been a valuable employee with a good work history, an employer may willingly make job and environmental modifications, if necessary.

Assuming his former job is no longer physically suitable or available, alternative jobs within the client's former work setting may ideally permit transfer of previously acquired skills or knowledge. Employers may be invited to participate in team conferences. As the employer provides input regarding the demands of the client's former job, he will be gaining positive education concerning cancer. Education of the lay community and employers about cancer is a responsibility of rehabilitation professionals. Attitudes of pity or revulsion toward persons with cancer, based on misinformation and fears, will create an employment barrier for the client.

Sound vocational counseling practices utilize a study of the client's interest patterns, based on the valid assumption that one performs better vocationally in occupations that compliment one's interests. This principle is applicable to vocational planning with cancer clients. However, selective job placement techniques, particularly with the severely disabled population, must include a realistic consideration of barriers in the community that may affect the client's job placement potential. Architectural barriers, e.g., a narrow doorway or a flight of stairs, may prevent the employment of a client in a wheelchair. Attitudinal barriers, e.g., employer resistance or public revulsion toward deformity, may limit the employment possibilities available to a cancer client who has had disfiguring head and neck surgery. Thus, while interest patterns of a client with head and neck cancer may point toward working with the public, it becomes the counselor's responsibility to honestly evaluate with

TABLE 28-4

GUIDE TO OCCUPATIONAL DEMANDS FOR CANCER PATIENTS AFTER REHABILITATION SERVICES

(x indicates patient usually cannot meet occupational demands)

OCCUPATIONAL DEMANDS	Breast	Head & Neck	MUSCULOSKELETAL AMPUTEES Upper	MUSCULOSKELETAL AMPUTEES Lower	Colo-rectal Digestive	Leukemia Lymphoma	Brain	NERVOUS SYSTEM Spinal Cord Paraplegia	NERVOUS SYSTEM Spinal Cord Quadriplegia	Peripheral	Lung	Genito Urinary	Skin
Cosmesis		x	x										
Writing							x		x	x			
Speech		x					x						
Employer resistance		x	x				x	x	x	x			
Sedentary													
Light lifting									x	x			
Moderate lifting			x	x			x	x	x	x			
Heavy lifting	x	x	x	x	x	x	x	x	x	x	x	x	
Prolonged standing				x		x	x	x	x	x			
Bending, squatting, stooping				x			x	x	x	x			
Climbing				x			x	x	x	x			
High-speed performance						x	x		x	x			
Manual skills			x				x		x	x			
Balancing skills				x			x	x	x	x			
Environmental stresses			x	x		x	x	x	x	x			
Visual-motor skills		x					x		x	x			
Intellectual skills							x						

the client the possible need to sacrifice interest patterns and accept a work environment without public contact.

Specific jobs can be broken down into groups of physical and environmental demands that should correlate with the client's physical status and tolerances to assure appropriate vocational placement. Table 28-4 lists factors that, singly or in combination, describe the work demands of many occupations. Utilizing this table, it is possible for the counselor to determine how closely the client may meet the occupational demands of a specific job. Clearly, table 28-4 is intended only as a guide, and individual clients may present exceptions to many of these generalizations regarding particular functional capacities attributed to each cancer group. By combining factors listed in table 28-4 under Occupational Demands, more complex activities can be projected.

As working tools, tables 28-2, 28-3, and 28-4 should provide answers to many of the questions counselors ask. For many of the remaining questions, there are no absolute answers.

BIBLIOGRAPHY

American Cancer Society: *A Cancer Source Book for Nurses.* New York, American Cancer Society, 1975.
This book is an excellent reference, not only for nurses but for all allied health professionals. It discusses the basic aspects of cancer and problems regarding cancers of various anatomic sites, with emphasis on rehabilitation and continuing care. It contains a good glossary and bibliography.

Brooke BN: *Understanding Cancer.* New York, Holt, Rinehart, and Winston, 1971.
This easy-to-read book describes in simple terms what cancer is and how it spreads. Various kinds of cancer are discussed and a section on treatment is included. The treatment section may be somewhat outdated at this time, but the material on the nature of cancer is still current.

Burdick D: Rehabilitation of the breast cancer patient. Cancer **36**:645–648, 1975.
Briefly describes the roles of the rehabilitation team members in treating a breast cancer patient, including the use of Reach to Recovery. Emphasis is placed on the team effort to provide complete rehabilitation.

Goldberg RT: Vocational and social adjustment after laryngectomy. Scand J Rehabil Med 7:1–8, 1975.
Sixty-two persons with laryngeal cancer (mean age = 56.3) were interviewed with respect to educational, work, and social history prior to cancer. The best predictors of adjustment and return to work are discussed.

Healey JE Jr (ed): *Ecology of the Cancer Patient.* Washington, DC, The Interdisciplinary Communication Associates for the Interdisciplinary Communication Program, 1970.
A condensation of three interdisciplinary conferences on the rehabilitation of the cancer patient. Participants included oncologists, rehabilitationists, educators, and consumers. Discussions dealt with the totality of relationships between cancer patients and their physical, biological, social, occupational, emotional, and cultural environments.

Healey JE Jr., Villaneuva R, Donovan ES: Principles of rehabilitation. *In* Holland JF, Frei E (eds): *Cancer Medicine.* Philadelphia, Lea & Febiger, 1973, pp. 1917–1929.
This presentation highlights some of the major physical restorative problems that may result either as a consequence of cancer or treatment of the disease.

Nealon TF Jr., (ed): *Management of the Patient with Cancer.* Ed. 2, Philadelphia, Saunders, 1976.
The text describes a comprehensive approach to the management of the cancer patient. General considerations are outlined, and descriptions of management of cancer of specific anatomic sites are given. Although directed to physicians, there is much management and statistical material which would be of assistance to a vocational counselor.

Orces H, Feldman J, Gardner B, Alfonso A: Analysis of patient disability after curative resection for colonic and rectal cancer. Am J Surg **131**:98–102, 1976.
Colorectal cancer patients were studied for 4 years to determine the degree of disability occurring postoperatively. Seventy percent of patients were not disabled and were employable after surgery. Of those who died, 73 percent had no disability until 3 months prior to death. The authors conclude that waiting 5 years to determine cure is wasteful and unnecessary.

Proceedings of the American Cancer Society's National Conference on Human Values in Atlanta, Georgia. American Cancer Society, 1973.
The humanistic approach to the care of the cancer patient was the theme of this conference. The papers presented cover topics related to the preparation of the patient for treatment and efforts toward the care of the patient with more advanced cancer.

Stone RW: Employing the recovered cancer patient. Cancer **36**:285–286, 1975.
Written by the Medical Director of Research at ATT, this article presents the employer's point of view and changing attitudes due to better disability insurance and health plans and longer survival rates.

University of Texas M.D. Anderson Hospital and Tumor Institute: *Rehabilitation of the Cancer Patient.* Chicago, Year Book Medical Publishers, 1972.
This is a compilation of selected papers and panel discussions relating to the rehabilitation of the cancer patient.

29 BLINDNESS AND VISUAL IMPAIRMENTS

Richard E. Hoover, M.D.
C. Warren Bledsoe

INTRODUCTION

Blindness means anatomic and functional disturbances of the sense of vision of sufficient magnitude to cause total loss of light perception. *Visual impairment* refers to any deviation from the generally accepted norm which affects (a) central visual function; (b) peripheral visual function; (c) binocular visual function; or (d) color perception. The deviation may be anatomic or functional, partial or total, and temporary, reversible, progressive, or permanent. Chapter 3 describes the normal visual apparatus and function, which the reader should review to understand more fully the issues discussed in this chapter.

Most countries and many states have created their own definitions of "blindness" that deviate from the factual one. Hence we have "legal blindness," which may not mean a total loss of light perception. The most widely accepted definition of "blindness" in the United States was established by the American Medical Association in 1934. It states, "a person shall be considered blind whose central visual acuity does not exceed 20/200 in the better eye with correcting lenses or whose visual acuity, if better than 20/200, has a limit to the central field of vision to such a degree that its widest diameter subtends an angle of no greater than 20 degrees." This definition therefore includes two distinct groups: (a) the blind, who have total loss of the sense of vision, and (b) those who are severely visually impaired, but nevertheless do have remaining visual function.

There is little scientific evidence to support attempts to classify levels of visual ability or inability. Nevertheless, almost every country has realized the need for such categorizations, and has therefore created a definition to isolate the "blind." Out of compassion perhaps, the "almost blind" (i.e., the "almost seeing") have been included in the "legally blind" category.

Severe visual impairment is a phenomenon only the impaired can realize fully. It defies any one specific measurement or set of measurements to determine the level of visual ability. As a practical concept, severe visual impairment is a loss of visual function of such magnitude that special aids and the use of the other senses are necessary to achieve performance ordinarily directed by visual clues. The difficulty in describing the severely visually impaired who are not totally blind has produced no simple term in general use. The most compact and exact word in classic English is *cecutiency*.

In the eyes of the law and in agencies for the blind, visual disability determination is an administrative responsibility. It requires an appraisal of the individual's present and probable future ability to engage in activity as it is affected by nonmedical factors as well as by the visual impairment. Nonmedical factors involved in visual inability have proven very difficult to measure. Too often they are neglected and the medical factor alone is used as the sole criterion for evaluation.

The occurrence of a 30 percent increase in the totally blind and cecutient population has been predicted for the years 1965–1985. The increase for those over 65 will be about 35–40 percent, while for those under 65, an increase of only 25–30 percent is expected. Rates of increase will also vary according to etiology. A 25–30 percent increase in blindness and cecutiency from diabetes and a 35–40 percent increase from senile macular degeneration are predicted. Infectious disease causes are likely to decline.

Absolutely accurate statistics of new cases are not available. The best data are from the National Society for the Prevention of Blindness, using information from state registers published last in 1966. Figure 29-1 indicates the following causes of new cases of "legal" blindness for 1962: (a) unknown specific causes made up 39 percent; (b) general diseases caused 25 percent; (c) prenatal factors caused 20 percent; (d) 6 percent were due to miscellaneous causes; and (e) 10 percent were undetermined.

Glaucoma (14.5 percent), diabetes (14.3 percent), and cataract (13.7 percent) led the list of diseases in 1962 and are probably similarly dominant today. They account for about one half of all *new* cases each year amongst people with a previous history of normal vision. Cataract and glaucoma are associated with the

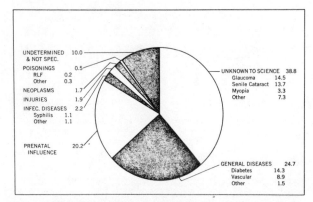

FIGURE 29-1. Percentages of new cases of legal blindness in the United States in 1962 by cause. (From *National Society for the Prevention of Blindness Fact Book,* 1966).

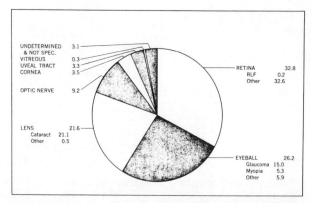

FIGURE 29-2. Percentages of new cases of legal blindness in the United States in 1962 by site and cause of eye affection. (From *National Society for the Prevention of Blindness Fact Book,* 1966).

aging process. Diabetes and other diseases that affect the vascular system also tend to be more prevalent among older persons.

Prenatal influences are responsible for about 10 percent of cecutiency. These include conditions which are hereditary (e.g., Friedreich's ataxia) and those present at birth (e.g., retinitis pigmentosa). The increasing prevalence of cecutiency and blindness caused by prenatal influences suggests the importance of specific genetic counseling as well as vigorous maternal and prenatal care.

Figure 29-2 indicates the anatomic location of the defect for the new cases reported in 1962 as follows: (a) retina, 33 percent; (b) eyeball, 26 percent; (c) lens, 22 percent; (d) optic nerve, 9 percent; (e) cornea, 3.5 percent; and (f) other structures, less than 7 percent.

Knowledge of etiologies suggests the structuring of prevention, research, and development programs. In addition, for any single client, knowledge of etiology suggests additional impairments which may exist and which often determine rehabilitation potential. For example, diabetes (see chap. 24) is also associated with vascular insufficiency of the limbs, neuropathy, and severe kidney disease (see chaps. 22, 7, and 25, respectively).

Important diseases to be discussed later in some detail are cataracts, glaucoma, myopia, senile macular degeneration, diabetes and the other vascular diseases, and corneal, prenatal, degenerative, and CNS diseases.

CHARACTERIZATION OF THE SENSE OF VISION

Central Vision

Visual acuity is determined by the smallest retinal image whose form can be appreciated. It is measured by the smallest object that can be clearly seen at a certain distance by the *fovea* (see chap. 3) or its surrounding retinal structures. The most convenient standard to be adopted is the size of the visual angle; that

is, the size of the angle formed by an object on the retina (see fig. 29-3). The standard of normal visual acuity has been accepted as subtending a visual angle of one minute (1/60 of a degree). This principle has been embodied in Snellen's Test types, a series of letters in lines of decreasing size which are almost universally accepted in testing visual acuity. The results of the testing are expressed as a fraction. The numerator denotes the distance of the subject from the chart (20 feet, or 6 meters). The denominator denotes the distance from the chart at which a person with normal vision would be able to read the same line. The nine lines on a Snellen chart, therefore, represent acuities of:

	In meters	In feet
1	6/60	20/200
2	6/36	20/120
3	6/24	20/80
4	6/18	20/60
5	6/12	20/40
6	6/9	20/30
7	6/6	20/20
8	6/4.5	20/15
9	6/3	20/10

Thus, an acuity of 20/100 means that the particular line the subject sees at 20 feet can be seen by a person with normal vision at 100 feet. Readings of 20/15 and 20/10 represent better than "normal" acuity.

Peripheral Vision

Peripheral vision is mediated by the retinal cells away from the fovea area. It allows the eye to perceive objects not directly in the visual axis. It is designated as a *visual field* and may be examined by a technique called *perimetry*. The purpose of perimetry is to detect defects within the visual field, as well as to define the outside limits of the visual field. Sensitivity is highest in and near the fovea. If different sized and colored test objects are used, it is possible to map contours of retinal sensitivity for each of these. The fovea represents only a small fraction of the entire visual

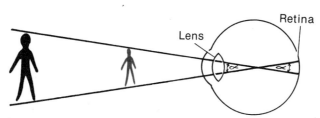

FIGURE 29-3. The visual angle (α) used to characterize visual acuity is the smallest angle made by light rays from the "edges" of the object. Note that the closer in to the eye an object may be, the smaller it must be to subtend the same angle.

field, and the periphery accounts for 95 percent of the total light-sensitive surface.

Two visual systems have been recognized, the "what" system in the foveal region and the "where" system in the periphery. In the normal course of visual processing, peripheral stimulation provides information about the presence of an object (i.e., "where" it is) to be fixated by the fovea (i.e., "what" it is). Peripheral vision is thought to be very important in tasks that call for large areas to be monitored, such as in driving, flying, and searching. Visual function analysis determines which system is critical to the particular task faced by the individual, whether there is selective impairment of one or the other or both systems, and, if possible, how the impairment can be alleviated. The defects in peripheral vision are sensitive indices of ocular and neurological pathology, and therefore examination by perimetry can reveal significant information about function and diagnoses.

Binocular Vision

Binocular vision results from the coordinated use of the two eyes to produce a single cortical image. At the peak of its highest development, the blending of the two images into one results in the heightened perception of depth (*stereopsis*). Additional advantages of binocular vision are that (a) optical defects in one eye are less obvious if the other eye is normal; (b) visual field defects in one eye are often masked, since the same defect is not likely to occur in identical parts of the two retinas; and (c) the peripheral visual field of both eyes is larger than either field alone.

To achieve binocular vision, the following conditions must be met: (a) fixation on the object by each eye must be possible; (b) the visual fields of the two eyes must overlap to some extent; (c) approximately the same size and quality image must be formed on each retina; (d) the retinas must possess physiologically corresponding parts; and (e) the eyes must be coordinated so that retinal receptors which have a common visual direction will at all times receive the same image. Awareness of depth is the result of a number of physiological mechanisms, most of which are not innate but are learned by experience (see chap. 3). There are both monocular and binocular clues.

Color Vision

Most objects have color in bright daylight but will lose their color when the illumination falls below a certain level. This is because the physiological mechanism responsible for color perception only functions above certain light intensities (see p. 47).

Little is known of the physiology of color perception and color blindness, but the ability to distinguish colors may be lost as a result of heredity or as a result of disease to the retina or optic nerve. Persons with hereditary forms of color deficiency may have no other abnormal visual function. Color deficiency is transmitted by the female but appears mostly in the male.

Total color blindness, *achromatic vision*, is rare and can be associated with decreased visual acuity. It is thought to be a simple recessive character or, in some instances, may represent a male sex-linked character. When it is total, there is associated nystagmus and severe photophobia in addition to decreased vision.

Night Vision

Night vision is the ability to see in the dark. In night blindness there may be a pronounced deficiency in dark adaptation as well as a defect in the appreciation of different light intensities. It may be congenital or acquired. The most commonly encountered night blindness is due to a hereditary disease resulting in pigmentary degeneration of the retina (retinitis pigmentosa).

Eyeball Movement

Normal eyeball movement is a complex neurophysiological mechanism (see chap. 3). If there is any disease, mechanism, or abnormality affecting the extraocular muscles or their integration, visual function can be impaired. For example, double vision (diplopia) or loss of binocular vision may occur.

DISEASE LOCALIZATION BY SITE

Some of the common diseases that can cause cecutiency or total blindness are identified in table 29-1. In addition, the table shows the possible

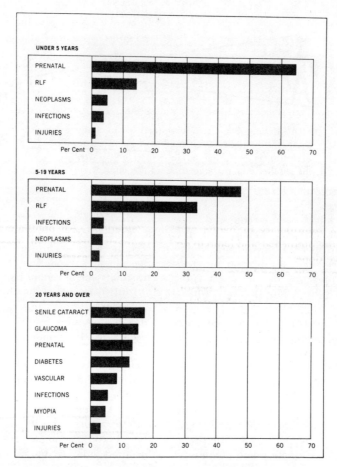

FIGURE 29-4. Percentages of leading causes of legal blindness in the United States in 1962 by age groups. (From *National Society for the Prevention of Blindness Fact Book,* 1966).

anatomic site of affection for each disease and whether involvement is also possible at other sites. The first two columns indicate either the probable or possible likelihood of cecutiency or blindness. As the table shows, many diseases can involve several sites at the same time or at different times in individual patients. Evaluations and therapy may therefore vary from one patient to another.

TOTAL BLINDNESS

Causal Diseases

Figure 29-4 shows the causes for legal blindness determined for 1962, and table 29-2 indicates the estimated prevalence in percent of legal blindness by cause and age group in the United States for the years 1960 and 1962. Table 29-3 summarizes the most probable causes of total blindness at the current time.

Functional Disabilities

The totally blind (no light perception) lose the ability to manage by visual means. This means they must learn new techniques for such skills as mobility, communication, eating, dressing, shaving, grooming, sewing, ironing, housekeeping, and organization of clothes, money, valuables, and food without visual clues.

In addition to the functional losses, there are other important social and psychological losses. Carrol has identified these losses, and the counselor is referred to his book *Blindness* for an in-depth study. Among the possible psychosocial disabilities of blindness, Carrol cites the following:

1. Loss of physical integrity
2. Loss of confidence in the remaining senses
3. Loss of reality contact with the environment
4. Loss of visual perception of the pleasurable
5. Loss of light security
6. Loss of visual perception of the beautiful
7. Loss of recreation
8. Loss of career choices
9. Loss of job opportunities
10. Loss of financial security
11. Loss of personal independence
12. Loss of social adequacy
13. Loss of self-esteem

14. Loss of anonymity
15. Loss of total personality organization

While the above list is formidable, it is unlikely that every patient will have major concerns in each area. These losses are interrelated, however, and a rehabilitation program must address the whole complex of problems associated with blindness, including problems unique to an individual patient which may further complicate the reorganizational process.

Individual temperament undoubtedly plays a part in determining reaction to blindness. Adjustment can be equally difficult for those who lose their sight as adults and those who are born blind. Those with acquired blindness must change a multiplicity of habits and relearn many skills, drawing on the ear and hand to do many things the eyes have done.

Those who lose sight in a split second (e.g., soldiers in battle, hunters blinded by gunshot, or a person blinded in a car crash) experience not only sudden initial emotional shock, but further shock when they realize they must begin all over again on a par with a child learning to walk and feed himself. Nevertheless, they may have an advantage over persons who lose their sight gradually by disease in a long, slow therapeutic battle fraught with doubt and hope over chances of keeping what sight remains.

Even when the disease process is leading inevitably to total blindness, the patient may resist any service or aid which carries, however subtly, the dreaded label "for the blind" and may gradually slip into expedient habits for dealing with less and less vision. Accepting a guide dog, a cane, Braille, or other aids and training necessarily means a step toward the crucial experience of "accepting blindness." The patient must relinquish hope of returning sight and alter his self-concept from that of a sighted person to that of a blind person before he can make a successful adjustment to blindness and proceed with a rehabilitation program.

Standards of Evaluation

To designate blindness in an individual, only the ophthalmologist can be relied upon to determine if there is any residual of the sense of vision or light perception, or if any particular "legal blindness" definition has been met. Additional medical review is essential if the disease causing the blindness affects other body systems. Examination of table 29-1 reveals that many of the causal conditions require medical review by a knowledgeable internist. These include infectious diseases, poisonings, neoplasms, and systemic diseases. The internist or ophthalmologist might also suggest review by a neurologist, orthopedic surgeon, or physiatrist, depending on the other nonvisual disabilities that may exist.

In addition, the extent of functional and psychosocial disabilities requires evaluations by mobility instructors (peripatologists), occupational therapists or others skilled in personal care training, and by psychologists and social workers trained or experienced in the problems of the blind. Functional and psychosocial evaluations are often best achieved in centers where evaluations are conducted within a comprehensive setting.

Total Treatment

Restoration of vision is naturally the primary concern of any blind person and his ophthalmologist. Exclusive management by an optometrist is not recommended, although he may perform some evaluations. An ophthalmologist should provide the primary direction of treatment because so many medical diseases may be involved (see table 29-1). The ophthalmologist will determine the need, type, and extent of medical care, including concern for freedom from discomfort and the realistic appreciation of the need for proper cosmetic presentation. Tearing, pain, and unattractive appearance will require special care and possible referral to such specialists as a plastic surgeon, otolaryngologist, internist, or allergist.

If blindness is certain, when medical treatment is complete, the ophthalmologist has the additional responsibility of informing the patient. Advice concerning normal activities and function should be substituted for hope of sight. The physician should exert his influence to encourage the patient to accept professional training in developing the skills of mobility, communication, and employment.

No matter how fine a program of blind rehabilitation may be, it must always wait on the readiness of the individual to grant that he is blind. A psychologist with knowledge of all the emotional, physical, and practical aspects of blindness may be very helpful in facilitating the patient's adjustment to blindness and acceptance of the aids and training necessary for learning new skills to overcome the losses associated with blindness. In addition, a social worker can help identify family problems resulting from the patient's disability, and work with family members to assist them in overcoming any adjustment problems and financial difficulties.

Professional knowledge and skill are also necessary for prescribing and training in techniques of self-care, mobility, reading, writing, and educational and vocational planning. Few blind persons have been successfully rehabilitated by gaining expertise in just one phase of the adjustment complex. Most are successfully rehabilitated by mastery and understanding of all aspects of retraining to cope with all the losses resulting from the state of blindness. A comprehensive rehabilitation center for treatment and retraining is likely to provide the best approach to the solution of these multiple problems.

Treatment includes the development of not only

TABLE 29-1
TYPES AND SITES OF OCULAR INVOLVEMENT
Pr = probable (more than 50% of time);   Po = possible (less than 50% of time)

Types	Total Blindness	Cecutiency	Cornea	Lens	Vitreous	Uvea	Retina	CNS Pathways	Cortex
Infectious Disease									
Toxoplasmosis		Pr				Po	Pr		
Histoplasmosis		Pr				Pr	Po		
Syphilis	Po	Pr	Po	Po	Po	Po	Po	Po	Po
Herpes		Pr	Po						
Cytomegalovirus	Pr	Po				Po	Pr		
Ophthalmia neonatorum	Po	Pr	Pr						
Measles		Pr				Po	Pr		
Trachoma	Po	Pr	Pr	Po					
Injuries									
Mechanical	Po	Pr	Pr	Po		Po	Po	Po	Po
Chemical	Po	Pr	Pr	Po		Po	Po		
Sympathetic ophthalmia	Po	Pr				Pr	Po		
Poisonings									
Retinopathy of prematurity	Po	Pr					Pr		
Methanol	Pr	Po			Pr			Pr	
Lead	Pr	Po						Po	Po
Drugs	Po	Po					Pr	Pr	Po
Neoplasms									
Retinoblastoma (bilateral)	Pr	Po			Po		Pr		
Melanoma	Po	Pr				Pr	Po		
Metastatic tumor	Po	Pr				Pr	Po		
Glioma	Po	Pr						Pr	
Meningioma	Po	Pr						Pr	
Craniopharyngioma	Po	Pr						Pr	
Astrocytoma	Po	Pr						Pr	
Pituitary tumor	Po	Pr						Pr	
Systemic General Disease									
Diabetes	Po	Pr		Po	Po		Pr	Pr	
Other metabolic		Pr							
Vascular	Po	Pr			Po				Pr
Sarcoidosis		Pr	Po			Pr	Po		
Vitamin deficiency	Po	Pr	Po				Pr	Po	
Prenatal									
Hereditary	Pr	Pr	Po	Po		Po	Po	Po	Po
Toxins	Po	Pr	Po	Po	Po	Po	Po	Po	Po
Maternal infection	Po	Pr	Po	Po	Po	Po	Po	Po	Po
Unknown	Po	Pr	Po	Po	Po	Po	Po	Po	Po
Diseases of Unknown Causes									
Glaucoma	Po	Pr					Pr	Po	
Senile cataract		Pr		Pr					
Myopia	Po	Pr				Po	Pr		

substitutes for sight but also an awareness of the stimuli the person is receiving through all his senses. Such sensory training must first arouse awareness and then help the person achieve correct interpretations and develop successful correlations with purposeful behavior.

Blind persons also require training in self-care.

Although it is now commonplace to expect blind persons to function as regular members of society, this is seldom accomplished without rigorous training in special skills for living without sight. The needs of those whose sight is so limited as to be negligible are far more clearcut than those of the cecutient. For those born blind, or who develop blindness while of school age, the acquisition of necessary skills is a normal part of development, either in a residential school for the blind or in a public school program. Not all those blind at birth or at school age receive adequate education, and rehabilitation programs may therefore have to include educational components.

Persons gradually blinded by disease have the use of some sight over a longer time. They also have more time to shun and put off any service labeled "for the blind" and to gradually slip into expedient habits for dealing with less and less vision. Treatment must therefore continue periodically to reduce maladjustment and facilitate adaptation to decreasing vision.

The devices for self-management which have been developed by isolated blind individuals have been many and varied, and it is a truism of the field that sophisticated work for the blind is very largely the assembly and organization of devices and ideas originating with blind persons. However, the average individual's single-handed attack on each of his day-to-day techniques of living, compared with skills taught in an up-to-date rehabilitation center for the blind, is like the hunt-and-peck system of typewriting compared to properly taught touch typing.

In the United States, treatment of the blind has a distinct personality of its own apart from general rehabilitation, although it plays a key role in general rehabilitation. Two groups of trained workers for the blind, *orientation and mobility instructors* and *rehabilitation teachers*, have permeated agencies for the blind and perform a large part of the solid prevocational work which readies the client for the services of the vocational counselor.

The first graduate training program in orientation and mobility instruction (or peripatology, as it is sometimes designated) was established in 1960. Concurrently, grants from the Vocational Rehabilitation Administration were made to modernize and strengthen the traditional function of the home teacher for the blind. Ultimately, a graduate course in this specialty was also established in a number of universities, and the home teacher was redesignated the rehabilitation teacher.

The province of these professionals includes all the basics of living without sight and written communication. Rehabilitation teachers primarily work with blind persons in their homes, teaching self-care, indoor mobility, home-maintenance skills, such as cooking and cleaning, and other skills in the activities of daily living. They may also teach Braille and writing, and they offer some counseling in functional and personal problems. Orientation and mobility instructors teach the whole range of mobility skills, from limited indoor mobility to the use of sophisticated electronic aids. They can also train blind persons in the use of electronic reading devices, and are usually qualified to teach Braille.

These two groups of professionals are very valuable colleagues of the rehabilitation counselor. They have access to the client at the earliest stage in the rehabilitation process and thus the earliest opportunities to influence and observe him. The nature of their professions gives them intimate knowledge of the problems of blind persons before they reach the vocational counselor.

Initially, the two most basic losses, mobility and written and printed communication, must be faced, evaluated, and accepted before vocational adjustments can be considered. These losses require an individualized prescription in every case. The blind person's needs, desires, capabilities, limitations, and life style all need to be considered in prescribing mobility and communication aids.

Some blind persons, because of temperament, physical circumstances, and life style, require the help of a sighted guide when venturing into public places. The blind person walks beside or slightly behind the guide, and grasps the guide's relaxed arm a bit above the elbow. Dog guides are a distinct emotional and mobility asset to many, but the percentage of blind persons for whom they are truly suitable is small.

The long cane is relatively widely used as a mobility aid. The cane has an aluminum shaft with a nylon tip and a small crook for gripping. With proper training in its use, the long cane provides the blind person with information about the environment ahead of him which, combined with other sensory cues, enables him to be safely mobile. He may, however, be subject to some hazard from obstacles at head or chest height if they are not perceived through other sensory cues. Long canes equipped with an electronic sensing device have been developed to diminish these risks. The electronic device emits an audible warning signal and/or tactile stimulation in the cane's crook when an obstacle is detected in the pathway ahead of the blind person. The signals vary depending on the height of the obstacle.

Other electronic devices, designed to be used in combination with a long cane, have also been developed to detect objects in the blind person's pathway and emit an audible or tactile warning signal. These various devices, though experimental and not in wide use, can increase the safety and ease of independent mobility for the blind person trained in their use.

Some printed material is accessible to blind persons in the form of records, tapes, and Braille transcription. Braille is helpful, but in some cases impractical due to loss of sensitivity of touch in the fingertips from the peripheral neuropathy often associated with diabetes. These aids all require production of the materials by other persons. More sophisticated reading devices which allow the blind person independent access to written materials are now used by highly motivated individuals. These reading devices consist of a small

TABLE 29-2
ESTIMATED PREVALENCE OF LEGAL BLINDNESS BY CAUSE AND AGE GROUP

Etiology	1960				1962			
	Total	Under 5	5–19	20 & over	Total	Under 5	5–19	20 & over
	Percentage				Percentage			
Infectious diseases	5.2	3.6	3.8	5.4	5.2	3.8	3.9	5.4
Ophthalmia neonatorum	0.3	...	0.3	0.3	0.3	...	0.3	0.3
Syphilis	2.1	...	0.3	2.3	2.1	...	0.3	2.3
Other	2.8	3.6	3.2	2.8	2.8	3.8	3.2	2.8
Injuries	2.9	1.1	2.4	3.0	2.9	1.1	2.4	3.0
Poisonings	3.6	21.6	33.7	0.3	3.5	14.1	33.3	0.4
Retrolental fibroplasia	3.3	21.6	33.7	*	3.2	14.1	33.3	0.1
Other	0.3	...	*	0.3	0.3	...	*	0.3
Neoplasms	1.4	4.3	3.5	1.2	1.4	5.0	3.5	1.2
General diseases	20.3	1.4	1.6	22.4	20.4	1.5	1.6	22.4
Diabetes	11.1	...	...	12.4	11.2	...	...	12.4
Vascular	7.6	...	...	8.4	7.6	...	...	8.4
Other	1.6	1.4	1.6	1.6	1.6	1.5	1.6	1.6
Prenatal influence	16.7	59.0	47.4	13.2	16.7	64.6	47.7	13.2
Unknown to science	38.0	2.5	1.4	42.0	38.0	2.7	1.4	41.9
Glaucoma	13.5	...	...	15.0	13.5	...	...	15.0
Senile cataract	15.6	...	...	17.3	15.6	...	...	17.2
Myopia	4.3	...	...	4.8	4.3	...	...	4.8
Other	4.6	2.5	1.4	4.9	4.6	2.7	1.4	4.9
Undetermined & not specified	11.9	6.5	6.2	12.5	11.9	7.2	6.2	12.5
Total	100.0	100.0	100.0	100.0	100.0	100.0	100.0	100.0

*Less than 0.1 percent.

hand-held camera, or probe, which the blind person moves across a line of print. The printed image is converted to either a tactile image or some specific audible tone pattern which the blind person learns to recognize. Good short-term memory is required because letters are perceived one at a time and the blind person must mentally form the letters into words. Although these reading methods are slow and require extensive training and practice, they do afford the blind person privacy and access to a much broader range of reading materials than would otherwise be available to him. Rapid advancements are making such devices more versatile and useful.

Vocational Implications

The primary vocational need of blind persons is a working concept of what they can do. Certain fundamental realities concerning blindness, often covered up or distorted, must be considered. Briefly, these realities are:

1. There are very few situations in which blindness itself is an asset, but there are some occupations where performance may be more irksome to the sighted worker than it is to the blind one, as in a darkroom. In other occupations, the development of the remaining senses which blindness occasions becomes a distinct advantage. Many occupations of blind persons have been built on this sensory keenness which was developed of necessity.

2. There are a large number of things blind persons can do as well as the sighted with a little more concentration or some special arrangement. Usually these activities are either highly intellectual or involve the fashioning or manipulation of the tangible. In the latter case, spoken language usually plays an important part. In this general category are, for example, computer programmers, musicians, politicians, public relations specialists, teachers, vending stand operators, judges, clergy, and masseurs.

To formulate these categories is easy; to apply them specifically requires both aptitude and experience. This means finding out to what extent the blind person can make the fullest use of other-than-visual resources in doing things.

In developing the vocational plan for a blind client, the counselor will take the realities discussed above into consideration. Other factors which must also be

TABLE 29-3
MOST PROBABLE CAUSES OF TOTAL BLINDNESS BY APPROXIMATE AGE OF ONSET

0–5 Years	5–19 Years	20 & Over
Prenatal influences	Prenatal influences	Glaucoma
Anophthalmos	Retinopathy of	Diabetes
Cortical blindness	prematurity	Vascular disease
Congenital glaucoma	Neoplasms	Myopia
Hydrocephalus		
Congenital		
Retinopathy of prematurity		
Neoplasms		

considered include: (a) the client's educational and intellectual abilities; (b) the client's personality, temperament, and interests; (c) the client's social and family responsibilities; (d) the ultimate skill level achieved in functional abilities; and (e) the current and future job market. Prevocational exploration of the available alternatives may be necessary. In a sense, the vocational rehabilitation process for blind clients is the same as for clients with other disabilities.

The counselor should maintain a meticulous and scrupulous accuracy in his education of potential employers, trainers, or educators, with particular care to dispel any lingering unconscious superstitions about blindness they may have.

There is every reason to promote dispersal of blind persons and cecutients in as many occupations as possible, not only for their own self-development, but also so that the general public will grow accustomed to encountering these workers in "ordinary" settings and not only in settings "for the blind."

CECUTIENCY

Causal Diseases

The most probable causes of cecutiency and their approximate age of onset are listed in table 29-4. Table 29-1 also lists more specifically those diseases capable of causing cecutiency.

Functional Disabilities

There are many degrees of cecutiency, ranging from light perception to vision which is recorded as 20/200 or better (i.e., better than legal blindness). The cecutient may lose the ability to perform from visual clues under many circumstances as a result of his basic impairment coupled with variations in the environment. Some environments, depending on lighting, terrain, and familiarity, may be more incapacitating than others. Nevertheless, when possible, the cecutient will use the remaining sense of vision for certain purposes no matter how frustrating, tiresome, or inefficient it is.

Some will only be able to distinguish the presence of light and dark, which is important in itself because it tells when lights are on or off or whether it is night or day. Others will be able to see colors. There are a few who will organize their remaining vision so well as to read, write, drive, work, and play without appropriate rehabilitation treatment.

It is difficult for social service workers, physicians, friends, colleagues, the public, and many others to understand the cecutient's anomalous circumstances. Sometimes he needs the special aids and appliances which common sense would seem to indicate his visual problems would necessitate, and in other situations he is able to function quite well by dispensation of the little "peeping" capacity peculiar to his unique pathology.

This variation in visual ability may lead to frustration, embarrassment, anger, or confusion. The cecutient may also be defensive about the misunderstandings of others that arise as a result of his living in both a sighted and a blind world. In addition, cecutiency is often accompanied by uncertainty about the future stability, improvement, or progression of the visual impairment. His psychosocial adjustment may consequently be more difficult than the adjustment required for one totally blind.

Cecutients may develop a tendency to operate continually in a safe, familiar, and unchanging environment. This is not always possible. Therefore, if they are to succeed, they must be prepared for the humiliation of being labeled "fakes," "drunks," or "malingerers." They must maintain an objective view of the restrictions and assets they still possess. As a partial explanation of their behavior, it is helpful to the counselor to know the causes and site of the affection (see table 29-1) since these can be useful guides in appreciating possible responses to visual stimulation.

The losses affecting the cecutient, with the exception of light security, are the same as for the blind, but the degree of the losses, and hence their impact, will be less.

Standards of Evaluation

Those characteristics of the visual sense needing measurement and analysis by the ophthalmologist are:

TABLE 29-4
MOST PROBABLE CAUSES OF CECUTIENCY BY APPROXIMATE AGE OF ONSET

0–5 Years	5–19 Years	20 & Over
Prenatal influences	Prenatal influences	Glaucoma
Congenital glaucoma	Congenital glaucoma	Diabetes
Hydrocephalus	Hydrocephalus	Vascular disease
Retinopathy of prematurity	Congenital optic atrophy	Myopia
Neoplasms	Neoplasms	

visual acuity for distance and near, with the best correction and with the best low-vision optical aids; field of vision; color vision; accommodation; the effects of unbalanced eye movements; and binocular vision. Visual acuity alone is not the sole index of visual impairment and all aspects of the remaining vision must be analyzed. The counselor should consider meeting with the ophthalmologist to achieve a full understanding of the client's residual visual acuity, peripheral vision, color vision, and binocular vision. Specific questions directed to the ophthalmologist about optimum environments for the individual client's type of impairment might improve the counselor's understanding of how useful the residual vision may be for certain job settings.

Other medical and psychosocial evaluations discussed above for the blind also apply to the cecutient.

Total Treatment

The ophthalmologist's role requires regular review for restoration, prevention of further loss, and alleviation of discomfort and disfigurement. While some of these functions might also be performed by the optometrist, exclusive management by the optometrist is not recommended because, as in blindness, multiple medical diseases are potentially involved. In addition to medical evaluation, regular review and examination are required to provide the best possible aids available to produce better performance. Low-vision aids include contact lenses, small telescopes mounted to spectacles, microscopes, prisms, closed-circuit television, and electronic aids. New aids become available frequently. Periodic review, therefore, may lead to enhancement of function. The ophthalmologist and counselor may enlist the aid of the specialized optometrist, the knowledgeable optician, and the paraprofessionals skilled in teaching the use of such aids.

The past decade has seen marked progress in the development of low-vision clinics. These clinics usually have ophthalmologists, orientation and mobility instructors, low-vision specialists, and psychologists. There are approximately 114 such clinics scattered widely throughout the United States. For a complete listing, the counselor is referred to the most recent survey conducted by the American Foundation for the Blind.

A cecutient need not be rehabilitated as if he were totally blind. Instead, the maximum use of his remaining resources should be developed. No matter how severe the impairment, it is not dangerous to use any of the remaining sense of vision. Therefore, all treatment should be directed toward incorporating the remaining vision into as effective a system of personal management as possible.

The cecutient who has insidiously suffered the loss of visual function over a long period of doubt and waiting creates a special problem for treatment. He has had more time to fumble and develop expedient methods of his own without benefit of the programs for the blind that have been developed. These expediencies may have to be replaced with more effective methods. Such an individual is seldom cordial toward the skills of blindness, for he, his family, and often his physician had hoped the course of his disease might have been arrested. This is an event calling for a little more patience and understanding on the part of the rehabilitation team.

The additional therapeutic approaches discussed above for blindness apply to a variable degree to the cecutient.

Vocational Implications

Impairments of distant and near acuity, visual fields, accommodation, color perception, binocular function, and combinations of these in varying degrees of severity may occur. The meaning of these with regard to employment requires close interaction of counselor and the ophthalmologist. Probably no two cecutients are exactly the same in the various functions.

Many cecutients indulge in a certain amount of "play" regarding what they can and cannot see. This "play" not only plagues the inventor, but also confounds counselors and employers. A prevocational setting and job sampling techniques performed in known environments can help prevent "play" from interfering with planning.

In vocational planning and in job placement, resources must be directed to helping the cecutient function as fully as possible with impaired sight. With regard to low-vision aids, the simplest devices remain the best. Once an aid is chosen, even if it is specific to a single job, implementation may require a good deal of drill and practice. The training component of a new job may therefore take longer.

The Bureau for Blind and Visually Handicapped of the Rehabilitation Services Administration estimates that of the 32,000 jobs listed in the Dictionary of Occupations, 80 percent can be managed by the "legally blind" and cecutient if a proper survey of job requirements is made by a trained placement counselor and the individual is equipped with adequate aids and training.

The above discussions apply to the blind and cecutient regardless of cause. The remaining sections will deal specifically with individual causal diseases.

CATARACTS

A cataract is an opacity or clouding of the crystalline lens. By far the most common type is the so-called senile cataract, causing nucleus clouding (see chap. 3). The usual age of onset is from the fifth decade onward. Congenital and hereditary cataracts are either present at birth or come on in the first or second decade. The opacity may be at any position within the lens or may occupy the entire lens.

Cataracts may also be caused by or be a result of ocular trauma or inflammation at any age, and may be associated with certain systemic disorders, such as arachinodactyly (Marfan's), diabetes (see chap. 24), electric shock (see chap. 31), maternal rubella (German measles), hypoparathyroidism, Down's syndrome, myotonic dystrophy (see chap. 6), retinitis pigmentosa (see below), scleroderma, and certain therapeutic drugs such as steroids (cortisone preparations).

By far the most effective method of treatment of cataract is surgical removal. This may be extracapsular (small portions of the lens may remain) or intracapsular (the entire lens is removed). The choice depends on age and the plan for use of glasses, contact lenses, or intraocular prosthesis.

The ophthalmologist has the final responsibility for deciding with the patient when surgery is indicated and what method should be employed. When recommending surgical intervention, the examiner will consider age, type and location of the opacity, visual requirements, general health, bilateral or unilateral affection, and his own skill. Each case must be decided on individual characteristics, requirements, and indications.

Occasionally, by either constriction or dilation of the pupils, the visual ability will be improved, thus obviating the necessity for immediate surgical intervention. There are no drugs or medicines presently available which will remove or lessen the opacity once it has formed.

The formation of cataracts can be prevented by exact therapy of certain metabolic diseases, such as hypoparathyroidism, juvenile diabetes, and galactosemia. Judicious use of systemic steroids may prevent cataracts caused when their use is necessary for the control of disease (e.g., rheumatoid arthritis or lupus erythematosus).

In the majority of routine cataracts of the senile variety, good visual acuity will result from successful surgery. However, absence of the lens (aphakia) itself carries a significant amount of impairment, such as loss of accommodation, impairment of binocular vision, sensitivity to ultraviolet light, and, when glasses are worn, a significant peripheral field impairment. Often depth perception is impaired. With training and practice, some of the difficulties can be overcome.

An interpretation of the significant aphakic impairments as they apply to vocational opportunities and goals cannot be generalized but must be made by the ophthalmologist in each individual case.

GLAUCOMA

Glaucoma exists when the degree of pressure within the eye is sufficient to cause damage to the nerve fiber layer of the retina. The damage to the retina is similar in all types of glaucoma. It causes loss of peripheral vision first and central vision much later in the course of the disease. The exact cause of increase in pressure is not always known. It probably results from an absolute increase in the volume of aqueous humour in the anterior chamber due to a block of the outflow of the aqueous humour in the anterior cavity at the canal of Schlemm (see chap. 3).

Symptoms and signs vary with type of glaucoma but can include an apparent "fogging" of sight, a rapid failure of sight, a halo of rainbow tints around lights, mild or severe pain, dilated pupils, a clouded cornea, and an inflamed conjunctiva.

The most common of the many types of glaucoma is *primary open angle glaucoma*. This is a chronic, insidious, painless disease. Severe impairment may therefore be present before the process is detected. Once the nerve fibers are damaged, they cannot be regenerated and thus impairment is irreversible.

As part of a routine eye exam, the intraocular pressure should be measured. The optic discs (see chap. 3) should be examined for evidence of glaucomatous cupping or excavation. A peripheral field examination should be performed to detect subtle early evidence of field loss indicating inadequate pressure control.

Treatment of glaucoma varies with cause. For most patients with primary open angle glaucoma, eye drops or oral medications are used to control the intraocular pressure at safe levels. These medications constrict the pupil. For some types of glaucoma, or when pressure is not controlled by medication, surgical intervention may be necessary. Treatment usually is palliative and not curative, so patients will require regular medical care to monitor intraocular pressure and visual fields and to alter therapy as needed.

The medications used for glaucoma may themselves cause considerable impairment. For example, the pupil-constricting (miotic) drugs may cause visual problems in dim light and accelerate cataract formation. They will also severely reduce visual acuity in those with posterior subcapsular cataracts.

Rehabilitation of the client with glaucoma requires an individualized approach based on the degree of disability produced by the disease because glaucoma can produce all degrees of cecutiency as well as total blindness. If peripheral vision is lost first, occupations making use of good peripheral vision would obviously not be possible.

DIABETES

Diabetes (see chap. 24) affects the eye in numerous ways. It contributes to the formation of cataracts and to a type of severe glaucoma. Its most devastating effect is to the vasculature of the retina.

The most serious type of retinal vascular disease is *proliferative diabetic retinopathy*, in which new blood vessels form in ischemic areas of the retina. These fragile new vessels also extend into and cloud the vitreous and tend to bleed easily. The blood clot may then be replaced by opaque fibrous tissue which contracts and detaches the retina either partially or totally from the pigment epithelium (retinal detachment).

In addition to measurement of visual acuity, the ophthalmologist examines the eye with a special ''slit'' lamp. A thorough retinal examination is necessary to detect changes. Fluorescein angiography, in which a fluorescent dye is injected into the bloodstream to delineate the retinal vessels, is helpful in demonstrating new vessels and areas of leakage.

The patient with diabetes should be under the supervision of his physician to assure control. Regular ophthalmological examinations are also necessary to detect the retinal changes early and allow for timely therapy. In recent years, various forms of destruction of new vessels by laser beams (photocoagulation) have been found to be effective in controlling new vessel growth.

Once hemorrhage into the vitreous has occurred, treatment is more difficult and prognosis worse. Mechanical vitrectomy is a new surgical technique to remove the blood-filled vitreous. Controlled studies are under way to evaluate its efficacy and determine the optimum time after hemorrhage for this procedure.

Once fibrous proliferation and traction retinal detachments have occurred, prognosis is very poor, since these types of detachments are very difficult to repair even if the traction bands can be broken. Thus,

effective treatment in diabetic retinopathy depends on early detection of disease and appropriate therapy.

Diabetes may cause all degrees of cecutiency, as well as total blindness. In general, it is the chronicity of the disease that influences the severity of the retinopathy, nephropathy, and neuropathy. Therefore, vocational goals should be carefully considered and planned in anticipation of what disabilities may occur with time.

OTHER VASCULAR DISEASES

There are many other types of vascular diseases which affect the eye. These may be divided into two main groups, those causing ischemia of the retina and those causing ischemia of the optic nerve. The first group includes sickle cell diseases (see chap. 27), central retinal artery occlusion, central retinal vein occlusion, and leukemia. The second group includes ischemic optic atrophy and temporal arteritis. With both groups, the end result is similar: cecutiency or blindness.

Evaluation will include assessment of the underlying systemic disease by the appropriate specialist and by the ophthalmologist. The retinal picture in the diseases of retinal ischemia is of engorged tortuous veins with exudate, edema of the optic disc, and hemorrhages. There may be new vessel growth. With diseases causing optic disc ischemia, the optic nerve disc shows pallor and the retinal vessels may be narrowed.

Therapy varies according to the nature of the systemic disease and, as in diabetes, photocoagulation may control neovascularization. In temporal arteritis, a disease of patients over 60, early steroid therapy may prevent further loss of sight.

In many of these diseases, central or macular vision may be lost early. Employment requiring close direct vision will therefore be affected, as will activities in bright light. Peripheral fields may be constricted as well, thus impairing scanning activities in dim light.

MYOPIA

Myopic persons are ''nearsighted'' and in most cases the myopia is caused by an increase in the axial length of the eyeball. The increased length may be present at birth or may evolve with age and development. If present at birth, it may be associated with other ocular developmental defects, particularly of the foveal region. Degenerative changes from stretching of the choroid and retina can involve both the macula and the optic nerve and might cause retinal detachment.

Ophthalmoscopic examination at routine intervals to detect early retinal degeneration will often allow for early therapy for detachments and the avoidance of total blindness. Accurate optical correction of the refractive error, in most cases with glasses, alleviates the visual problem in myopia. If retinal detachments are present, photocoagulation or more extensive detachment surgery may be necessary. If there is foveal involvement, low-vision aids may be indicated.

This condition often allows quite good visual acuity for in-close objects and it is not harmful to the eye to make use of this asset by highlighting desk or bench type activities.

CORNEAL DISEASES

Any corneal disease causing clouding or opacification in the central area of the cornea may produce cecutiency or blindness. Corneal disease may be hereditary, degenerative, or caused by trauma, particularly chemical burns, and the opacities or cloudings take many forms.

Ophthalmologic examination with the slit lamp is used to assess the cornea. In addition, the eyes must be examined for associated anomalies. Visual acuity can often be improved by the use of contact lenses.

When the eyes are otherwise healthy and there is a good visual prognosis, corneal transplant is performed. This may either be partial thickness (lamellar), when the clouding opacity is superficial, or full thickness (penetrating). Because the cornea is avascular, rejection of the graft is less likely than with other organ transplants. If rejection does occur, it can be managed medically with steroids. If this fails, further transplants may be performed. Banks of corneas taken from cadavers exist in most major cities.

The purpose of a corneal transplant is to give the patient good vision, removing him from the population of the visually disabled. Once the wound has healed, there are no particular contraindications or restrictions. If, for some reason, a transplant cannot be done successfully, occupational counseling would take into account the diffuse impairment of vision with normal peripheral fields and perhaps an intact fovea.

HEREDOFAMILIAL AND DEGENERATIVE DISEASES

The heredofamilial and degenerative diseases often involve the central nervous system, in addition to the eye, and are often associated with anomalies of the fingers and toes. All of them have a profound bearing on vocational ability and placement. The inheritance and variety of these diseases are complicated and numerous, so only two of the more important ones will be mentioned.

Friedreich's ataxia (see chap. 6) and related conditions occur at age 7 to 8 years and extend into adult life. Clumsiness in walking and hand use are usually the first symptoms. The cecutiency results from optic atrophy and nystagmus. Also, pigmentary degeneration of the retina may occur.

Retinitis pigmentosa is a bilateral progressive hereditary disorder usually commencing in childhood and often producing marked peripheral visual field constriction in late youth and early adult life. Night blindness is usually the first symptom. Complaint of loss of vision often comes late in the disease. Almost total bilateral loss of all useful peripheral fields occurs around age 50. Posterior subcapsular cataracts are frequently present, thus eliminating the useful vision in the small remaining field. Deafness can be associated (Usher's syndrome). Polydactyly, hypogenitalism, and obesity may accompany the pigmentary changes (Laurence-Moon-Biedl syndrome).

In addition to examination by an ophthalmologist, audiological, orthopedic, and internal medicine review may be necessary. There is no satisfactory treatment for these heredofamilial diseases. However, cataract extraction in some persons with retinitis pigmentosa can be helpful.

These diseases are progressive, and multiple motor, sensory, visual, and cerebral effects will take place. A knowledge of the individual disease and its usual course will therefore be necessary to guide the vocational planner.

CENTRAL NERVOUS SYSTEM DISEASES

The more important central nervous system diseases are the demyelinating diseases, including multiple sclerosis, which can affect vision by involving the optic nerve, optic tract, or optic pathways (see chap. 3). They can also cause nystagmus and paralysis of the extraocular muscles.

Neoplasms are also important causes of both blindness and cecutiency (see chap. 28). Pituitary adenomas, meningomas, craniopharyngiomas, gliomas, dermoids, and astrocytomas are among the most common. Their locations and size will determine their effect on visual function. Neurological, ophthalmological, and neurosurgical examinations are usually necessary to determine site of involvement and to decide on proper therapy. For the neoplasms, therapy may include radiation, chemotherapy, surgery, or a combination of any or all three.

Since many of these conditions affect the age groups who are active vocationally, and since they may cause visual impairment as well as impairments in sensory, motor, and cerebral function, a complete evaluation of all these factors will be important in determining vocational potential. One cannot be specific since these disease processes very seldom affect any two individuals in exactly the same way.

SENILE MACULOPATHIES

From a provocation not understood, the retina and choroid respond to aging in a way which causes retinal or choroidal changes ultimately affecting the macula or foveal regions of the eye. Thus, central direct vision is most affected, peripheral vision less. This is most commonly referred to as senile macular degeneration or maculopathy. The etiology is not understood. It accounts for the largest number of cecutients age 45 and above but seldom causes blindness. It is a significant causative factor in the total population of those over 40 years of age whose central visual acuity drops to 20/200 or below but not to total blindness. These aging factors are not easy to analyze or predict. Why maculopathy affects some at an early age, others later, and some not at all is not explainable.

Evaluation of residual function is performed by the ophthalmologist. All functions, including acuity, color, accommodation, field of vision, binocularity, and eye movement, need to be assessed. Treatment generally involves magnification and learning techniques to compensate for failing vision. Low-vision clinics are helpful. Occupations requiring direct examination of objects are most affected.

OTHER DISEASES

There are several other congenital diseases, some with established hereditary patterns, which are commonly seen, seldom cause blindness, and are associated with retention of useful vision for most or all of the patient's life.

Congenital nystagmus is one of these disorders. Nystagmus is defined as involuntary oscillating movement of the eyes when the gaze is fixated in any direction.

There are several clinical types of *albinism*, but only the generalized type seems to have severe ocular involvement. There is a lack of pigment throughout the body, and the ocular anomalies are varied. There is constant photophobia and nystagmus. Another type of albinism affects the eye only. This is often accompanied by nystagmus and is inherited as a sex-linked recessive.

In *achromatopsia*, there is a complete lack of color vision. There is also low visual acuity, which is better in dim illumination. Horizontal nystagmus, which increases with attempted fixation and tends to disappear with age, also occurs.

In *aniridia*, absence of the iris except for a small rim occurs. It is transmitted as an autosomal dominant and is usually bilateral. Poor vision and progressive glaucoma and cataracts usually, but not always, accompany this defect. Also, since kidney tumors have been reported in association with aniridia, regular examinations should be performed.

The direction and type of nystagmus in the above diseases should be recorded in all fields of gaze because occasionally the nystagmus is less in a certain field. The proper refraction in glasses or contact lenses suitably tinted for protection from light should be given for best vision and to reduce the bothersome

photophobia. Low-vision aids are often helpful for near vision. Most of these patients can attain good visual ability, especially for in-close viewing.

SUMMARY

Varying sites and types of diseases may result in the same recorded visual acuity measurement. For example, two individuals with 20/200 recorded visual acuity may differ in site and type of affection in ways which will determine visual function and they thus will not be impaired to the same degree. The underlying diseases and all visual functions, namely, visual acuity, color, accommodation, visual field, binocularity, and eye movement, must be evaluated and understood to plan effectively.

With the totally blind, the visual difficulty is clear-cut, and performance depends exclusively on the integrity of other-than-visual functions, whereas the cecutient's performance can be influenced by remaining visual function, as well as by other sensory and motor capacities. Planning with the cecutient may therefore be more difficult than planning for the blind. The counselor can exert influence in several areas of responsibility in addition to organizing the rehabilitation process. When visual impairment is already severe, prevention of additional impairment through regular programs of prevention and ophthalmological care should have the highest priority.

Since those who are not totally blind have the potential for increased visual function, every effort should be made to assure the proper prescription and use of optical and other aids to increase the use of the remaining sense of vision. Several examinations and special devices, as well as supervised training in the use of aids, devices, and residual vision may be needed.

The role of genetic counseling has never been adequately developed as part of prevention and is an area where prevention could be certain and long lasting. The counselor who arranges for effective genetic counseling programs will do much for the rehabilitation process. He will need expert professional help, but such programs could be worthwhile.

Professional medical care on a continuous basis must never be omitted from a treatment plan. There is no such thing as a final examination or a final evaluation. The dynamics of life, diseases, and disorders demand a routine program of continuous care. This is never more true than in visual and ocular disorders.

A number of great divides occur with respect to the ideal ways and means of helping the visually handicapped to meet their needs. One approach is by law, the other by custom or what Helen Keller called "public habits." What blind persons need as much as anything is a courteous nation, capable of social maturity.

BIBLIOGRAPHY

Bull Prosthet Res, BPR 10-26, Fall, 1976.

This issue is almost entirely devoted to vision impairments and research being done on new aids and prostheses. Of special interest are articles on low-vision mobility and mobility aids for the severely handicapped.

Carrol TJ: *Blindness: What It Is, What It Does, and How to Live With It*. Boston, Little, Brown, 1961.

This book describes the carefully worked out rehabilitation theory and practice of a Roman Catholic priest whose life was devoted to the visually impaired. It describes their problems in terms of 20 losses, followed by a detailed account of means for restoration.

Blindness Annuals of the American Association of Workers for the Blind. American Association of Workers for the Blind, Washington, D.C.

Since 1964, this annual has published articles with the expressed purpose of "tracing the movement of human thought with respect to blindness." A section is devoted to detailed listings of government research programs, including those of the Rehabilitation Services Administration, National Eye Institute, and the Veterans Administration.

Hardy RE, Cull JG: *Social and Rehabilitation Services for the Blind*. Springfield, IL, Thomas 1972.

This book brings together the opinions and experiences of 22 leaders of American work for the blind, and demonstrates the wide range of disciplines and skills included in a comprehensive program to meet the needs of the blind.

Hoover RE, Freiberger H, Bliss JC, Bach-y-Rita P, Brindley GS: Symposium: Prosthetic aids for the blind. Trans AA00 **78**:711–746, 1974.

The most recent information on all mobility aids and practical reading devices. Also includes a summary of tactile vision substitution systems and implantation of stimulators in the visual cortex.

Keegan DL, Ask DD, Greenough T: Blindness: Some psychological and social implications. Can Psychiatr Assoc J **21**:333–340, 1976.

Description of a study to determine some aspects of psychological and social adjustment to vision loss and blindness. Factors affecting adjustment and rehabilitation potential are discussed.

Koestler FA: *The Unseen Minority: A Social History of Blindness in America*. New York, McKay, 1976.

This is an astute, well-written, and detailed account of the development of work for the blind in the United States. It relates the movement of thought in work for the blind to national and world events and identifies the causes of ebb and flow of resources for blind rehabilitation.

Neu C: Coping with newly diagnosed blindness. Am J Nurs **75**:2161–2163, 1975.

Discussion of the phases of coping with recent-onset blindness for both the blind person and his family. Losses suffered are described briefly, and recommendations are made for helping the person and his family to adjust.

Sloan LL: *Reading Aids for the Partially Sighted: A Systematic Classification and Procedure of Prescribing*. Baltimore, Williams & Wilkins, 1977.

The most recent book dealing with the prescription of reading aids for the visually impaired. Covers basic optical principles, information required prior to selection of an aid, special equipment necessary, special problems, types of magnification, and nonoptical aids which may be useful in visual rehabilitation.

Walsh FB, Hoyt WF: *Clinical Neuro-Ophthalmology*. Vol 3. Baltimore, Williams & Wilkins, 1969.

The most comprehensive book of its kind. It has detail of the anatomy, pathology, and functional disturbances of all conditions and diseases affecting vision and the visual system. It is superbly indexed and contains interesting case histories to illustrate functional pathology.

30 HEARING IMPAIRMENTS AND DEAFNESS

Jerome D. Schein, Ph.D.

DISEASE DESCRIPTION

Hearing impairment refers to a reduction in sensitivity to sounds, which may be accompanied by some loss in the ability to correctly interpret auditory stimuli, even when amplified. Hearing impairments vary by degree, locus of pathology, and cause. They may be permanent or transient. This chapter considers only those that are permanent.

Since hearing impairments lack a common etiology, confusions in terminology are difficult to avoid. *Hearing impairment* means any degree and type of auditory disorder, while *deafness* means an extreme inability to discriminate conversational speech through the ear. Deaf persons, then, are those who cannot use their hearing for communication. Persons with lesser defects are called *hard of hearing*.

Hearing impairments fall into three categories: conductive, sensorineural, and mixed. *Conductive impairments* arise from defects in the auditory system (see chap. 3) which interfere with sound waves reaching the cochlea. The locus of the lesion in conductive losses lies in the outer or middle ear (e.g., external auditory meatus, tympanic membrane, auditory (Eustachian) tube, auditory ossicles), while *sensorineural impairments* are caused by defects to the auditory pathways within the central nervous system, beginning with the cochlea and auditory nerve, and including the brain stem and cerebral cortex. Lesions in these locations prevent or disrupt interpretation of the auditory signal. *Mixed impairments* involve both conductive and sensorineural defects. As will be seen, this tripartite classification, though oversimplified, has considerable value for the rehabilitation counselor because the client's type of impairment is an important factor in determining the direction of his rehabilitation.

In the United States, more persons have a hearing impairment than any other chronic physical disability. The most recent National Health Survey (for 1971) reports that 13.2 million persons would respond "yes" to the question, "Do you have any trouble hearing in one or both ears?" The number of positive responses yields an estimated rate for hearing impairment in the civilian, noninstitutionalized population of 6.6 percent. Almost exactly half that number (3.4 percent) have a hearing impairment in both ears (bilateral impairment).

Table 30-1 summarizes these data, as well as those for deafness, and distributes them by reported age at onset. Hearing impairments are relatively uncommon in childhood and early adulthood. By senescence, however, hearing impairments affect more than one of four adults. Of the latter, about 10 percent are deaf, so for the population 65 years of age and older, nearly 1 of 40 cannot use their hearing for communication. In contrast, congenital deafness occurs at a rate near 1 per 1,000 live births.

The later in life hearing loss occurs, the less severe are its consequences. In general, born-deaf persons tend to present the greatest challenge to rehabilitation

TABLE 30-1

PREVALENCE RATES PER 1,000 FOR HEARING IMPAIRMENTS IN THE CIVILIAN, NONINSTITUTIONALIZED POPULATION 3 YEARS OF AGE AND OVER, BY DEGREE AND AGE AT ONSET: UNITED STATES, 1971

AGE AT ONSET	ALL DEGREES	UNILATERAL	BILATERAL	
			Hard of Hearing	Deaf
All ages	66.0	32.5	24.8	8.7
3–16	14.7	7.6	6.4	0.7
17–24	24.7	16.9	7.3	0.5
25–44	42.0	29.0	12.0	1.0
45–64	96.1	51.9	41.0	3.2
65 and over	265.9	92.9	148.5	24.5

because, in addition to being unable to hear, they usually have poor or absent speaking ability and serious deficiencies in language. Once speech is established, it usually can be maintained despite loss of hearing. Hearing impairments after 19 years of age do not seem to severely affect speaking ability and language. Those hearing losses occurring from birth to 19 years of age are now referred to as *prevocational deafness*, while those occurring before 3 years of age are termed *prelingual deafness*.

Etiology

Our knowledge of the causes of hearing impairments is incomplete and in some dispute. New explanations and new causes of hearing loss continue to be uncovered. For example, before 1950, maternal rubella ("German measles") was unknown as a cause of deafness in the neonate. Another instance was the discovery of the ototoxicity of aminoglycoside antibiotics (such as dihydrostreptomycin, gentamycin, and neomycin) soon after their introduction, which resulted in their more careful use in medical practice. In addition, more thorough genetic studies have identified previously unsuspected familial strains of hearing impairment. More insights into etiology like these can be expected.

Heredity. Perhaps as many as half the cases of congenital deafness have a genetic basis. The comparable rate for hard-of-hearing persons has not been calculated because few cases of milder losses are detected at or near birth. Mildly hearing-impaired children tend to blend into the general population until audiometric screening in school detects them, by which time establishing etiology is made very difficult by the children's exposure to numerous potentially damaging diseases and accidents.

Literally dozens of anomalies familially associated with hearing impairment have been identified. One of the most prominent is *Waardenburg's syndrome*. When fully expressed, it consists of a combination of auditory, ocular, and pigmentary anomalies. Only the auditory feature is disabling. The pigmentary anomalies consist of a white forelock and different colored irises (heterochromia). A broad nasal root and odd-shaped eyelids complete the syndrome.

In *Alport's syndrome*, the hearing loss is usually only in the high frequencies and often detected only by audiometry. Nephritis with hematuria also occurs and may result in complete renal collapse, possibly leading to death in males in their second decade.

Another important hereditary condition is *Usher's syndrome*, manifested by retinitis pigmentosa and deafness. Affected individuals progressively lose central vision and become functionally blind by early adulthood. Night blindness and a reduction in the visual field leading to "tunnel vision" occurs. The accompanying hearing loss is present at birth and ranges from severe to profound. For such individuals, diagnosis in childhood is crucial so that rehabilitation may be undertaken before the inevitable loss of sight.

Not all authorities agree that *otosclerosis* has a hereditary basis, but all hold hope that its disabling effects can be overcome. In its common form, otosclerosis develops insidiously as a spongy lesion around the stapedial footplate. The result is a slowly progressive conductive hearing loss manifested in early to middle adulthood and sometimes in childhood. Rarer forms involve the cochlear capsule as well. Otosclerosis in the United States affects two females to one male and almost exclusively the white population.

Infections. Diseases may attack the auditory system at every developmental stage. A mild attack of measles in a pregnant woman (*maternal rubella*) may lead to severe hearing impairment or deafness in the child.

In early childhood, middle-ear infections (*otitis media*) commonly occur during the winter months. Earaches, like the common cold, do not threaten life and are often neglected as a minor health problem. If untreated or incompletely treated, serious complications may result, leading to a conductive hearing loss and, if the disease is allowed to invade the inner ear, even to a sensorineural loss. Damage to the auditory apparatus continues as long as the disease remains uncontrolled.

Cerebrospinal meningitis formerly caused much hearing impairment. Whether due to the high fever accompanying the disease or to action of the offending organism, the losses tended to be profound, with major destruction of inner-ear tissue and accompanying vestibular damage. Meningitis is a potential complication of measles, scarlet fever, and mumps. The advent of antibiotics, however, has lessened the incidence of hearing losses from these complications.

Acoustic nerve tumors. These tumors usually are diagnosed in the third or fourth decade of life. Their growth is typically slow and continues into the sixth and seventh decade if untreated. Early diagnosis can be critical, since the smaller the tumor, the less the risk of complications and, of course, death.

Accidents. Among accidental causes of hearing impairment, noise doubtless ranks first. The cochlea is the site of the lesion in hearing losses induced by noise. Early in this century, chronic, persistent exposure to loud sound was known as a factor contributing to hearing impairment (e.g., boilermakers' deafness). Exposure to acoustic trauma has greatly increased and, with that increase, there will probably be a decrease in hearing acuity for a sizable portion of the population. A potential cause of hearing loss indicated by recent studies is frequent attendance at concerts where popular music is played at very high sound pressures. Listening to loud music through head-worn speakers can also result in decrements in auditory sensitivity. Sources of industrial noise, such as diesel truck motors and jet engines, added to the much higher environmental sound level in most cities, also mean more hearing impairment.

Blows to one side of the head can affect the ear on the opposite side by causing the stapes on the opposite side to be driven so violently inward that it damages the cochlea. Explosions can similarly cause sensorineural damage. Ruptures of the ear drum (tympanum) may be caused by head trauma and changes in air pressure, resulting in conductive hearing loss.

Presbycusis. Presbycusis literally means "old hearing." As already discussed, hearing impairments are common in later life. But while sharing a common label, these impairments do not have a single etiology. Some may be due to cumulative effects of noise; others to various illnesses; others may have a hereditary component; and still others may be due to vascular disease. The list could go on, adding to the picture of complexity. What seems clear is that presbycusic impairments are largely sensorineural. It is also probable that many cases of presbycusis result from a mixture of pathologies.

A symptom common in many of the above conditions is *tinnitus*, a sound arising within or about the cochlea of the patient's ear. The sound may be heard by the patient, by an observer, or both. When severe, tinnitus can disturb sleep and precipitate emotional disturbance. Even in a mild form, it is annoying. Its etiology is usually unknown.

The examples of the major causes of hearing impairment discussed here are summarized in table 30-2. The majority of the causes are associated with sensorineural impairments. Conductive losses are often lesser in degree (usually not exceeding moderate impairment) and far less in quality. Sensorineural losses involve distortion in the capacity to interpret auditory signals as well as reduced acuity. Hearing may continue to decline due to new pathology or progression of an untreated or untreatable ongoing condition. In general, conductive losses are potentially reversible, while sensorineural losses are not. Both types of losses can be helped by aural rehabilitation.

FUNCTIONAL DISABILITIES

The extent to which a hearing impairment disables an individual depends heavily upon two factors: the degree of impairment of auditory discrimination in the speech frequencies (500–2000 Hz) and the affected individual's age at onset of the impairment. Of course, in assessing a particular handicap, other information about the individual and his milieu must be considered. In general, the greater the loss of the ability to distinguish single words (speech discrimination) and the earlier the onset of the loss, the greater the rehabilitation problem. Thus, clients born deaf may require the most effort to rehabilitate and those who become hard of hearing in senescence may require the least effort.

Communication Disorders

Hearing impairment produces a communication disorder which may be manifested in both reception and expression. Serious impairment of expressive communication mostly occurs in cases of severe, early impairment.

Hearing. Complete loss of hearing ability is exceedingly rare. Even deaf persons frequently have some capacity to hear, though they lack the discrimination that enables correct identification of sounds, particularly speech. Impairments in the speech frequencies interfere with the reception and interpretation of spoken communication. The counselor must remain aware that clients may respond to loud noises and yet be unable to understand even loud conversation. Furthermore, a particular hearing loss may permit discrimination of some, but not all, speech sounds. A thorough evaluation will establish how useful an individual's remaining hearing will be for communication.

The deaf client is always handicapped when information is only delivered auditorially. For example, deaf travelers do not hear announcements of gate changes or cancelled flights. When "all passengers" are instructed solely over a loudspeaker to do something, those who are deaf do not know what to do, or even that something is to be done. If they are in an airplane, they will observe the other passengers and then seek the answer to why the others are acting as they do. In the terminal, however, deaf passengers often lack such clues, so they must remain close to airline personnel in order to receive any information applicable to themselves.

Similarly, in a vocational setting, a supervisor may obscure his face while giving instructions. Dependent in some measure on speechreading, the hearing-impaired person's communication is disrupted by the speaker who holds a hand in front of his face, turns away from the listener, or smokes. The speaker may be seated at a desk with a large object, such as a vase of flowers or a framed picture, blocking the hearing-impaired person's view.

Speech. When deafness occurs prelingually, speech does not spontaneously develop. Prelingually deaf persons can learn to speak, but their speech is usually difficult for most people to comprehend. The later deafness occurs, the more likely speaking ability will be retained. Effort by teachers and speech pathologists is required to correct dysfluencies due to disruption of auditory feedback. The effect of hearing loss on speech declines with increase in hearing ability. However, hard-of-hearing children often need speech therapy to overcome problems due to their attenuated hearing.

Language. Until recently, linguists did not distinguish between speech and language. Now most concede a distinction. For our purposes, language is a sizable set of symbols combined in systematic ways and

TABLE 30-2

SELECTED CAUSES OF CHRONIC HEARING IMPAIRMENTS BY USUAL TYPE OF HEARING IMPAIRMENT

Cause	Type
Heredity	
Waardenburg syndrome	Sensorineural
Alport's syndrome	Sensorineural
Usher's syndrome	Sensorineural
Otosclerosis	Conductive
Infections	
Maternal rubella	Sensorineural
Meningitis	Sensorineural
Otitis media	Conductive and mixed
Acoustic nerve tumors	
Accidents	
Noise	Sensorineural
Cephalic trauma	Conductive and mixed
Barotrauma	Conductive
Presbycusis	
Specific etiology usually not diagnosed; most cases probably multiply determined	Sensorineural and mixed

used by two or more persons to convey ideas and emotions. Languages may be transmitted by speech, hand signals, or print. Thus, American Sign Language (Ameslan) is indeed a language, though it is not spoken. It has a large vocabulary (signs), a syntax, and is used by many persons.

Deficits in language are common among prelingually deaf persons. Consequently, the average deaf adult in the United States obtains reading scores on standardized tests below fourth-grade level. Their written language is frequently unintelligible, containing constructions that confuse the reader unaccustomed to "deaf English."

Deaf adults who are illiterate in English are frequently fluent in Ameslan, having little or no difficulty communicating in the latter language. Yet Ameslan is seldom taught in schools for deaf children. The students learn it from each other and from deaf adults.

Since prelingually deaf persons have great difficulty learning English and considerable success learning Ameslan, the conclusion seems inescapable that our schools have not found adequate means of teaching English visually. The average deaf person scores at or near the mean on performance tests of intelligence. This fact, coupled with demonstrated ability to learn sign language, obviates the argument that failure to learn English is a *necessary* consequence of prelingual deafness.

As with deficits in speaking ability, the later the onset of deafness, the less the language deficit. The degree of hearing impairment is also related to language learning, though less markedly so. Hearing-impaired children, properly fitted with hearing aids, may have more success acquiring good language than

good speech. The deficit in English competence which accompanies hearing impairment reflects the present lack of expertise in special education.

The communication disabilities of deaf persons are diminished by sign language, fingerspelling, and speechreading (lip reading). However, deaf persons do not automatically learn these techniques. Instruction is required if the person is to become proficient. Therefore, the counselor cannot assume that deaf persons will understand sign language or be able to speechread simply because they are deaf.

Psychosocial Disabilities

Pediatricians unfortunately too often fail to correctly identify deafness, leaving many born-deaf children's condition undetected until they are past 3 years of age. By that time, the family often has erroneously concluded that the deaf child is autistic or mentally retarded. Because of this, the child is deprived of essential early remedial measures, and his special needs are not met.

The overwhelming majority (90 percent) of deaf children have normally hearing parents and siblings. The parents are therefore generally unprepared emotionally for their deaf child and have no particular knowledge of what steps to take when the diagnosis of deafness is made. Counseling for the parents will not only help them, but can also aid the child, who might otherwise be deprived of prompt remediation as parents go from place to place seeking assurance that earlier diagnoses were mistaken.

As with most childhood disabilities, the occurrence of deafness often arouses severe guilt feelings in the parents. Left without effective help in resolving the emotional upheavals accompanying the diagnosis of deafness, many parents reject the disabled child. Parents of born-deaf children frequently reject their child's deafness even after he has attained adulthood. It is thus common to find young deaf adults who cannot communicate effectively with their parents and siblings. This lack of acceptance and communication within the family may profoundly affect the deaf child's emotional and social adjustment.

For those born deaf or deafened during childhood, the marital partner chosen is usually deaf (80 percent) or hearing-impaired (7 percent). Thus, communication between spouses and acceptance of each others' disabilities is usually excellent. When the deaf or hearing-impaired person's spouse is not disabled, tension and hostility may be aroused because of lack of acceptance of the hearing impairment by the spouse or by the disabled person. The spouse may become impatient with repeating missed or misunderstood portions of conversations. The disabled person may complain that everything would be all right if only the spouse would speak up.

Intellectual deficits are frequently associated with deafness. However, these deficits do not necessarily accompany hearing impairment. Rather, deaf children may be viewed as having a low intellect because our culture places a high premium on verbal facility, and deaf children often speak unintelligibly or not at all. Yet, surveys comparing large samples of deaf persons to their peers in the general population show essentially equal performance on nonlanguage tests of intelligence. When the deaf child is considered less intelligent than he is, his learning opportunities and social development may be unnecessarily restricted. In fact, deafness need not prevent a person from high intellectual achievement nor from professional employment.

Like intellectual deficits, emotional problems are not necessarily associated with deafness. No evidence shows mental illness to be more or less prevalent among deaf adults. Unfortunately, few psychiatrists and psychologists can communicate with a prelingually deaf person. They frequently overlook even fairly severe hearing impairment if the patient has speech.

On a day-to-day basis, deaf persons may be avoided by colleagues at work and neighbors at home unless they can communicate easily. Social contacts generally depend upon swift, easy interchanges. When conversations must be repeated frequently or written out, frustration ensues. From childhood on, deaf persons learn to smile and nod yes when they are asked if they understand in order to avoid the hostility often aroused and poorly disguised in the person who is asked to repeat again and again.

Persons who lose their hearing early in life tend to associate with other deaf persons. They are sometimes accused of being clannish and of rejecting others, but the isolation of deaf persons from general society is at least by mutual action. Indeed, deaf persons as a group appear no less gregarious than any other group. They simply socialize with other deaf persons because the severity of their disability prevents easy integration into general society. Instead, deaf persons congregate in their own minority group, one in which communication uniquely depends upon Ameslan. They have many social organizations, service groups, and athletic clubs whose members are all deaf. The existence of the deaf community is an important reality for the rehabilitation counselor serving deaf clients. To be successful, the counselor should become familiar with the deaf community, its folkways, and its resources.

Hard-of-hearing persons seldom join the deaf community, especially if their loss occurred in adulthood. The immediate consequence of their hearing impairment is a period of mourning when they become depressed and isolate themselves. With proper rehabilitation, they receive the necessary prostheses and training assistance which enhances their reintegration into their milieu. However, as with any physical or sensory handicap, acceptance of deafness does not emerge simultaneously with the diagnostic pronouncement. Until a person with an irreversible hearing loss stops believing that tomorrow his hearing will be restored, he is apt to resist adaptive measures, such as learning sign language, as signifying the surrender of hope. Many rehabilitation plans are frustrated by the client's lack of cooperation because he is not emotionally ready to accept his hearing loss and the necessary ameliorative measures.

Rehabilitation Potential

The rehabilitation counselor must assiduously avoid stereotyping the deaf or hard-of-hearing client. Prelingually deaf persons, in particular, may seem very much alike in the severity of their handicap and the limitations on employment potential, but this is not the case. Consideration must be given to each individual's ability and potential for further education and vocational training. Long-term planning is appropriate, and every effort should be made to overcome the educational and vocational deficiencies caused by previous underestimation of the abilities of hearing-impaired persons and the consequent discrimination against them.

Educationally, prelingually deaf persons have succeeded at every level. Many have completed high school, some have graduated from college, and a few have earned doctorates. While in each instance the proportions of academic success are lower than for the general population, the fact must be kept uppermost that early deafness does not preclude highest academic achievement. It does make such achievements more difficult, but not impossible, to attain.

Occupational achievement also has not been limited

TABLE 30-3
PERCENTAGE DISTRIBUTION OF PRINCIPAL OCCUPATIONS OF EMPLOYED DEAF[a] PERSONS 16 TO 64 YEARS OF AGE,
COMPARED TO THE GENERAL POPULATION: UNITED STATES, 1972

Occupations[b]	Deaf[a]	General
All	100.0	100.0
Professional and technical	9.2	14.0
Managers and administrators, nonfarm	1.9	9.8
Sales	0.3	6.6
Clerical	8.1	17.4
Craftsmen	29.0	13.2
Operatives, nontransit	31.1	12.7
Operatives, transit	1.9	3.9
Nonfarm laborers	8.2	5.2
Service workers	8.1	13.4
Farmworkers	2.3	3.8

[a]Includes only persons who became deaf before 19 years of age
[b]Categories as defined by the U.S. Bureau of the Census

by deafness. Table 30-3 compares the distribution of employed deaf and general populations by occupational categories. Three facts emerge: (a) deaf persons are represented in every occupational category; (b) they are underrepresented in the higher categories (professional, technical, managerial); and (c) they are overrepresented in the middle categories (nontransit operators and craftsmen). The latter disproportion places the deaf community heavily at risk to automation. Continued emphasis by vocational counselors on machine-tending jobs for deaf persons, despite excellent past performance, cannot be justified in the face of the projected composition of the labor market, which anticipates relatively fewer and fewer such jobs. Keeping in mind that there are deaf lawyers, dentists, physicians, actors, sculptors, counselors, teachers, clinical psychologists, corporation executives, chemists, and others, all of whom have lost the ability to discriminate speech at an early age, should provide an antidote to any counselor's premature rejection of a deaf client's high vocational ambitions.

STANDARDS OF EVALUATION

For the deaf client who has been disabled since childhood, the requirement of a physical examination, especially re-examination of hearing ability, before initiating rehabilitation may seem irrational. The counselor should take time to explain why medical evaluation is necessary and to prepare the client for the psychological assessment. This preparation will smooth the evaluation process and may prevent a client's failure to return after the initial contact.

Audiological/Otological Examination

The clinical evaluation of hearing should include both otologic and audiologic examination, with thoughtful merging of the results from each. Etiology is often difficult to establish, but the general location of the damage is not. Present clinical techniques classify the nature of the impairment as to sensorineural, conductive, or mixed with high reliability. The examination should attempt to establish site of the lesion and probable cause, degree, onset, and progression of the impairment. The examination can usually provide a good estimate of prognosis and recommendations regarding the next step in rehabilitation, such as surgery or prescription of a hearing aid. Furthermore, the audiologist and otologist can inform the rehabilitation counselor about the likely functioning of the client in various work settings. This information adds significantly to the total evaluation of the hearing-impaired client.

In addition to tuning-fork tests in the office, the otologist (otolaryngologist, ENT specialist) visualizes the outer and middle ear with an otoscope. Then, the medical history and related tests, as indicated, are combined by the otologist with the audiologist's findings to arrive at a diagnosis.

The audiologist (usually Ph.D. level) administers various tests under carefully controlled conditions. These tests determine the intactness of the sensorineural apparatus, the presence of conductive impairments, the degree of loss at specific frequencies under various circumstances, and the ability to discriminate speech. Audiologists also evaluate the client's potential benefits from different types of hearing aids.

One of the more common audiological reports is the pure-tone audiogram, which graphs the client's responses to calibrated stimuli presented under controlled conditions. The stimuli are words and pure tones (a sound having a simple vibration at a constant rate). These stimuli may be presented through earphones directly into the patient's ears or by a loudspeaker (air conduction). Hearing may also be measured by placing a vibrator on the skull to test conduction of sound that bypasses the middle ear (bone conduction).

Testing is done in sound-treated booths to ensure that the client is not distracted by any sounds other than those generated by the audiologist. To generate

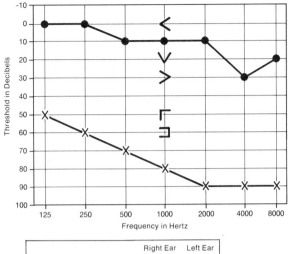

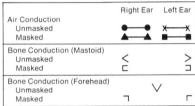

FIGURE 30-1. Sample pure-tone audiogram showing air-conduction and bone-conduction thresholds for a hypothetical hearing-impaired person. The lefthand axis is the threshold for hearing scaled in decibels (dB). Across the bottom, the audiogram is divided into frequencies in Hertz (Hz).

The air-conduction threshold for the right ear (X) is much lower than for the left ear (O). The pure-tone average for the right ear is 10 dB, and for the left ear, 80 dB (see text). The better-ear (right) average (BEA) is 10 dB. When the better ear is masked, the mastoid bone-conduction threshold for the left ear (⊐) is lower than when the right ear is unmasked (>) because some sound is picked up by the right ear when it is unmasked. Similarly, the unmasked forehead bone-conduction threshold (∨) is higher than the threshold for the left ear when the right ear is masked (⌐) because the right ear picks up sound when it is not masked.

the test signals, the audiologist uses an *audiometer*, an electrical instrument for producing vibrations at a specific rate, shape, and intensity, and on which the intensity of voice signals can be monitored. The audiologist instructs the client to respond by raising his hand when the signal is first heard or by repeating the words which are spoken to him. If the client is unable or unwilling to cooperate, the audiologist can use other techniques that measure physiological changes in the client as a function of the test signal.

Figure 30-1 shows a pure-tone audiogram for a hypothetical hearing-impaired person. The symbols used on this audiogram are those adopted by the American Speech and Hearing Association and are most widely used. When encountering other notations, the counselor should request an explanation.

Decibels are logarithmic units expressing the relative intensity of sound. On the decibel scale of the audiogram, zero represents normal hearing, i.e., the threshold for healthy young adults. Larger numbers on the decibel scale mean more power is needed to cross the hearing threshold. Hence, the higher the number on the audiogram, the greater the pathological deviation from normal. A negative score means better than average hearing.

Frequencies, expressed in cycles per second (Hz), represent tones from low to high, paralleling the octaves on a musical scale. A 250 Hz pure tone lacks the overtones of a musical note, but its position would be a little below that of middle "C" on the piano. The 500 and 1,000 Hz pure tones are, respectively, one and two octaves higher than the 250 Hz pure tone. For understanding connected discourse, the critical range of frequencies (the *speech frequencies*) is 500, 1,000, and 2,000 Hz. Significant hearing decrements (increased thresholds) among these frequencies will affect understanding of spoken communication. Sometimes audiometry is limited to testing these frequencies. However, testing at 125, 250, 4,000, and 8,000 Hz should also be done because impairments at these frequencies are in themselves important and because they have diagnostic and prognostic value for rehabilitation.

A quick summary of hearing in either ear is the *pure-tone average*, the arithmetic mean of the air conduction thresholds at 500, 1,000, and 2,000 Hz for each ear independently. The *better-ear average* (BEA) is the pure-tone average for the ear with the lower mean threshold.

Bone-conduction thresholds are obtained by placing a vibrator on the right or left mastoid process of the skull (see p. 34), or by placing the vibrator on the forehead to measure both ears. Even when the vibrator is placed behind one ear, the response may be to sensation felt in the opposite ear because the skull transmits vibrations to both. An ear can be isolated by masking the opposite ear with noise. This is accomplished by delivering a buzzing sound that contains all frequencies to the ear through earphones.

The audiologist's examination will also include measures of speech-hearing ability. One such measure is the *speech-reception threshold* (SRT), obtained by asking the patient to repeat words presented through earphones at varying intensities and finding the loudness at which correct identifications are made half the time. In the other test, for *speech discrimination*, the words to be identified are delivered at a listening level significantly above the patient's threshold. This latter measure is particularly useful in predicting how well the hearing-impaired individual will function in everyday situations.

Additional Physical Examination

As noted previously, other physical disabilities often coexist with hearing impairments. Whenever examining a deaf client, the otologist and the counselor should be alert to these other conditions, since they complicate rehabilitation and may even threaten life. The following additional organ system examinations may also be necessary.

Visual system. The deaf person is almost totally dependent on his eyes for receptive communication. A refractive error or imbalance of eye muscles (strabismus) which would be minor for otherwise normal persons can severely handicap a deaf person who must read the minute, fleeting changes of a speaker's lips and the swift, small movements of fingerspelling. All deaf and hard-of-hearing persons should therefore be examined by an ophthalmologist or by an optometrist to optimize the visual function. Clients with deafness due to Usher's syndrome should receive continuing ophthalmological care because they also have severe visual impairment due to retinitis pigmentosa (see Chap. 29).

Vestibular system. Persons deafened by meningitis frequently suffer disturbances of the vestibular system (see chap. 3) and may have problems with balance. A neurologist or otologist is able to assess this system.

Other organ systems. Children deafened in utero by maternal rubella have a high probability of additional defects. Among these are visual problems, cardiac deformities, and a wide range of motor defects. Examination by an ophthalmologist, a cardiologist, and a neurologist may therefore be required.

Since the genetically transmitted syndromes involving hearing impairment also involve other systems, other additional evaluations are appropriate. Clients with Alport's syndrome, for example, should be evaluated by a nephrologist to assess renal function.

Psychosocial Evaluation

The hearing-impaired client challenges the skills of the social worker and the psychologist, who depend heavily for assessment on the client's language behavior. Even moderately hearing-impaired persons may be incorrectly assessed because of their tendency to guess at spoken instructions rather than to admit they cannot understand. When the person's speech is also impaired, the consultant unfamiliar with such cases may be unable to function properly. When possible, the counselor should therefore ensure that he refers hearing-impaired clients to consultants with manual-communication competence and experience working with hearing-impaired persons.

A social worker should evaluate the client's family supports to identify problems of parental rejection, lack of communication between the client and other family members, and stresses associated with a lack of acceptance or understanding of the client's hearing impairment by parents, siblings, or spouse. Analysis of the family relationships involves observation of the family members as they interact, plus independently discussing the relationships with each family member.

These observations can assist in planning the family's role in the client's rehabilitation.

Evaluation by a clinical psychologist is particularly important for the person whose hearing has recently been impaired. The psychologist can evaluate the client's adjustment to his new disability and can recommend additional counseling, when appropriate, to help the client accept his hearing impairment and the aids and training necessary for his rehabilitation.

Persons deafened early in life do not become aware of a sudden change, and therefore do not go through the same process of adjustment as those whose hearing becomes impaired later in life. Personality assessment of these early-deafened clients requires unusual proficiency because the psychologist needs a broad experiential base for understanding prelingually deaf persons and because of the reduced ability to communicate with them fluently. It may require a psychologist who is able to sign and read sign language. The emotional maturity of these clients is consequently often misassessed by psychologists inexperienced with deaf persons. When given a negative personality assessment of a deaf client, the counselor should seek further assessment unless the consultant has demonstrated ability in dealing with this rare client group.

In assessing intelligence, the psychologist will use one or more of several nonverbal tests, such as the Performance Scale of the Wechsler Adult Intelligence Scale (WAIS), the Chicago Nonverbal, the Hiskey-Nebraska Test of Learning Aptitude, and the Leiter International Performance Scale (Arthur Revision). The latter two tests have norms and procedures of administration for deaf persons and are therefore recommended.

Recent surveys of psychologists who have tested deaf persons show, however, that the WAIS is most commonly used, despite the lack of published accounts of its validity with deaf persons. The wide acceptance of using the WAIS with the general population seems to have convinced many psychologists that it will be equally valid for those who are severely hearing-impaired. The counselor would be better advised to ask for substantiation of the deaf client's assessed mental ability by a second test, preferably the Leiter, whenever the assessment places the client at the extreme ends of the range or does not accord with other observational and psychometric data. The likelihood of underestimation of a deaf client's mental ability is far greater than that of overestimation. For rehabilitiation purposes, then, *the counselor should probe vigorously for areas of potential strength and be reasonably skeptical of imputed weaknesses.*

In recognition of the great need for a new test of academic achievement, the 1974 revision of the Stanford Achievement Test (SAT) has been standardized on a large sample (15,000) of deaf students in a variety of educational settings. The revision includes new procedures for administration as well as new norms. The procedures virtually eliminate errors due to the "floor effect," i.e., assigning an inferred minimum level of achievement to anyone taking the test. Thus, persons who are given an advanced form would score about the fifth-grade level, even if they did not answer a single item correctly. Before administering the revised SAT for deaf students, the evaluator administers pretests that indicate the proper form for that individual, regardless of chronological age or years in school. The pretest also helps to overcome mistakes due to lack of familiarity with the test format.

Another valuable aspect of the revision is the availability of norms for both deaf and hearing populations. Such readily made comparisons help the counselor keep the client's achievement in proper perspective, recognizing how much may have been accomplished in comparison with the other hearing-impaired persons and how little in comparison with the general population.

Speech should be assessed by a speech pathologist, not only to determine present functioning but also to indicate rehabilitation potential. Similarly, reading and writing must be independently tested. A manual-communication specialist can assess the client's ability to communicate in sign language. As previously stated, sign language competence cannot be taken for granted, nor is skill in American Sign Language necessarily predictive of skill in using English. A highly competent deaf signer may have poor English and vice versa. Knowledge of the client's communication abilities will strongly influence the counselor's decisions on how to proceed with a rehabilitation plan and what the objective of the plan should be.

TOTAL TREATMENT

Surgery

Conductive impairments arise from defects in the outer or middle ear which interfere with the sound waves reaching the cochlea. These obstructions can usually be removed. Failure to develop an external opening of the ear (congenital atresia) can be corrected by surgery. Impactions in the external auditory meatus (e.g., wax in the ears) can be removed. A ruptured tympanic membrane, which may be the result of otitis media or injury caused by pressure (barotrauma), can be surgically repaired. Surgery can also correct immobility of the auditory ossicles resulting from otosclerosis by freeing them (mobilization) or replacing them (e.g, stapedeoplasty). While recurrence of hearing impairment after stapes mobilization or stapedeoplasty is more frequent than would be desired, the procedures appear well worth the risks of recurrence in return for the periods of restored hearing.

Hearing Aids

The purpose of a hearing aid is to amplify sounds so they become audible to the user. Basically, this is accomplished by first changing sound waves (acoustic energy) into electrical energy. The electrical energy is amplified and converted back to acoustic energy. The resulting sound waves are therefore more intense than the original input.

The main components of a hearing aid are the microphone, the amplifier, the receiver, the battery, and the earmold. The *microphone* converts the sound waves into electrical energy. The *amplifier* increases the electrical signal coming from the microphone, and the *battery* supplies the energy for this purpose. The *receiver* converts the amplified electrical signal into sound waves, which the *earmold* carries into the ear canal.

The earmold is a custom-made part of the hearing aid. An ear impression is obtained by inserting a special material into the ear canal, the concha, and the helix of the external ear. When the impression material has hardened slightly, it is removed and sent to a laboratory where a finished earmold is produced. The earmold must fit securely into the ear to prevent the amplified sound from feeding back into the microphone, causing "squealing."

Persons with conductive losses receive the greatest benefit from the electronic hearing aid. The obstacles to sound transmission causing these losses can usually be overcome by the hearing aid. However, recent advances in hearing-aid technology have made it possible for persons with sensorineural losses to derive benefit from amplification as well.

The prescription of a hearing aid is not yet an exact procedure. The interactions between the hard-of-hearing person, the hearing aid, and environmental noises create exceedingly complex situations. The audiologist or otologist works with hearing aid dealers to select the instruments most likely to be optimal for a particular individual. Considerations include whether one (monoaural) or two (binaural) aids should be prescribed, and whether the battery and amplifier are attached to the temples of eyeglasses or carried in a clothing pocket. Since various makes of hearing aids amplify the frequencies differently, the choice of model is important to the user.

Selection of a hearing aid tends to be by trial and error. The client decides between aids offered after wearing them and being tested to determine the benefits from each. At least a 1-month trial period should always be allowed a client before finalizing the hearing aid purchase.

Dispensing hearing aids without accompanying orientation reduces their effectiveness. Since hearing aids amplify selectively, the resulting output sounds strange to the person who has had hearing. The first reaction to the new sound may be irritation. In addition to being annoying, the sounds may be difficult to distinguish. The client needs to learn to discriminate auditory stimuli filtered through the new appliance. Also critical is instruction in maintenance of the hearing aid. Fittings must be periodically checked and cleaned, and batteries replaced as they lose power. The hearing aid is a fairly delicate electronic prosthesis demanding care to retain its effectiveness. Authorizing a program of auditory training for the hearing-impaired client makes good rehabilitation sense.

Facilities and procedures for hearing-aid evaluation vary widely across the country. The roles of audiologists, hearing-aid dealers, and otologists differ from place to place. The counselor's agency will usually have an established procedure for hearing-aid evaluation if many hearing-impaired persons are served. If the agency has no established practice, the counselor should seek the best available consultation from audiologists and otologists in the area. In addition to hearing-aid evaluation, these consultants will advise on essential followup and maintenance programs.

Educational Services

Deaf persons generally require special instructional programs in which the content is visualized. Such programs can be found throughout the United States at the elementary education level, and high school programs for deaf students are available in many states. Postsecondary programs, however, are relatively scarce. Only 41 such programs were identified in 23 states in 1975, of which only 1 devotes itself solely to deaf students. Gallaudet College in Washington, D.C. is the only liberal arts college in the world exclusively for deaf students. Other postsecondary programs are housed within existing institutions, such as the National Technical Institute for the Deaf, which is situated within Rochester Institute of Technology. The principal characteristics of these specialized programs are the availability of sign-language interpreters, notetaking facilities, and counselors and tutors prepared to work with deaf students.

The range of educational opportunities for the postsecondary education of deaf persons will very likely be greatly expanded as a result of the Rehabilitation Act of 1973. Under Title V of this act, educational facilities receiving Federal funds must make reasonable accommodations for the instruction of disabled students.

Speech instruction is part of the special education program for prelingually deaf children at the elementary level and usually continues into the secondary level as well. Teaching speech to prelingually deaf children requires great skill and patience. Lacking auditory feedback, these children must use visual, tactile, and proprioceptive cues to match the sounds they make to an unheard spoken model. Despite heroic efforts by teachers and pupils, few prelingually deaf children develop good speech. Nonetheless, the effort to teach speech should continue. Present failures only mean that educators have as yet not developed adequate methods. The successes, though far too few, support the proposition that born-deaf children *can* learn to speak well.

Speech will also be affected when hearing is present but imperfect. Hearing-impaired children should be given corrective speech instruction as soon as possible after the loss is diagnosed. The nature and extent of remediation will depend largely upon the extent of the loss and the age at onset.

Any hearing-impaired person can benefit from learning manual communication, provided he will be in contact with others who use it. The use of manual communication by children and adults is increasing rapidly, judging by the number of classes being offered for its study.

Ameslan and Manual English (ME) are two different forms of manual communication. Ameslan has its own grammar which deviates from English, and ME follows English syntax, substituting signs for words. Most schools for deaf children do not formally teach Ameslan, but it is used in classes or in the dormitories. Thus, Ameslan has many variants typical of languages that are passed from person to person without direct education. It takes as much time to learn as it would take to learn any foreign language. Adults usually study ME, which can be acquired in a matter of months.

Other communication skills, such as reading, writing, typewriting, and speechreading, can also be maintained or improved by educational programs designed for hearing-impaired persons. The amount of information that can be accurately conveyed by speechreading alone is limited. Only 16 different lip shapes are available to represent the 43 phonemes in English. Hence, the speechreader must guess at the probable word being spoken. Further, the ability to speechread depends heavily on one's knowledge of the language being spoken. Since prelingually deaf persons tend to have the poorest command of English, they are likely to be the poorest speechreaders.

Psychosocial Treatment

Social services to help hearing-impaired and deaf persons with family problems are often required. A social worker can aid the family in adjusting to one family member's hearing loss. Since few social workers are skilled in working with deaf persons, the counselor should urge an inexperienced social worker to use an interpreter when needed to overcome the communication barrier.

The major psychosocial treatment for persons with irreversible sensorineural impairments is directed toward teaching them how to live with their disability. The psychologist's first consideration should be given to emotional factors if the person has recently suffered a hearing loss. Taking positive remedial steps often constitutes good, though indirect, therapy for the accompanying emotional upset. For those clients who persist in hoping their hearing will soon be restored despite explanations that the loss is irreversible, this technique will not help. These clients will usually not cooperate in a rehabilitation plan until they have been helped to accept the reality of their irreversible disability.

VOCATIONAL IMPLICATIONS

Equipment

It is ironic that Alexander Graham Bell invented the telephone to assist deaf persons. In fact, the telephone has become a major impediment to the vocational advancement of deaf workers because much commerce involves the rapid communication at a distance that the telephone makes possible for those who can hear. The deaf person can, however, surmount the telephone barrier in one of two ways. If he has clear speech, he can have a hearing person instantly interpret an incoming message and respond in his own voice. This method is employed by some deaf executives. An alternative is the teletypewriter (TTY) coupled through the telephone to a similar machine at the other end. Whatever is typed on one machine is transmitted via telephone to the receiving machine, which types the message. This hookup can operate overseas, between states, and locally. It is limited by the expense and availability of the equipment and by the typing ability of the user. The TTY does, nonetheless, contribute significantly to increasing the deaf person's vocational potential.

Other equipment can also help the deaf person adjust vocationally and socially. Devices are available that replace audio signals with flashing lights or vibrators. For example the doorbell can be wired to the lights in one or more rooms so that, when it is pressed, the room lights go on and off. Similarly, a flashing light can replace the buzzer on an alarm clock, or a vibrator attached to an alarm clock can be placed under the pillow to awaken a deaf sleeper.

In a vocational setting, it is essential that a hearing-impaired person have access to information essential to his work. If loudspeakers, buzzers, or other auditory devices are used regularly and exclusively to impart such information, the counselor needs to ensure that the client can receive the information in a nonauditory manner.

Special equipment may not be necessary in job tailoring for deaf clients. The alert counselor can frequently overcome objections to hiring a deaf person by showing that restrictive elements in a job description actually need not be retained. For instance, ability to use a telephone was a requirement at one time for a claims adjuster in a government agency. A work analysis showed that virtually all pertinent communication was done in writing, and thus the requirement that barred a deaf person was removed. Similarly, specifications for a stockroom clerk included the need to converse fluently. When the company's own policy to fill only *written* orders was pointed out, along with the loss of time when workers used the stockroom as a place to chat, the position was opened to a deaf person.

Opportunities abound for job tailoring by careful analysis and, when appropriate, restructuring tasks or using various equipment to substitute visual signals for auditory signals. Title V of the Rehabilitation Act of 1973 should also help the counselor combat discrimination against the employment of hearing-impaired persons.

Environment

In vocational planning for hearing-impaired clients, there are a number of environmental factors the counselor needs to consider. One critical factor is lighting. Being visually dependent, the hearing-impaired person requires better lighting than a person who can add reliable auditory cues to the available visual information. Speechreading demands a well-lit face. Good lighting does not necessarily mean bright lighting. Indeed, overly bright lights increase visual fatigue. Trying to observe a person standing in front of a highly luminous surface induces negative afterimages. Since deaf persons develop the habit of inhibiting their eyeblinks when concentrating on a speaker, doing so can be counterproductive when lighting deviates markedly from optimum.

Another important environmental factor is noise. It is not true that a person who already has a substantial hearing loss would be a likely candidate for work in a noisy environment. Deaf persons are usually uncomfortable working in a noisy environment because the noise source assaults their vibratory sense. Any person who has a hearing loss, especially one that is noise-induced, should avoid further prolonged exposure to loud sounds which would only add to the loss. All hearing-impaired persons should use ear protection when using noisy power tools or when riding in a noisy vehicle, such as a subway train, to prevent further hearing loss induced by noise.

It is important to consider room acoustics for the

client using a hearing aid. Harsh surfaces, like uncarpeted floors and unadorned plaster walls, create echoes that lower the effectiveness of the hearing aid. Reducing reverberations by adding sound-absorbent materials, such as rugs and drapes, to a room will help the hearing-impaired person's comprehension of speech. In noisy environments, rather than turning up the hearing aid's volume, the wearer should move as close as possible to the speaker. This will increase the signal-to-noise ratio effectively.

The rehabilitation counselor who attends to these environmental factors in the workplace can greatly aid deaf clients. They are unlikely to complain about these conditions. Their early training, particularly if they are prelingually deaf, teaches them to adjust to the environment as they find it. Seldom do they encounter the reverse—the environment being adjusted to them. This insight into the early training of prelingually deaf children can serve the counselor well. He must test the deaf client's understanding constantly and not rely on his nodding affirmatively. The counselor should rather request the client to restate the message the counselor wants him to understand.

Use of Interpreters

To overcome the communication impasse, counselors who do not specialize in work with deaf clients will find an interpreter essential. Counselors unaccustomed to using interpreters may be bothered by a third person joining the usually private one-to-one relationship, and the situation may be awkward at first. The counselor's discomfort will be relieved by experience with qualified interpreters. Their ability to smoothly speak for the speechless client and to convert the counselor's speech to sign language soon seems commonplace rather than an amazing intervention. Further, interpreters who have been trained by the National Interpreter Training Consortium or who have been certified by the Registry of Intepreters for the Deaf accept a stringent code of ethics which requires, among other things, that all transactions in which they participate must be kept strictly confidential. The assurance of confidentiality should also ease the counselor's concern about the use of interpreters. Of course, it would be better if the client and counselor could communicate without an intermediary. However, the client should not be denied service or be given inadequate treatment because the counselor does not have sign-language ability.

Interpreters will also be needed at other points in the rehabilitation process. From intake through assessment, training, and placement, interpreters may be essential for some deaf clients. Providing an interpreter for a job interview can smooth a deaf worker's entry into the new position. The employer has a demonstration of how effectively he and the deaf person can communicate, thus making a good initial impression. However, this arrangement can give the employer the idea that an interpreter will be required on a full-time basis at heavy expense. With care, the counselor can prevent such an erroneous notion from developing. The knowledgeable counselor will explain to the employer that, once familiar with the surroundings, the deaf worker will usually manage very well.

The counselor can then, or at a later time, provide information on how to optimize communication with deaf employees. Of course, the deaf person should participate in these discussions to the extent he is able. Otherwise, the counselor may leave the employer in doubt about the deaf applicant's competence. The counselor should ensure that employers and co-workers understand that, when speaking to the hearing-impaired person, their mouths must be clearly visible to facilitate speechreading. Therefore, it is important for them to know that they should not smoke, sit or stand in a shadow or behind a visual obstruction, or turn away while speaking to the hearing-impaired person.

Finally, the counselor should bear in mind the variety of individuals who lose or have never had hearing. Nothing in this chapter should be construed to imply that hearing impairment homogenizes behavior. On the contrary, differences among hearing-impaired persons are as wide as among the general public. Intellectually, emotionally, volitionally, and physically, hearing-impaired persons retain their individuality. They share many minor characteristics and some may have important traits in common. To the rehabilitation counselor, the client's individuality should predominate. The general propositions discussed above offer useful points of entry into the counseling relationship; they should not merge into stereotypes. A knowledge of what to expect from ''typical'' deaf and hard-of-hearing persons should aid the counselor in appreciating the uniqueness of each client.

BIBLIOGRAPHY

Bolton B: A behavior-oriented treatment program for deaf clients in a comprehensive rehabilitation center. Am J Orthopsychiatr **44**:376–395, 1974.

After a brief description of the psychosocial and vocational problems of the deaf, this article describes a training program that includes training in personal adjustment, vocational skills and adjustment, independent living, and personal hygiene. Followup studies indicated that two-thirds of those completing the program were competitively employed.

Bowe FG Jr: Non-white deaf persons: Educational, psychological and occupational considerations. Am Ann Deaf **116**:357–361, 1971.

A literature review indicating a general lack of research

using a nonwhite population. Those studies that have been done indicate that the nonwhite deaf are less educated, have lower IQ (which may be culturally biased), higher unemployment, lower incomes, and hold less desirable jobs than their white peers.

Cook L, Rossett A: The sex role attitudes of deaf adolescent women and their implications for vocational choice. Am Ann Deaf **120**:341–345, 1975.

A short article describing a study of 20 deaf and 42 hearing women (mean age 15.7 years) who were tested to determine their sex-role views. Hearing women were shown to have significantly less traditional views of sex roles, which also applied to the types of employment they were seeking.

Davis H, Silverman SR: *Hearing and Deafness*. Ed. 4. New York, Holt, Rinehart and Winston, 1978.

A comprehensive treatment of the anatomy, physiology, and pathology of the auditory system. In addition, sections are devoted to the education and rehabilitation of deaf persons.

Furth HG: *Deafness and Learning: A Psychological Approach*. Belmont, CA, Wadsworth, 1973.

This short book deals with the process of learning in the deaf. Education is thoroughly discussed, including the different approaches used in teaching language to the deaf.

Hardy RE, Cull JC (eds): *Educational and Psychosocial Aspects of Deafness*. Springfield, IL, Thomas, 1974.

This book, dealing with the psychosocial and educational aspects of deafness, has chapters on work adjustment, psychological adjustment, and education available both for the deaf and for those working with the deaf.

Northern JL (ed): *Hearing Disorders*. Boston, Little, Brown, 1976.

Multiply authored volume covering diagnosis, pathology, and treatment of hearing impairments. Especially thorough discussions of otitis media, presbycusis, and noise-induced hearing loss. Contains chapters on acupuncture and cochlear implants.

Schein JD: Model for a state plan for vocational rehabilitation of deaf clients. J Rehab Deaf Mongr No. 3: 1–4, 1973.

Endorsed by Rehabilitation Services Administration, National Rehabilitation Association, and National Association for the Deaf, among others, these guidelines have been accepted by all State VR agencies. The plan is presented in nine chapters: Philosophy, Population, VR Process, Manpower, State Advisory Councils, Interagency Cooperation, Special Facilities, Deaf Community Development, Communication—National-State-Local.

Schein JD, Delk MT: *The Deaf Population of the United States*. Silver Springs, MD, Natoinal Association of the Deaf, 1974.

Reports the detailed information about the deaf population gathered in the 4-year survey completed in 1972. In addition to the data on the size and distribution by age, sex, and geography of hearing-impaired persons, the report contains extensive details on education, rehabilitation, occupation, and economic aspects of this population. Also contains figures on morbidity and mortality.

Watson D (ed): *Deaf Evaluation and Adjustment Feasibility*. Silver Springs, MD, National Association of the Deaf, 1977.

Subtitled "Guidelines for the Vocational Evaluation of Deaf Clients," this book contains the combined wisdom now available on this topic. The discussions are ordered under these major headings: Vocational Evaluation Process, Initial Assessment, Work Samples, and Situational Assessment.

31 BURNS

Edward J. O'Shaughnessy, M.D.

DISEASE DESCRIPTION

Over 300,000 Americans are hospitalized each year because of burn trauma. Their stay is three times longer than that of the average patient in an acute hospital. The age of the burned patient is represented by all decades to include the extremes of old age, but the age group at greatest risk is from 20 to 30 years. The home is the highest risk area for thermal burns at all ages. Consequently, these individuals are not normally covered by the various occupational insurance programs in force, even though most burned patients are of working age. Table 31-1 details age and risk distribution common to a metropolitan center. Note that 66 percent of burn injuries occurred in the home, and 41 percent were suffered by persons 17 to 40 years of age.

The Skin

Skin is the major organ system which is exposed to excessive temperature. Its functions are to protect the body from the external environment and to maintain the stability of the internal environment (homeostasis). The skin protects the body from bacterial invasion and the ultraviolet rays of the sun, conserves and regulates body temperature, and protects the body from excessive fluid loss. Alteration in its anatomy and function forms the basis for the classification, treatment, and sequelae of burns.

The skin is composed of two structurally different cellular layers, the *epidermis* and the *dermis* (fig. 31-1). The outer portion, the epidermis, consists of densely packed epithelial cells, and is itself layered. The two main layers are the stratum corneum and stratum germinativum. The stratum germinativum, the deepest layer of the epidermis, is the major source for new skin cells. These cells contain the pigment melanin, which is responsible for the color of the skin. Newly formed cells migrate upward to the stratum corneum.

The stratum corneum, the most superficial layer, is composed of tough, dry cells which ultimately die and slough off with rubbing or pressure. The greater the irritation or pressure, the thicker the stratum corneum. This is apparent over the soles of the feet, palms of the hands, and in calluses.

The dermis, or inner portion of the skin, consists mostly of stout connective tissue. It is rich in capillaries, bundles of collagenous fibers, and elastic fibers. With increasing age, the elastic nature of the skin diminishes. Contained within the dermis are the skin appendages—the hair follicles and sweat and sebaceous glands. These structures are also made up of epithelial cells. Therefore, if only the epidermis is lost,

TABLE 31-1

AGE DISTRIBUTION WITH RELATION TO ENVIRONMENTS IN WHICH INJURY OCCURRED FOR PATIENTS AT HARBORVIEW MEDICAL CENTER, SEATTLE, WASHINGTON

Age Range	Home		Work		Other		All Environments	
	#	%	#	%	#	%	#	%
0–16	103	87	4	3	11	9	118	26
17–30	55	43	36	28	37	29	128	28
31–40	30	51	19	32	10	17	59	13
41–50	30	63	13	27	5	10	48	10
51–60	26	65	6	15	8	20	40	9
61–70	30	81	4	11	3	8	37	8
71 +	25	96	1	4	0	0	26	6
All Ages	299	66	83	18	74	16	456	100

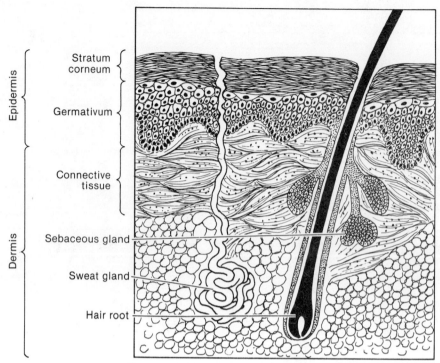

FIGURE 31-1. Cross section of the skin.

new epidermis can form from these glands. If epidermis and all glands are lost, no new skin can form and only scar remains.

Under the dermis is the subcutaneous layer containing loose connective tissue which ties the skin down to underlying muscle, tendon, or bone. It also contains varying amounts of fat cells and the glands described above. Nerve endings sensitive to pain, touch, heat, and cold are located in the epidermis, dermis, and subcutaneous layers.

Mechanism of Burn Injury

A burn is defined as the damage done to tissue cells by temperature incompatible with the life of a cell. The extent of damage is related to the intensity of the temperature and the duration of time the tissue is exposed. Temperature greater than 113 degrees F (45 degrees C) over a reasonable length of time can produce burns. The major causes of burns are thermal agents, such as flame, hot liquids, electrical current, and chemical agents. While the mode of inflicting damage may vary somewhat with each agent, the basic effect is sufficient heat to elevate the temperature of the tissues.

Classification of Burns

Burns are classified according to the depth to which the tissue is injured and the percentage of the body surface involved. The classification is the basis for therapeutic decisions and prognosis.

Burn depth. Burns had for years been classified into three degrees of severity according to the layers of tissue destroyed. However, as therapeutic options expanded, it became necessary to indicate the depth of the wound more precisely. At the present time, both the old and new nomenclature are in use. Table 31-2

TABLE 31-2
OLD AND NEW BURN CLASSIFICATIONS BY DEPTH

Old Nomenclature	Location of Damage	New Nomenclature
First degree	Epidermis only	Superficial
Second degree	Epidermis and dermis at varying depths	Partial thickness
Third degree	Epidermis, dermis and all appendages	Full thickness

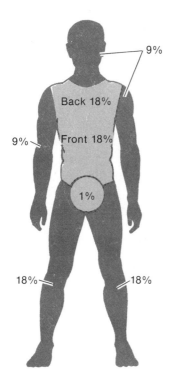

FIGURE 31-2. Skin surface of body divided into percent of total—the "Rule of Nines."

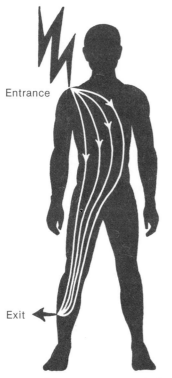

FIGURE 31-3. Path of electrical current in the body. Note spread of current within body. Visible damage will appear only at entrance and exit points.

relates the old and new terminology.

A superficial, or first degree, burn includes only the epidermis, and results in redness, edema, and pain. It is considered minor and does not usually require hospitalization.

A partial thickness, or second degree, burn involves the epidermis and dermis in varying amounts. This wound might result in blister formation and be painful, and still might well be in a minor classification requiring minimal outpatient wound care. However, it might involve the dermis to a greater depth and involve capillaries and appendages. The results can be infection, loss of body fluid, and the necessity for skin grafting. A partial thickness burn may be further identified as superficial partial thickness and deep partial thickness.

A full thickness, or third degree, burn involves the epidermis, dermis, and all skin appendages and, at times, deeper tissues. In the acute stage, it presents a charred painless surface known as *eschar*. Such a burn, even when involving only a small area, is a major burn and usually requires hospitalization.

Percentage of body burned. The greater the surface of the body deprived of its protective covering, the greater will be the damage to the entire support systems of the body. The patient will be at greater risk of cardiovascular collapse (shock) initially and more prone to overwhelming infection until the skin is replaced. Thus, the greater the extent of the burn, the greater the risk of complications and death. The percentage of body burned is used in calculating nutritional and fluid requirements during the acute treatment stage of burn trauma.

In order to standardize the method of estimating the surface area involved, the body has been divided into areas grossly equal to multiples of 9 percent of the body surfaces (fig. 31-2). This method is known as the "Rule of Nines." Thus, a person with partial thickness burns of the upper extremity would be classified as "superficial partial thickness, with 9 percent body surface burned."

The determination of the depth of the burn wound and the percentage of the body surface burned has proven an accurate method of determining the anticipated severity of the trauma. In cases of children and the elderly, age must also be taken into account in anticipating greater morbidity and mortality. Thus, a 2-year-old child with a full thickness burn with only 5 percent of body surface involved is still a severely burned child in danger of death, while in a young adult this type of burn would be minor. At the present time, all young adults should be admitted to a hospital who have suffered a partial thickness burn of more than 20 percent. However, if the partial thickness burn involves the face, hand, foot, or perineum, a young adult should be admitted regardless of percentage of body burned. With older and younger patients, admission with less than 20 percent of the body burned may be required.

Electrical Burns

Electrical burns, because of their frequent association with severe postburn disabilities, warrant special consideration. Electrical burns are almost entirely associated with occupational accidents. The peak of occurrence related to age is in the working-age group from 17 to 40 years.

All electrical burns are full thickness burns and are extremely deceptive in their presentation, since they appear to involve only a small area of the body surface where the electric current entered and exited. Beneath the skin, however, there may be considerable tissue damage (fig. 31-3).

Electricity produces heat as it passes through a conductor, such as the body. The amount of heat is directly proportional to the square of the current strength, times resistance of the tissue, times the duration of the current flow. The current strength itself is directly proportional to the voltage, and inversely proportional to the tissue resistance.

The higher the voltage and the lower the resistance, the greater the current that enters and exits through the skin at the contact points. Between these two points, the current spreads in the body over a wider area and generally where blood flows, since blood is a low-resistance conductor. If the skin resistance is high, less current flows through the body and internal damage is less. If skin resistance is low, as it is when the entrance or exit points are wet or immersed in water, internal currents are higher and the internal damage is greater.

Skin resistance concentrates the heat damage at the site of both entrance and exit. After the skin has been penetrated, the electricity will flow along paths of least resistance, the blood vessels. There is massive and immediate clotting of the blood, producing necrosis of the tissue supplied by the vessels involved, and frequently resulting in the necessity of amputation of limbs involved, excision of areas of the trunk, and resection of organs within the body cavity. In a small number of electrically burned patients, there is even a delayed spinal cord damage that may become apparent within a year of the injury. Immediate death from electrical burns is usually secondary to heart stoppage or paralysis of respiration.

Complications

During acute treatment, while damaged tissue is removed or treated and skin covering again finally achieved, a number of complications may occur. Some of these are discussed under Total Treatment. Of importance to rehabilitation, however, are the long-term secondary complications that persist after acute treatment is over. The most important of these are discussed here.

Contractures. Contractures result from joints having to remain in an abnormal position for a long period,

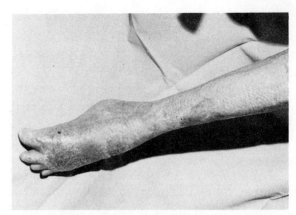

FIGURE 31-4. Contracture caused by allowing foot and ankle to remain in plantar flexion, which interferes with walking.

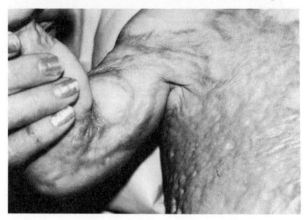

FIGURE 31-5. Hypertrophic scar, anterior thorax and axilla, causing an adduction contracture of the shoulder and an inability to raise the arm overhead.

causing shortening of the supporting structures, namely, muscles, tendons, and joint capsule. The functional result of such contracture is the loss of the range of motion of the joint involved. The limb cannot be voluntarily moved through the normal degree of rotation about the joint. For example, if the knee is allowed to rest in a semibent position in bed, it can contract in that position. The patient will then be unable to straighten the knee, thus effectively shortening the limb on that side. Similar contractures can occur at the hip and ankle. Figure 31-4 illustrates an ankle contracture. All of these may either inhibit or prohibit walking. Involvement of the upper extremities can cause functional impairments which can reduce the person's reach or interfere with the dexterity of the wrist and fingers and affect dressing, eating, and various employment skills.

Positional contractures are most likely to occur during the acute and subacute phases of burn treatment when the patient is allowed or forced to assume a position for maximum comfort or treatment, or is positioned to accommodate some necessary resuscitative equipment. The functional loss is thus indirectly related to the burn injury.

Hypertrophic scars. Hypertrophic scars are almost universally confined to the burn patient. The cause for this heaped up, florid, cord-like scar formation is not known, but it results from an increased production of collagen fibers which take on an abnormal configuration. Instead of the usual stratified appearance (fig. 31-1), the skin develops a whorl and nodular configuration, with an increase in capillary formation and fluid retention in the scarred tissue.

This peculiar formation begins with the healing process and reaches its peak in 2 months, but may remain as long as 2 years before it resolves. When this scarring involves a joint, it causes contractures, and when it involves the face, an unsightly cosmetic effect. Disfigurement anywhere in the body may result (fig. 31-5).

Pruritus. Itching (pruritis) is a complaint frequently voiced by the burn patient during the first year after burn trauma. It will disappear in time, but can be controlled by the use of topical ointments, such as hydrocortisone, and oral medications, such as antihistamines (e.g., Benadryl or Temaril). Frequently, incessant scratching of new skin itself causes damage.

Eye injuries. The eye is involved in some way with about 7 percent of hospitalized burn patients. The most common complication occurs when the eyelids are burned, causing them to invert (ectropion), so that the person cannot close his eyes, thus increasing the risk of corneal damage. Surgical release and suturing the lids temporarily closed with split thickness grafting over the released area will eliminate this complication.

The next major eye complication is scarring or clouding of the cornea resulting from trauma or burn. Actual severe burn of the cornea is rare, representing less than 1 percent of all burns. Most of these can be treated conservatively with medication applied to the eye. In the few cases in which there may be sufficient scarring to interfere with vision, a corneal transplant can be accomplished.

Loss of facial members. Certain burns about the face may cause the loss of the nose and ears. The destruction of the cartilage of the ear is a fairly frequent complication of burn plus infection. These burns present cosmetic problems that respond to reconstructive surgery and prostheses.

Hair loss. Those who suffer a full thickness burn of the scalp lose their hair permanently. A split thickness graft, which will not be hair bearing, is required to cover the area. The cosmetic defect can be remedied, if the patient feels it is necessary, either with a hair piece or hair transplants at a later date.

FUNCTIONAL DISABILITIES

Physical Disabilities

Burn trauma is not a progressive disease. Functional impairments will not worsen over the years, and many are remediable in a year or two postburn. The impairments which may initially be present after discharge from the hospital do not, in the majority of cases, preclude simultaneous return to a vocational environment and intermittent reconstructive procedures.

Contractures, caused either by positional shortening of the tissues surrounding the joints or by hypertrophic scarring, will cause loss of range of motion of the involved part. In practical terms, this may interfere with normal ambulation, requiring aids such as crutches or canes and, in many cases where the foot and ankle are involved, specially constructed shoes.

For those patients who have contractures involving the upper extremities, which may cause difficulties in dressing, self-feeding, and activities of personal hygiene, adaptive equipment will frequently be required on a temporary basis and, in a few cases, permanently. The occupational therapist can assist these patients with clothing adaptations and train them in the use of appropriate adaptive equipment.

The resolution of such contractures, depending on their severity and duration, will require intensive physical therapy or reconstructive or orthopedic surgical intervention.

Psychosocial Disabilities

The period of hospitalization associated with the treatment of an acute burn is extremely stressful. The patient is placed in a status of enforced dependency and, frequently, isolation. There are extended periods when the patient's waking hours are dominated by pain, associated not only with the burn itself, but also with frequent wound cleaning and dressing changes. The patient may exhibit periods of severe depression, regression to infantile behavior, hallucinations, and delirium. Despite these stress reactions during hospitalization, the long-term prognosis is good.

In the majority of cases, the patient makes a good readjustment to his former life style. When he does have difficulty following burn injury, it does not appear to be associated with duration of hospitalization, extent of burn, or physical or cosmetic deformities, but rather with the patient's previous ability to adjust to stress.

The members of the burned patient's family are subject to severe psychological stress as well. Initially, they are faced with a life-threatening trauma to a family member. When it is obvious that the patient will survive, there is the overwhelming anxiety of seeing him experience the various stressful situations described above. In their anxiety, the family members are likely to attempt to intervene in the treatment in a manner which would be detrimental to the patient.

A social worker who is attuned to the burn treatment environment should be in constant touch with the family to explain to them the rationale of treatment procedures they may see, and to help them with problems caused by the patient's hospitalization. In many cases, the family is involved in a financial crisis if the patient has been the major source of income. The social worker can act as an effective advocate for the family in reducing the impact of the sudden loss of funds.

Rehabilitation Potential

Return to gainful occupation within 6 months of hospital discharge is usually accomplished by 85 percent of burned patients who were employed at the time of injury.

Of the remaining 15 percent, some require extensive intermittent cosmetic or reconstructive surgery for a period of about 2 years. These patients need a complete vocational assessment and vocational plan, since their prior jobs will probably be lost.

The vocational potential for those who may have lost limbs or who have sustained spinal cord injury are discussed in chapters 13 and 5, respectively.

When physical problems are significant and psychosocial problems are also present, evaluation and management by a rehabilitation center where total team coordination exists may be appropriate.

STANDARDS OF EVALUATION

The rehabilitation couselor is most likely to meet the burn patient just prior to discharge from the hospital, or later if the patient has residuals of the burn that interfere with his return to his prior employment.

As mentioned earlier, the disabilities most likely to influence vocational potential are caused by the reduction of range of motion due either to positional or scar contracture, the presence of hypertrophic scar under treatment, loss of limbs, or cosmetic disfigurement.

Loss of range of motion due to contractures should be evaluated to determine the extent of functional deficit it entails. The deficits may be in ambulation, self-care, dressing, or dexterity of hand function.

Medical evaluation can be accomplished by the staff of a burn treatment facility. Lacking such a facility, a physician who has access to physical therapy, occupational therapy, and orthotic support should be consulted.

If physical therapy proves ineffective or is considered inappropriate, then the opinion of a reconstructive surgeon or an orthopedic surgeon should be sought. Physical therapy can be anticipated as part of the postsurgical status in any case.

Hypertrophic scarring should be treated as subsequently discussed under Total Treatment. If, however, there is not evidence of a progressive improvement during the period of conservative

treatment, the advice of a reconstructive surgeon should be sought. Cosmetic deficits should also be evaluated by the reconstructive surgeon.

Persistent psychosocial adjustment problems suggest premorbid problems which may require psychological or social review of the patient and his family.

The evaluation of the amputee is discussed in chapter 13.

TOTAL TREATMENT

Less than a decade ago, death from a partial thickness burn of 35 percent or more of the surface of the body was the rule rather than the exception. Now the survival rate for burns of 65 percent of the body surface in patients over 7 years old and under 45 is 70–80 percent. It is also not unusual for a person with a burn of 85 percent of body surface area to survive.

The factors that have so improved survival expectations are a greater understanding of the total body effects of burns, better monitoring and treatment of the accompanying infection which is always present, and newer methods of covering the wound. The knowledge leading to this change has come primarily from facilities dedicated to the care of the burned patient.

A burn facility usually consists of a staff of specially trained surgeons, pulmonary specialists, nurses, physical therapists, occupational therapists, medical social workers, and surgical technicians. However, there is no official definition of what constitutes a burn center or facility. For that reason, there is currently no list of such facilities available. The American Burn Association has been formed for those who are interested in burn care, and its membership consists of health professionals who are engaged in the care of the burned patient. This organization maintains lists of educational materials that can be utilized in the care of the burned patient and in the prevention of burns. It is the essential public advocate of the burned patient.

An insight into the acute and postacute treatment of burns will aid in understanding the stress the patient experiences.

Acute Treatment Phase

The immediate burn period involves an extensive loss of fluid from the body. The capillaries are so damaged that there is a massive escape of fluid to the surrounding tissues and evaporation from areas no longer protected by skin. Large volumes of electrolyte solutions containing the proper salts in the same ratio normally found in the body must be given within the first 24 hours to combat ensuing shock. For example, fluid replacement for a 125-pound (57 kg) person may be in the realm of 10 to 11 liters. During the next 24 hours, there is a loss of protein, which also must be replaced. The major loss of fluid after this period is from evaporation at the burned site, which is devoid of the protective skin covering.

Complications. Major acute complications of burn injury are smoke inhalation, sepsis, weight loss, urinary tract infections, gastrointestinal disturbances, and thrombophlebitis.

Smoke inhalation accounts for 18 percent of deaths. Inhaled minute carbinaceous particles lodge in the narrowest of the terminal branches of the bronchi. They cause extensive irritation, resulting in a massive outpouring of fluid into the lung tissues and the closing down of bronchi which, if not treated immediately, causes death by asphyxiation.

Treatment of this condition must be accomplished in an intensive care unit of a hospital where the patient's status can be monitored continuously. Sometimes, if the inhalation problem is severe, a chronic lung impairment may develop.

Widespread infection (sepsis) develops because dead tissue on the burned area (eschar) is a fertile field for the rapid growth of bacteria, which can spread to adjacent areas and invade the blood stream. Such an overwhelming growth of bacteria, together with their toxic products, combine to produce a major threat to the life of the patient. To remove all the eschar at once would require an extensive surgical procedure which, in patients with large burned areas, would further denude the body surface and would have to be covered immediately. Such a method, while theoretically possible, is accomplished only in a few centers on an experimental basis.

The common method now employed is to gradually remove the dead tissue (*debridement*), either by shaving multiple thin sections of smaller areas with specialized instruments or, more commonly, by washing the area and gradually removing the separating dead tissue manually or with specialized dressing techniques.

Since the areas of burn are colonized with bacteria within 24 hours after the trauma, a method must be utilized that will control the spread of the bacteria. In deep partial or full thickness burns, the blood vessels at the burn edges are occluded. Antibiotics therefore cannot reach the area via the bloodstream. This has led to the present three-pronged approach to combat sepsis. The bacteria are identified by surface culture, by biopsy of the eschar, and from blood samples. A surface antimicrobial ointment (such as Sulfamylon) is used on the burn surface, and the antibiotic to which the offending organism is sensitive is introduced into the undersurfaces of the eschar and is also given intravenously. Thus, antibacterial medication is delivered to the surface, into the burned tissue, and through the bloodstream.

Since patients may be easily contaminated by organisms carried by the staff caring for them, they are usually isolated during the early period of treatment until the burned areas can be covered by some protective method. This period, which may last for several weeks, is very stressful to the patient, both physiologically and psychologically. It is characterized by immobilization, painful debridement, and social isolation. After the skin is covered, infection and sepsis cease to be a problem.

Weight loss is secondary to marked energy loss. The destruction of skin results in heat being lost from the body. In compensation for this loss of insulation from the exterior, the body uses up an excessive amount of energy to produce heat to maintain body temperature. The weight loss may be as much as a pound per day. The patient is essentially in danger of starvation. Formulas have been derived from which the appropriate caloric requirement can be determined. For the average 125-pound (57 kg) person, the requirement for the patient lying at rest in bed is the same as that required by a soldier undergoing the rigors of basic training: 3,600 calories per day! Since this is too great an amount for a debilitated patient to ingest, it is necessary to use intravenous as well as oral routes for nutrition.

Urinary tract infections may develop because a catheter to continuously drain the bladder is usually required during fluid replacement therapy. These infections rarely produce problems after the acute phase.

Gastrointestinal disturbances related in part to feedings by nasal tube can also occur, but rarely require surgery. Electrical burns may cause gastrointestinal problems that require surgery and may produce some later disturbances.

Thrombophlebitis, particularly of superficial veins, is also of life-threatening importance in the acute phase, especially if major burns in the lower extremities have occurred. Postacute chronic vein insufficiency may also exist (see chap. 22).

Skin replacement. The goal of the acute treatment phase of burn care is to replace skin lost by the burn trauma. Prior to grafting the patient's own skin on the denuded area, there must be a bacteria-free, healthy base of tissue. After the wound has been completely debrided of dead tissue, it can be temporarily covered to allow the deeper tissue to recover from the effects of the burn. Coverage can be accomplished with the "biologic dressing."

There are two such dressings presently in use, the *xenograft* and the *homograft*. The xenograft is skin obtained from domestic animals; pig skin is the type most commonly used. This is harvested commercially, and one can receive a shipment by air of fresh pig skin graft on order from several commercial facilities. Homograft is skin harvested from cadavers. This skin can be maintained in a frozen state and used as required. The biologic dressing, whether xenograft or homograft, is usually removed every day or so, the wound cleaned, and a fresh dressing applied.

When the wound has developed a healthy tissue

base, the patient's own skin is removed from an uninvolved area (the donor site) as a partial thickness graft and placed over the wound. Depending on the surface area to be grafted and the amount and location of healthy skin, the same donor sites may have to be used repeatedly.

Postacute Treatment Phase

Contracture is mostly a problem after the acute phase. However, right from the time of injury until discharge from the hospital, and in some cases for a time after discharge, the patient must be exercised either actively or passively with the assistance of a physical therapist to maintain a normal range of motion in all joints in an effort to inhibit contracture formation. The patient must be positioned in such a way to prevent contractures over joints and consequent loss of function. In the case of burned areas, the body part must be held in the position opposing the direction a scar contracture is most likely to occur (figs. 31-5 and 31-6). These positions require the fabrication, usually by occupational therapists, of splints that must conform to each individual patient.

If contractures have developed, they will frequently yield to intensive physical therapy and such modalities as dynamic splinting or serial casting and ultrasound diathermy (high frequency sound which produces heat to increase the pliability of the joint). Contractures not yielding to these treatment modalities may require surgery (see chap. 32). Contracture complications may occur for about 2 years, the length of time it takes scar to mature.

Hypertrophic scars can be inhibited by pressure over the healing burn area before and following grafting. Since scar formation may well continue for a long period, it is necessary to use compressive dressings continually for a period of 1 year or more. Elasticized garments to achieve this are made by the Jobst Company. These garments must be fabricated from careful measurements of patients obtained either by representatives of the company or by personnel of the burn facility who have been specially trained. Since they must be worn continually, they are ordered in pairs and will have to be replaced several times during the period in which they must be worn. The company maintains a "hot line," which one can use to obtain the garment in 5 days from the reception of the order. These garments are especially tailored for the body part to be treated, as shown in figures 31-7, 31-8, and 31-9.

All burned patients with disfigurements, even if not functionally limiting, deserve review by a plastic surgeon for possible correction whether they are as severe as loss of facial members or simply unsightly scars or hair loss.

Chronic venous insufficiency secondary to severe

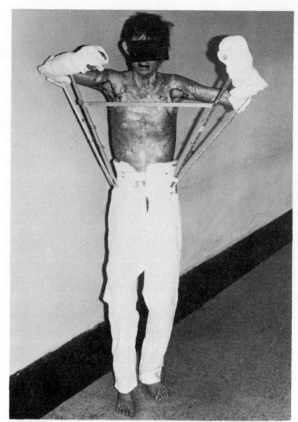

FIGURE 31-6. Bilateral abduction splint to prevent postgrafting adduction contracture in the underarm area.

lower extremity burns can be helped somewhat with elastic stockings similar to the garments discussed for control of hypertrophic scars.

VOCATIONAL IMPLICATIONS

Compressive garments, which are required for up to 2 years after burn injury, may represent a vocational barrier that deserves some consideration. The garments must be worn 24 hours a day. They are extremely warm, and hence work or rest in environments with high temperatures is not only uncomfortable for the patient, but shortens the life of the garments because of perspiration absorption. When worn as gloves, these garments prevent the wearer from using oily substances that will be absorbed into the garment. Therefore, the patient will have to wear rubber or protective gloves over the compressing fabric and this will reduce his dexterity. The use of the opaque face mask, which resembles a ski mask, frequently is unacceptable in certain occupations in which the person must deal with the public.

Cosmetic disfigurement, while temporary, may extend over a period of 2 or 3 years while plastic surgery is accomplished in stages. Vocational planning for proper placement of the burn patient may be

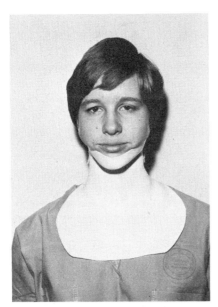

FIGURE 31-7. Neck conformer made from Orthoplast to prevent neck contracture in which chin would be fixed to the chest.

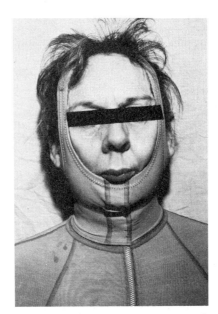

FIGURE 31-9. Jobst vest with neck and chin mask to control hypertrophic scar formation on neck and face.

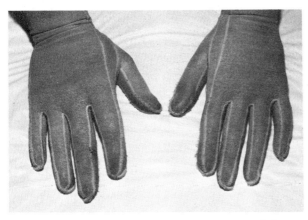

FIGURE 31-8. Compression Jobst gloves to control hypertrophic scar formation of hands, particularly between fingers.

required during this period. Burn patients rapidly become desensitized to their appearance, but the public frequently does not, and this presents a barrier to returning to work requiring interpersonal relationships.

The pigment cells found in the epidermis are lost in burn injury and require about 1 year to reconstitute; hence, patients should not expose the previously burned area to the sun for that period of time.

Since covered burned skin is not always as strong as normal skin, it may also be necessary to avoid occupations likely to produce trauma and irritation to the skin if the burned area is sufficiently extensive and exposed. Similarly, burned areas may not have as much fat insulation. If such areas are extensive, the person may not be able to tolerate environments which have very high or very low temperature extremes for

prolonged periods of time. Chronic pruritis may be exacerbated by extremely dry climates.

If there was a smoke inhalation problem with residual difficulty in the lungs, the person might not comfortably tolerate environments where there is much dust, smoke, or other particulate matter. However, problems from smoke inhalation are not likely to persist for more than 2 years after the injury.

Burn patients with a chronic insufficiency of the veins in their lower extremities may not be able to tolerate occupations requiring standing for prolonged periods without discomfort and development of edema.

Residual ambulation problems or contracture problems in the hands and shoulders may also restrict the range of occupations available to the severely burned patient. All of these must be carefully assessed and matched against available employment options. The same applies for persons with residual visual deficits.

The loss of limbs requires replacement with prostheses. The vocational implications of amputation are discussed in chapter 13.

BIBLIOGRAPHY

Abston S: Burns in children. CIBA Symposia 28, 1976. Provides an excellent description of the pathology and treatment of burns in children with descriptive illustrations. While the treatment is aimed at the pediatric population, the discussion forms a good basis for the understanding of burns in any age group.

American Burn Association, Office of Secretary, University Hospital and Clinics, University of Iowa, Newton Rd., Iowa City, IA 52240.

The Association is a good source from which educational materials can be obtained pertaining to the care of burned patients and the prevention of burns.

Andreasen NJC, Norris AS, Harford CE: Incidence of long-term psychiatric complications in severely burned adults. Ann Surg **174**:785–793, 1971.

An analysis of 20 severely burned adults seen from 1 to 5 years after injury. The results indicated that successful adjustment can be expected.

Andreasen NJ, Norris AS: Long-term adjustment and adaptation mechanisms in severely burned adults. J Nerv Ment Dis **154**:352–362, 1972.

Using a similar population to the above study, this study goes into more detail on such psychosocial aspects as family and social adjustment.

Chang FC, Herzog G: Burn morbidity: A followup study of physical and psychological disability. Ann Surg **183**:34–37, 1976.

A study of 51 patients who were interviewed about 2 years after burn injury to determine the effects of the injury on their ability to return to work or school, and on their social status.

Goldberg RT: Rehabilitation of the burn patient. Rehabil Lit **35**:73–78, 1974.

Discusses adult and child burns independently. Includes a summary of medical management, psychological, social, and economic aspects, as well as educational and vocational aspects.

Larson DL: *The Prevention and Correction of Burn Scar Contracture and Hypertrophy.* Galveston, TX, Shriners Burn Inst., 1973.

This is an easily read, copiously illustrated monograph on hypertrophic scar and methods of prevention.

Willis BA: *Burn Scar Hypertrophy, A Treatment Method.* Galveston, TX, Shriners Burn Institute.

A monograph explaining and illustrating the various types of Jobst Burn Supports.

32 PLASTIC AND RECONSTRUCTIVE SURGERY

Robert V. DeVito, M.D.

INTRODUCTION

Plastic surgery is the branch of surgery concerned with the correction or restoration of malformed, injured, or lost parts of the body. The earliest writings in plastic surgery (around 800 B.C.) recorded the rebuilding of noses amputated as punishment for certain crimes in India. Modern plastic surgery had its birth during World War I, when specialized units were established to care for facially wounded. Plastic surgery developed slowly for two decades and became a mature specialty during World War II, when centers were established throughout the world to care for wounded military personnel and civilians. Surgeons who worked in these wartime units subsequently established training programs, and the discipline has grown steadily since 1945.

If one takes a dictionary definition of rehabilitation—"to restore to a condition of good health, ability to work, or the like"—the indication for all plastic and reconstructive surgery is rehabilitation. The scope of procedures performed ranges from those obviously necessary for function to those which are purely "cosmetic" but nonetheless helpful for certain patients.

Plastic surgery plays a very important role in the rehabilitation of clients with many of the severe disabilities covered in other chapters of this text. For example, extensive skin grafting by a plastic surgeon is part of the primary treatment of severe burns and for complications of burns, such as contractures or hypertrophic scars. Contractures severe enough to require surgical correction may also be a complication of spinal cord injury, cerebral palsy, multiple sclerosis, and stroke. Plastic surgery is often required to correct various deformities secondary to cancer and its treatment, and also to repair decubitus ulcers in spinal cord injured clients. Hand deformities causing significant disability can often be corrected by plastic surgery, thus restoring hand function and greatly increasing the client's vocational opportunities. Because so many severely disabled persons have had rehabilitative plastic surgery or could benefit from such surgery, it is important for the counselor to understand the range of problems addressed and resolved by this specialty.

The counselor should also be aware that there may be some residual effects of plastic surgery that he should take into account in vocational planning with a client. For example, the site of surgery may be more tender and susceptible to re-injury; restricted joint range of motion may require therapy and may limit vocational choices; skin sensitivity may be affected; or there may be cosmetic considerations affecting vocational choice. The counselor should always obtain an evaluation of these residual effects from the plastic surgeon before proceeding with vocational planning with a client who has undergone plastic surgery.

Unlike most other surgical specialists, plastic surgeons do not confine their activities to a certain part of the body or to a given organ system, but rather use special techniques in many parts of the body. These special techniques and concepts include wound repair to promote optimal healing; grafts; flaps; use of certain synthetic implants (allografts); repositioning or remodelling of tissues; and reconstruction of body parts.

WOUND REPAIR

Incisional injury through skin or mucous membrane initiates an orderly sequence of cellular and chemical events. These events result in the production of fibrous tissue, or scar, which acts to heal the wound. All human wounds heal by scar tissue; hence all wounds produce scar.

If the wound edges are held close together by suturing or taping, the amount of scar is less and healing to a reasonably functional tensile strength more rapid than if the wound is left unrepaired. An unrepaired wound that is permitted to heal in by vascular, immature scar tissue (granulation tissue) may require several weeks to months to close completely. Wounds that "granulate in" heal by a process of scar contraction which slowly pulls the surrounding tissues together. Healing is particularly slow when the defect is large or when the adjacent tissues are tight. Such open wounds are painful, restrict activity, may require hospitalization, and are threatening by virtue of fluid and protein loss, possible bleeding, and possible destructive infection.

When wounds do finally heal by contraction, the end result is less satisfactory than if proper wound repair had been done. The excessive mass of scar tissue produced is often unsightly and is always inelastic compared to normal skin or mucous membrane. This inelastic property of fibrous tissue may produce contracture bands, which reduce or prevent motion of joints (see fig. 31-5, p. 412); strictures, which obstruct viscera; adhesions which interfere with joint or tendon action; and skin surface areas that break down with slight trauma because there is no cushioning "give" by the firm underlying scar.

Excessive, or hypertrophic, scar will develop in certain circumstances even when primary wound repair is performed. First, any wound subjected to persistent tension will tend to develop hypertrophic scarring. This is seen in contracture bands developing over flexor surfaces of joints and thick scars in vertical midline abdominal incisions (as compared to the fine scars of transverse abdominal wounds). Second, any wound subjected to an intense inflammatory reaction early in healing will tend to produce more scar. This inflammation may be caused by infection, harsh chemicals, foreign debris left in the wound, or irritating suture material.

Hypertrophic scarring is usually not apparent for 3 to 4 months following wound repair. Although sutures may be removed when the wound tensile strength is sufficient to resist disruption (usually in several days), the collagen of fibrous tissue continues to be deposited and continues to change in its chemical and physical nature. It usually reaches its peak of volume in 3 to 4 months. Subsequently, collagen matures and shrinks in mass, so that hypertrophic scar may slowly reduce to an acceptable level over 6 to 24 months. For this reason, attempts are rarely made to correct scar problems until a year or more after the original wound repair.

The plastic surgeon uses these data constantly to promote optimal wound healing without excessive scar. Incisions and lacerations are repaired as quickly as possible with gentle technique to avoid tissue damage, reduce infection, and minimize inflammation by foreign material, caustic antiseptics, or inappropriate suture material. Wound tension is reduced or avoided by correct orientation of incisions and by mobilization of adjacent tissues. When necessary, skin can be transplanted into the wound to provide safe closure without tension or disfiguring distortion.

GRAFTS

Free Grafts

Skin may be transplanted into wounds as a free graft. A *skin graft* is completely separated (i.e., free) from its source, or *donor site*, and transferred to the wound requiring coverage (the *recipient site*). Such grafts have no initial blood supply. They must survive for 2 to 3 days simply by osmosis or transudation of nutrients into and waste products out of the skin. Later, circulation develops between the graft and its recipient bed. It is therefore obvious that skin grafts must be thin (consisting of skin only, without fat) and that an intimate contact must be maintained between the graft and an adequately vascular bed without gross pus during this critical time period.

All skin grafts require that the donor site be protected from infection, and that the graft be meticulously held in firm contact with the recipient bed. Small grafts can be done as outpatient procedures, but most skin grafts require hospitalization of several days to ensure success. Activity levels depend on the degree of immobilization required to protect the skin graft.

Split-thickness grafts. A skin graft comprised of only part of the skin layers is called a split-thickness graft. (For a discussion of the structure and function of the skin, see chap. 31, p. 409.) Because the epidermal cells of the dermis have the capability of forming a new epidermal layer when that layer is removed, it is possible to remove large sheets of skin as split-grafts. The donor site will reconstitute itself by re-epithelialization, without scar.

Several hundred square inches of skin can be taken, using special cutting instruments of diverse design called *dermatomes* and used, for example, to cover large burn areas. Split-thickness skin grafts may be sliced off as extremely thin sheets (8/1,000"-10/1,000") where rapid successful wound coverage is necessary (fig. 32-1). Thicker split-grafts (16/1,000"-20/1,000") would be more suitable for isolated large skin defects, such as hand or face wounds (fig. 32-2).

Full-thickness grafts. Full-thickness grafts contain all of the dermis and hence leave a donor site wound which must be small enough so that it can be sutured closed, or must be grafted with split-thickness skin. Full-thickness grafts are therefore generally only several square inches in size and used only for specific purposes. Thin skin grafts generally "take" better because nourishment is better assured prior to vascularization, and because they conform better to irregular wound contours. The thicker the graft, the more like normal skin it is with respect to elasticity, texture, color, and hair growth. Full-thickness skin grafts are used to cover small wounds, particularly where elasticity is important, such as in eyelid replacement.

Flap Grafts

A *flap* consists of a segment of skin and subcutaneous fat that is elevated from its donor site but left attached

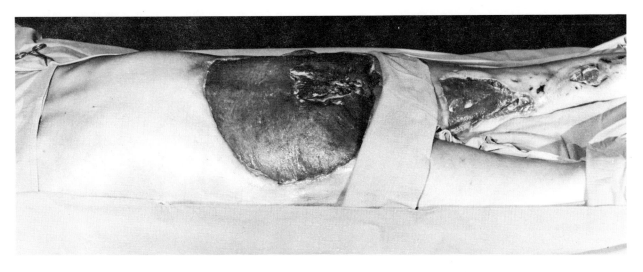

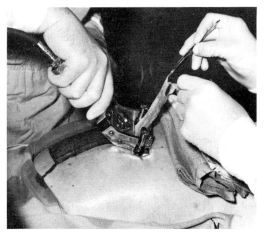

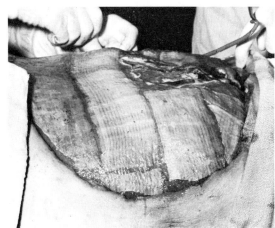

FIGURE 32-1. *(Above)* Granulating defect over sacrum and buttocks of middle-aged man, ready for skin grafting. *(Below, left)* Thin split-thickness grafts are taken with the Brown dermatome from the donor site on the patient's back, 3 inches wide and approximately 10/1,000 inches thick. *(Below, right)* The thin grafts laid in place, requiring no sutures or dressings.

at one margin so that an intact blood supply (arterial and venous) is preserved to nourish the freed-up portion of the flap. This free end is then sutured into the recipient wound and is maintained by the donor site circulation.

Flaps are used for wound closure when subcutaneous fat as well as skin is necessary for adequate repair. Examples are contour defects; wounds exposing joints, major vessels, nerves, and tendons; and wounds that would not stand up to abrasive wear and tear or pressure unless fat padding is provided. Flaps are also required to reconstruct defects with poor circulation, such as radiated tissues which would not nourish a free skin graft, and to reconstruct portions of the oral cavity.

Local flaps. A *simple* local flap is produced when the subcutaneous tissues adjacent to an open wound are loosened or detached (*undermined*) from their deep connective tissue attachments overlying muscle so that the skin can be more easily sutured closed (fig. 32-3).

When undermining does not free up the tissue sufficiently to permit moving it into the open wound, incisions are made around most of the perimeter to produce a *pedicle flap* (fig. 32-4). The flap must remain attached at one margin, the pedicle, so that blood supply is adequate to keep the mobilized skin and fat alive. Examples are transposition and rotation flaps used to repair decubiti (see chap. 5).

In designing flaps, it is of paramount importance that an adequate base, or donor site continuity, be maintained for circulation while mobilizing sufficient tissue to permit wound closure. When a discrete arterial and venous system is identifiable, large blocks of tissue can be transferred with an extremely narrow base containing essentially only the single artery and vein (axial blood supply). In other circumstances, an axial blood supply does not exist and the flap is based on random circulation. In this case, the length of the flap that can be adequately perfused by the base circulation available may be much less. For these reasons, flaps of different types must be used for specific purposes.

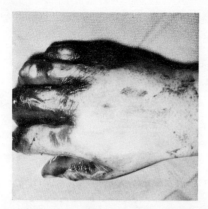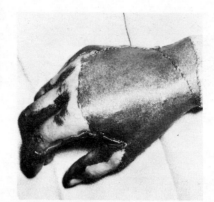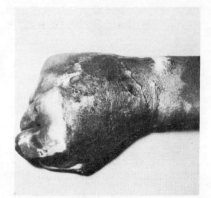

FIGURE 32-2. *(Left)* A hand burn 2 hours after injury; obviously total thickness in extent, as shown by total loss of pigment of burned area on black male. *(Center)* A thick split-thickness skin graft (24/1,000 inch thick) from the thigh sutured carefully into place after excision of the burn on the day of injury. Thick grafts contain elastic tissue and must be sutured to hold them in place. *(Right)* The totally healed hand with full range of flexion 6 weeks after injury.

Regional flaps. Regional flaps are elevated from parts of the body close to the defect, and span an intervening area of uninvolved tissue to be sutured into the defect (fig. 32-5). As the flap heals in place, a capillary circulation develops between the recipient site and the flap, sufficient to nourish the flap itself. The pedicle can usually be amputated within 3 weeks and the unused portion of the flap returned to its donor bed. Examples of regional flaps are forehead flaps to build the nose or reconstruct cheek defects, and chest flaps brought up to the neck.

Distant flaps. Distant flaps are transferred to one part of the body from another. As in the regional flap, the pedicle is divided when circulation is adequate at the recipient site. Examples of distant flaps are cross-leg flaps (fig. 32-6) and abdomen-to-hand flaps.

When a direct transfer from donor site to recipient site is not possible, indirect transfers are done. A common example of indirect flap transfer involves raising an abdominal pedicle and suturing it into the wrist as a temporary recipient site. Three weeks later (after wrist circulation is established), the base of the abdominal flap is sectioned and the arm is then used as a carrier to transport the now-free pedicle to the scalp, face, leg, or wherever the defect might be. After an additional 3 weeks of healing, the wrist pedicle can be divided, leaving the abdominal flap in its distant recipient site.

The donor site wound created by elevation of a flap can sometimes be closed by undermining and primary suture, but often must be closed by split-thickness skin grafting. Local and regional flaps are used whenever possible, but when suitable donor tissue is not available close to the wound, distant flaps must be used, even though the prolonged immobilization required is uncomfortable and requires hospitalization.

Special Grafts

Island flaps. Tissue, including skin, can be

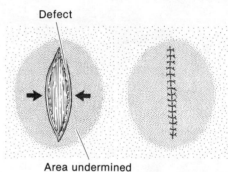

FIGURE 32-3. Simple local flap. *(A)* The subcutaneous fat under the skin in region of arrows is freed from deeper tissues. *(B)* The freed edges are brought together over the wound and sutured.

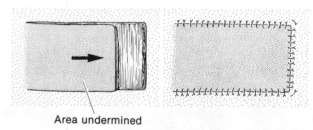

FIGURE 32-4. Pedicle flap. *(A)* A "tongue" of skin and subcutaneous fat under arrow is freed from the deeper tissues. *(B)* It is then moved over the wound defect and sutured.

transplanted as an island flap when it has a discrete blood supply. The blood supply of the tissue to be moved does not come from neighboring skin, but rather from deeper vessels. These vessels, and sometimes the sensory nerves serving the tissue, can be freed from their original bed and moved. Thus, a precise block of tissue (the island) can be cut free from the donor site and moved with the freed blood supply and nerve, sometimes subcutaneously, to the defect to be closed.

An example of an island flap that is transferred subcutaneously is the movement of hair-bearing

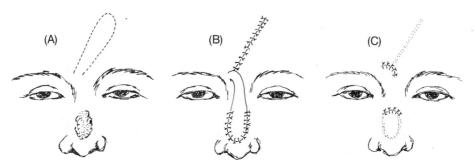

FIGURE 32-5. Regional flap. *(A)* To cover the defect over the nose, a "tongue" of skin and subcutaneous tissue is lifted off forehead. *(B)* The end of the "tongue" is sutured onto the defect, but its base is left attached to supply blood. The forehead wound is closed by a simple local flap (fig. 32-3). *(C)* When the "tongue" has developed a blood supply from neighboring nose tissue, its base is cut and discarded and all edges are sutured.

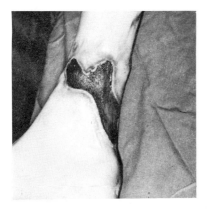 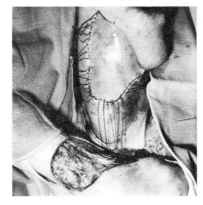 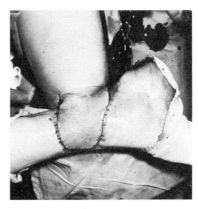

FIGURE 32-6. *(Left)* A chronic ulcer over the right ankle, medial aspect, after several unsuccessful attempts at split-thickness skin grafting. Split-skin grafts in such areas do not stand up to wear and tear. Local flaps are not available, so a cross-leg flap is used. *(Center)* The right ankle ulcer has been excised, and the right foot lies over the left knee area to receive a large thigh flap raised above the left knee; the flap donor site has been repaired with a split-thickness skin graft. *(Right)* The left thigh flap has been sutured into the ankle defect. The patient will be maintained in this position by plaster casts for three weeks, when the flap will have healed into the ankle sufficiently to permit division of the flap base from the thigh.

temporal skin in front of the ear with its vascular pedicle to reconstruct eyebrows. Similarly, sensation can be provided to a denervated index finger tip by elevating an island flap from the ring finger (where loss of sensation is less crippling) and passing it subcutaneously, together with its digital vessel and nerve pedicle, to the index finger tip.

More than skin and fat can be transferred with the island flap technique. Thumb reconstruction for amputation or congenital absence can be accomplished by mobilizing an entire digit (usually the index finger), including bones, joints, tendons, and covering skin, with the neurovascular pedicle intact, and transferring it directly to the thumb position *(pollicization)* with remarkable success (fig. 32-7).

Free flaps. Advances in microvascular surgery permitting successful anastomosis of vessels in the 1.5 –2.0 mm range are now permitting free transfers of flap tissue to all parts of the body, as well as successful replantation or transplantation of digits. Arteries and veins which are cut at the donor site are sutured to

vessels at the recipient site. The transferred flap then is nourished directly from the vascular system of the recipient site. This is an exciting new technique in plastic surgery which should continue to develop and be more widely used.

Other Grafts

Homografts and heterografts. A skin graft taken from an individual's own body is called an *autograft*. Sometimes skin taken from other humans (*homografts*) or skin taken from other species (*heterografts*) are used as temporary biological dressings in certain large wounds, such as burns and areas where skin has been torn off (avulsions). Unlike autografts, homografts and heterografts will not establish an effective circulation with the recipient wound because of immunological rejection. Therefore, they will not survive for more than a short period of time. They can be, and are, used as temporary dressings, however, to reduce fluid loss, to clean up or reduce infection in the wound, and to

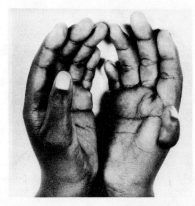
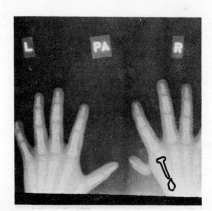
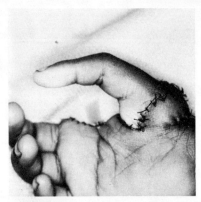
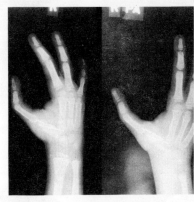
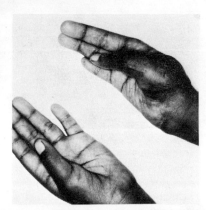

FIGURE 32-7. *(Above, left)* This youngster was born with a congenitally deficient right thumb. *(Above, right)*X-rays showing the bony deficiency of thumb structures on the right, as compared to the left, with bone-peg to be fashioned from the index metacarpal drawn in. *(Below, left)* The right index has been transposed into thumb position as an island flap—completely separated from all skin attachments but with nerves, blood vessels, and tendons left intact. *(Below, center)* X-ray of reconstructed right hand, showing the index now in thumb position. *(Below, right)* Function of the new thumb. Good opposition is provided by a ring finger superficialis tendon transfer to the thumb.

prepare the wound for autografting.

Cartilage grafts. Cartilage grafts are used to correct contour defects and to reconstruct ears. Autogenous grafts survive as living tissue and show little loss in volume after transplantation. Homografts are not completely rejected, as in skin, but the chondrocytes die and are replaced, so that there is always significant shrinkage and distortion in cartilage homografts. Cartilage heterografts are slowly but totally absorbed and hence are never used. Rib cartilage is a ready source for cartilage autografts. After removal, it can easily be carved to shape for subcutaneous implantation where needed.

Bone grafts. Bone grafts are used extensively in plastic surgery to aid in healing of fractures, to repair nonunited fractures, to restore contour defects of the facial skeleton, and to immobilize repositioned bony parts in major facial reconstructive procedures. The bone graft may serve only as a matrix and as a source of calcium salts so that osteogenesis in the graft area is potentiated. In certain circumstances, the osteoblasts of the graft do survive and participate in the remodelling osteogenesis that occurs, so more rapid and effective incorporation occurs.

Autografts survive as viable grafts better than homografts, and autografts of cancellous bone function better than autografts of dense cortical bone. The iliac crest is a favorite donor site because of its large amount of cancellous bone. The ribs are also a large "bone bank," since several ribs can be removed subperiosteally in a single patient. The remaining "tube" of periosteum forms a new rib. However, ribs have restricted use because they are mainly cortical bone. A bone-grafted area is treated as a fracture, and the part must be immobilized for several weeks so that solid union occurs.

Fat grafts. Fat can be transplanted as an autograft to improve soft tissue contour defects. For ease in handling, the fat is removed from its donor site with an intact layer of dermis over it, so it is often referred to as a dermal-fat graft. A 30–50 percent overcorrection is usually performed in anticipation of some reabsorption of fat, which always occurs in these grafts.

Tendon grafts. Tendon grafts are used to restore

continuity of destroyed or damaged tendons, usually in the hand. The tendons of the palmaris longus muscle in the forearm (when present) and the plantaris muscle in the calf are the most common donor sites. Because tendon heals slowly, prolonged immobilization followed by protected motion is required in tendon graft surgery.

Nerve grafts. Nerve grafts are used to bridge gaps in nerves secondary to trauma or cancer excisions. These grafts function as a conduit along which regenerating nerve fibers grow to reach the distal nerve stump and hence reach the muscle or sensory organ the nerve serves. They are autografts, usually taking less important nerves to replace the missing nerves.

Allografts

A wide diversity of nonliving materials have been and are being used as implants to correct contour defects and as structural members to bridge gaps in tissues. Metal pins, screws, rods, and plates are used in facial fracture repairs, and plastic materials are used to correct contour defects in many areas. Specially shaped implants are used as a subcutaneous framework to reconstruct missing body parts. Silicone is the most widely used implant material because it stimulates minimal inflammatory response and because it is available in a wide range of forms—gel, semigel, soft to hard rubbers, sheets, sponges of various densities, and preformed prostheses of all types. The allograft materials have the advantage of not requiring additional surgery to obtain graft material, but all are more susceptible to infection (and hence failure) than are grafts of living tissue. Since they never become totally incorporated, they are susceptible to motion, change in position, and even extrusion.

REMODELING AND REPOSITIONING PROCEDURES

Plastic surgeons do many reconstructive procedures by simply repositioning tissues into a more functional or acceptable position. In certain acute injuries, such reconstruction may merely be a repositioning of displaced tissues into their previous anatomic location, as is done in fractures of the face and jaws, for example.

In other circumstances, the reconstruction involves "taking apart" operations so that body parts can be totally reshaped and restructured. A deformed ear may be corrected by resculpturing the ear cartilage, and an old nasal fracture corrected by taking the nasal bones apart with chisel and saw and then repositioning them in normal position. Grotesque congential deformities of the facial skeleton are repaired by multiple bone cuts (*osteotomies*) of the facial bones. The bones may be moved to normal position and held by direct wiring

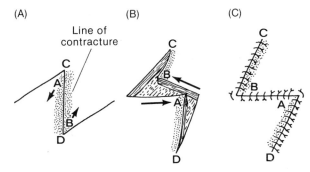

FIGURE 32-8. Z-plasty. *(A)* Cuts made through the skin and subcutaneous tissue are of equal length, and the diagonal passes through the middle of scar contracture (CD). Triangular flaps A and B are freed up and pulled back (arrows indicate movement of flap). *(B)* Flaps A and B are now transposed. Arrows now show direction of flap movement after transposition. *(C)* After suture, the length of skin between points C and D is now 1.8 times increased and the contracture is relieved.

plus autografts of bone. Tendon transfers are performed to put less necessary tendons to work serving the function of destroyed important tendons, as would be done when, for example, the tendon that flexes the middle phalanx of the ring finger (flexor digitorum superficialis) is detached from the phalanx and attached to the thumb to produce thumb opposition (fig 32-7).

SPECIFIC PROBLEMS AND PLASTIC SURGICAL MANAGEMENT

Plastic surgery can provide direct help for many specific rehabilitation problems. These, together with the reconstructive techniques used to correct them, are discussed below.

Hypertrophic Scars

Wounds that heal with excess scar may require reconstruction if the scar is unsightly, restricts motion, or is unstable and repeatedly breaks down, or ulcerates. Scar revisions should not be done until the collagen has matured, usually 12–24 months after initial healing.

When the scar is a narrow band (1 cm or less), repair usually involves a Z-plasty, which is simply a pair of triangular local flaps raised on either side of the central scar and then transposed across this central line (fig. 32-8). The Z-plasty reorients the scar lines, and inserts normal elastic tissue into the line of tightness so that contracture is relieved.

When the scar area is wide, it must be excised totally. The fresh wound so created is then reconstructed by either a thick split-thickness skin graft or by flap tissue, depending on the needs of the local area for elasticity, contour filling, and fat padding. Local flaps are always used in preference to distant flaps if adequate tissue is available.

Open Wounds and Tissue Defects

The simpliest, quickest, and surest way to manage chronic open wounds is to apply a split-thickness skin graft. A healed, sterile, pain-free wound is obtained in a matter of days with successful grafting. Split-grafting is the definitive procedure of choice whenever a healed graft will be acceptable cosmetically, will not restrict motion, and will tolerate daily wear and tear of the part involved. On occasion, a split-thickness skin graft should be used to get a healed sterile wound quickly as an intermediate stage prior to definitive flap procedures.

Certain wounds are better treated definitively by full-thickness grafts. Examples are eyelid defects where elasticity is important and palmar skin loss where toughness and resiliency of the graft are necessary.

When the wound bed does not have sufficient vascularity to nourish a skin graft, or indeed may require additional blood supply to survive (as when bone, tendon, or joints are exposed), coverage requires an appropriate pedicle flap. Pedicle flap coverage is also required when the wound area is subjected to repeated trauma or pressure and the padding effect of fat is necessary. Examples are ulcers on the ankle or in front of the tibia, wounds on the sole of the foot, and pressure sores.

Specific Deformities

Plastic surgery is involved in correction of many deformities of various body parts, using the techniques already described. Such malformations may be congenital, developmental, or acquired. *Congenital deformities* are present at birth, and usually represent incomplete or inappropriate development of body parts. *Developmental deformities* become manifest as growth or maturation of an originally normal body part is modified or interfered with by things such as muscle imbalance, denervation, external pressure by tumor masses, or tissue destruction by infection or trauma. *Acquired deformities* are secondary to direct destruction or distortion of tissue by infection, trauma, or surgery. The list of specific deformities that might be tabulated is almost endless. Certain deformities are of specific importance in rehabilitation, however, and will be briefly considered.

Deformities of the lips and oral cavity. A relatively common defect is *cleft lip and palate*, which occurs in 1 per 750 live births. While definitive repair is often totally accomplished in infancy and childhood, residual problems may require later reconstruction.

When initial lip repair has not been optimally successful, the cosmetic disfigurement is obvious and poor muscle anatomy may affect speech. Reconstruction requires redoing the lip repair, taking it apart and reshaping the local tissue to restore muscle continuity and produce symmetrical lip appearance. Such reconstruction can usually be done with local anesthesia and very brief hospitalization.

Persistent cleft palate problems usually involve oral-nasal fistulae, malpositioned gum segments with secondary malocclusion, and speech problems. Speech problems are due either to dental abnormalities or to continued leakage of air into the nose because the repaired palate is scarred or of insuffient length.

Fistulae are repaired by local flap techniques. Dental malpositions not correctable by orthodontics are reconstructed by osteotomies which permit repositioning of the bony segments and stabilization with the aid of bone grafts. Speech problems related to incompetent palate, if not responsive to speech therapy, require either palate lengthening surgery or partial closure of the pharyngeal space. In palate lengthening surgery, the entire soft palate is mobilized as a large flap and repositioned closer to the pharyngeal wall (palate pushback). To partially close the pharyngeal space, a flap is raised from the posterior pharynx and brought forward to be sutured into the edge of the soft palate (posterior pharyngeal flap).

Cleft lip patients often have associated nasal deformities that require plastic surgery of the nose (rhinoplasty) after adolescence, and cleft palate patients may have retarded development of the cheek bone that requires specific correction.

Some acquired deformities of the lips and oral cavity are secondary to treatment for cancer. Appropriate treatment of malignancies of the lips, cheeks, and tongue frequently entails surgical excision. Small cancers of the lip can be treated by total thickness "wedge" excision and primary closure. When more than one-third of the lip width must be removed, good function and appearance can be obtained by use of local flaps from the opposite lip or adjacent cheek for reconstruction.

Cancer of the tongue treated surgically often requires removal of one side of the tongue (hemiglossectomy). If the resultant defect were simply closed by direct suture, the remaining tongue would be so "tied down" that speech and swallowing would be restricted. Therefore, such defects are best reconstructed using regional flaps from the forehead, neck, or upper chest, performed at the time of the hemiglossectomy to promote rapid healing and return of function.

Similarly, cheek cancers often require excision of the total thickness of the cheek. The resultant hole into the mouth requires immediate closure by appropriate regional or local flaps.

Deformities of the jaws. Congenital jaw deformities

may be due to inadequate, excessive, or unequal growth of the upper or lower jaw. Apart from the cosmetic defect produced by such abberations, irregular contact of opposing upper and lower teeth (malocclusion) is a severe problem.

Correction involves preliminary orthodontics to determine the degree of malposition and the direction of surgical treatment necessary, plus initial realignment of teeth by "bands." The plastic surgery involved requires appropriate osteotomies to permit repositioning the jaw structures, often with bone grafts added to stabilize the new position or to augment surface contours of the bones.

Acquired jaw deformities usually involve loss of bone, so that replacement of the missing bone may require large blocks of bone graft from the ribs or iliac crest. Fractures of the jaw may result in persistent deformities requiring that the bones be "rebroken" (in actuality, requiring specific osteotomies) to realign the structures in the normal position, supplemented by bone grafts where necessary.

Deformities of the face. Congenital and developmental defects of the face include a number of syndromes eventuating in abnormal growth of the mid-face, orbits, and nose. Some include abnormal growth of the skull as well, and are called craniofacial defects. The maxilla, or cheek bone, may be underdeveloped or malpositioned. The orbits may be incompletely developed (hypoplastic), or widely separated so that the eyes are in a "wall-eye" position. In all of these malformations, surgery can be performed to "take apart" the facial bones, reposition them, and stabilize the structures with bone grafts. The dramatic improvement in appearance of such grotesquely affected patients can be the most important rehabilitation effect.

Acquired deformities of the mid-face often require bone grafts to recontour or replace missing bone. At times, overlying soft tissue deficiencies require appropriate local or regional flap reconstruction.

Deformities of the trunk. Congenital deformities of the trunk include breast asymmetry due to unilateral underdevelopment (hypoplasia) or overdevelopment (hypertrophy). Breast size can be augmented by implantation of a soft silicone prosthesis, and can be reduced by partial mastectomy with incisions and flaps designed to produce normal breast contour on closure. Developmental malformations include hypermastia, or breast enlargement of severe degree. Patients with hypermastia have significant problems due to the excessive breast weight producing neck and shoulder discomfort, and occasionally even brachial plexus (see p. 27) injury due to traction on neck structures. Correction is by reconstruction of the breast to reduce its size (reduction mammoplasty).

Acquired breast deformities include those related to childhood trauma (usually burns) destroying the breast, and those secondary to operation for cancer or premalignant disease. When reasonable skin cover remains, plastic surgery to enlarge the breast (augmentation mammoplasty) using a silicone prosthesis may be all that is required. When significant skin deficit exists, a local skin flap will be required prior to augmentation.

Ischemic ulcers (decubiti, pressure sores) are common trunk problems in paraplegics and quadriplegics. Patients with spinal injuries are more susceptible to such pressure sores than normal people, simply because they lack sensation and mobility to perceive and avoid pressure. Such defects require excision of all damaged tissue, with reconstruction by appropriate local or regional flaps to provide good tissue coverage capable of tolerating pressure.

Deformities of the hand. Reconstructive surgery of the hand is of extreme importance because hand function is so critical. The scope of hand surgery is very diverse, but generally involves the following concepts. Wounds are managed with meticulous technique to minimize scar hypertrophy which would limit motion and be hypersensitive. Soft tissue defects are appropriately resurfaced by grafts or flaps to reduce contractures, protect vital structures (nerves, tendons, joints), and to provide a durable skin surface. Nerves are repaired or reconstructed to provide sensation. Broken bones are anatomically reduced to preserve strength and function, and tendons are repaired, grafted, or transferred to maintain functional motion. Neurovascular skin pedicles are transferred to important parts of the hand when required. Entire digits can be moved from one part of the hand to another, and amputated parts can be reimplanted with microvascular surgical techniques.

COSMETIC SURGERY

Aesthetic, or cosmetic, surgery is a much misunderstood part of reconstructive surgery. While almost all reconstructive surgery involves some modification in appearance of the operated part — and hence could be considered cosmetic — few people question the validity of such correction when the affected body part is "abnormal." When the body part operated upon is within the broad range of "normal," reconstruction is considered to be totally cosmetic, and unfortunately often considered to be unnecessary.

Many persons are markedly affected by cosmetic defects, and operations to improve their appearance are extremely valuable in restoring such individuals to more complete function. Since the only valid test for a successful cosmetic result is a patient who is ultimately happier and hence more effective in daily activity, it is imperative that the patient's defect, expectations, and potential benefit be carefully evaluated preoperatively. The defect must be real and apparent, not imagined.

The expectations for benefit must be confined to an improved appearance only. Secondary potential benefits, such as a better marriage or job promotion, should not be anticipated. Finally, the surgeon must be able to perceive the result desired and be technically capable of performing the necessary operation.

Commonly performed cosmetic procedures include *rhinoplasty*, to improve appearance of the nose; *rhytidectomy* (or ''face-lift'') to reduce the wrinkles and sagging skin associated with premature aging; *blepharoplasty* to remove excess eyelid skin; *augmentation mammoplasty* to enlarge breast size; and *otoplasty* to correct protruding ears. There are many other cosmetic operations available for specific problems. They should not be dismissed as being done only for vanity. Those individuals who are less able to cope adequately with daily living because of concern about their body image are often totally rehabilitated by such procedures.

BIBLIOGRAPHY

Grabb WC, Smith JW (eds): *Plastic Surgery: A Concise Guide to Clinical Practices.* Ed 2, Boston, Little, Brown, 1973.
This textbook is a comprehensive guide to clinical practice of plastic surgery, designed for the medical student and house officer. It is well organized and illustrated and terminology is simply used and well defined so that even the most complex procedures can be understood.

Kazanjian VH, Converse JM: *Surgical Treatment of Facial Injuries.* Ed 3, Baltimore, Williams & Wilkins, 1974.
A comprehensive text covering the acute and reconstructive management of all facial injuries; it is therefore a wealth of information.

Longacre JJ: *Rehabilitation of the Facially Disfigured: Prevention of Irreversible Psychic Trauma by Early Reconstruction.* Springfield, IL, Thomas, 1973.
A collection of a large number of case reports with long-term followup of one surgeon's extensive experience with facially disfigured patients. Psychosocial aspects of reconstructive surgery are well discussed.

McGregor IA: *Fundamental Techniques of Plastic Surgery and Their Surgical Application.* Ed 6, Edinburgh, Churchill Livingstone, 1975.
This small volume is well described by its title and provides a valuable source for medical students and general surgical house staff. It does not pretend to cover specific operations, but superbly clarifies basic techniques used in all plastic surgery.

Sabiston DA (ed): *Textbook of Surgery: The Biological Basis of Modern Surgical Practice.* Ed 11, Philadelphia, Saunders, 1977.
The broad area of surgical practice is covered in this textbook. Excellent chapters are devoted to wound healing, burns, and basic plastic surgical techniques and would therefore be of value.

GLOSSARY

ABDUCTION The movement of an extremity (an arm or a leg) away from the midline of the body. The muscles that perform such a function are generally called *abductors*.

ACIDOSIS An abnormal condition in which the blood is more acid than normal.

ACUTE A sudden change, generally used to characterize a change in health.

ACUTE TUBULAR NEPHROSIS See VASOMOTOR NEPHROPATHY.

ADENOCARCINOMA A malignant tumor of glandular origin or with a glandlike cell arrangement.

ADDUCTION A movement that draws a displaced body part, usually an arm or a leg, toward the center or midline of the body. The muscles that perform such a function are generally referred to as *adductors*.

ADHESIONS The joining together, by fibrous tissue, of bodily parts or tissues that are normally separate.

AFFERENT NEURON A nerve that transmits sensory impulses from the periphery toward the central nervous system.

AGRAPHIA Inability to write.

ALEXIA Inability to read.

ANALGESIC Causing a painless, although fully conscious, state.

ANASTOMOSIS A joining together of two separated but similar tissues, such as skin, blood vessels, or nerves.

ANEMIA A decrease in red blood cells or amount of hemoglobin, or both, in the bloodstream, resulting in paleness and generalized weakness.

ANESTHESIA Loss of sensation. May be limited to a specific area (local anesthesia) or involve a loss of consciousness (general anesthesia).

ANEURYSM A sac formed by the "ballooning out" of the weakened wall of an artery or the wall of the heart.

ANGIOGRAPHY Process of visualizing blood vessels with X-rays after first injecting a radiopaque substance.

ANTAGONIST A muscle or drug that acts in opposition to or counteracts another.

ANTERIOR HORN CELL The motor neuron cell body located in the ventral (anterior) horn of the spinal cord; the nerve cell of the motor unit.

ANTIBODIES Proteins produced in the body in response to the body's contact with an antigen, and having the specific capacity of neutralizing the antigen and hence creating immunity to it.

ANTIGEN An enzyme, toxin, or other substance, usually of high molecular weight, to which the body reacts by producing a specific antibody.

APHAKIA Absence of the lens in an eye.

AORTA The largest artery in the body. It distributes blood to the lower part of the body as the thoracic aorta and abdominal aorta, and sends branches to the upper extremities and head from the ascending aorta.

APHASIA A general language deficit affecting the ability to read, write, listen, and talk, usually secondary to stroke or traumatic brain damage to the left cerebral hemisphere.

APRAXIA The inability to voluntarily perform a learned motor movement in the absence of paralysis or paresis.

APTITUDES Natural abilities or skills.

ARTERIOLES The smallest branches of an artery.

ARTERIOSCLEROSIS Hardening, thickening, and loss of elasticity of the walls of the smaller arteries (arterioles).

ARTHROPLASTY Surgical repair of a joint.

ASPHYXIATION Suffocation.

ASSOCIATION AREAS Areas of the cerebral hemispheres that connect the different parts and are concerned with higher mental function. Also contribute to interpretation of related information.

ASTERIXIS A motor disturbance marked by inability to hold a fixed posture or position, usually involving the hand.

ASTROCYTOMA A malignant tumor, usually of the brain, derived from a central nervous system connective tissue cell.

ATAXIA Total or partial inability to coordinate voluntary bodily movements, especially muscular movements.

ATELECTASIS   Collapse of all or part of a lung.

ATHEROSCLEROSIS   Extremely common form of arteriosclerosis in which deposits of fatty substances are formed within and beneath the innermost layer (intima) of arterial walls.

ATHETOSIS   Constantly recurring series of purposeless motions of the hands and feet, usually the result of a brain lesion.

ATRIUM   The upper chamber on either side of the heart. The right atrium receives venous blood from the inferior and superior vena cava; the left atrium receives arterial blood from the pulmonary veins.

AUDITORY EVOKED CEREBRAL POTENTIAL   The interval between production of a sound and the brain wave produced by it.

AUTONOMIC DYSREFLEXIA   Sudden increase in blood pressure, with profuse sweating and flushing, usually caused by overdistension of bowel or bladder in quadriplegic patients.

AUTONOMIC DYSTONIA   Dysfunction of the autonomic nervous sytem, giving rise, in patients with kidney disease, to postural hypotension, impotence, and lack of sweating.

AUTONOMIC NERVOUS SYSTEM   Divided into the sympathetic and parasympathetic systems. Functions automatically and controls the motor functions of the heart, lungs, intestines, glands, and other internal organs, and the smooth muscles, blood vessels, and lymph vessels.

AUTOSOME   Any chromosome that is not a sex chromosome.

AUTOSPLENECTOMY   Disappearance of the spleen through progressive fibrosis and shrinkage; occurs in sickle cell anemia.

AXON   Central core that forms the essential conducting part of a nerve fiber. It is a long nerve cell process that carries impulses from the cell body.

BIOFEEDBACK   The process whereby an instrument is used to inform a subject of the magnitude of a particular function, such as muscle activity, to assist the person's control of that function.

BIOPSY   Removal and examination under the microscope of body tissue, usually for diagnostic purposes.

BOECK'S SARCOID   A chronic and benign infectious disease of unknown cause involving various structures, such as the lungs, salivary glands, lymph nodes, bones of the hands and feet, skin, and eyes.

BRAIN SCAN   A test used to visualize brain damage. After injection of a radioactive substance into the blood, a special counter scans across the skull and records where the radioactivity is localized.

CALCULUS   A stony mass or deposit formed in the body, as in the kidney. The plural is *calculi*.

CARDIAC CATHETERIZATION   A diagnostic procedure in which a thin tube is passed through an artery or vein until it reaches the inside of the heart to record the pressures in the various chambers and to inject radiopaque dyes for X-ray visualization.

CARDIOTONIC   Usually refers to a drug that can affect the force of contraction of the heart muscle.

CAROTID   Designating, of, or near either of the two principal arteries, one on each side of the neck, which convey the blood from the aorta to the head.

CARTILAGE   A gristle or elastic substance attached to articular bone surfaces. It is a kind of dense connective tissue, usually at the joints.

C.A.T.   An abbreviation for computerized axial tomography, a special X-ray technique for visualizing the cross-section of various structures in the body, in particular the brain.

CEREBRAL ARTERIOGRAM   X-ray of cerebral arteries after injection of a radiopaque substance into the vessels.

CENTRAL NERVOUS SYSTEM   Comprised of the brain and the spinal cord, as well as the nerve trunks and fibers connected with them; also known as the cerebrospinal system.

CHONDROCYTE   The specialized connective tissue cell present in cartilage.

CHRONIC   Persisting for a long time.

CIRRHOSIS   A disease of the liver in which there is progressive destruction of the cells and excess formation of connective tissue. Usually associated with chronic alcoholism and malnutrition.

COGNITIVE ABILITY   The ability to accumulate and retain new knowledge.

COLLAGEN   The main supportive protein of skin, tendon, bone, cartilage, and connective tissue.

COLLAGENOUS   Pertaining to or producing collagen.

COLOSTOMY   Surgery to create an opening between the colon and the outside of the body; also refers to the opening itself. Made to divert the feces from exiting at the anus.

CONDYLES   Prominences of the long bones, usually at the ends close to the joints.

CONTRACTURES   Shortening of the tissues surrounding a joint, preventing full range of motion of the joint.

CORONARY   A left or right artery that arises from a coronary sinus in the heart and distributes to either the left ventricle and atrium or the right ventricle and atrium.

CORONARY ARTERIOGRAPHY   An X-ray technique for visualizing the coronary blood vessels of the heart.

CORTISONE   One of the steroids elaborated by the adrenal gland. The term is sometimes used to indicate the whole family of corticosteroids, simply called steroids. Can also be given as a drug.

CRANIAL NERVES   Nerves that originate in the brain, including the 12 cranial nerves proper, their branches, and their ganglia.

CRANIOPHARYNGIOMA A tumor of the pituitary gland which produces symptoms of reduced pituitary hormone function.

DEBRIDEMENT Removal of dead tissue and foreign matter from a wound until healthy tissue is exposed.

DECUBITUS ULCER Bedsore or pressure ulcer caused by prolonged bed rest, with vascular compression.

DENERVATION Loss of nerve supply to a muscle (axon disrupted).

DEPRESSORS Muscles that draw some part of the body down, usually the shoulders.

DERMOID Resembling skin.

DIATHERMY A technique for heating body tissues using high-frequency electromagnetic radiation or sound vibrations (ultrasound).

DIPLOPIA Double vision.

DISTAL Situated away from a point of origin or attachment, such as of a bone or a limb; opposite of proximal. For example, the shoulder is proximal and the hand is distal.

DIURETIC Increasing the secretion and flow of urine. Also applies to a drug that increases urine secretion by drawing water out of the blood and the tissues.

DORSAL Pertaining to the back or a position toward or on the back side of a structure (posterior).

DORSIFLEXION Backward bending of a part, such as a hand or foot. The muscles that perform this function are called *dorsiflexors*.

DYSARTHRIA An incoordination of the muscles of respiration, phonation, articulation, and resonation, leading to slurred and imprecise speech. Sometimes also accompanied by swallowing problems.

DYSEQUILIBRIUM SYNDROME A condition following renal dialysis, resulting from rapid removal of water and/or electrolytes, giving symptoms of headaches, low blood pressure, fainting, weakness, and sometimes convulsion or coma.

DYSPHAGIA Difficulty in swallowing.

DYSPHASIA Same as aphasia, although generally used for a less severe speech and language disturbance.

DYSPNEA Difficulty in breathing.

DYSPRAXIA A disturbance in the motor patterns for speech, resulting from an inability to voluntarily select, organize, and/or sequence the speech musculature. Same as apraxia.

DYSURIA Painful urination.

ECHOCARDIOGRAM A noninvasive technique for visualizing the thickness of the walls of the heart and the character of the heart valve by measuring the reflection of sound waves directed at the heart.

ECHOENCEPHALOGRAPHY A diagnostic technique in which ultrasonic waves are beamed through the head from both sides. The echoes from the midline structures of the brain are recorded on a graph. Shifts from the midline may indicate a centrally placed mass.

ECLAMPSIA Convulsions and coma occurring late in pregnancy or during childbirth, associated with edema, elevated blood pressure, and/or proteinuria. Also called toxemia of pregnancy.

EDEMA Swelling, resulting from an excessive accumulation of fluid in the tissue.

EFFERENT NEURON A nerve that transmits motor impulses from the central nervous system toward the periphery.

ELECTROCARDIOGRAM (ECG, EKG) Graphic tracing of the electrical voltages produced by the heart muscle during contraction.

ELECTROENCEPHALOGRAM (EEG) Graphic tracing of the electrical voltages developed in the brain (brain waves).

ELECTROLYTE SOLUTION A solution of ions, usually sodium, potassium, chloride, and bicarbonate.

ELECTROMYOGRAPHY (EMG) A technique for recording muscle action potentials for the detection of nerve and muscle disease.

ELEVATORS Muscles that raise a body part; usually refers to the shoulder.

EMBOLUS Undissolved material, such as a clot, a fat globule, or an air bubble, carried by the blood from one vessel into a smaller one which is thereby obstructed.

ENDOTHELIUM Single layer of epithelial cells lining the cavities of the heart, blood vessels, lymph vessels, the pleura, and the peritoneum.

ENTERITIS Inflammation of the intestine.

EOSINOPHIL CELLS White blood cells that are readily stained with eosin. Their number greatly increases in certain allergic and parasitic diseases.

EPITHELIUM Epithelial tissue covering the external and internal surfaces of the body and lining the digestive, respiratory, and urinary tracts. It may be ciliated (fringes of hair on a free surface), columnar, simple, squamous, or transitional.

EVERTER A muscle that turns a part, such as a foot, out.

EXPECTORATION The act of coughing up and spitting out material from the lungs, bronchi, and trachea.

EXTENSION Straightening or unbending of a joint. This movement is the opposite of flexion.

EXTRAVASATED Discharged, as of blood, from a vessel into the tissues.

FISTULA An abnormal passage between two internal organs or between an internal organ and the surface of the body.

FLEXION Bending at a joint, such as the elbow or knee. Opposite of extension.

GAIT, FOUR-POINT A walking pattern using two crutches. In sequence, the right crutch, left leg, left crutch, and right leg are advanced. Used by lumbar-level paraplegics and others with very weak lower extremities.

GAIT, SWING-THROUGH A walking pattern using two crutches. In sequence, the two crutches are simultaneously advanced and then the two legs are lifted and swung through and past the two crutches. Used mostly by thoracic-level paraplegics.

GLIOMA A tumor made up of the supporting structure cells of nervous tissue, usually within the central nervous system.

GLOMERULONEPHRITIS Infection or inflammation of the capillary loops in the glomeruli. It occurs in chronic, subacute, and acute forms, and is usually secondary to an infection, especially with a hemolytic streptococcus.

GLOSSOPHARYNGEAL BREATHING A technique for breathing which, when taught, can be used for short periods by patients with weak or totally paralyzed respiratory muscles. The technique literally involves the swallowing of air into the lungs utilizing the throat and tongue muscles.

HEART MURMUR An abnormal sound heard through a stethoscope between the regular heartbeats. It is caused by turbulence in the blood flow through the heart, secondary to defects in heart valves.

HEAVY WORK Maximum lifting requirement of 100 pounds (45 kg). Usual lifting requirement of 50 pounds (22.5 kg).

HEMATOCRIT (HCT) The volume percentage of red blood cells in whole blood. Useful to assess if anemia is present.

HEMATOMA A local swelling or tumor filled with blood.

HEMATURIA Presence of blood in the urine.

HEMIPARESIS Muscular weakness of one side of the body.

HEMOGLOBINURIC NEPHROSIS See VASO-MOTOR NEPHROPATHY.

HEMOSTASIS Stoppage of bleeding.

HOMEOSTASIS The tendency of the physiological system to maintain internal stability.

HYPERPLASIA Abnormal increase in the number of cells in a tissue, causing enlargement of the tissue.

HYPERTENSION High blood pressure.

HYPERTHYROIDSM A condition in which there is overfunctioning of the thyroid gland, with consequent enlargement of the gland and excessive secretion of thyroxine hormone.

HYPOCALCEMIC TETANY A condition of excess muscle twitching and irritability brought about by a low concentration of calcium in the blood.

HYPOGENITALISM A condition resulting from, or, characterized by, abnormally decreased functional activity of ovaries or testes, with retardation of growth and sexual development.

HYPOPARATHYROIDISM A condition of reduced activity of the parathyroid gland, with reduction in the secretion of parathyroid hormone and a subsequent disturbance in bone metabolism, leading to osteoporosis.

HZ (HERTZ) One cycle per second; the unit used to measure frequency.

ILEOSTOMY Surgical creation of an opening through the abdominal wall into the ileum, the lowest portion of the small intestine.

INFARCTION The formation of an infarct, i.e., an area of coagulation necrosis in a tissue, caused by local anemia resulting from the obstruction of circulation to the area. May be embolic or thrombotic.

IMMUNOGLOBULINS Special high molecular weight proteins produced by the body's defense systems; they are essentially antibodies and circulate in the blood.

IMMUNOTHERAPY A specialized chemical used in the treatment of cancer and other conditions to counteract either antigens or abnormal immunoglobulins.

INCIDENCE The number of new cases of a disease occurring during a certain period.

INNERVATE Furnish with nerves; grow nerves into.

INNERVATION Distribution or supply of nerves to a body part.

INTENTION TREMOR Involuntary trembling or quivering that arises or is intensified when a voluntary, coordinated movement is attempted.

INTERCOSTAL Between the ribs.

INTERSTITIAL NEPHRITIS Inflammatory disease involving the supporting tissue of the kidney and caused by numerous agents, including certain antibiotics, antipyretics, and analgesics, as well as bacteria.

ISCHEMIA Deficiency of blood in a part of the body, caused by constriction or obstruction of blood vessels.

LIGHT WORK Maximum lifting requirement of 20 pounds (9 kg). Significant walking or standing requirements. Heavy requirement for pushing, pulling, or leg control while seated.

LIMBIC SYSTEM A region deep within the cerebral hemispheres containing several nuclei and many tracts, which interconnect with the deeper brain structures as well as with the cortex. This region is concerned with functions such as memory and the emotions.

LOWER MOTOR NEURON Pathway from the anterior horn cell to the muscle fiber.

LOWER NEPHRON NEPHROSIS Old name for vasomotor nephropathy.

LUPUS ERYTHEMATOSIS A disease of unknown cause associated with involvement of many organs with inflammatory-like lesions. In the kidney, it produces glomerulonephritis. It most often affects young women.

MALINGERING The willful, deliberate, and fraudulent feigning or exaggeration of the symptoms of illness or injury, usually done to escape duty or work.

MEDIUM WORK Maximum lifting requirment of 50 pounds (22.5 kg). Usual lifting requirement of 25 pounds (11.3 kg).

MENINGIOMA A tumor in the meninges, the covering layers of the brain and spinal cord.

MENINGITIS Inflammation of the membranes covering the brain and spinal cord.

METABOLISM The sum of all physical and chemical processes by which living organized substance is produced and maintained. Also, the transformation by which energy is made available for the organism's use.

MORBIDITY Level of sickness; suffering.

MOTOR END PLATE A specialized structure, usually in the middle of a single muscle fiber, to which a single nerve fiber attaches. It serves to transmit the nerve action potential into a muscle action potential, which results in contraction of the muscle fiber.

MOTOR NEURONS Usually refers to the lower motor neurons that carry action potential impulses from the spinal cord to the muscles.

MOTOR TRACTS Usually refers to a bundle of nerve fibers within the spinal cord which carry impulses from the brain that will ultimately synapse with anterior horn cells and result in muscle movement.

MOTOR UNIT Consists of a single anterior horn cell, its axon cylinder, the motor end plate, and all the muscle fibers innervated by that neuron.

MYELOGRAM X-ray of spinal cord after injection of radiopaque medium.

MYXEDEMA A disease associated with diminished functional activity of the thyroid gland, characterized by lethargy and dry, waxy swelling of the skin.

NECROSIS Death of a cell or group of cells.

NEPHROSCLEROSIS Arteriosclerosis of the medium and small arteries of the kidney. Frequently associated with hypertension.

NERVE ROOT Usually means spinal nerve root, and refers to the bundles of nerves leaving the spinal cord at each of the spinal levels to carry messages out to the periphery or to bring information from the periphery back into the central nervous system.

NERVE TRACTS A bundle of nerve fibers having common origin, function, and termination.

NEUROMA A tumor consisting of nerve cells and nerve fibers.

NYSTAGMUS Rapid involuntary movement of the eyeball.

OBSTRUCTIVE UROPATHY Usually a disturbance of the urinary tract system that mechanically interferes with the flow of urine. It can occur in the urethra, prostate, or the bladder itself.

OPHTHALMODYNAMOMETRY A technique for measuring the pressure within the eyeball when searching for glaucoma, or for increasing the pressure in the eyeball to determine the pressure level of the arteries in the retina.

ORTHOTIST Specialist in orthopedic appliances and their use (usually braces and corsets).

OSMOSIS Diffusion of fluids through a membrane or porous partition.

OSTEODYSTROPHY Defective formation of bone.

OSTEOMYELITIS Infection of bone.

OTOTOXICITY The quality of having a deleterious effect on the acoustic nerve or the organs of hearing and balance. Some antibiotics can be ototoxic.

PARENCHYMA A general term referring to the functional elements of an organ, as distinguished from its connective tissue and blood vessels.

PATHOLOGY All the conditions, processes, or results of a particular disease.

PECTORAL Pertaining to the breast or chest.

PERIPATOLOGY The discipline involved with orientation and mobility instruction of the blind.

PERIPHERAL NERVOUS SYSTEM The part of the nervous system that consists of nerves and ganglia outside the spinal cord and brain.

PERIPHERAL VASCULAR DISEASE Term used for disease of arteries and veins in the limbs (periphery), but usually meaning peripheral *arterial* disease.

PHYSIATRIST A medical specialist in physical medicine and rehabilitation.

PITUITARY ADENOMA A tumor of the pituitary gland, with resultant disturbance in hormone function.

PHOTOPHOBIA Abnormal visual intolerance of light.

PLASTICITY Quality of being conformable or capable of being molded.

POLYCYSTIC DISEASE A hereditary disease of the kidney tissue. The disease becomes evident in early middle age when the amount of normal kidney tissue remaining begins to become insufficient.

POLYDACTYLY Presence of extra fingers or toes, caused by a developmental anomaly.

PREVALENCE The total number of cases of a disease in a given area at a particular time.

PROGNOSIS A prediction of the probable course of an individual's disease and chances of recovery.

PROLIFERATIVE RETINOPATHY Development of new blood vessels and connective tissue growing from the blood vessels of the retina forward into the vitreous.

PRONATION A turning down or downward. For example, turning the palm of the hand downward. The muscles used to perform this function are called *pronators*.

PROXIMAL Situated nearest to the center of

the body. Opposite of distal. Thus, the shoulder is proximal and the hand is distal.

PYELONEPHRITIS Inflammatory disease involving tubular structures of the kidney, usually caused by bacteria. See INTERSTITIAL NEPHRITIS.

QUADRICEPS The large muscle at the front of the thigh just above the knee, which extends (straightens) the leg.

RESECTION Excision of a portion of an organ, bone, or other structure.

RETINITIS PIGMENTOSA A group of diseases, frequently hereditary, of the retina, causing contraction of the visual field.

RETROGRADE PYELOGRAM Specialized X-ray technique for visualizing the urine-collecting system that leaves the kidney and carries urine to the bladder.

ROTATION Movement that turns a body part on its own axis; for example, the turning of the head. The muscles that perform this function are called *rotators*.

SCIATICA Any painful condition in the region of the hip and thighs, especially neuritis of the long nerve (sciatic nerve) passing down the back of the thigh.

SCLERODERMA A chronic disease in which the skin becomes hard and rigid.

SEMIPERMEABLE Permitting certain molecules to pass through and preventing other molecules from passing through. Usually refers to the character of a membrane.

SEPSIS The presence of pathologic micro-organisms or their toxins in the blood or other tissues.

SCAT (SHEEP CELL AGGLUTINATION TITER) Same as heterophil agglutination. A special diagnostic test for infectious mononucleosis ("mono"). Sheep red blood cells are mixed with the patient's blood serum.

SEDENTARY WORK Maximum lifting requirement of 10 pounds (4.5 kg). Work largely done sitting. Some standing or walking may be required.

SEPTICEMIA A systematic disease caused by the presence of pathogenic bacteria and their toxic products in the blood.

SHOCK KIDNEY See VASOMOTOR NEPH-ROPATHY.

SLIDING BOARD A highly polished slab of wood about 2 to 3 feet long and 1 to 2 feet wide, used by some patients with leg paralysis for transfers from a bed to a wheelchair and vice versa.

SOLUTE A substance dissolved in a liquid.

SPASTICITY A condition usually associated with stroke or spinal cord disease whereby stretch reflexes are exaggerated and may even occur spontaneously, producing involuntary muscle contractions.

SPHINCTER A ring-shaped muscle that surrounds a natural opening in the body and can open or close the opening by expanding or contracting.

STEROIDS Commonly used term to indicate a family of compounds similar to hormones elaborated by the cortex of the adrenal gland (e.g., prednisone, cortisone, decadron).

STRICTURES Decrease in the caliber of a canal, duct, or other passage, as a result of scar contraction or the deposition of abnormal tissue.

SUBCUTANEOUS Beneath the skin. Usually refers to the region between the skin and underlying fat layer.

SUBDURAL HEMATOMA Accumulation of blood in the space between the arachnoid and dura mater (coverings over the brain) due to a break in the wall of a blood vessel, usually caused by head injury.

SUPINATION A turning upward; for example, turning the palm upward. The muscles that perform this function are called *supinators*.

SYNCOPE A faint.

SYSTEMIC Pertaining to or affecting the whole body.

TOWER SKULL (OXYCEPHALY) Condition in which the top of the head is pointed.

TEMPORAL ARTERITIS Chronic vascular disease of older persons, largely confined to the carotid arterial system, in particular the temporal arteries just in front of the ears.

THROMBOSIS Coagulation of the blood in the heart or a blood vessel, forming a clot.

THROMBUS The fibrinous clot attached at the site of thrombosis.

TOXEMIA Literally, the presence of toxins in the blood. Specifically used to explain an abnormal condition in the mother during pregnancy, i.e., toxemia of pregnancy, also called eclampsia.

TRANSUDATION Process of passing or oozing through pores or interstices, especially blood serum through the vessel walls.

TRAUMA Wound or injury.

TRENDELENBERG TOURNIQUET TEST A physical examination technique whereby a physician assesses the competency of the superficial and deep veins of the legs.

ULTRASOUND TREATMENT A technique whereby ultrasound energy is directed into the body and converted into heat energy for purposes of temperature elevation of localized pathology.

UPPER MOTOR NEURON All of the descending fibers in the brain and spinal cord that can influence and modify the activity of the lower motor neuron.

VASOMOTOR NEPHROPATHY Acute failure of kidney tubular function following shock, trauma, certain toxins, and mismatched blood. Preferred term.

VENTRAL Of, pertaining to, or situated on the front or lower side or surface (anterior).

VERY HEAVY WORK Maximum lifting require-ment greater than 100 pounds (45 kg). Usual carrying capacity of 50 pounds (22.5 kg).

VISUALLY EVOKED CEREBRAL POTENTIAL The interval between the onset of a light flashed on a screen and detection of the brain wave produced by it.

VISUOMOTOR Pertaining to the performance of a function in response to visual input.

INDEX

Vertebral column, 34, 205–209

Vestibular system, 51–54

Vineland Social Maturity Scale, 266, 271, 276

Visual impairments: as complication of cerebral palsy, 143; as complication of diabetes mellitus, 324; as complication of multiple sclerosis, 111, 115; as complication of sickle cell disease, 356, 360. *See also* Blindness and visual impairments.

Visual system: characterization of the sense of vision, 378–379; and eye movements, 50–51; and nerve pathways to the brain, 48–50; structure and function of, 45–48. *See also* Blindness and visual impairments.

Vocational Evaluation and Work Adjustment Association (VEWAA), 270, 271

Vocational Information and Evaluation Work Samples, 271, 277

Vocational Interest and Sophistication Assessment, 271, 276–277

Von Willebrand's disease. *See* Hemophilia.

Waardenburg's syndrome, 396

Wallerian degeneration, 102

Wechsler Adult Intelligence Scale, 266, 271, 276, 403

Wechsler Intelligence Scale for Children (revised), 266, 271, 276

Werdnig-Hoffman disease. *See* Spinal muscular atrophy.

Wernicke's area, 23

Wheelchair, use of: in amputation, 179–180, 185; in multiple sclerosis, 113, in spinal cord injury, 70–71, 76–78, 80–81; in spinal muscular atrophy, 91, 92

Work, classification of levels, 8, 298–299

Wrist disarticulation (W/D) amputation, 170, 176, 178